salon
FUNDAMENTALS™
NAILS

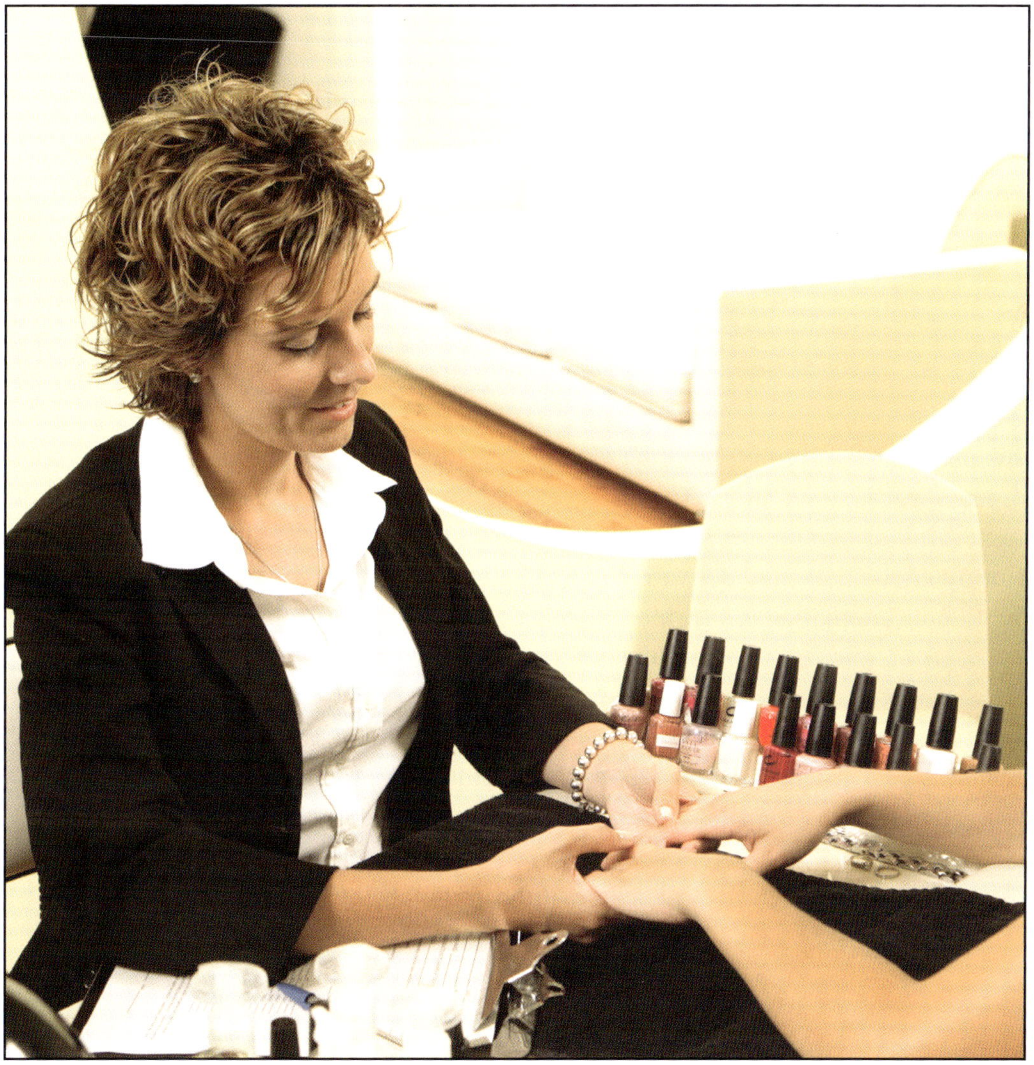

A Resource for Your Nail Care Career

Pivot Point International, Inc.
World Headquarters
8725 W. Higgins Road, Suite 700
Chicago, IL 60631 USA

847-866-0500
pivot-point.com

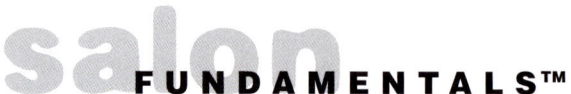

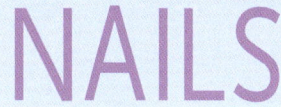

salon
FUNDAMENTALS™
NAILS

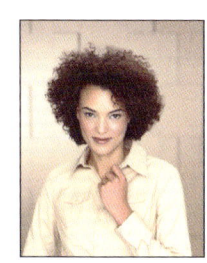
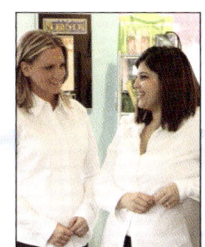

Career Essentials

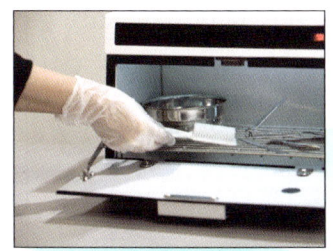
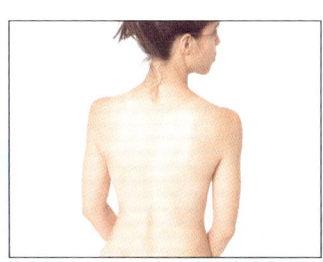
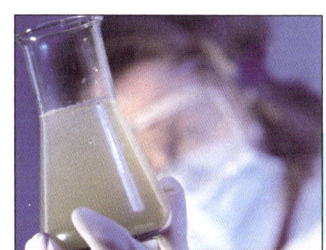
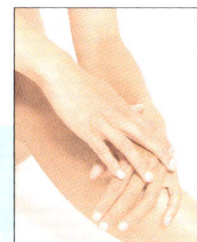

The Science of Nail Care

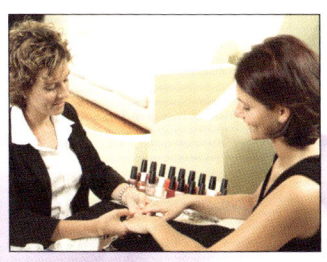
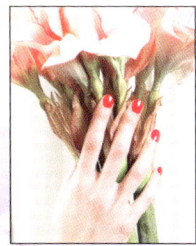
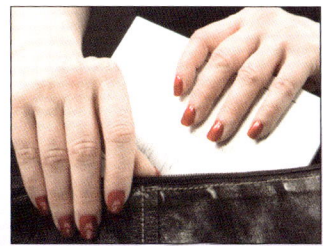
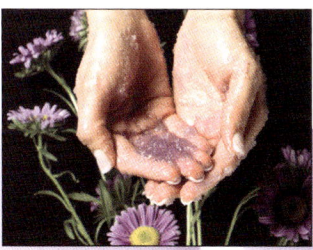

Nail Services

A Resource for Your Nail Care Career

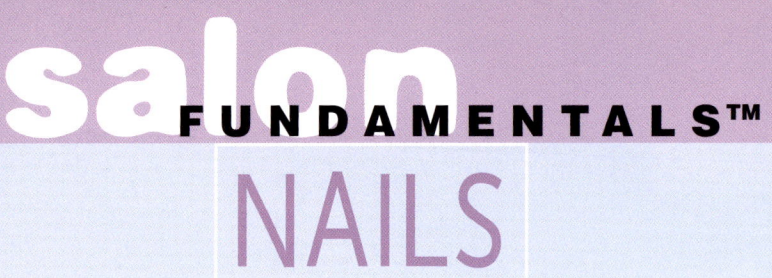

salon FUNDAMENTALS™

NAILS

DEAR NAIL TECHNOLOGY STUDENT:

CONGRATULATIONS! By enrolling in a school that utilizes *Salon Fundamentals™ Nails, A Resource for Your Nail Care Career,* you have taken important steps in ensuring your future success as a nail technician. This in-depth program will provide you with fundamental concepts and techniques that will help prepare you for state board licensure and entry-level positions within the industry. As you may already know, *Salon Fundamentals™ Cosmetology* and *Salon Fundamentals™ Esthetics* have set very high standards in hair and beauty education. Now we're doing it again in the nail care industry! By utilizing pertinent material, vivid imagery and an unrivaled learning system, you will find that the *Salon Fundamentals Nails* program makes learning easy and fun.

Best of luck to you as you embark on the fascinating journey of a *Salon Fundamentals Nails* education. The journey will ultimately lead you into a growing industry with limitless possibilities.

Sincerely,

The Staff of *Salon Fundamentals Nails*

salon FUNDAMENTALS™
NAILS

CONTENTS
SALON FUNDAMENTALS™ NAILS

NAIL CARE HISTORY

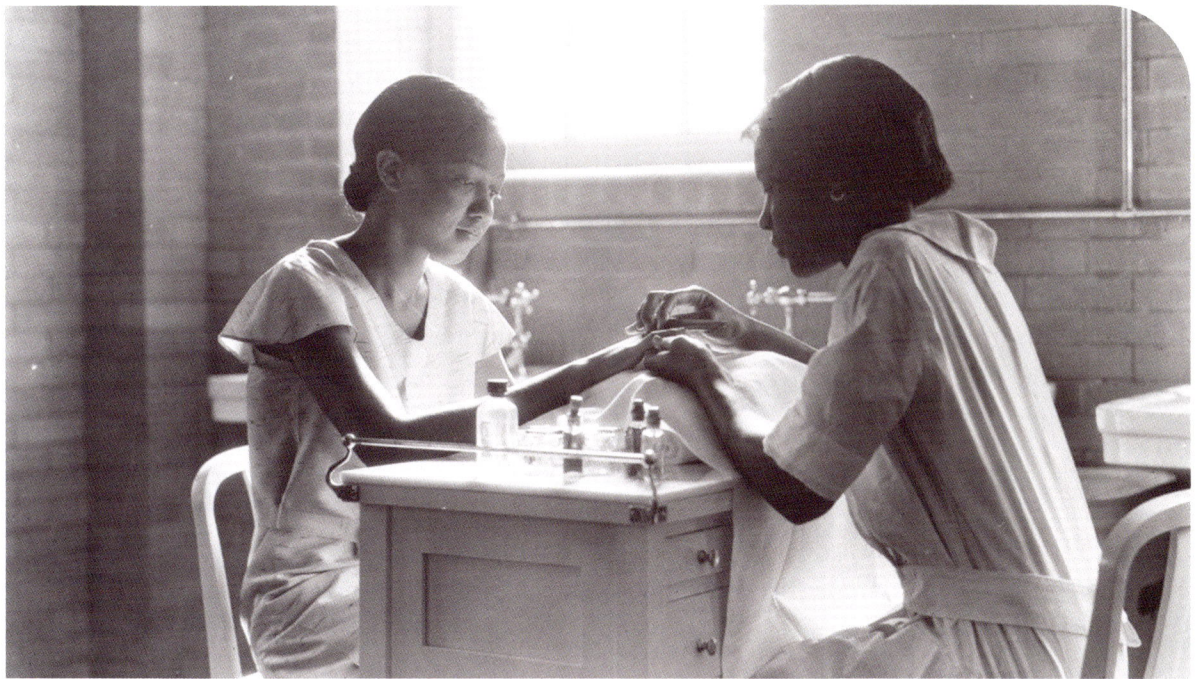

A young woman receives training in manicuring in a 1910 beauty course. Image courtesy of NAILS Magazine.

For thousands of years, a wide range of natural and manufactured products has been used by different cultures and classes to enhance and sustain the beauty of hands and feet. For example, in some cultures, attractive hands and nails were simply seen as a part of good hygiene. In other cultures, well-manicured hands were set apart from the upper class and high society, or were a necessity for women who wanted to attract attention from the opposite sex. Of course, the tools of the trade have changed over time as products for the hands and nails have evolved and become more sophisticated.

Ancient Beginnings

Much like the esthetics industry, the practice of nail art and design has been around for centuries. The Chinese wore nail art as early as 3,000 B.C. as did the Egyptians since around 3,500 B.C. The Chinese found ways to use gum arabic, egg whites, gelatin, and beeswax to create varnishes and lacquers for the nails, while the Egyptians used henna to stain them.

Archaeologists have found Egyptian palettes for grinding eye paint dating from about 10,000 B.C. They also used perfumed oils and ointments to soften the skin as well as paints and dyes to color it. Men and women regularly used makeup, and when they went to their final resting place, they were supplied with cosmetics for the next world.

Meanwhile, color played an important role in representing the status of one's social class. The Egyptians used red to show the highest social class. It is said that while Cleopatra's nails were painted a deep red, Queen Nefertiti sported a flashier ruby shade. At the same time women of lower rank were only permitted to wear pale tones. In fact, the wearing of royal colors without being royalty was punishable by death.

Excavations in the Middle East, particularly at Mohenjo-Daro in the Indus Valley, have turned up numerous cosmetic pots of clay, stone, ivory and alabaster in a variety of shapes and sizes that are more than 4,000 years old. The fourth and fifth centuries B.C. were considered a time of "opulence and luxury." The wealthy used cosmetic sticks made of gold and silver and kept their cosmetics in special boxes. A common practice of this period included staining the tips of the fingers and the soles of the feet with the coppery-red lac-dye.

Advancements in Nail Care

In the 18th century, there was wide debate about whether it was appropriate for women to use cosmetic aids to enhance their natural look, specifically paints for the face and nails. In

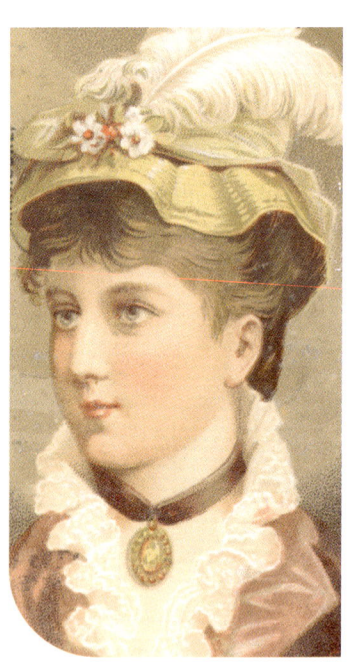

An 1880 business card advertising Madame Robison's Manicure and Cosmetic Parlors in San Francisco. Image courtesy of NAILS Magazine.

some areas of Europe, prostitutes were more often associated with the use of cosmetic products. Some argued that single women should be allowed to use the paints and beauty enhancers to attract a husband. However, the English Parliament, taking notice of how popular cosmetic paints had become, expressed its alarm and disapproval by passing a law stating that:

"All women, of whatever age, rank, profession or degree, whether virgins, maids, or widows, that shall from and after this act impose upon, seduce or betray into matrimony any of His Majesty's subjects by the use of scents, paints, cosmetics, washes, artificial teeth, false hair, Spanish wool, iron stays, hoops, high-heeled shoes, or bolstered hips, shall incur the penalty of the law now in force against witchcraft and like misdemeanors, and that the marriage, upon conviction, shall stand null and void."

In spite of this law, women continued to use various beauty agents that were increasingly becoming readily available to them.

Men and women in 19th century Persia went to the royal baths for special attention to their hair, skin and nails. Persian women, who also dyed their nails red with henna, regarded the bath as a place of amusement and made appointments to meet friends there. They would sometimes spend seven or eight hours together telling stories, relating anecdotes and eating while they received a variety of beauty treatments.

Americans and Nail Care

In the United States, until the early 1800s, fingernails were largely overlooked, although women and men began to polish their nails with scented oils. Short, almond-shaped nails with a slight point were the norm. In 1830, a foot doctor in Europe used a dental tool to develop the orangewood stick to aid in manicuring nails. Before this, people used metal tools, acid and scissors to perfect their nails. The technique reached the United States around 1892 and the service was offered to women, regardless of income. Almost 20 years later, Flowery Manicure Products, established in New York City, manufactured metal nail files and eventually invented the emery board.

Before long-lasting lacquers became available in the 20th century, Western women who

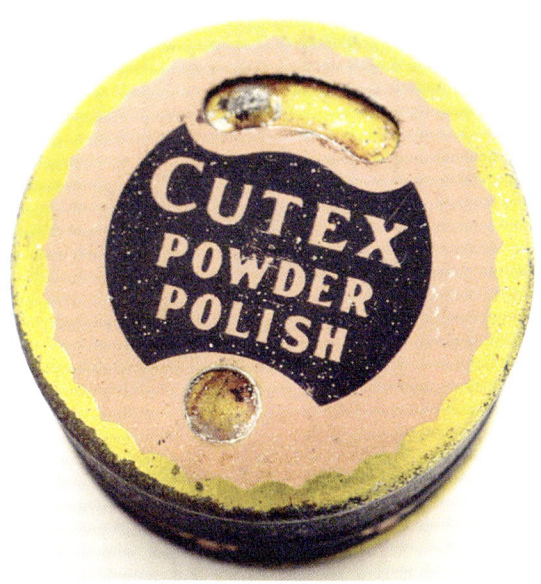

Cutex Powder Polish, circa 1917. Image courtesy of NAILS Magazine.

wanted a manicured look turned to either powder or cream polish, which had a base of beeswax, tin oxide or a form of silicon dioxide. These would make the nails shine and produce a slight pink shade when buffed onto the nails with a chamois cloth.

Nails and Cars

In 1921, 17 factories in the United States, were producing 5 million kilos of lacquers. Just four years later, the U.S. had 85 such factories producing 40 million kilos. Henry Ford's automobile assembly-line production system might not have been possible without the creation of rapid-drying automobile lacquers. In 1923, Dupont came out with Duco, a fast-drying pigment. These new types of lacquers were first used to varnish automobiles, golf balls, pianos and billiard balls. It can be said that during the 1920s, the lacquer business grew with the automobile industry. Yet, no one could have predicted that the coming development of automotive paint would pave the way for today's nail polishes. Without lacquers, "the manicuring art would not have been able to

turn ordinary nails into the flawless colored and brilliant jewels that they are today," said cosmetics historian Gilbert Vail.

Think Pink

A sheer, rosy red nail polish entered the market around 1925 and was applied only to the center of the nail. The "moon manicure" was popular in the mid-1920s and '30s. With this technique, the cuticles were cut, the free edges were filed into points and polish was applied to the nail but not to the moon. Max Factor provided the masses with his newest product, Max Factor's Society Nail Tint. When buffed into the nail plate, this cream gave nails a natural rose hue. In fact, Max Faktor *[sic]*, born in 1870 in Poland, is considered the father of modern makeup. The idea behind his company's brand was that every girl could look like a movie star by using Max Factor products.

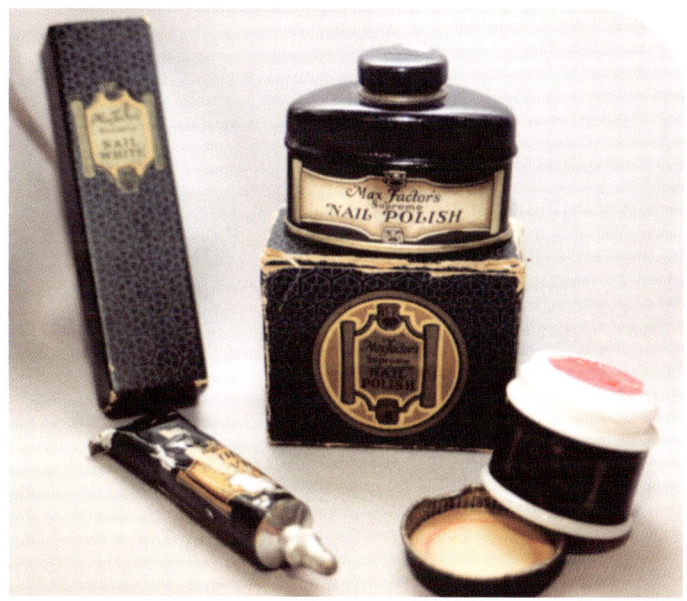

Max Factor produced a product called Supreme Nail Polish, a beige powder in a metal pot. Later, Max Factor introduced a pink nail tint. Image courtesy of NAILS Magazine.

Not long after Max Factor nail tint hit the market, Charles Revson *[sic]* created the first pigment-based nail polish with help from his brother and a chemist. The Revlon company was founded in 1935 and offered women an opaque nail enamel in a wide variety of never-before available shades. The company suceeded in selling its long-lasting nail enamel to salons through department stores and selected drugstores. With the end of World War II, the company produced manicure and pedicure instruments. Following the war, Revlon launched twice-yearly nail enamel and lipstick promotions tied to seasonal clothing fashions. Shortly after that, Max Factor introduced its

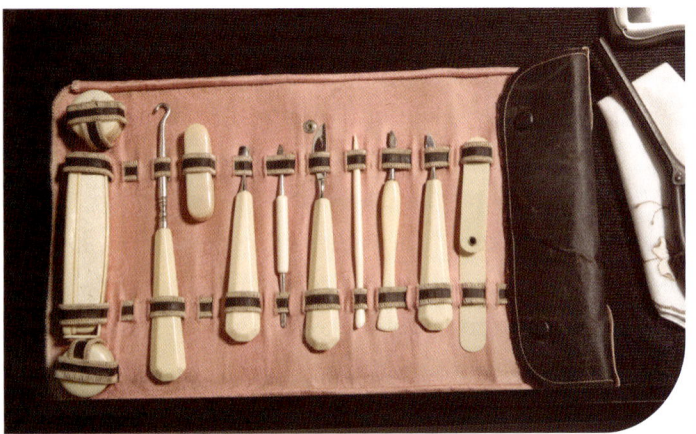

A manicure kit from the 1940s. Courtesy of Janet Hansen.
The Look Salon and Spa, Palatine, IL.

Liquid Nail Enamel, which is similar to nail polishes of today. The company used a limited number of pigments, and the enamel was available only in red, dark red, vermilion and crimson. The fashion then was to cover the entire nail with polish.

A World of Color

During the first half of the 20th century, men who frequented barbershops often received a manicure as well as a haircut, shave and shoeshine. Meanwhile, as women began to enter the workforce, part of their earnings was spent on manicures and nail polish. Bright colors for women, such as Schoolhouse Red Nail Polish from Elizabeth Arden, were $.75 a bottle. Clear polish brushed over and under nail enamel made manicures last longer. By the 1950s there was an explosion of colors on

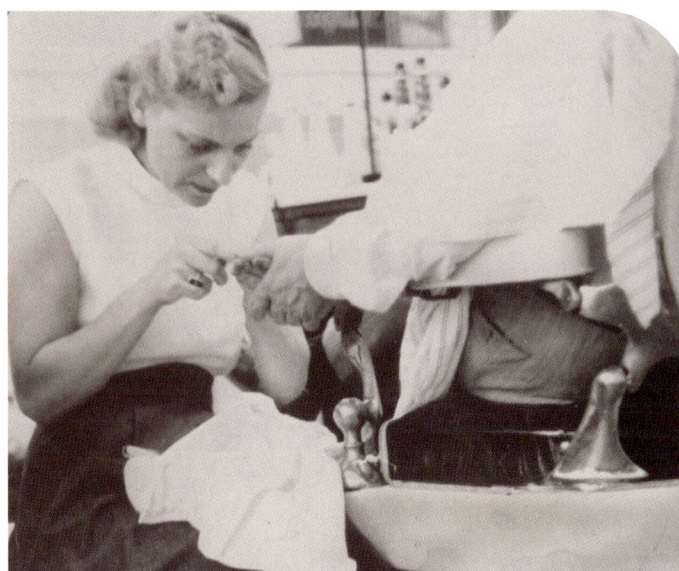

A manicurist from the 1940s gives a manicure in a barbershop
Courtesy of Janet Hansen. The Look Salon and Spa, Palatine, IL.

the market, and women began to grow longer nails with oval shapes and use softer colors modeled by Hollywood starlets and other famous women.

Length Matters

In 1957, Thomas Slack was issued a patent for a "platform" that fit around the nail edge. Acrylic polymer that was originally invented to fill cavities in teeth was used to create the first false nails in the form of acrylic extensions. However, these early compositions made typing almost impossible and dishwashing completely out of the question for women who wore false nails. During the 1970s, long nails were seen as a sign of wealth, much like in ancient Egypt. For those with less to spend, temporary glue-on and press-on nails were available. These artificial nails were inserted under a lifted cuticle to make them look as if they were growing out of the finger. The glue that held the nails could be dissolved with water.

Around this time, perm papers reinforced with airplane glue replaced teabags and coffee filters which were used for strengthening natural nails as women began to favor a square-shaped nail.

These innovations made possible the rise of artificial nails known as tips and overlays. Specialized brands and products that emerged during this time included Lee Press-On Nails by Lee Pharmaceuticals, and the "French manicure" kit, a term coined by Orly International.

Nail Design as an Art Form

As the number of two-income households grew in the 1980s and '90s, women began to spend more disposable income on nail care. Industry experts estimated that nail care generated $3.2 billion in 1990, and that figure doubled and rose to $6.4 billion in 1998. Nails-only salons popped up and more products were created to boost the nail industry. The use of nail drills (adapted from dental, hobby and jewelry drills) was more common when working with acrylic nails, and fiberglass became the newest wrap system—light, strong and flexible.

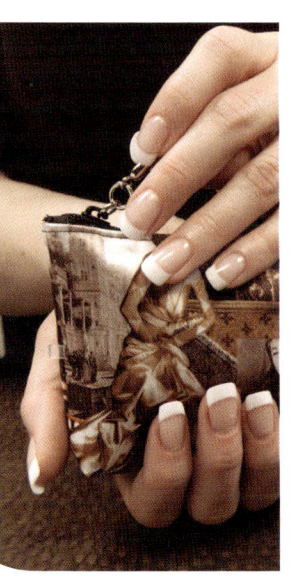

Gel form nails were introduced in 1985 and it was predicted that they would wipe out acrylics. It didn't, but it was noted that consumers were seeking out the gels and purchasing the home systems directly, so professional nail technicians began to make them one of the fastest-growing services in the salon. Once again, shorter nail lengths were preferred and quieter colors could be seen on hands. Today, French manicures and natural-looking nails dominate the business world and airbrushed looks have become more popular.

Airbrushing was originally introduced in Australia. The equipment consisted of industrial-

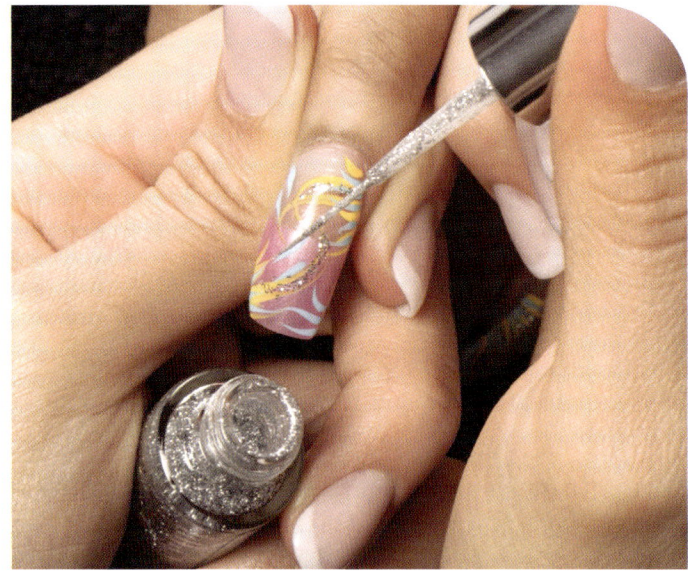

sized compressors, poor-quality paints and airbrushes not especially designed for the working nail technician. Today, small compressors with little noise, airbrushes especially for the nail technician, and paints of top quality made for fingernails have made this service a quick and easy design technique for both technicians and clients alike.

Looking Forward

Knowing that nail care had its beginnings more than 3,000 years ago speaks to its long-lasting popularity. The demand for professional nail care continues to grow at a steady rate. The amount of money spent in this industry can provide a successful and rewarding lifetime career if your client care skills match the technical skills. Clearly, professional nail care has entered into the mainstream to become an integral part of good grooming. It goes without saying that a well-groomed person will have well-groomed nails. As it once signified rank, status and wealth in the past, today it is very much part and parcel of fashion, design and looking great. The nail industry will continue to flourish as it has over thousands of years, with many new and exciting opportunities that you can be part of.

ACKNOWLEDGEMENTS

Salon Fundamentals™ Nails, A Resource for Your Nail Care Career is designed to provide nail care education to undergraduate students to help prepare them for licensure and an entry-level position in the nail care field. An undertaking of this magnitude requires the expertise and cooperation of many people. The *Salon Fundamentals Nails* staff wishes to take this opportunity to acknowledge with gratitude and respect, some of those many contributors.

Thank you to the reviewers across the country, models, outside consultants, individual and chain nail salons, industry manufacturers, Pivot Point's Educational Advisory Board and the dedicated Core Development Team that made this course possible.

In addition, we give special thanks to the North American Regulating agencies whose careful work protects us as well as our clients and thereby enhances the high quality of our work. These agencies include OSHA (Occupational Health and Safety Agency), EPA (Environmental Protection Agency) and ADA (Americans With Disabilities Act). The *Salon Fundamentals* programs makes extensive use of their policies and procedures.

The following is a listing of the many individuals and organizations that made this program possible.

Core Development Team

Editorial

Maureen Spurr
Editorial Manager

Deidre Glover
Editorial Associate

Benjamin Polk
Editorial and PR Associate

Production and Design

Tim Davis
Production Director

Chris Cote
Creative Manager

Csaba Zongor
Graphic Design/Illustration Associate

Joanna Jakubowicz
Graphic Design Associate

David Placek
Photography/Videography Senior Associate

Rick Russell
Graphic Design Associate

Denise Podlin
Illustration

Tina Rayyan
Production Administrative Manager

Marriell Marquette
Administrative Production Associate

Program Development

Sabine Held-Perez
Program Development Director

Eileen Dubelbeis
Program Development Associate

Markel Richards
Program Development Associate

Research and Development

Mia Kim
Research Associate

Clif St. Germain, Ph.D.
Educational Consultant

Jane Wegner
Educational Research

DVD Production

John Bernin
FrameOne Communications

Mandy Burton
Educational Content Expert

Brian Fallon
Educational Content Supervisor

Janet Fisher
Senior Director
Research and Development

Mary Jo Lofstrom
Educational Research

Renée Taylor
Art and Design Research Associate

Anna Fehr
Educational Technology Manager

Reviewers

Dr. Dennis Arnold, DPM, FACFAS
International Pedicure Association
Granbury, TX
www.pedicureassociation.org

Deborah Carver
Stephanie Yaggy
Nailpro Magazine/Creative Age
Van Nuys, CA

Cyndy Drummey
Nails Magazine
Torrance, CA

Jean Harrity
Pivot Point International
Bloomingdale, IL

Nicole Passage
Pivot Point International
Evanston, IL

Paul Bryson, Ph.D.
OPI Products Inc.
North Hollywood, CA

Gerri Cevetillo
Ultronics
Cuyahoga Falls, OH

Michelle D'Allaird
Aesthetic Science Institute
Latham and Syracuse, NY

Teresa Lewis
OPI Products Inc.
Chicago, IL

Debbie Mack
Pivot Point International
Evanston, IL

Executive Management Team

Leo Passage
Founder
Chairman Emeritus

Corrine Passage
Senior Vice President
Production and Systems Development

Judy Rambert
Vice President
Research and Development

Sarah Pirok
Vice President
International Academies

Karen Wilkin-Donachie
Chief Executive Officer

Robert Sieh
Senior Vice President
Finance and Operations

Ron Beible
Vice President
Sales and Marketing

OVERVIEW

The *Salon Fundamentals™ Nails* program is a valuable resource for successfully launching your nail care career. This basic nail care course utilizes proven instructional strategies that enhance learner understanding, involvement and retention, and contains a system of integrated learning tools that are unrivaled in the nail care industry. Designed to prepare nail care students for licensure and an entry-level position in the nail care profession, the *Salon Fundamentals Nails* program consists of the following educational tools:

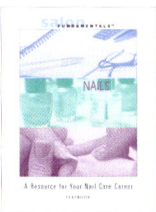

- ### Salon Fundamentals™ Nails Textbook
  A theoretical and practical reference book complete with objectives, key points, step-by-step technical procedures, interactive writing exercises and index.

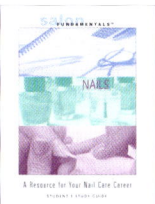

- ### Salon Fundamentals™ Nails Study Guide and Glossary
  The companion to the textbook, the *Study Guide* draws your attention to the important ideas in each chapter and helps you organize and manage the information you need to know for future licensure and employment success.

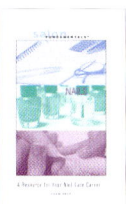

- ### Salon Fundamentals™ Nails Exam Prep Book
  Another support tool created to improve test-taking skills; includes questions for each chapter in a multiple-choice format, sample final exams, page-referenced answer key and "Did You Know?" statements that provide a summary and checklist for the questions for each chapter.

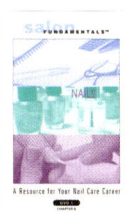

- ### Salon Fundamentals™ Nails Instructional DVD
  A classroom tool designed to provide reinforcement for theoretical knowledge and a close look at the step-by-step technical procedures using the latest in visual technology.

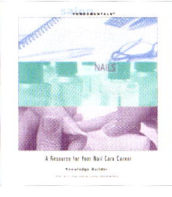

- ### Salon Fundamentals™ Nails Knowledge Builder CD-ROM
  A teacher's tool for building assessments that allows teachers to create custom and randomized tests and study guides easily in both print and electronic formats.

Add the detailed Teacher's Support Manual used by the teacher and you have the latest in learning systems. Developed and reviewed by a highly acclaimed panel of experts within the education and nail care professions, *Salon Fundamentals Nails* will help you build self-confidence as you embark on your professional journey.

As you begin working with the information found in this textbook, you might be reminded of how difficult studying can be some days. You'll be trying to learn and do new things. Sometimes you may get just plain discouraged. All learners experience this—it's part of the learning process. That's why every attempt has been made to clarify difficult concepts and offer hints, study tips and memory enhancers that make learning easier. This support, created with you in mind, begins on the first two pages of each new chapter. There you will find a sneak preview of the whole chapter.

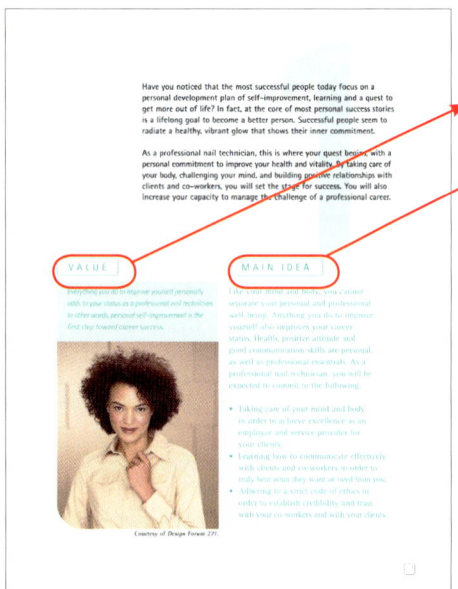

On the first page of each chapter after the introduction there is a VALUE statement, which answers the question, "What's in it for me?" The MAIN IDEA of each chapter is written in an inspirational style designed to paint a picture of the important concepts found within the chapter. On the second page, a PLAN for making your way through the chapter is listed. Think of the Plan as an outline of the chapter contents with the major sections indicated.

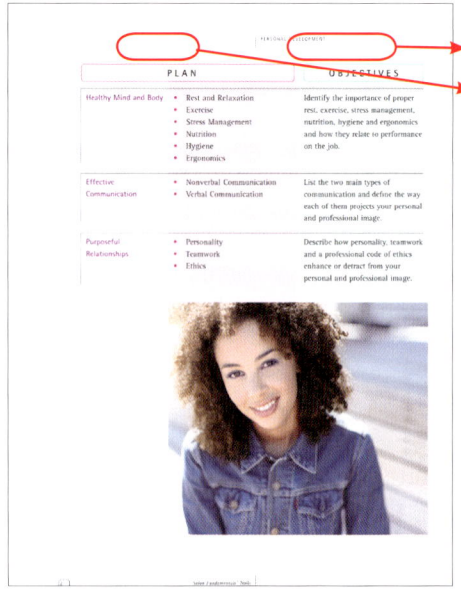

The major OBJECTIVES of the chapter are presented, following the PLAN, giving you a checklist to know what you will be expected to do after you complete the chapter. These objectives or expectations are based on best-practice indicators from within the nail care profession.

Chapter numbers appear on the right-hand side of each spread to help you quickly open the book to a selected chapter. Each chapter offers ways to help call your attention to key points as shown below.

LOOK FOR:

- Bullets

Color-Coded Headings

Numbers

Bold print

PLACED IN A CHART

or shaded box

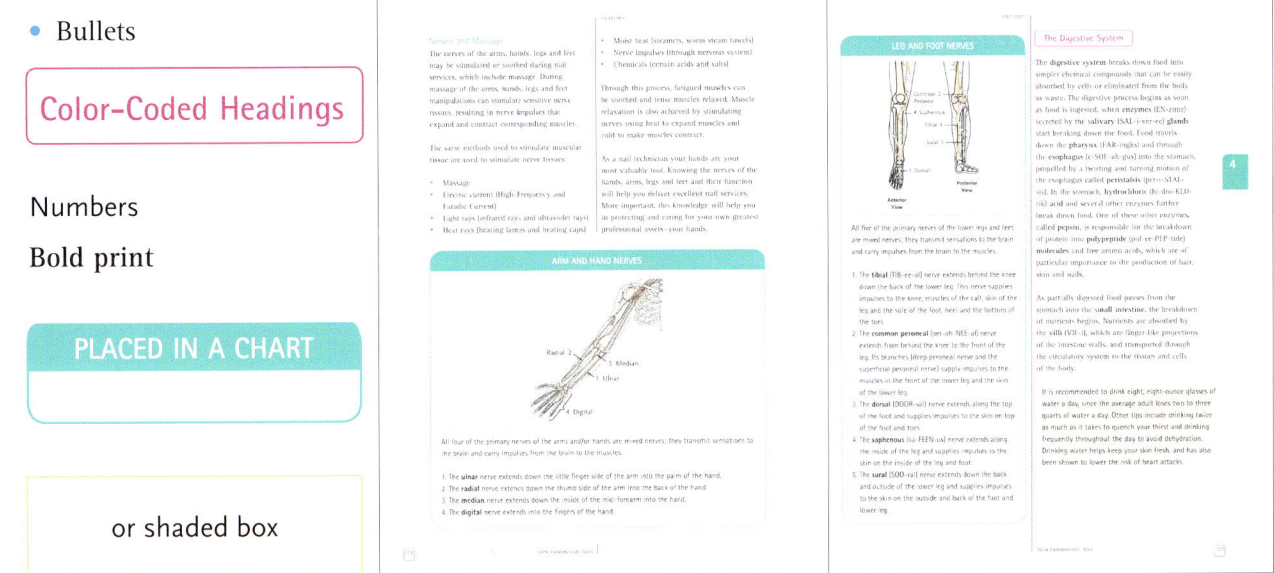

These tools have been designed to help you recognize the theory points to remember.

At the close of each major section you will find a

REFLECTIVE QUESTION

that helps you summarize what you have learned,

indicate your feelings and offer a personal opinion.

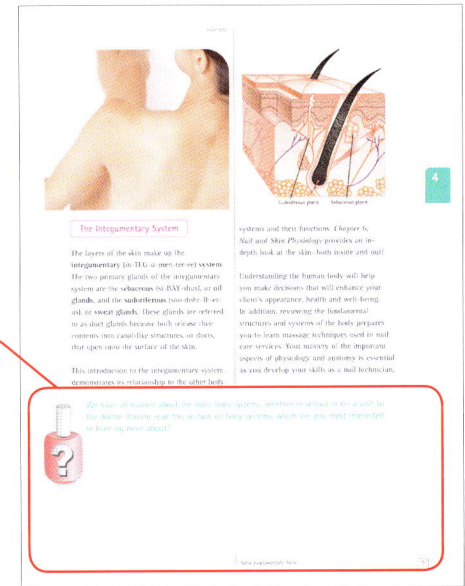

UNIT 3 NAIL SERVICES contains procedures which all have a standard format consisting of three components, which include the **PREPARATION** (announcing what needs to be done before you begin the service), **PROCEDURE** (the actual techniques you will perform during the service) and **COMPLETION** (the important final steps you do at the end of the service).

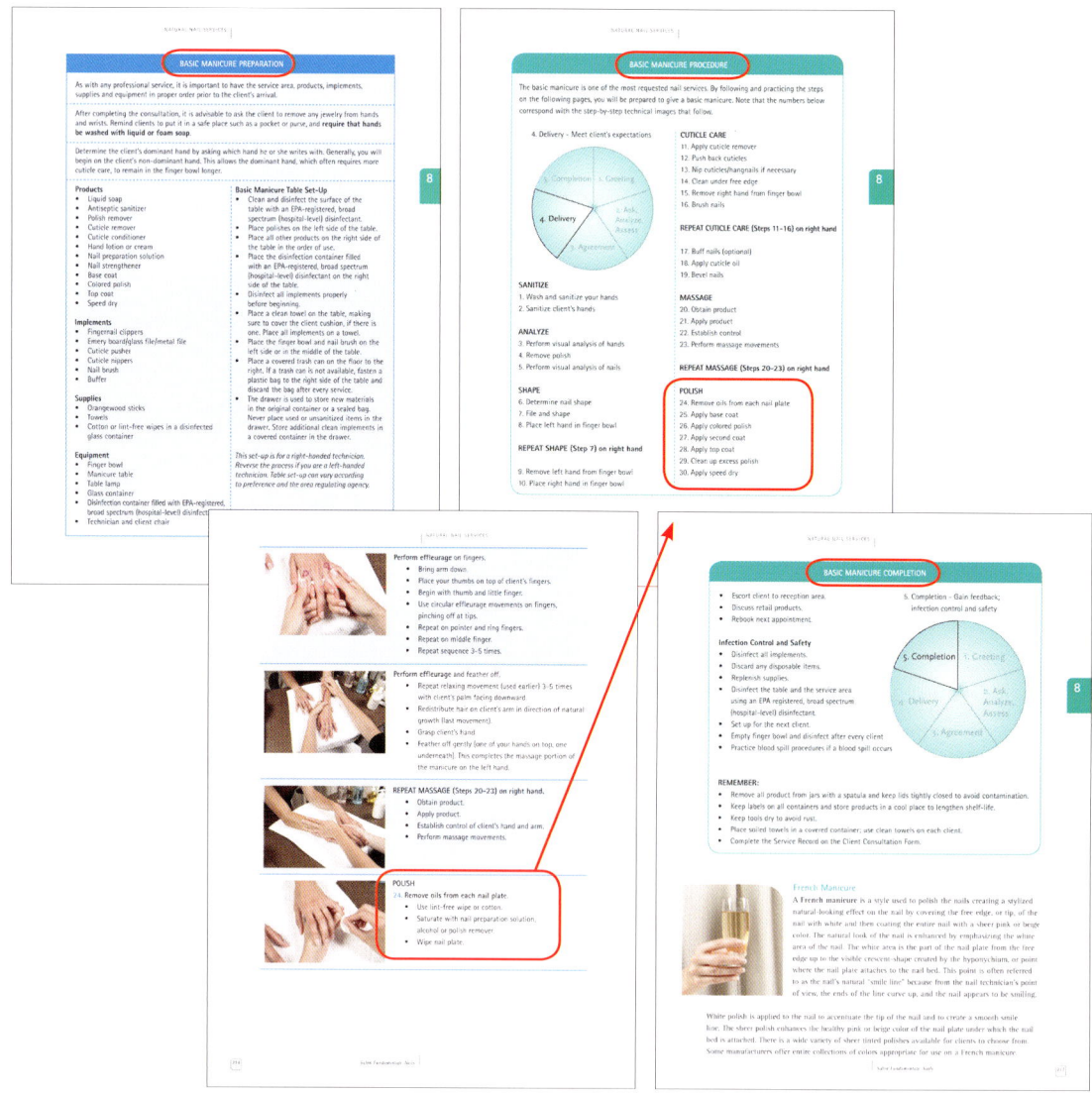

Within the procedures, techniques have been placed in bold print. These are the steps that are related to the Rubric, found in your *Salon Fundamentals Nails Study Guide,* described on the next page.

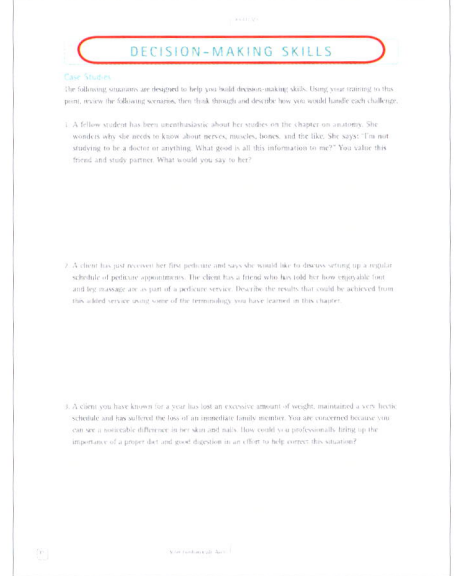

On the last page of each chapter you will find a section entitled

DECISION–MAKING SKILLS .

It is here that you will find real-life situations that give you an opportunity to utilize the content you are learning and apply it to possible future situations. This is your opportunity to show that you mastered the information found in the chapter and can now meet the expectations that have been established for the professional nail care industry.

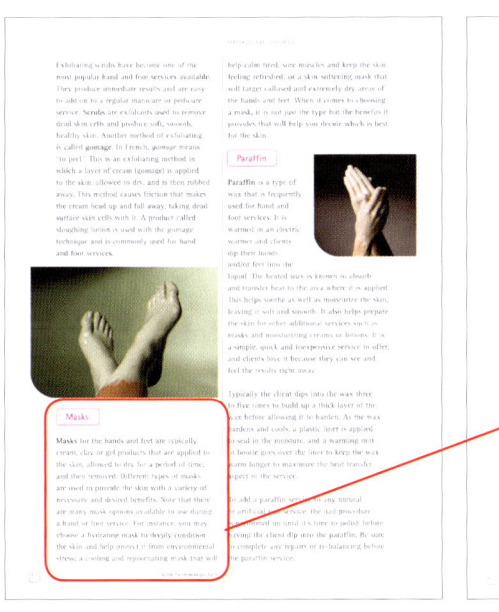

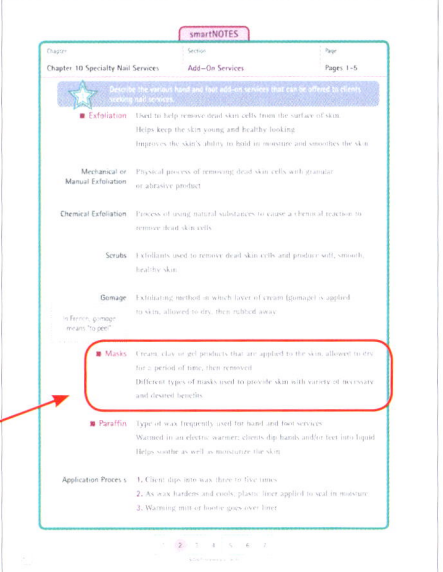

The *Salon Fundamentals™ Nails Study Guide* is your personal notebook that goes right along with this textbook. The Study Guide will help you direct your thinking, manage the information presented in the chapter and assist you in tapping into your own natural intelligence. It will become your best friend and personal tutor! Remember, when it comes to learning, effort is as important as ability. By completing the learning prompts in your Study Guide you are actually learning what you need to know. You are also teaching yourself to become a better learner in the future.

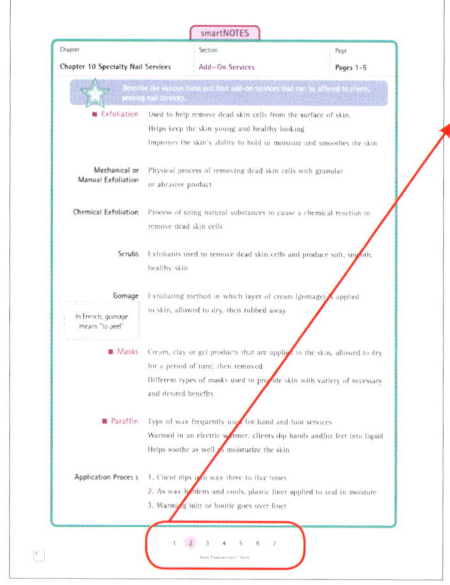

See the front section of your *Study Guide* for more detailed information about the learning strategies included within this valuable companion guide. Each strategy, called a M I N D F R A M E, gives you a different way of understanding the content. These Mindframes capitalize on your natural intelligence. Use them and you will become a stronger, more successful learner.

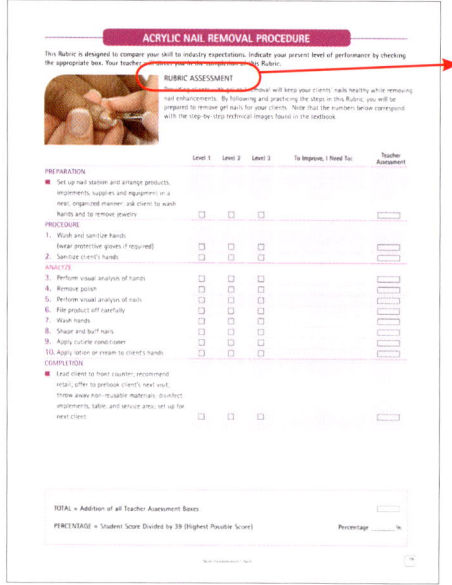

Here is a sample R U B R I C from your *Study Guide*. A Rubric is a level-by-level description of how your performance will be assessed. As a learner you will want to use these Rubrics to determine how well you are doing and what you must do to improve. Your teacher will also use these Rubrics to guide their assessments of your performance. See the front section of your *Study Guide* for more detailed information about the learning strategies included within this valuable companion guide.

You can count on your *Salon Fundamentals Nails* tools as you move from lesson to lesson. This textbook will remain a natural reference tool throughout your career. Your *Salon Fundamentals Nails Textbook, Study Guide* and other companion tools will help focus your thinking and effort as you learn to become a successful nail care professional.

Good Luck and Good Learning!

salon FUNDAMENTALS™
NAILS

Unit 1: Career Essentials

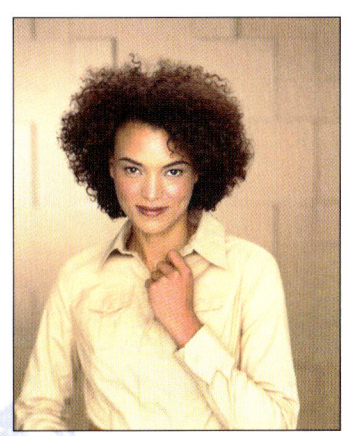 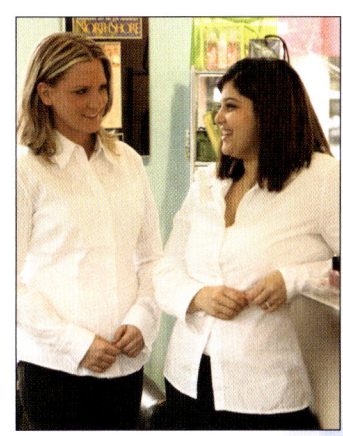

CHAPTER 1, PERSONAL DEVELOPMENT

CHAPTER 2, BUSINESS BASICS

UNIT 1 CAREER ESSENTIALS provides the entry-level nail technician with the practical knowledge and wisdom geared toward professional growth and success in the nail care industry. These two chapters present both personal and professional encouragement for nail technicians who are aiming for a well-rounded beginning in the nail care industry.

salon FUNDAMENTALS™

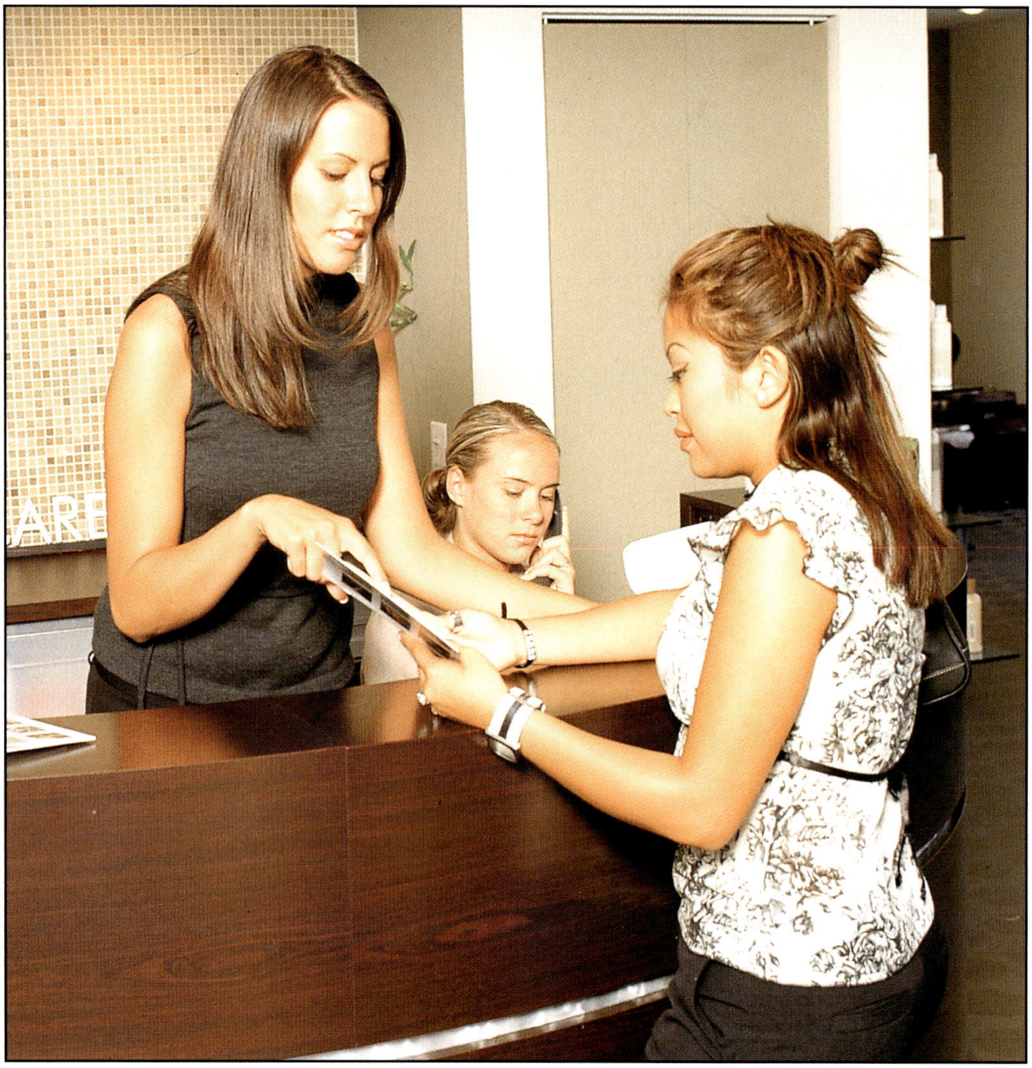

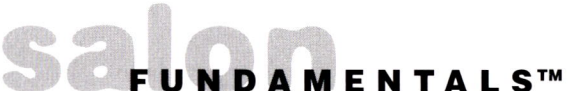

Have you noticed that the most successful people today focus on a personal development plan of self-improvement, learning and a quest to get more out of life? In fact, at the core of most personal success stories is a lifelong goal to become a better person. Successful people seem to radiate a healthy, vibrant glow that shows their inner commitment. As a professional nail technician, this is where your quest begins, with a personal commitment to improve your health and vitality. By taking care of your body, challenging your mind, and building positive relationships with clients and co-workers, you will set the stage for success. You will also increase your capacity to manage the challenge of a professional career.

VALUE

Everything you do to improve yourself personally adds to your status as a professional nail technician. In other words, personal development is the first step toward career success.

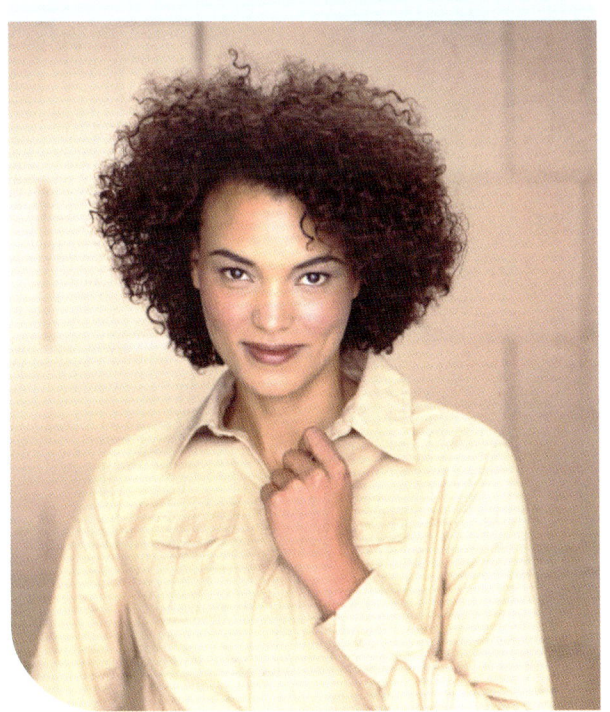

Courtesy of *Design Forum 271*.

MAIN IDEA

Like your mind and body, you cannot separate your personal and professional well-being. Anything you do to improve yourself also improves your career status. Health, positive attitude and good communication skills are personal, as well as professional essentials. As a professional nail technician, you will be expected to commit to the following:

- Taking care of your mind and body in order to achieve excellence as an employee and service provider for your clients;
- Learning how to communicate effectively with clients and co-workers in order to truly hear what they want or need from you;
- Adhering to a strict code of ethics in order to establish credibility and trust with your co-workers and with your clients.

PLAN		OBJECTIVES
Healthy Mind and Body	• Rest and Relaxation • Exercise • Stress Management • Nutrition • Hygiene • Ergonomics	Identify the importance of proper rest, exercise, stress management, nutrition, hygiene and ergonomics and how they relate to performance on the job.
Effective Communication	• Nonverbal Communication • Verbal Communication	List the two main types of communication and define the way each of them projects your personal and professional image.
Purposeful Relationships	• Personality • Teamwork • Ethics	Describe how personality, teamwork and a professional code of ethics enhance or detract from your personal and professional image.

HEALTHY MIND AND BODY

Personal development involves changing your habits and making decisions about how to attain and maintain a steady sense of well-being. This requires establishing routines to maintain a healthy mind and body. A well-balanced mind and body give you a more positive outlook on life. Focusing on each of the following health-related areas will help you stay on the track to success in your career.

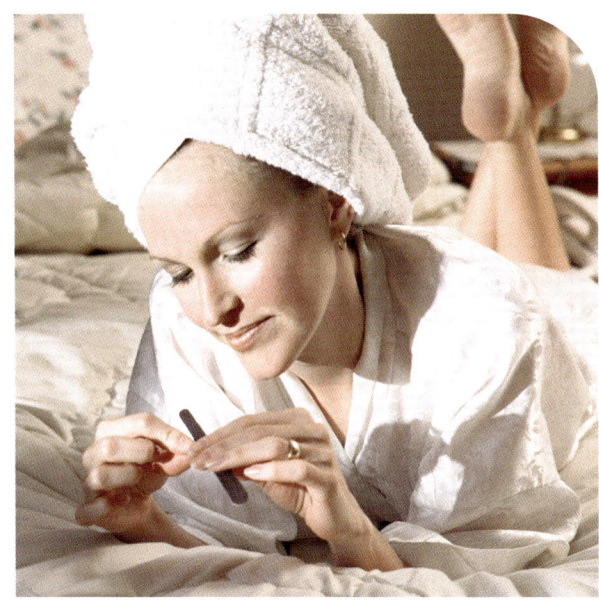

Rest and Relaxation

A restful night's sleep can actually prevent poor health and disease. The well-documented therapeutic effects of sleep include renewed vigor, reduced tension and time for the body to repair. Most people need six to eight hours of sleep nightly, or they suffer fatigue and cannot function properly. Research also shows that inadequate sleep slows reaction time, lowers IQ, disrupts normal body functions (hormone levels, heart rate, blood pressure) and weakens the immune system's ability to protect the body from disease. Lack of sleep also contributes to low energy and headaches, as well as poor job performance. Staying out late can have a negative effect on your ability to manage those early morning appointments that require you to be at your best.

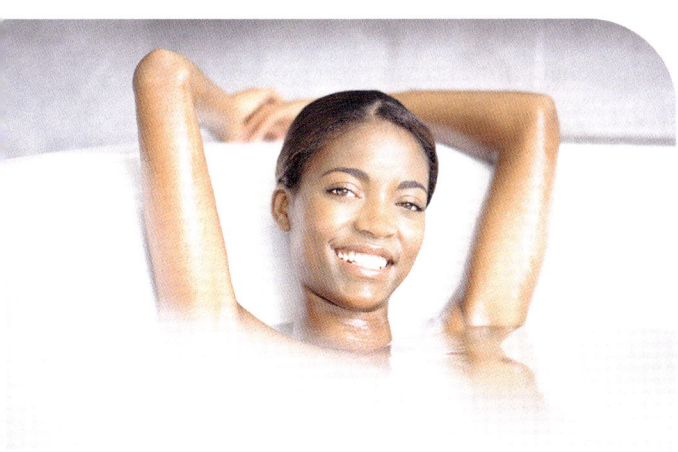

Being able to relax and "get away from it all" also helps maintain a healthy mind and body. Reading a good book, listening to music, watching TV or going for a walk can all provide a chance for the body and mind to clear, relax and refocus so that you can return to work refreshed.

Exercise

A regular exercise program will help you feel, look and work better. Your muscles—heart muscles included—need to be in the best possible condition in order to be healthy. Exercise helps develop and sustain muscle tone, priming your body to work, look and feel better. Exercise also helps stimulate the blood circulation and metabolism, allowing your body to function at optimal performance.

In medieval times, mattresses were secured on bed frames by ropes. When you pulled on the ropes, the mattress tightened, making the bed firmer to sleep on. Hence we have the phrase "good night, sleep tight."

A well-balanced exercise routine includes three disciplines: cardiorespiratory fitness, strength training and flexibility. Take the time to set up your own personalized exercise program, optimally striving for all three. For cardiorespiratory fitness, try aerobic activity, such as brisk walking, running, cycling, rowing or skating. These activities strengthen the heart and lungs to improve blood circulation, lower blood pressure, build endurance, boost your immune system and reduce stress. For strength training, use free weights, weight machines or elastic bands to build muscle mass, increase muscle tone, lose weight and strengthen the entire musculo-skeletal system.

Weight-bearing exercises, such as yoga, running or brisk walking are also effective for strength training. Flexibility training, an often overlooked part of the fitness formula, may include yoga or tai-chi, as well as more basic stretches. These movements will increase range of motion, improve posture, alleviate muscle spasms, decrease stress and maintain agility. Just getting out a few times a week to enjoy the fresh air will make an incredible difference in your health and outlook.

Remember that you have chosen a profession that is not only mentally, but physically challenging. The better you condition your body, the easier it will be to sustain good health in your physically demanding career. Health and vitality will help you along the path to success.

Round out your exercise program by exercising your mind. Reading can be a relaxing way to learn, stimulating brain activity. It is an excellent way to exercise the mind.

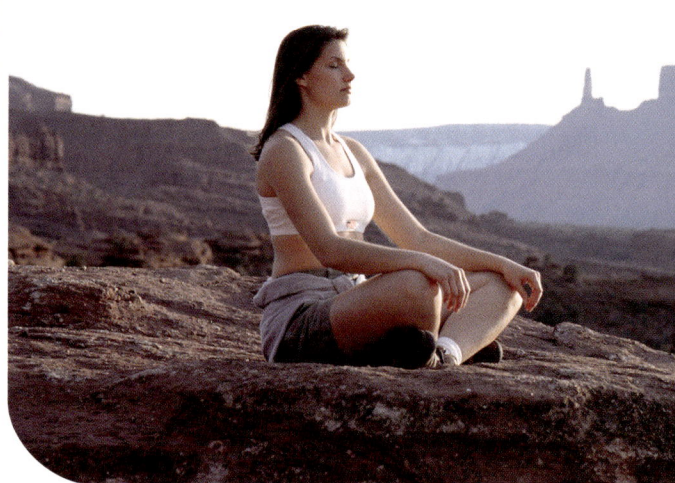

Stress Management

Stress is the tense, "tied-up-in-knots" feeling we get when life's circumstances become challenging. Believe it or not, there is good stress or bad stress. As a positive influence, the feeling of stress can compel us to action or result in a new awareness that helps us solve a difficult problem. For example, you might remember a time when you were "pumped up" or "psyched" for an exam or competition; that is the good stress that helps you to perform. As a negative influence, stress results in feelings of frustration, anger, helplessness and even depression. For example, you might remember a time when you were running late for an important appointment or interview, or a time when you could not focus or think straight and everything seemed to be going wrong; that is the bad stress that can take a toll on your mind and body.

Your ability to manage stress and live in moderation and balance works wonders for your mental health. Sound mental health practices begin with an awareness of the physical and mental consequences of your emotional life. Anger and depression harmfully affect and weaken body functions, especially those of the heart, arteries and glands. Angry thoughts, for example, may cause the heart rate to increase. It is also widely known that many illnesses are related to unrelieved periods of stressful living. Because stress is unavoidable these days, it's best to try to reduce stress as much as possible and learn to manage it. This means becoming aware of what causes you stress and adopting a personal set of coping strategies for those things you cannot change.

Nutrition

As the saying goes, "You are what you eat." In other words, nutritional habits greatly influence health and well-being. **Nutrition**, the process of converting raw materials in the form of carbohydrates, fats and proteins into energy, is another health consideration.

Almost all foods contain a combination of these energy-producing substances. The energy they produce is measured in units of heat called calories and used by the body in three essential ways:

- To regulate body temperature
- To build and re-build structures
- To move and think

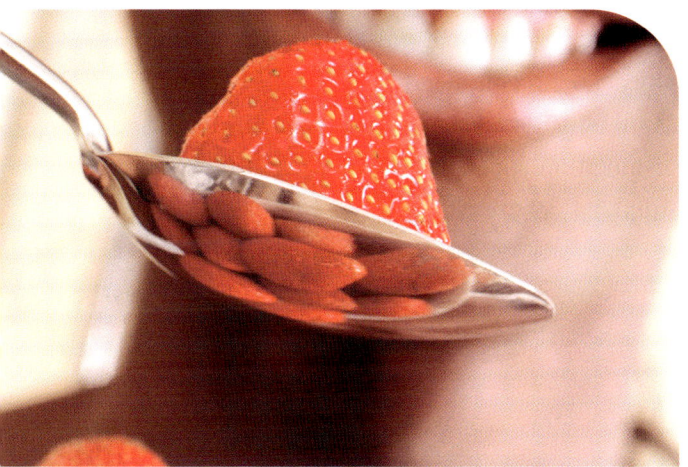

RDA Guidelines

You may have heard the term **RDA**, which means Recommended Dietary Allowance. The U.S. Government established the RDA as appropriate nutrient intakes for people in an effort to help them select an adequate daily diet from the array of available foods. The human appetite cannot always be trusted to choose the best foods. The following are basic RDA Guidelines for calorie intake:

- Calories: 2,300-3,000 for men; 1,900-2,200 for women
  - Carbohydrates: 45-65% (complex)
  - Proteins: 10-35%
  - Fats: 20-35%

Calories

The fact is, few people really eat what's best for them. With options such as fast food, packaged foods, snacks and desserts, it's very tempting to eat only what you like or crave. This type of impulse eating is at least one explanation for the serious health problems in industrialized countries across the world. For example, statistics have shown that more than 50% of the population in the United States is overweight.

Another explanation for the growing problem of obesity is lack of exercise. The same agency that established the RDA system also recommends a certain number of calories per day, approximately 2,300-3,000 for men, and 1,900-2,200 for women. If you consume more than that amount, you risk gaining weight.

Runners are known to eat a big serving of pasta, which is loaded with carbohydrates, before a race. The carbohydrates serve as a major source of energy.

Additionally, if you do not burn an adequate number of calories through exercise or daily activity, you will also gain weight since "left over" calories are converted to fat. The energy may be stored as body fat for use at a later time.

Carbohydrates

Carbohydrates serve as a major energy source and are found in whole grains, vegetables, fruits, legumes, nuts and seeds. They should account for 45-65% of your daily nutrient intake. These foods increase energy levels and calm you while providing the fiber necessary for regulating digestion.

Proteins

Proteins are the body's building blocks. Skin, hair and nails, along with brain, muscle and connective tissue, consist primarily of protein. A good diet includes approximately 10-35% protein that is low in cholesterol and saturated fats. This means lean meats, poultry, fish and low or no-fat dairy products along with plant proteins like grains, legumes, nuts and seeds.

Fats

Believe it or not, fats are an important part of a healthy diet. They are a source of concentrated energy that provide the body with necessary fatty acids. A healthy daily diet includes approximately 20-35% unsaturated fat. Essential fatty acids (EFAs) produce hormones and protect against heart disease, cancer, autoimmune diseases and skin diseases. Excellent sources for EFAs include the following: fatty fish, cod liver oil, flaxseed oil, beans, nuts, seeds, black currants and evening primrose.

Other Essential Nutrients

In addition to appropriate nutrients that the RDA Guidelines recommend, the body also needs water and essential vitamins and minerals.

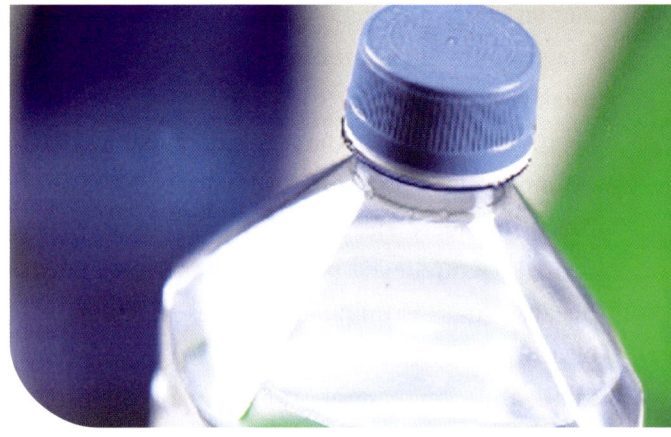

Water

The body is 2/3 water. The body's need for water is second only to its need for oxygen. Water is a clear, colorless, odorless, tasteless liquid essential for almost all living things. It helps regulate body temperature, transports nutrients and hormones throughout the system and flushes out toxins via the kidneys. Lack of sufficient water can cause a decrease in mental performance, aches and pains, dry, sallow skin, irritability and fatigue. Recommendations from the Mayo Clinic recommend 12 cups of water a day for the average man and 9 cups a day for the average woman. This water can be from all sources, including foods that contain water.

Vitamins and Minerals

Vitamins and minerals are organic substances essential for normal growth and activity. A wide variety of healthy foods will provide you with many of the essential vitamins and minerals; however, some nutritionists and primary-care physicians recommend a daily multivitamin as an added source. Speak with your doctor or nutrition specialist to see if vitamin supplements are right for you.

The word vitamin was coined in 1911 by Warsaw-born biochemist Casimir Funk (1884-1967). The letters A, B, C, D and so on were assigned to the vitamins in the order of their discovery.

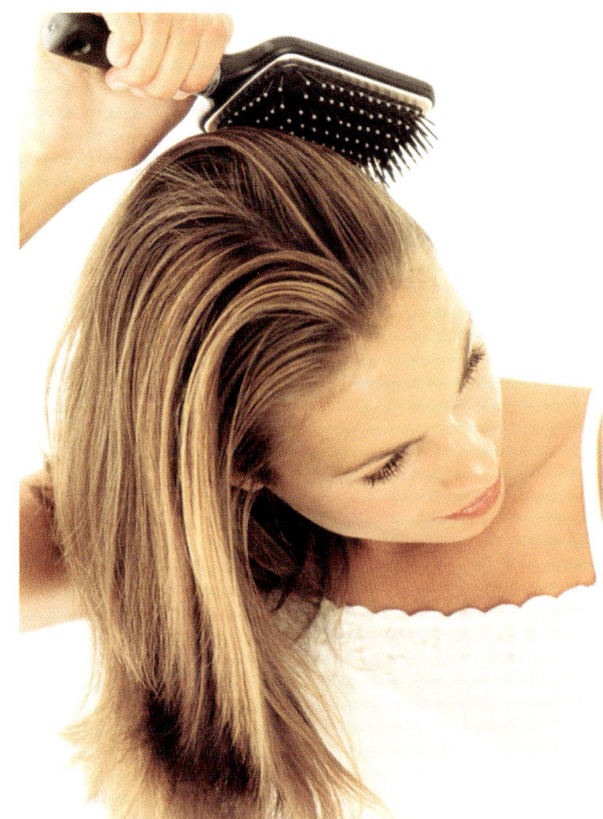

Hygiene

Hygiene is the applied science that deals with healthful living. The practice of **public hygiene** (also referred to as public health) significantly helps promote and preserve the health of the community. As you train to be a licensed professional, you are learning that your clients depend on you to protect them from health and safety hazards in the salon or spa environment. Impure air from poor ventilation, inadequate lighting, improper disinfection practices and improper storage or use of food are the primary health hazards against which health officials expect you to protect clients. In essence, it is your job to protect and serve the public.

Personal hygiene is your individual system for maintaining your cleanliness and health. Cleanliness is the single most important aspect of personal hygiene. In your work, you will constantly be in close proximity to your clients. Scents that would ordinarily go unnoticed or soil that would normally go undetected can be offensive. If you expect your clients to enjoy your company and want to come back, establish and maintain a personal hygiene routine. To prevent body odors from becoming offensive, bathe regularly using soap and water, apply deodorant or anti-perspirant and wash clothing regularly. Avoid excessive use of cologne or perfume because some clients are sensitive to certain fragrances.

The early Egyptians used scented baths followed by an underarm application of perfumed oils. The early Greeks and Romans followed the Egyptian example and created perfume that acted as deodorant to mask body odor.

The food you eat and the state of your health also affect the condition of your breath. One way to prevent bad breath, or **halitosis** (hal-eh-TOH-siss), is by taking good care of your teeth and gums. Good dental care, also referred to as oral hygiene, requires brushing your teeth two to three times a day—generally after every meal—and using mouthwash. Your clients will be grateful. Consider all of these potential hygiene problems and establish a personal hygiene plan that addresses them daily.

Image

The beauty care business is a service business that focuses on image; therefore, close attention to personal grooming and professional appearance is a must. Personal hygiene and good grooming add to your self-esteem and raise your image in the eyes of clients. The better you care for your hair, skin, hands, feet and clothing, the more positively you will be perceived. Your image is a direct representation of who you are and of the professional impression that you wish to make. Basic guidelines listed in the next section will help you maintain your professional image.

Hair Care

A daily hair care program is essential for nail technicians. The professional nail care business recommends that hair be neatly groomed and pulled back from the face if it is shoulder length or longer. A good guideline is that if your hair touches your face when you tilt your head forward, it should be pulled back.

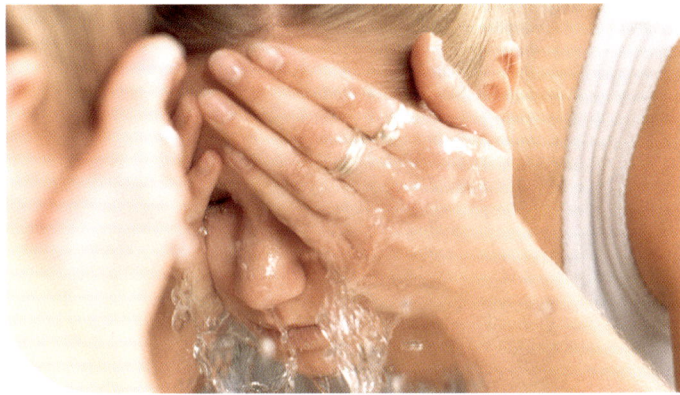

Skin Care and Makeup

Take advantage of your industry to care for your own skin. By networking with a skin care professional, you can determine how best to care for your skin. Healthy, glowing skin is dependent on good nutrition, exercise, rest and, most of all, the products you use. Remember, for most of the day you will be sitting face to face with your clients and you want to professionally portray the beauty industry.

Artfully applied, makeup can enhance facial features. As a nail care professional, you will want to keep your makeup application minimal. The majority of your day will be spent with a warm light near your face. Too much makeup can end up running down your face if you sweat. The most professional approach to your own makeup is to choose neutral colors in light applications. At the same time, it is important that you put some effort into a neat makeup application in a way that communicates to your clients that you are a professional.

Hands

Maintaining attractively manicured, well-cared-for hands can be challenging for nail technicians since their hands are exposed to a wide variety of chemicals throughout the day. It is important to use your own expertise in nail and hand care in order to keep your hands smooth, soft, immaculately clean and well-manicured. Remember you are your own best advertisement, and your beautiful hands and nails will represent the results that you can help your clients achieve.

Feet

In order to feel your best and maintain a cheerful attitude, it's important to take proper care of your feet. Practicing good posture and wearing properly fitted, low, broad-heeled shoes that give the body support and balance are great ways to be comfortable, even though you may not spend too much time on your feet throughout the day.

To keep your feet at their best, you also should schedule regular pedicures that include cleansing, exfoliation of callused skin, massage and toenail trims. At home, it's important to thoroughly dry your feet after bathing to prevent fungus infections like athlete's foot. If you develop bunions, corns or ingrown toenails, see a podiatrist (also known as a chiropodist or foot doctor).

Clothing

Looking and feeling your best is also reflected by your clothing. Freshly washed or cleaned and pressed clothing are a part of good hygiene. Unsightly rings around the collar or the armpit are unacceptable. The fit around the shoulder should be loose enough to allow easy movement. No article of clothing should be uncomfortably or unflatteringly tight. Shoes must always be clean and polished.

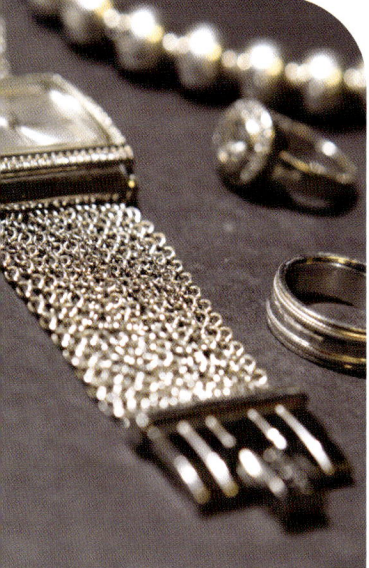

Jewelry

Pay attention to your choice of jewelry. Be aware that large, flashy pieces of jewelry can detract from your professional image, so it is best to keep necklaces, earrings and watches very plain and simple. Avoid bracelets and rings. They may be cumbersome when gloves are required or as you perform services. Most schools and salons have a dress code for their students or professionals. Follow the code with careful consideration of your personal sense of style, and you'll look great!

Dress well first. Make money second. Some people think they can't dress well until they make enough money. What they don't understand is that to make more money, they need to dress like those who do!

Posture

Good posture enhances both physical and mental well-being. Correct posture reduces fatigue and helps the internal organs function properly. As you perform nail care services, you'll bend and stretch and stoop. As you restock inventory, you may need to lift boxes as heavy as 50 pounds. Maintaining good posture and moving your body properly will prevent muscle strain and potential injury, reduce physical fatigue and present an attractive professional image.

Good posture begins with sitting correctly while providing services. Sit with your back against the back of the chair, with your feet flat on the floor.

First impressions count! These impressions are made based on your clothes, jewelry, makeup, speech, posture, voice and any other apparent feature. Present an image that generates a positive impression. Always dress and act like the professional that you are.

DO's AND DON'Ts FOR GOOD POSTURE

DO

- Do use the height adjustments provided on the technician chairs. Most chairs and stools are designed to be raised and lowered so you can reach your client properly without stooping over or tensing your shoulders.
- Do keep your feet and knees together, feet on the floor when sitting, and sit squarely on the seat of the chair.
- Do use a mirror to note any posture defects you may have and work diligently to correct them.

DON'T

- Don't slump over in an attempt to reach a client. Instead, bend forward at the waist holding your shoulders straight.
- Don't bend at the waist when lifting objects from the floor. Instead, bend at the knees to lower your whole body.

Ergonomics

A science called "ergonomics" is used to study the relationship between people and their work environment. The body movements, positions, tools and equipment involved in completing a task affect a person's overall health and comfort. This growing science continually develops new tools and equipment to support these health issues, and help increase productivity.

ERGONOMIC RECOMMENDATIONS FOR NAIL TECHNICIANS

A correct seated position will allow you to provide services to your clients with less strain on your feet, legs, shoulders and back. Sit with your back straight and both feet on the floor directly below your knees. Pulling in your stomach muscles helps to support your back. If you find your back, shoulders or arms are uncomfortable when you are trying to reach your client's hands or feet, then adjust the height of your chair.

You will be spending long hours sitting, bending, reaching and repeating the same motions. Any repeated activities can cause fatigue and pain in various parts of the body—especially the back— and can sometimes even result in serious injury. Some aches, pains and injuries develop slowly over a long period of time. In many cases, health challenges can be prevented by improved posture, better work habits and proper equipment.

HAND AND WRIST

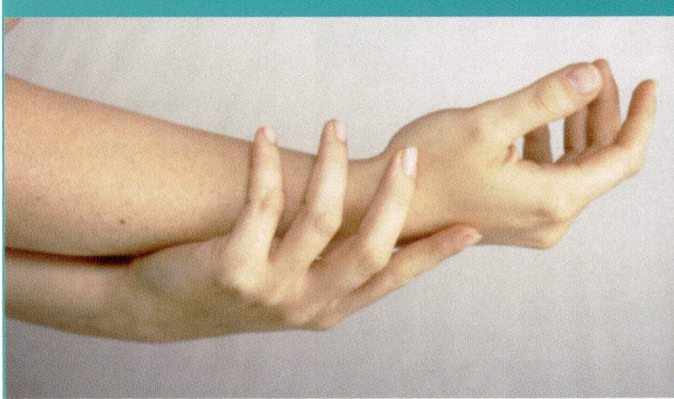

Most of the muscles that move your hands and fingers are actually in your forearms. These muscles are connected to the hands and fingers by tendons, which are like cords passing through your wrists. Tendonitis occurs when the tendons become inflamed. The carpal tunnel is a tunnel in the wrist surrounded by bone and tissue. A nerve and several tendons pass through this tunnel. When tendonitis develops, the tendons swell and the nerve in the tunnel becomes pinched. This condition, called **Carpal Tunnel Syndrome,** can make your hands numb and weak and can eventually affect your career and ability to work. The main causes of tendonitis and Carpal Tunnel Syndrome are:

- Bending your wrist often
- Pinching or gripping with force
- Repeating a motion over and over

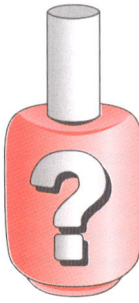

What can you do to improve your overall personal health, hygiene and appearance?

EFFECTIVE COMMUNICATION

Communication is an exchange of thought. This can take place verbally or nonverbally, but in today's fast-paced world, use of technology means that much communication is now transmitted through a system, such as a telephone, e-mail or fax. However, your profession is one of the few that still requires face-to-face contact and involves touch!

Every time you exchange ideas, thoughts or feelings with someone, you are communicating. Therefore, your communication skills are every bit as important to your success as are your technical skills.

As a nail technician, your primary responsibility is to use your knowledge and skills to help your clients look and feel their best. Your professional advice and services are measured by your ability to communicate with your clients. Most of your interaction will involve face-to-face communication, which is where your expert interpersonal skills come into play.

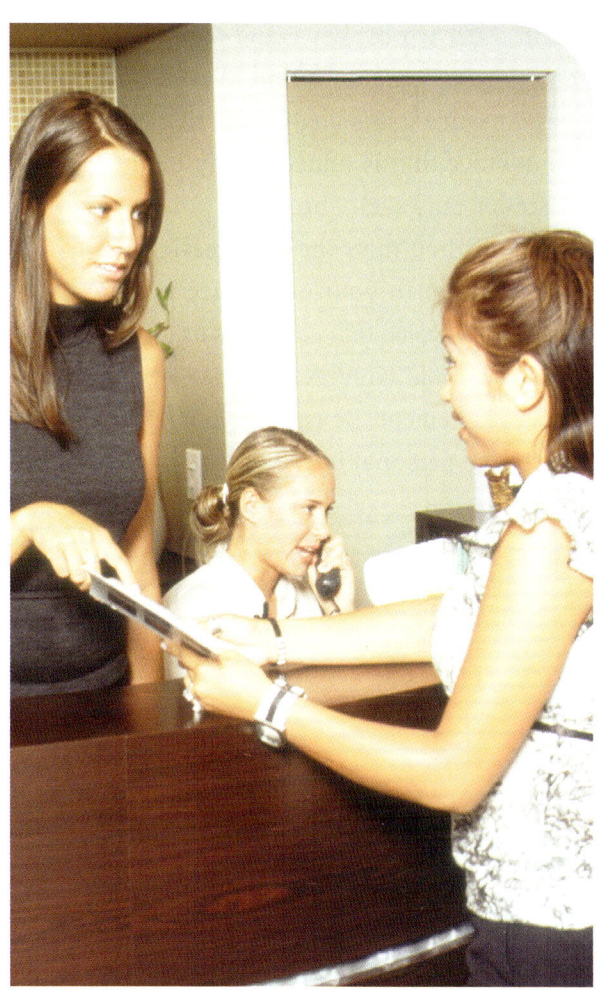

1

Nonverbal Communication

In **nonverbal communication** (sometimes called "body language"), messages are exchanged without speaking. Appearance, posture, poise, touch, facial expression, eye contact, gestures and silence often "speak more loudly than words." For example, a smile is a universal sign of approval. Another example is the peace sign. Additionally, one who stands up straight with shoulders squared and head held high, and extends a hand to greet, communicates self-confidence. Bowed shoulders and sloping body posture convey uncertainty and low self-confidence.

Eye contact tells your client that he or she has your full attention. Simple eye contact can validate and reassure. It is a universal sign of acknowledgement and attention.

Become aware of the subtle ways posture can communicate your feelings about yourself and those around you. Be sure your posture conveys confidence and your movements indicate interest in what your client is saying.

Verbal Communication

How you speak is as important as what you say. In other words, voice and tone are very important in communication. A well-modulated, pleasant voice gains greater positive attention than a voice that is unnecessarily high or shrill. A listener may well "tune out" an irritating voice and then miss the information being shared. Listen to your own voice in various situations. A voice that can carry harmonious tones in normal conversation may become shrill during excitement. Be certain your voice always reflects the personal image you want to project.

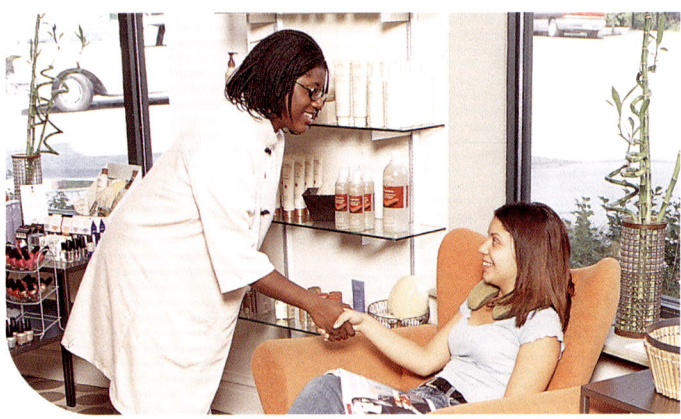

How you speak can also influence the meaning of what you say. The level and tone of your voice, inflection and rate of speech all play an important role in verbal communication. For example, think of a time when someone has said one thing but the tone of his or her voice certainly meant something else.

Grammar

Your language, if used correctly, can clearly and beautifully communicate all of your thoughts and needs. Used incorrectly, however, the beauty of the language may be marred and your level of communication can diminish. The choice of words that you use is vital to the art of conversation and will impact the listener's understanding.

When poor grammar is used, your intended message may not be clear. For example, the use of double negatives and certain slang can detract from the thought you are attempting to communicate. The listener can be confused by such communication and be left with a completely incorrect understanding of what you meant to say.

The use of poor grammar can begin accidentally as you copy poor speech patterns used by those around you. It can also begin intentionally, when you choose to use it to imitate certain peers or to create particular effects.

The use of poor grammar may become a habit, and you might not notice it while speaking. Ask people close to you to point out any words you may misuse and speech patterns you have that aren't appropriate. A great way to improve your communication skills is to tape record yourself during a client consultation, then later replay the tape and evaluate what you said and how you said it. This allows you to instantly recognize what you may need to change in your style of communication.

Two-Way Communication

Your success in providing your clients with the exact service they require and desire depends on how well you are able to understand and interpret their initial request.

There is an easy method for accomplishing this. First, encourage your clients to give you enough information so that you understand their desires. Ask questions that require more than a simple "yes or no" answer. Then be sure to *listen* to what is said, not just hear what is said. To hear something is to perceive the sound, which is the function of the ear. To listen means hearing with intention to understand.

Second, repeat back to the client, in your own words, what they have expressed as their needs or concerns. Then, follow through by telling them what you can and will provide in order to meet those needs or concerns.

For example:
Technician: "How have your nails been since I last saw you?"

Client: "My cuticles are still dry and I have a lot of hangnails."

Technician: "Judging from the look of your cuticles and what you are telling me, you could try using a cuticle oil every morning and night. My recommendation is a hot oil manicure today to give you some added moisture."

When you have finished your explanation, always ask your clients if they understand what you will be doing and if they would be interested in receiving the service and purchasing the product for home care. Encourage the client to ask questions. If you can communicate comfortably, your job will be much easier. Several suggestions that will help you become a better communicator include the following:

Present a Pleasant Greeting

- Always greet a client by using the last name (Mrs. Brown, Mr. Smith, Ms. Johnson) unless the client offers permission to be on a first-name basis and that practice is acceptable in the school or salon.
- Use a pleasant tone of voice that projects your professionalism and maturity as well as your eagerness to offer your services. Smiles and warm words of welcome indicate graciousness.

Use Tact

- Tact requires that you learn to be truthful without being offensive. This skill requires sensitivity.
- Tact is a very important communication skill to use in building honest and professional relationships with your clients.

For example, a client may insist that your product caused her nails to break, yet you suspect that the problem is more likely the harsh household cleansers that she uses without wearing gloves. It is your responsibility to educate her about product ingredients and tactfully suggest otherwise.

Client: "We need to use a different base coat. This one caused my nails to break."

Technician: "I'm so sorry to hear that. Is it possible that it could be a cleaning product that you are using at home? This base coat is formulated to promote nail strength. Perhaps we can try it for one more week and you can try using gloves to do your chores at home, to see if that could be the problem. If you are still having a problem, I will certainly have another base coat for next week."

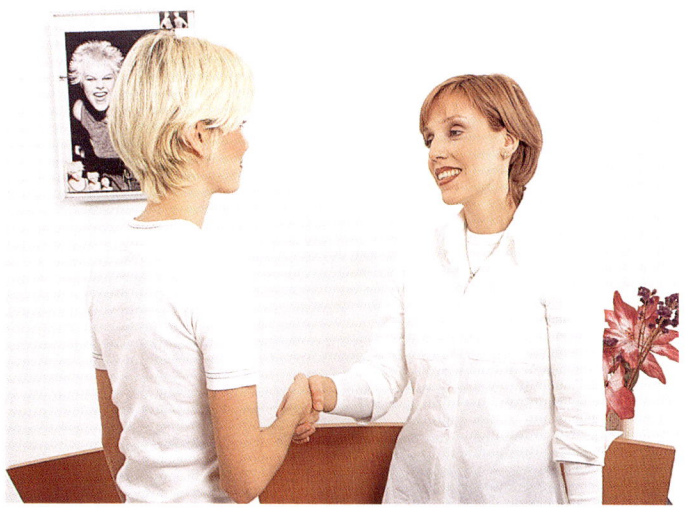

1

Express Your Ideas Clearly

- Think an idea through completely before you talk about it.
- Many good ideas are not realized because they are not thought through before they are expressed.

Define the Purpose of Your Communication

Before you begin to express your idea, determine the purpose of your communication. Is it to:

- Gain information?
- Change an attitude?
- Seek support?
- Motivate?

Know the Importance of Your Ideas

Be certain that the communication is valuable to others. When speaking:

- Consider the listener's needs and desires.
- Ask yourself, "How will the listener benefit from what I'm saying?"

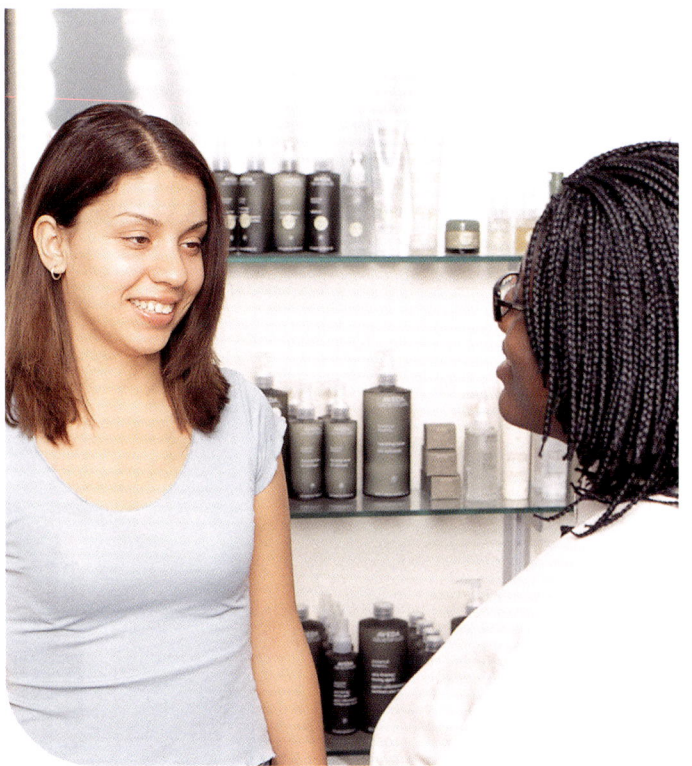

Be Aware of Your Environment

- Be sure the timing is right for your communication.
- Decide whether your ideas or feelings should be expressed in public or private.
- Decide who should be the recipient of your communication.

Watch Your Overtones

An overtone occurs when your tone of voice, inflection, expressions and reactions do not match your words. For example, if you say, "I'm so happy to see you today," but you are not smiling or extending your hand in greeting, you convey a negative overtone.

- Be careful that your overtones aren't saying something entirely different from the words you speak.
- Be sure you are communicating the idea you want to convey.

> To find out how others hear you, try recording your own voice and playing it back. Ask yourself, "Do I need to change the level, tone or speed at which I speak?"

Consult With Others When Necessary

- Be certain you have all the facts and information available.
- When in doubt, consult with others to gain new insights, ideas, opinions and support.

Active and Reflective Listening

The most successful business people and the best communicators are those who have learned to listen, both actively and reflectively. Active listening involves the whole body. Good listeners give nonverbal and verbal signs that they are listening. They sit in an attentive posture, nod in acknowledgement, make good eye contact, convey a positive, encouraging attitude and give feedback.

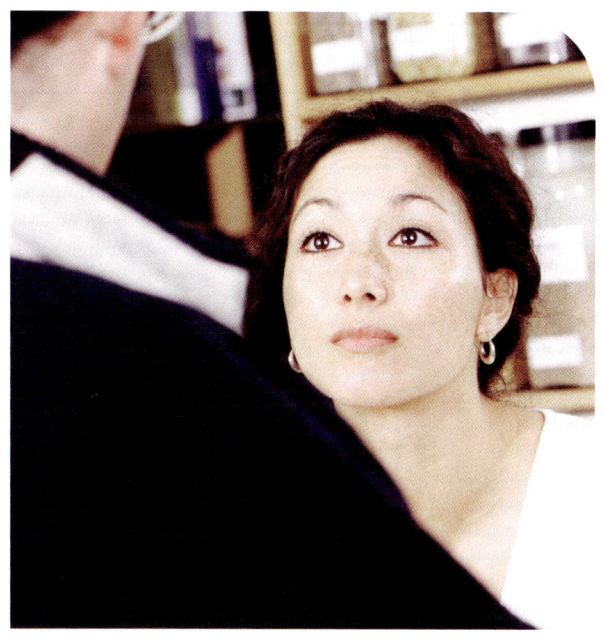

Reflective listening involves reporting what you heard. The act of repeating out loud what you heard and processed inside your head helps you to remember the information. It also provides a way to confirm what was actually said.

The topics you select to discuss with your clients should be chosen with care. Many nail technicians rely on the weather, current movies and famous personalities to provide neutral topics to discuss with clients. Avoid controversial topics such as politics or religion. Also avoid talking continuously since some clients prefer to relax peacefully during a nail service. As a true nail care professional, you'll want to focus your conversation on your client's nail care needs. Professional recommendations will help to meet those needs. Personal conversation must be kept to a minimum, and gossip about other clients or colleagues should definitely be avoided. It is acceptable to let your clients share information about their personal lives—that is often a way for them to vent frustrations—but it is not acceptable for the professional nail technician to share his or her personal life with clients.

Always try to bring the conversation back to the current task—nails. Throughout the entire service, explain what you're using and why. This explanation provides you with a "selling" technique. Your client will expect to receive your full attention while in your care and to receive the full benefit of your professional expertise. Your responsibility is to meet the needs of each of your clients. This means delivering results that are accomplished through the services and products that you offer. Whenever a client approaches you with a complaint, handle it calmly and judiciously. Fulfill your responsibility, and your success will be guaranteed.

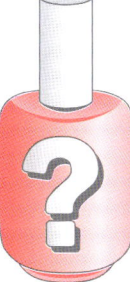

Experts tell us that the best communicators are also the best listeners. What can you do to improve your listening skills?

PURPOSEFUL RELATIONSHIPS

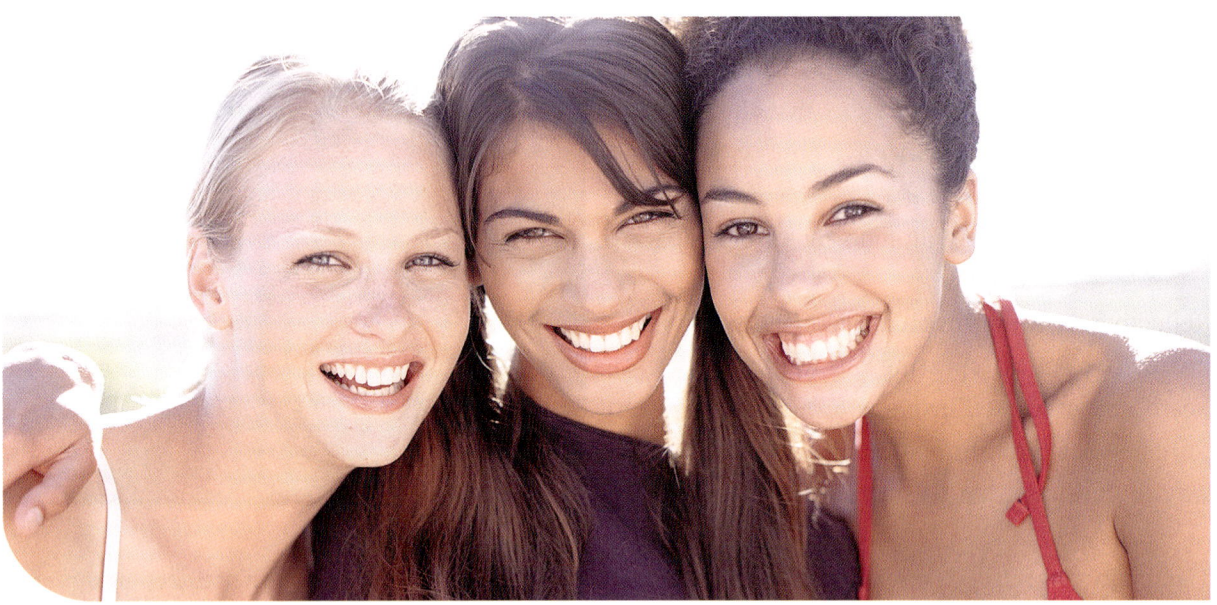

The ancient Greeks believed that health and vitality were rewards for organizing inner thoughts, feelings and attitudes. Today we know that self-knowledge is an essential to developing meaningful relationships. Self-knowledge includes understanding and accepting different personalities, the importance of working with others and asserting a personal code of ethics.

Personality

Personality is a complex set of characteristics that distinguishes individuals from others. It is also the outward reflection of inner feelings, thoughts, attitudes and values. Carl Jung, a famous psychologist, was fond of saying that people are only alike in those ways that are different from other types of people. In other words, sharing common differences is what makes us similar to others. Therefore, your personality is the sum total of the emotional and behavioral characteristics that make you unique. Many experts tell us that although personality is influenced by our experiences, it is rarely changed, only modified over time.

Imagine it is your last day on a job. Your co-workers have surprised you with a going-away party. What do you want people to say about you as they stand and converse?

Attitude

An **attitude** is a feeling or emotion toward something or someone. Because your attitude is projected, it will have an effect on those around you. "Positive" and "negative" are the two adjectives most often used to describe attitudes. A negative attitude, obviously, can have a negative impact on others. Conversely, projecting a positive attitude can have an uplifting effect on the people with whom you come into contact. Other adjectives that describe attitude include enthusiastic, caring, confident, defensive, aggressive or fearful.

People are not born with attitudes. Attitudes, like habits, are learned. Therefore, attitudes, like habits, can be unlearned, changed and modified. As parts of your personality, they are very resistant to immediate change; however, they can be altered. A good attitude is quite often the key to being successful personally and professionally.

All of us have attitudes. Some are so deeply ingrained that they've become accepted as unchangeable parts of our personalities. Too often, when questioning someone who constantly complains, you'll hear, for example, "Oh, don't mind me. That's just the way I am." Not true! It's the way that person has, consciously or unconsciously, chosen to be. Allowing yourself to project negativity in any form because "it's just the way I am" is unfair to everyone around you. In the long run, you will gain the most by projecting a positive attitude.

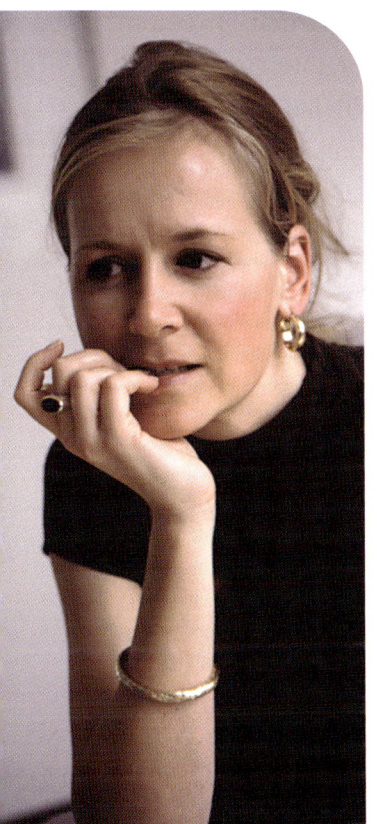

Habits

Some people bite their nails; others bite their lips. Some people drum their fingers; others tap their feet. The only thing all these actions have in common is that the people performing them are probably not aware of their actions. These actions are very likely all habits.

Habits are "learned" behaviors that are reinforced through events in your environment. Like attitudes, habits become ingrained and are difficult to change. Most habits are harmless, inoffensive actions that others barely notice. But some habits are annoying and unattractive. You're entering a professional service business and cannot allow yourself to keep those habits that others may find annoying. Unattractive habits will limit your potential for success and detract from your professional image.

> Studies have shown that it takes at least 21 days to change a habit.

Developing a positive attitude and maintaining sound work habits are two essential elements of purposeful relationships. Additional elements that will help along the way to your success include maintaining attendance and punctuality, so try to:

- Manage your personal and professional schedule to avoid conflicts with time.
- Arrive at work on time. Fifteen minutes prior to starting time is preferred by most employers.

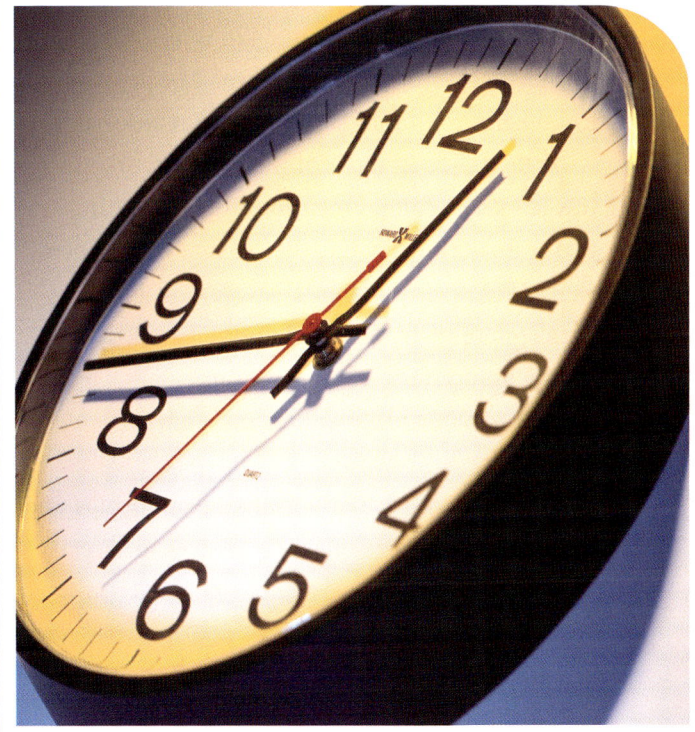

1

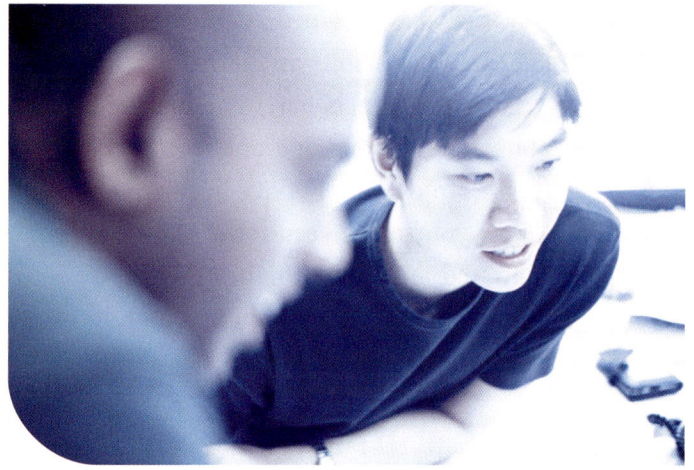

Teamwork

The emotional atmosphere of a salon or spa has a unique importance. The nail care business is a service business, and a part of that service is the creation of a relaxed, peaceful environment. The existence of a harmonious environment depends heavily on teamwork. Working together to create such an environment is also personally gratifying.

As an individual member of a team, you can bring certain valuable characteristics to it that will have a positive influence on the group. Your special behavior, skills and abilities all contribute to the success of the group. You can begin by establishing a rapport, or positive relationship, with each person and continuing to work toward good communication, understanding and teamwork every day. Respecting confidences shared by peers or clients is essential for an atmosphere of trust and sharing. The people with whom you work can become your friends as well as your professional associates.

However, be aware that personal relationships and the condition of personal workspace can greatly impact the professional environment. Keeping your service area clean with all your tools in place is a positive reflection of your professionalism, as well as that of the rest of your team.

Ethics

Over the years your parents and teachers may have taught you to live by the "Golden Rule": "Do unto others as you would have them do unto you." The Golden Rule may have been your first introduction to a code of ethics. As you grow older, you begin defining what is good or bad, right or wrong, according to the rules of society. These rules, or **ethics**, determine right and wrong conduct concerning relationships with others. As your personality develops, you establish your own personal system of moral principles and values, such as honesty and fairness, which become known as your **personal ethics**. The study and philosophy of human conduct known as **professional ethics** deals with proper conduct in relationships with your employer, co-workers and clients.

Most professions have associations that establish a "Professional Code of Ethics" for their individual members. It is important for you to familiarize yourself with the International Nail Technicians Association's (INTA) Code of Ethics or that of another association in your area. These codes, typically based upon high moral principles and values, are designed to protect the public and guarantee that they will be treated honestly and fairly.

Some of the responsibilities and work ethics that will help you earn respect and build solid professional relationships with your clients and co-workers are listed in the following sample points of a "Professional Code of Ethics."

- Show respect for the feelings and rights of others. Remember the Golden Rule.
- Be fair and courteous to your co-workers. Don't criticize other technicians or services or attempt to win clients away from your fellow nail technicians.

- Be fair and courteous to your clients. Be consistent in pricing your services. Don't show favoritism to certain clients.

- Suggest services that meet your clients' needs; never provide a service that may harm your client.

- If you leave the nail care industry, offer the names of other technicians you trust. Never abandon your clients.

- Represent yourself, your services and your products honestly to the public. Do not advertise a service that you cannot perform, and do not make extravagant claims or promises you cannot fulfill.

- Set a positive example of good conduct and good behavior. Always cherish a good reputation. It will carry you and your business a long way.

- Be loyal to your employer and co-workers. Keep your word and fulfill your obligations. Never break the confidence entrusted to you by a client or co-worker. Clients show loyalty and respect if you show dependability.

- Practice only the highest standards of infection control as provided by your regulating agency laws. Keep your work area and tools spotlessly clean.

- Believe in and be proud of your profession, just as you believe in yourself!

You have chosen to pursue a career that allows you to nurture others through the act of human touch. Caring sincerely and professionally for your clients will become your hallmark. What the sages say, however, is true: In order to care adequately for others, you must first care for yourself. Being a nail care professional, it is important to stay up-to-date in your industry, uphold the industry's code of ethics, and listen intently to your clients in order to know how best to serve them. It also means taking care of yourself, getting proper rest, exercise and nutrition in order to be at your peak of performance while on the job. You will also be responsible for providing a comfortable and restful environment for your clients, as well as for yourself to work in. And most important, it means developing a strong sense of self, inner strength, courtesy to others and personal integrity, which will enable you to be the best person—as well as the best professional—that you can be.

1

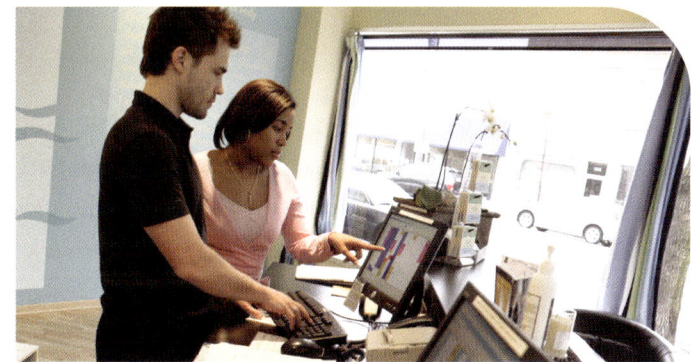

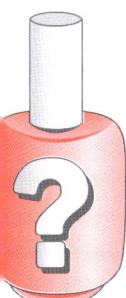

Can you have a great personality and a positive attitude, but behave unethically? Explain.

DECISION-MAKING SKILLS

Case Studies

The following situations are designed to help you build your decision-making skills. Using your training to this point, review the following scenarios, then think through and describe how you would handle each challenge.

1. Last night your best friend visited you, and it was 2:30 a.m. before you were able to go to sleep. That was the second night this week that you had fewer than four hours of sleep. Now, a new friend has just asked you to drive with her to see her brother's school play, which is being held in a city three hours from your home. If you go, it means that you will be home late again. You are booked completely tomorrow, and two are new clients who will require special attention during consultation. Your new friend is counting on you. What would you do?

2. Your boss has just asked you to work a double-shift because a new employee is absent again. You saw this new employee at the same party you attended last night. You were able to get up and come in for your work shift, but the new employee was not. This is the third time this has happened in a 30-day period. What would you do?

Success in business comes from an unquenchable desire to learn something new every day. This is particularly true in the beauty industry. By staying on top of new industry trends and educating yourself about the business you are in and how it operates, you are distinguishing yourself as an industry professional. Whether you are interested in business ownership or not, you can attain a new level of professional achievement by knowing the basics about the nail care business.

VALUE

An ongoing commitment to professional development will help you excel in your career, become a valued asset to your clients and colleagues, and help you achieve personal, professional and financial rewards.

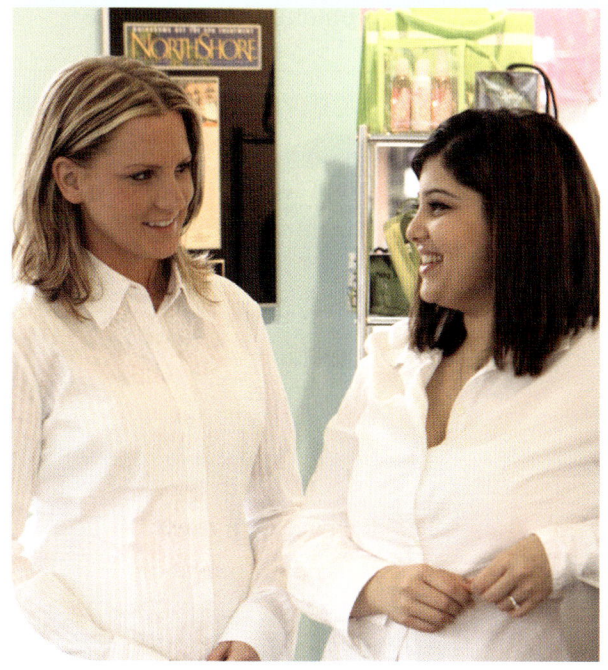

MAIN IDEA

A professional is someone who commits to higher standards of performance and continually seeks to improve. In this chapter on business basics you will learn about the essentials needed to keep improving professionally—from starting out in the industry to opening your own business. Ultimately, what is key to getting ahead in your industry? A commitment to lifelong learning!

PLAN	OBJECTIVES
Job Search • Finding a Job • Evaluating the Salon	Survey job search preparation skills to include resume and cover letter development, job interviewing skills and work environment evaluations.
Career Building • Professional Relationships • Building a Clientele • Lifelong Learning	Give examples of strategies that can be used to help you introduce yourself to other professionals in the nail industry. Describe strategies for building professional relationships with clients and staff. Formulate a lifelong learning plan to continue career and professional development.
Retailing • Professional Recommendation • Motivating Buyers • Sales Promotion	Describe the components of a professional product recommendation and how to motivate buyers. Identify the different types of sales promotions.
Business Ownership • Business Essentials • Plans for a Successful Salon • Expenses and Income • Nail Salon Philosophy, Policies and Procedures	Name the types of business ownership. List several factors to consider before opening a nail salon. Identify three types of taxes: • Withholding • Sales • Income State the components essential to a salon's daily operations. Describe advertising and promotion techniques that will increase sales.

JOB SEARCH

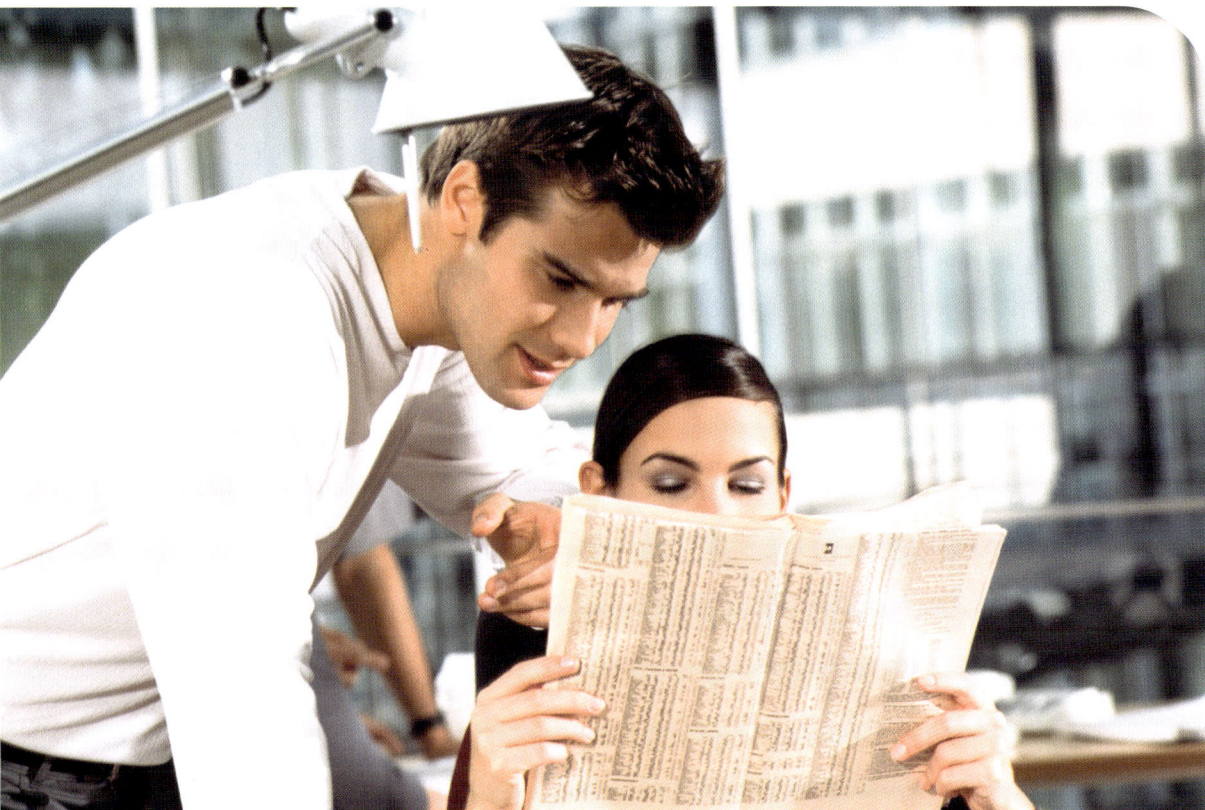

2

If you enjoy working with people and are especially interested in helping others look and feel their best, your career choice is perfect. Health, vitality and looking good are in—big time! People all over the world are becoming increasingly dedicated to "health-wise" lifestyles.

Professional industries that offer personal care services like nails, cosmetology, skin care, massage therapy and others are reporting record-breaking growth and profit statistics. These trends are predicted to continue well into the future. Career opportunities in these industries will go to the most prepared and dedicated individuals.

Successful people in any industry:
- Define goals
- Plan ahead
- Keep an open mind
- Continue to learn

THE NAIL CARE INDUSTRY WANTS YOU!
Take control of your life.
Take your choice of jobs.
Get an education.

...rching for a certi-...hnician with spa ...with gels, tips and ...ease fax resume to ...234. ATTN: Medical ...r.

...an ...et salon is ...technicians, ...nd hair stylist ...nt. Please ...to work in high-energy e- ...to: 312-555-1234. ...ronment. Excellent s- ...benefits. Sales e- ...a

...il Technician ...plus. Fax resu- ...R at ...lon & Day Spa has an ...312-555-123. ...ening for an ...ablished ...il technician ...st be a tea ...SEP\/ICE SAL ON ...er a grea ...ase fax ...5-1234.

...IL CA ...\/PT Busy ...Il. Please call Rachel at ...2-555-1234.

Nail Tech - Salon & Day Spa has an opening for an es-...lished Nail Technician. Candidate must be a team player. V-...offer a great salary and commission. Please fax resume to ...555-1234.

Nail Care Specialist
We are looking for an exp-...enced **nail care speci-**...to give facials and o-...care services. W-...service salon ...pride ...in the extr- ...d service ...we pro- ...r clients. W- ...are ...r someone to f ...staff. Must be inte-...in furthering their edu-...in this field and becomin-...part of our family. Call Susie ...312-555-1234.

Hair Salon & Day Spa has PT pos. for nail technician. Call 312-555-1234.

NAIL CARE PROFESSIONAL ...in

...E ...Makeup Artist. FT\/PTposition-

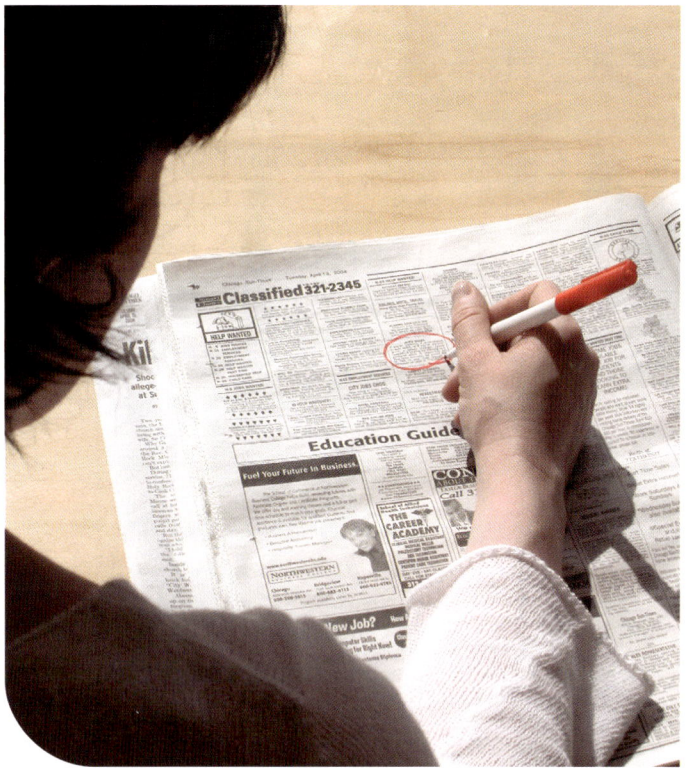

Finding a Job

As you look for a job, you will learn a lot about the inner workings of the industry and about yourself. Think about how your goals relate to the position you are considering.

To find out about nail care locations that are currently hiring or interviewing for future positions, consider several of these methods:

- Talk to nail technicians who are employed in the type of work environment you admire. They may know of positions that are about to become available.

- Check the classified sections of your local newspapers or trade publications on a regular basis. Be prepared to scout under several headings. You may discover an ad under "Nail Technician," "Manicurist" or other special headings, such as "Hotel" or "Resort."

- Talk to distributor sales consultants from companies that sell nail care products to schools, salons and spas. Also talk to representatives from nail product manufacturers or national nail care publications.

- Refer to your school's bulletin board for job postings and ask your instructors for some ideas about seeking employment.

- Check out different areas and make a list of those spas and salons where you would like to work. Call or visit the places that impress you the most and ask if they are hiring new employees or if they have a human resources department.

- Mail out your resumé (explained in the next section), always with a cover letter attached, to the companies you choose. Request that the owner or manager contact you for an interview if an opening is available.

- Check out the Web sites of nail product companies that interest you. Available positions are usually the "Employment Opportunities" button on any given Web site.

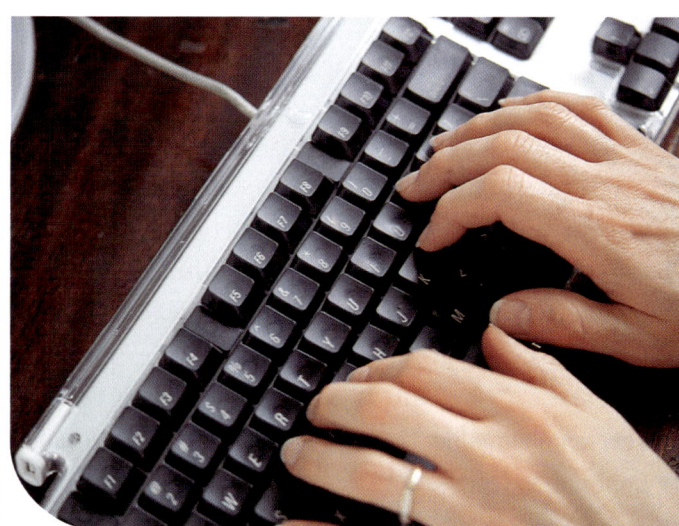

Resumé

Most prospective employers require a **resumé**, which is a one- or two-page outline that lists your educational history, work experience, additional skills and achievements. A resumé is usually submitted with an application and gives an employer an opportunity to quickly review your qualifications. A professional resumé describes personal and professional characteristics in a brief, concise manner. It includes:

- Personal data (name, address, phone, e-mail)
- Educational background (schools attended)
- Additional training (seminars attended)
- Previous employment (if applicable)
- Special skills or areas of expertise
- Special awards or recognition

Also include the following:
- References (professional/personal)
- Interests (hobbies, skills)
- Objective in seeking this position

It makes good sense to maintain a current, complete, error-free resumé throughout your career. Type your resumé neatly and check it thoroughly for grammatical and spelling errors. If you cannot do it at home, professional business services offer resumé creation and writing at a reasonable cost. You may also want to use their services for printing your resumé on professional paper stock with blank matching envelopes.

What Should My Resumé Look Like?

Most professionals recommend that you select white, ivory or a pale shade of beige, blue or gray paper (stock). These colors represent a professional image. In addition, be sure to use the same paper for the resumé, cover letter and envelope. Select a medium-weight paper stock that is not too transparent, but is light enough not to have unattractive wrinkles when folded. Business professionals recommend a 24-26 lb. classic laid or linen paper. Finally, select a legible font or type style for writing the letter and resumé.

The spellcheck feature on a computer might not catch every spelling error, so it is best to read over your resumé to avoid a mistake like this:

"Seeking a party-time position with potential for advancement."

An error like this might keep a prospective employer from calling you for an interview.

Your Name
Address, City, State, Zip
Phone
E-mail

OBJECTIVE
To obtain an entry-level position as a nail technician in the industry so I can use my knowledge, experience and skills to build a clientele and grow professionally.

EDUCATION
Nail Arts Academy, Evanston, Illinois—Certificate in Nail Technology, May, 2003
Hudson Valley Community College—AA, Liberal Arts, May, 2002
Chicago High School, Chicago, Illinois—Graduated, May, 1999

ACADEMIC & PROFESSIONAL EXPERIENCE
- State-Licensed Nail Technician since May, 2005
- Professional training in all areas of nails including manicures; pedicures; acrylic application; gel application; wrap application; client relations and retail sales.

2005-Present
Cosmetics and Nail Care Consultant—Oakbrook Mall, Oakbrook, IL
  Makeup consultations at a major department store representing a famous brand-name product line of cosmetics and nail care products. Required product application, demonstration and presentation skills. Worked extensively with clients on product recommendations. Familiar with cash register balance and close-out.

2002-2004
Server—Sam Maguire's Irish Pub & Restaurant, Orland Park, IL
  Duties included managing an entire service station; working extensively with the public and utilizing an electronic cash register.

ADDITIONAL ACCOMPLISHMENTS
1st Place in Nail Art Design Class, Chicago Midwest Beauty Show, March 2005

LANGUAGES
Spanish, Portuguese

PERSONAL INTERESTS
Reading; photography; studying trends in makeup design and traveling.

References available upon request

Date

Your Name
Address
City, State Zip
Phone
E-mail

Nail Care Center Owner or Manager
Name of Nail Care Center
Address
City, State Zip

Dear (Nail Care Center Owner):

As a highly motivated nail care professional, I am currently seeking employment with a nail care center such as yours. My objective is to find a position in which I can use and enhance my knowledge and professional skills, as well as further my education and technical abilities. I strive for every opportunity possible to learn the broad spectrum of services that the nail care profession has to offer.

Your nail care center appeals to me because it is highly regarded in the beauty industry and has a reputation for being a professional work environment. After visiting a few local nail care centers, yours stands out because of the professional and attractive environment I found when I walked through the door. I am particularly impressed with your retail section—the display is fresh, innovative and the product offering thorough!

I was so excited after my visit that I jotted down a few notes about ideas I have about how I might contribute to your nail care center. I'd like to share these with you. I have enclosed my resumé for your review and would like to schedule an appointment to meet at your earliest opportunity.

I look forward to speaking with you further and will contact you within the next week concerning a meeting.

Thank you so much for your time and consideration.

Sincerely,

Your Name

Your Name

TYPICAL INTERVIEW QUESTIONS

Write your answers to typical questions that an interviewer might ask you, such as:

Tell me a little about yourself.
How long does it take you to do a manicure? A pedicure?
What product lines are you familiar with?
What is your strongest professional characteristic in dealing with people?
What are your strengths and weaknesses?
In what areas do you feel you need improvement?
Give an example of your best experience with a client.
Give an example of your worst experience with a client and how you handled the situation.

Cover Letter

A **cover letter** is a necessary companion piece to your resumé. The cover letter is the "personality piece" that introduces you to your prospective employer. This letter offers a brief summary of why you would like to be employed at this spa or salon. It also provides a brief description of the skills and qualities you feel you could bring to the position.

This letter should be neatly typed in a standard business-letter format, such as in the example to the left. It should contain the date, your address, the employer's address, a greeting, the body of your letter, a closing and your signature with your typed name below it. Always address your letter and resumé to the owner or manager of the salon. If you don't know the owner or manager's name, call to find out. Always double-check your spelling. If you are applying to a large company, send a copy of your resumé to the attention of the human resources department (personnel department).

Job Interview

The impression that you make as a professional is your responsibility. You alone will have to promote yourself and your skills to the potential employer. Be sure to arrive early for the appointment and that you have confirmed the exact location, parking availability and travel costs.

The interviewer will be evaluating your personal qualities. The salon management may evaluate you on such qualities as your:
- Sincerity and honesty
- Motivation and enthusiasm toward the industry
- Obvious desire to work
- Ability to promote a new service or retail product
- Willingness to work as a member of the salon "team"
- Educational and professional goals

Your first job interview can cause some nervousness. Try to remember that you are interviewing the company as much as it is interviewing you. Try your best to stay calm and just be yourself. Take a moment to think before answering questions. You may wish to role-play with friends or family before your scheduled interview.

Evaluating the Salon

Correctly evaluating your future workplace is very important, for it is there you will be spending most of your days developing your career. Understanding what the salon can offer you is just as crucial as what you can offer the salon. Selecting the right salon environment for your employment will allow you to provide the best possible service and products to the clients you serve and will, in turn, allow you to feel proud of yourself and the profession you have chosen.

Work Environments

Before accepting a position, try to carefully assess the advantages and disadvantages of the particular work environment. Managers appreciate questions that show your interest in the business. Suggested questions include the following:

- What are the specific job responsibilities?
- Which product line is used and recommended to clients?
- What type of clientele does the salon serve (students, professionals, mostly women or men)?
- How large is the salon staff? How long have they been with you?
- How many new nail technicians have joined the staff in the last year?
- Does the salon have an active advertising and promotional program?

- What benefits are offered to employees (medical insurance, retirement, paid holidays, educational advancement, paid continuing education units)?

If any of these questions remain unanswered after your initial interview, be sure to find out the answers during your final interview.

Compensation

There are three common ways an employee can be paid:

1. A **commission** structure is based on a percentage of the dollar income the individual nail technician generates by serving clients. For example, if a nail technician earns a 50% commission and performs a $50 service, he or she will earn $25 for that individual service.

2. A **salary** structure is a compensation system that guarantees a set income on a weekly or monthly basis. The advantage is that the employee can count on receiving a set amount each pay period.

3. A **salary-plus-commission** structure guarantees the employee a certain amount of money per pay period and provides additional income when the nail technician meets a predetermined benchmark or goal. This system gives the technician a steady paycheck, while rewarding him or her for building a clientele.

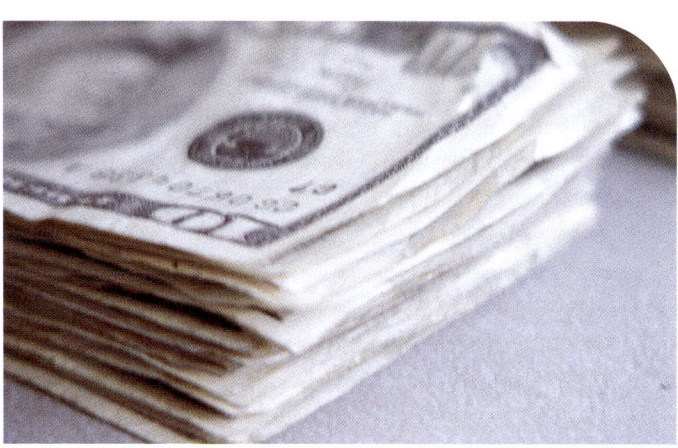

Job Benefits

Job benefits play a key role in determining which job you accept. Sometimes the amount of money you will earn may not be the most important issue. A position that pays less in salary may actually give you more by providing you with costly benefits or "extras." This is called a **"compensation package."** It includes your salary plus the benefits that would otherwise cost you money. For example, these could include insurance, paid sick or vacation time and educational repayment. The components of a total benefit package may include the following:

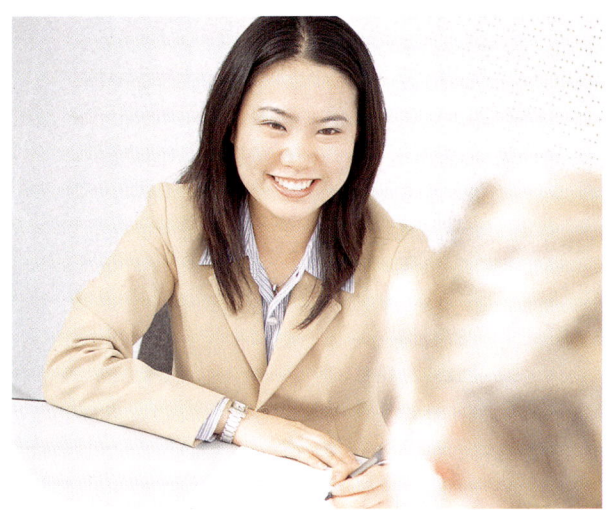

- Salary and/or commission for services performed.
- Sales commission for products purchased by clients.
- Paid holidays, vacations, bonuses.
- Number of sick days allowed each year (paid or not).
- Insurance benefits (health, accident, life).
- Retirement plan.
- Opportunities for travel, advancement, promotion, greater responsibilities.
- Educational seminars and events allowance, ongoing educational programs and guest speakers.

Before you accept employment with a salon, spa, or manufacturer, compare the benefits of each and how they relate to your goals.

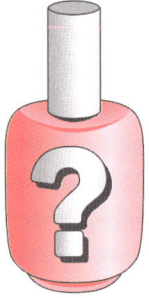

What kind of skills and personal qualities would you emphasize during a job interview?

CAREER BUILDING

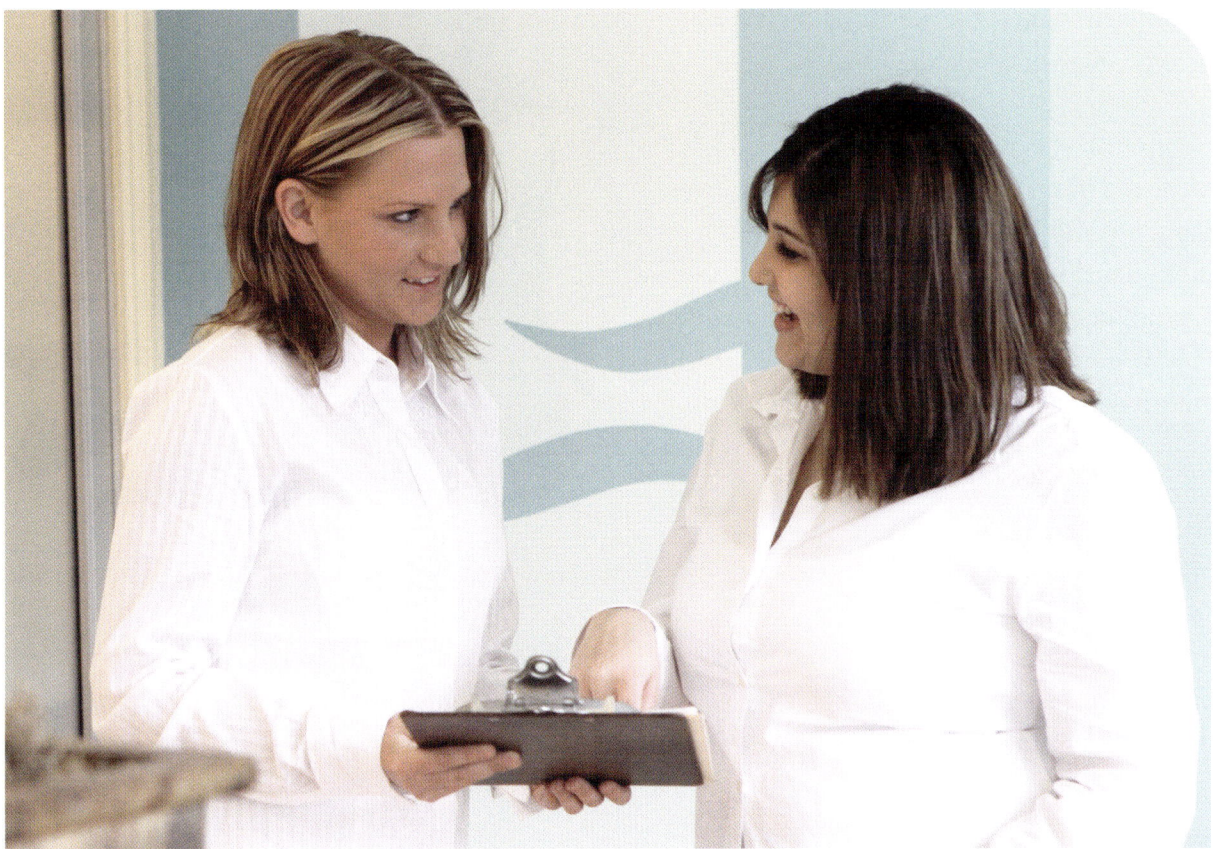

2

The ability to build and maintain professional relationships will prove invaluable to your career. Why? Because, no matter how technologically sophisticated the nail industry becomes, you will always need the ability to communicate and network with other people.

Professional Relationships

Networking means developing relationships with individuals who can put you in contact with potential customers or employers. You may think it's important to get to know the industry "stars." Actually, it's just as important to maintain professional relationships with your fellow students and peers. As you work in the industry, you and your colleagues will make many moves and career advances. Eventually,

you'll all be at higher levels and can utilize each other as valuable contacts and resources!

As these relationships grow, they form a unique support network of people. They can advise, answer questions, share knowledge, help build your clientele and introduce you to other industry professionals.

Client Relationships

Customer service is generally described as personal attention to the needs of the client and a willingness to show concern for his or her personal well-being. For example, remembering a client's specific physical needs, previous services, and unique requests are all important aspects of customer service. In its simplest form, it is building relationships.

Staff Relationships

All successful businesses depend upon a strong "team" approach involving all staff members. This "team" concept revolves around several factors, some of which are listed below:

Communication

Members of a successful team express ideas, thoughts and feelings. They create an open, professional relationship with others. Dreams and aspirations, as well as frustration and anger, may be expressed in a professional manner within a team that has open communication.

Sharing Knowledge

Have you ever heard the expression "two heads are better than one?" This serves to remind us that it is valuable to get input from someone you trust. Before making important decisions, most people ask for advice from the ones close to them, such as friends or family members.

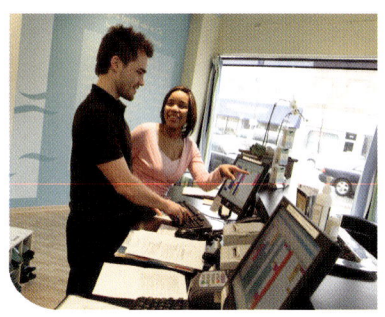

In salons, sharing knowledge helps everyone save time and continue to grow and develop professionally. For example, everyone may not be able to attend the latest workshop or educational event. However, if someone attends the event and shares the information upon his or her return, it helps keep everyone "in the know."

Helping Others

Although you have your own clientele to serve, teamwork encourages you to take the initiative and help co-workers when there is time. In return, they will help you when you need assistance. Co-workers can be professional associates and lifelong friends!

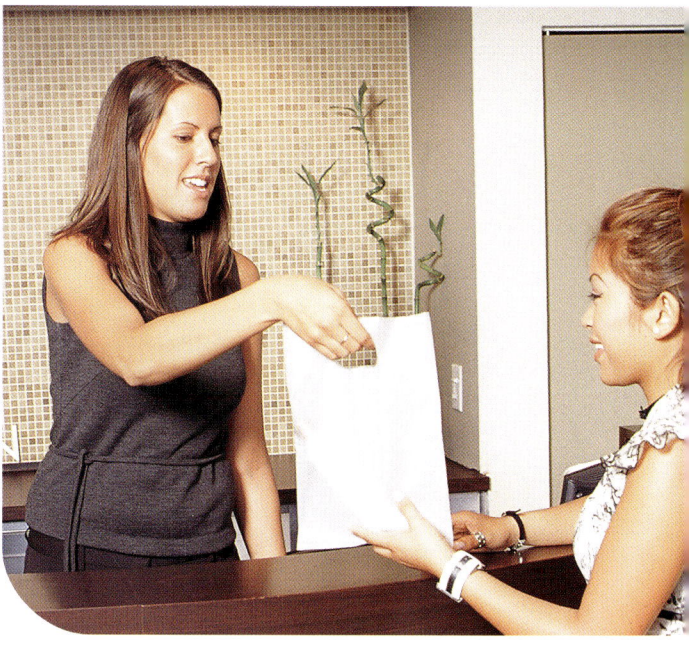

Building a Clientele

Nail technicians work to grow their client base; they learn about and sell professional products; they market, display and promote their services; and most of all, they continually challenge themselves to learn more about their profession. **Marketing** is creating awareness of products or services, but you can also market yourself.

A client scheduled for a hair service might be referred to a nail technician for nail care needs, or vice versa. This reinforces the salon's message that the overall well-being of the client is important. Working as a team, you can provide each new client with special care. Education + Skill + Confidence = SUCCESS!

Your clientele consists of both the clients you serve repeatedly, and those that you try to "recruit" as repeat customers. A satisfied client base shows that your skills and services meet or exceed customer standards. The following techniques are great for bringing in new clients.

Word-of-Mouth Advertising/Referrals

Positive word-of-mouth advertising is probably the most effective way to build your clientele. Satisfied clients will recommend your services to their friends.

Business Cards

Most employers have business cards printed with a company logo, name, address and phone number. Keep them on hand and give these cards to current and potential clients.

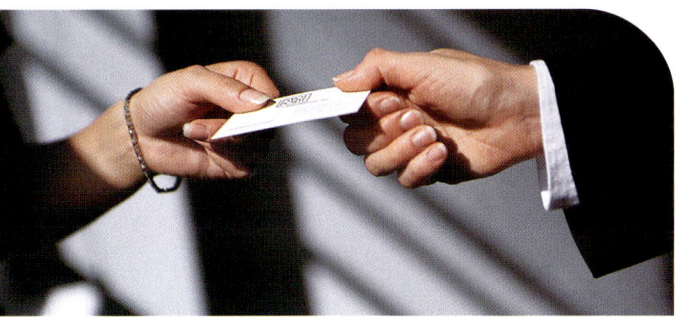

Rebooking

One of the simplest and most effective ways to build clientele is to ask clients to make a future appointment, or **rebook**, (also known as **pre-book**) before they leave the salon. It is a very powerful tool for building a clientele.

Promotional Literature

Distribute flyers, newsletters or postcards to people you meet. Offer a complete menu of all the services you provide. Itemize the services, list the costs and give an accurate description of each service.

Correspondence

Send thank-you cards to every new client after the first appointment or call these new clients after their first visit to follow up. Mail out reminder notes one week before each appointment or call the day before an appointment to offer a friendly reminder.

Lifelong Learning

The nail care industry is constantly evolving to better serve clients. If your goal is to become the best nail technician, commit yourself to lifelong learning. This means learning about the latest products, innovative treatments, new technologies and industry trends.

Many professionals, including lawyers and physicians, are required to continue their education in order to maintain their licenses. Some regulating agencies require continuing education hours/units (CEUs) for renewal of your nail technology license. After you finish school you may continue your education with seminars and classes; trade shows; current periodicals; salon and spa visits and Internet research.

Seminars and Classes

Manufacturers, distributors and industry organizations regularly conduct or sponsor educational seminars, clinics and training programs. These will upgrade your technical and business skills and product knowledge to help you stay ahead.

Trade Shows

At trade shows you will see a wide array of products, services and resources that you need to know about. Trade-show exhibitors include everyone from nail care distributors to spa-facility equipment manufacturers. Trade shows are also great networking opportunities.

Ads in industry publications that announce trade shows also usually feature a registration form or tell you where to acquire one. Most trade shows are open "to the trade only" meaning you must work in the industry.

Current Periodicals

You might be surprised at the wealth of information available in daily, weekly and monthly periodicals. Sections of your daily paper might also feature news and updates about spa openings, fashion and makeup reports and other information that could be useful.

Current fashion and beauty magazines also provide a wealth of information. These include new trends in services, new product releases shown in advertisements and editorial coverage, or even social trends that impact the beauty industry. The most valuable information can be found in the professional periodicals that are published by industry or trade organizations, medical associations or research centers. Find out how to subscribe to them as you are looking at the periodicals. You can also use the Internet to determine if they have publications and find out how to acquire them.

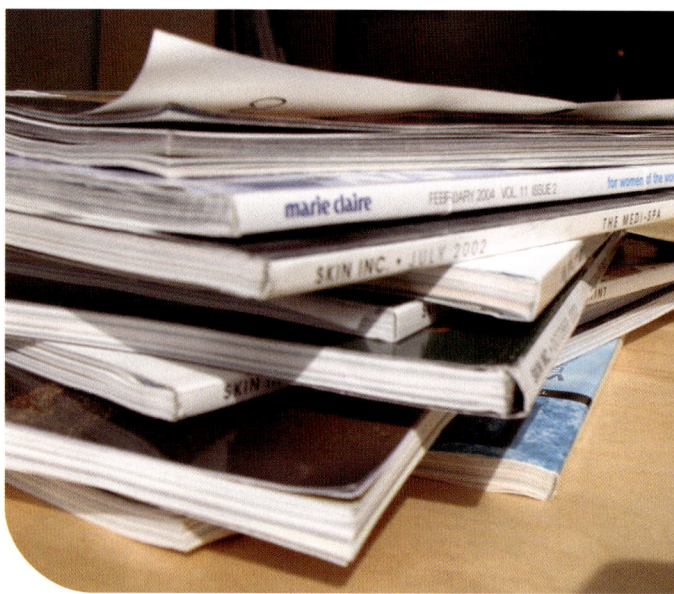

Some trade publications are available only to members of organizations that publish them. You may wish to consider joining one or several industry organizations. It's a great way to network and to stay informed about the industry.

Comparison Shopping

Comparison shopping is the practice of visiting competitors to compare their business practices to your own. First, decide what factors you want to compare. These might include how competitors market and sell their products and services, or how they book clients and guarantee quality.

Internet Resources

The Internet can serve as a starting point to learn more. Remember, the industry changes quickly and you need to be open to change.

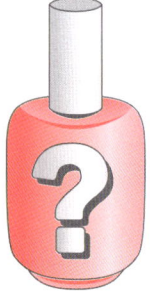

Can you predict what you will be doing in five years?
What will you need to learn to get there?

RETAILING

Retailing is recommending and providing the best products for client purchase. Product retailing benefits the nail technician as well as the client. Many salons pay a commission ranging from 8% to 15% of the nail technician's total retail sales. Some owners pay lower commission for lower dollar volume sales. A sliding scale creates the incentive to sell more.

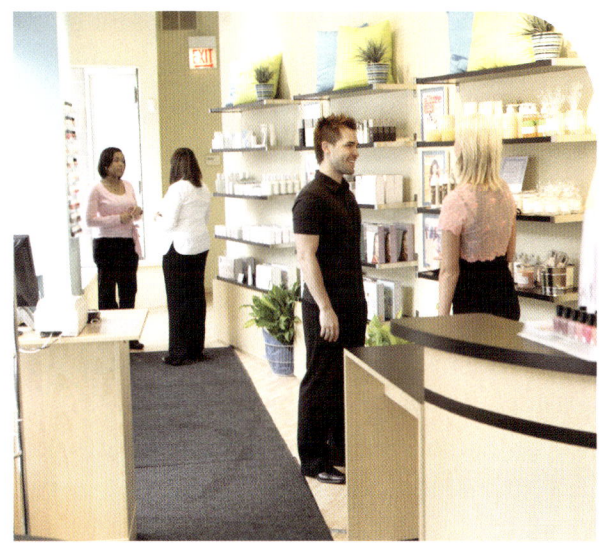

Professional Recommendation

As a professional nail technician, you will be persuading clients to:

- Trust your abilities, services, credibility and professionalism.
- Depend on nail care products that you, as a professional, know and believe to be of the finest quality.
- Understand the importance of a commitment to home care to achieve optimal results. Self-confidence is the foundation of good salesmanship. Thoroughly evaluate the key ingredients in each product and the benefits they provide, so you can convey information to your clients with confidence.

Research as many product lines as you can, to learn how various products perform. It's also a good idea to try products yourself first.

In most cases the salon owner or manager is in charge of the products that the salon sells. It is important to share information about new products and items that your clients request. This helps you to remain on the cutting edge of your profession and be aware of what is new on the market.

Professional Products

Salons have advantages over drugstores, department stores and supermarkets when retailing nail care and cosmetic products. Licensed professionals can demonstrate the use of a product in the salon while explaining its effectiveness.

Features and Benefits

Features of a product include its characteristics, such as the size of the container, the aroma or a specific ingredient. **Benefits** describe what the product does to enhance the appearance or improve the condition of the client's nails.

Involve Clients

While you are performing a service, tell your clients what you are using and why. This is actually the beginning of the selling process. Inform your clients about the proper product choices throughout the service. The actual demonstration speaks more loudly than words.

Motivating Buyers

All clients share similar motivations for buying, including need, desire to look good, profit or gain and impulse. **Need,** a want or necessity, is perhaps the easiest buyer motivation to recognize. For example, everyone needs a good cuticle conditioner. Creating need for a product means making clients aware of products that can benefit them.

Profit, or gain, represents the next major category of buyer motivation. People like to believe that they make intelligent purchases, no matter what the items.

Cosmetic products lend themselves to **impulse buying,** which is making a spur-of-the-moment decision to buy something. Manufacturers create the need for these products through print and television advertising and promotion. Statistics show that 45% to 65% of all purchases stem from impulse buying.

Sales Promotions

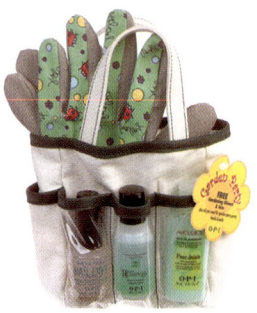

Sales promotions are important tools for accomplishing both short- and long-term benefits. In the short term, they are cost-effective, can attract new clients quickly, help reduce overstocked inventories or announce new services and products. In the long term, a sales promotion keeps your salon's name in mind. Clients associate a product brand with the logo, packaging or advertising tagline.

Selling is often called "the art of persuasion" or the "technique of recommendation." You will learn different ways to sell and gain new strategies for making recommendations as you progress through your training. Some of the most common types of promotions are listed below.

Types of Sales Promotions

Gift-with-Purchase (or Gift-with-Service)
Clients purchase a service or a product at full price and they receive a free gift or service, or a discounted product or service. It is a cost-effective method to introduce a new service or product.

Holiday and Seasonal Promotions
Holidays are year-round, and most businesses capitalize on these celebrations to sell their products. A change of season is also a great time to run a promotion.

Referral Promotions
Tell your existing clientele that if they refer a friend who comes in for a service or to purchase a product, they will receive a discount or free gift during the next visit.

Monthly Promotions
Special package kits or gift packs are a great way to allow clients to try new items and/or present your products as gifts to family, friends and neighbors.

Effective Displays
Most salons or spas allocate floor and wall space with display shelves to display retail merchandise. Use your imagination. Keep all of your displays updated and interesting. Change your displays often to create interest and excitement.

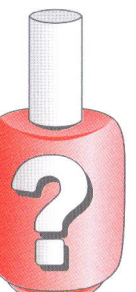

How will you explain the importance of nail and skin care products to your clients?

BUSINESS OWNERSHIP

If you have a desire to own a salon, it is important to know the fundamental principles of business ownership and operations. A successful nail salon owner must also be able to identify his or her own personal strengths and weaknesses, hire employees who complement their skills and recognize nail care trends and technical expertise.

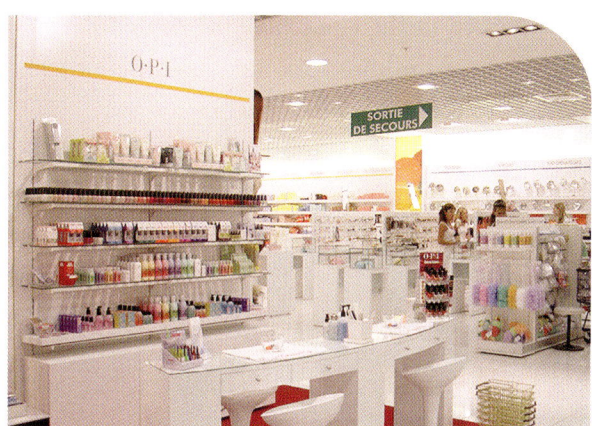

Business Essentials

To start a business you need to have a **business plan**. Basically, this is the central company document that you and your employees use to make decisions. Lenders often use business plans to help determine whether or not to loan a salon or spa money. There are many resources available to help you create a business plan, such as books, software programs or Internet sites that feature sample business plans. Just go to a search engine and type in "sample business plan."

BUSINESS PLAN ESSENTIALS

Elements of a Business Plan:

Executive Summary—Outlines goals and objectives.
Origin of Company—Describes how it began.
Company Goals—Lists short- and long-term goals.
Market Potential—Describes why your product or service would be in demand by a large market.
Marketing Strategy—Describes how you plan to tell the world about your product.
Three-to Five-Year Financial Projection—Summarizes your financial projections.
Exit Plan—Describes your strategy in case you decide to call it quits.

Types of Business Ownership

Investigate the various types of business ownership available. Understanding the differences between business types allows you to match your professional goals and start focusing all other decisions around the one you have chosen.

Finding the work style that you desire and reaching your professional goals begin with knowing your ownership options. There are four types of ownership:

1. A **sole proprietorship** is a business owned by one person. He or she is in complete control of the business, receives all profits from the business and is responsible for all debts and losses.

2. A **partnership** is a business owned by two or more persons.

3. A **corporation** is a legal entity, separate from its members, formed under legal guidelines. A corporation is actually owned by its shareholders (stockholders), or members who have funds invested in the company. The shareholders elect representatives known as the board of directors. The board of directors then appoints officers (such as the president, vice president and treasurer) to run the day-to-day business.

4. A **franchise** is more of a license for operation than a form of ownership. A franchise is simply an operating agreement in which a fee is paid to a parent corporation in exchange for fixtures, promotion, advertising, education, management techniques and, most important, the recognizable name.

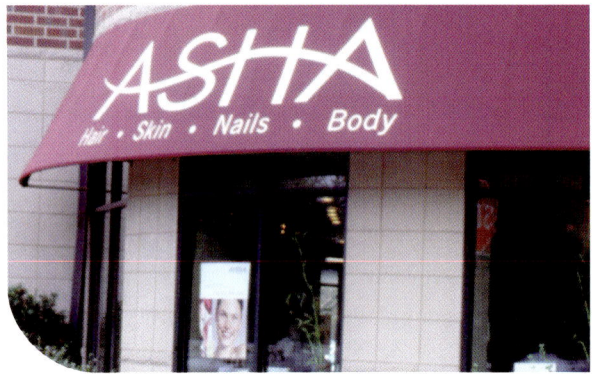

Plans for a Successful Salon

The first step is identifying three important factors to help you make choices that lead to success:

- **Location**
  Ever heard the expression "Location, location, location?" Location is one of the most important factors in planning to open a business. What are the available locations in your area? You need to assess parking conditions, high-traffic activity (walk-by, drive-in or bus service) and rental fees per square foot.

- **Market Need**
  Determining how many other salons and nail technicians are in the area is the first step in gauging the market need. Find out what services are offered, prices charged and what types of potential clientele (age, income and social groups) exist in the area. A 10-year forecast of the economic future of the community can usually be obtained from the local Chamber of Commerce or Economic Development Agency.

- **Cost of Necessary Improvements**
  Improvement costs are the amount of money that must be spent to meet a salon's unique needs, but does not include separate expenses for salon equipment. Improvements could include plumbing to accommodate the basins for foot services; electrical requirements for equipment; and upgrades to electrical wiring, heating, air conditioning and so forth. Landlords sometimes share in these expenses.

Floor Plans

Keep two primary goals in mind. First, the salon should be designed to function smoothly and efficiently. Second, the overall visual appeal or emotional impact should be pleasant.

Before trying to determine any details on cost of equipment or interior decorating, hire a developer or an architect to help you create a floor plan for a proposed location. If a potential location cannot be arranged to fit your floor plan without going over budget, look at other locations. Sometimes a location is priced right, with good traffic and the type of clientele desired, but the cost of installation is too high. Examine alternatives and then work out the design details.

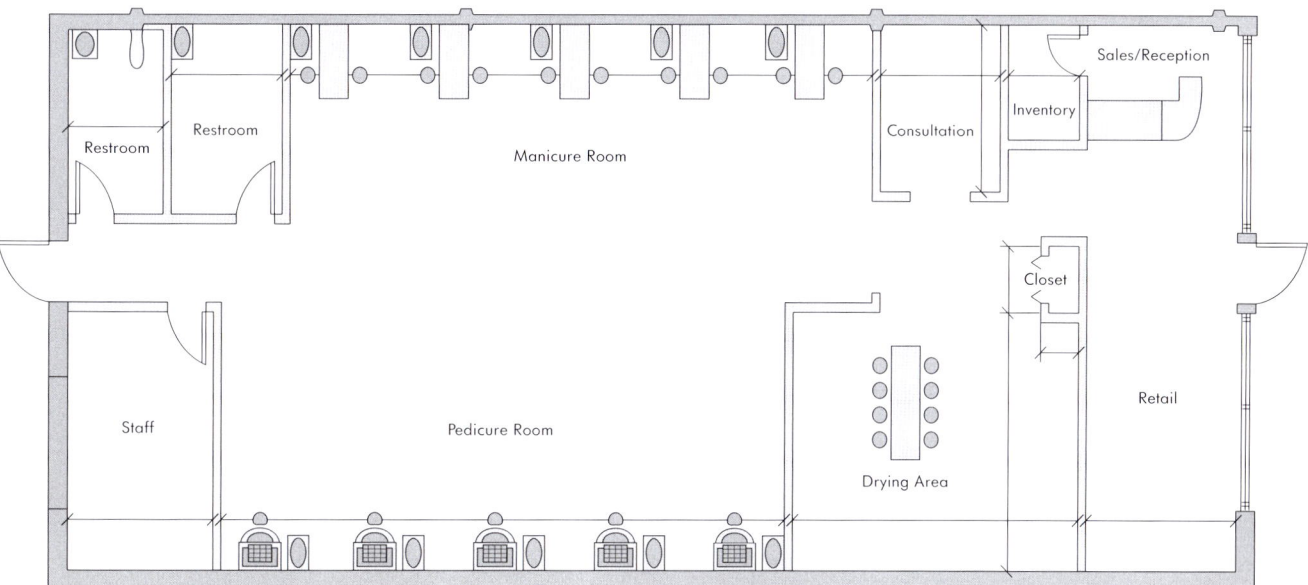

Equipment

The types and quality of the equipment are determined by the types of services you want to offer your clients. "Basics" that virtually every nail salon needs include:

- Manicure tables
- Pedicure basins
- Technician stools and storage cabinets
- Chairs for clients
- Smaller tools, such as table lamps and disinfection containers

Be sure to allocate enough space and a location for all of the equipment you need.

Another thing to consider is how to pay for the equipment. If you need to borrow money to design and construct your salon, you may wish to purchase the equipment outright. However, just as you can lease a car, you can also lease equipment. The same suppliers that sell the equipment may also be able to arrange a lease option for you. Otherwise, there are separate companies that arrange leasing for all types of equipment, including computers and furniture. Consult with your accountant, who will advise the best option for your business.

Borrowing Money

After you have found a location, designed a suitable and affordable floor plan, calculated the cost of fixtures and the capital improvements necessary, you must determine how much money you need to borrow. Generally, you must be willing to invest some of your own money in order for any lending institution to grant a loan. You will need many types of documents to prove that you are a worthy credit risk. One such document will probably be a "profit and loss projection" or "income and expense projection" (explained in more depth later in this chapter). Work with an accountant to prepare the projection; not only does it help you get a loan, but it also helps you determine how much cash you really need.

There are many ways to finance your business ventures. There are commercial lenders, venture capital companies and more. In business, it is usually best to avoid borrowing money from friends and family.

Operating capital is the reservoir of cash that you will need to stay ahead of your creditors. When applying for a loan to start your business, make sure you have enough money to operate for at least six months, or better yet, a full year.

Once your salon is open and you have an operating **track record,** which means a good relationship with your bank, and you have paid-down your debt, you can apply for a **line of credit** with your bank. A line of credit from the bank provides a reserve of cash that you can draw upon to meet operating expenses if you have a slow month or two. It is advisable to pay money you borrow from a line of credit back as quickly as possible.

Rental Agreements

Upon obtaining a loan, you can enter into a **rental agreement** also called a lease. As the renter, or lessee, you promise to pay rent and use the property according to the agreement. In order to avoid unexpected rent increases, a lease should extend for five years with an option for five more years. During the rental negotiation process, you should make sure that certain basic services will be provided by the landlord, which include:

- Maintenance to the building as well as any repairs to facilities.
- Adequate water capacity and pressure.
- Late night and/or weekend access to the building.

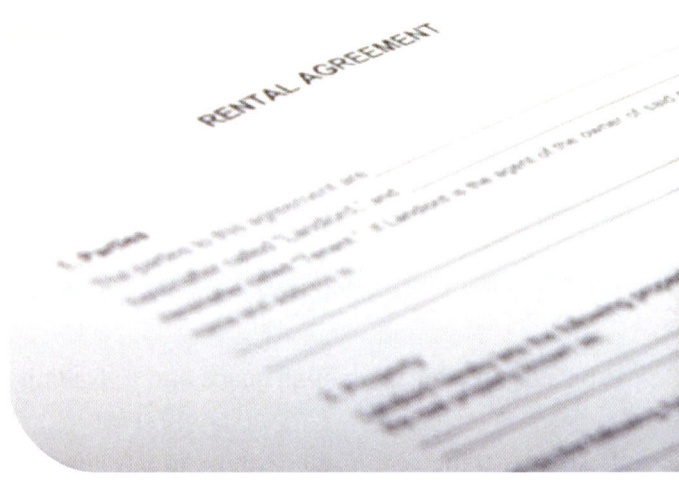

You should also negotiate for all or part of the capital improvements to be paid by the owner of the building, or lessor. Special features, such as extra water pipes or a larger water heater, will probably have to be paid for by the lessee (you). During the lease negotiation process, you, your lawyer and the landlord should sort out what improvements will be paid for by whom.

A large portion of the expense of the salon is the rent. There are two kinds of rent:

1. **Fixed**—A set dollar amount paid each month to the lessor. A fixed rent allows you to predict your monthly expenses carefully.

2. **Variable**—A set dollar amount paid per month plus a percentage of the total monthly income. Variable rents are common in malls and large shopping centers. Have an accountant predict the results of a variable rent system before signing a lease. Also, be sure to have a lawyer evaluate a tentative lease and make suggestions for change. You can negotiate changes in any lease. Remember, don't sign a lease unless you, your lawyer and your accountant are satisfied that it is fair and reasonable.

Insurance

There are several types of insurance to protect you from the financial difficulties that can follow the unexpected loss of property, income, health and/or life. This is known as risk management. The following types of insurance are recommended:

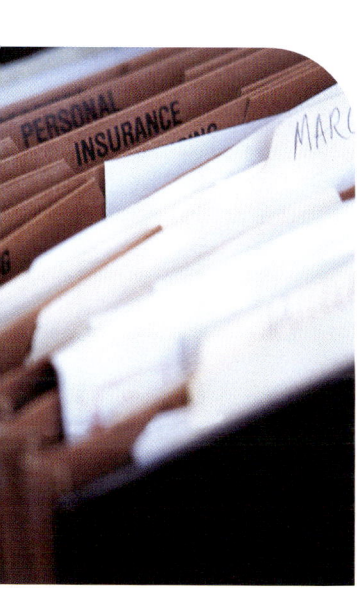

- **Malpractice**—A policy that protects the salon owner from financial loss that can result from an employee's negligence while performing services on clients. The owner must insure each technician in the salon.

This insurance covers the cost of a lawsuit or settlement resulting from damage inflicted on a client during any service.

- **Property or Premise**—A policy that covers the actual salon equipment and physical location in case of natural disasters, fire, theft or burglary, or accidents occurring at the business. It covers replacement of lost items and carries a liability clause that will pay a claim if someone is injured on the premises.

- **Product Liability**—A policy that protects the salon from lawsuits brought on by injury caused by a product that is recommended or sold in the salon. Although a nail technician thoroughly explains how to use a home nail care product, clients may misuse products and damage their nails. The salon, distributor and manufacturer can be sued for recommending, selling and producing the product. Insurance companies sometimes require an educational program in product knowledge for all staff before product liability insurance is granted.

- **Worker's Compensation**—A state-controlled insurance required by law. This insurance is paid directly to the state on a quarterly basis to cover any expense resulting from an injury to an employee working in the salon.

"It's better to prepare than to repair."—John C. Maxwell

Now that you are familiar with the steps required to open a salon, it is time to consider the many important aspects of day-to-day operation. These include learning about everything from costs of operation and pricing of services and products, to all matters pertaining to employees.

INCOME AND EXPENSE PROJECTION

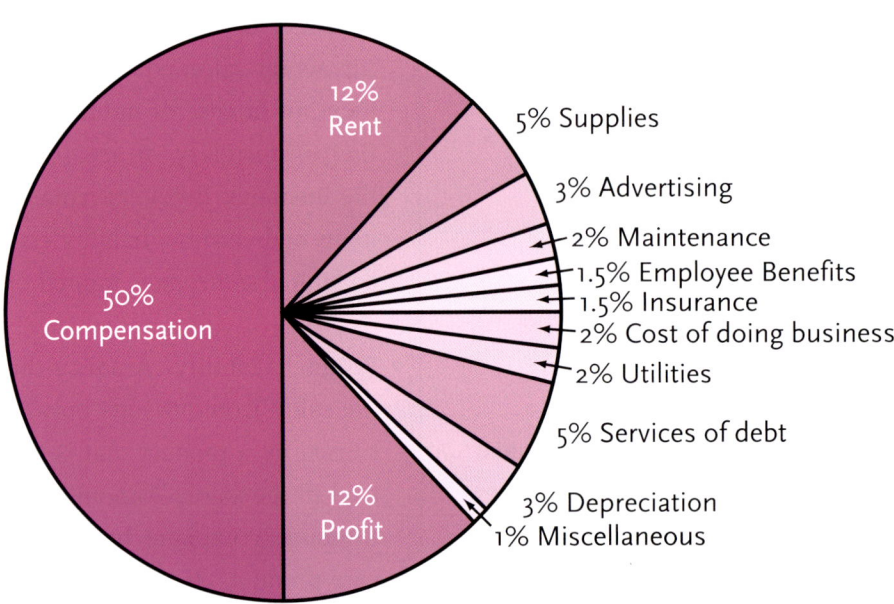

12% Rent

5% Supplies

3% Advertising

2% Maintenance

1.5% Employee Benefits

1.5% Insurance

2% Cost of doing business

2% Utilities

5% Services of debt

50% Compensation

12% Profit

3% Depreciation

1% Miscellaneous

Total Operating Expense (OE): 88%

The average cost of operating a business (by percentage of income) breaks down as follows:

- **Compensation (Payroll): 50%**
  Salaries or commissions for you and your employees, including payroll taxes

- **Rent: 12%**
  Fixed or variable

- **Supplies: 5%**
  Professional and retail products; miscellaneous equipment and tools

- **Advertising: 3%**
  Promotion of the salon

- **Maintenance: 2%**
  Repairs, laundry, cleaning and replacement of equipment

- **Employee Benefits: 1.5%**
  Education, paid vacations, pension plans or profit-sharing, health insurance

- **Insurance: 1.5%**
  All types

- **Cost of Doing Business: 2%**
  Accounting, legal, licenses, subscriptions, professional dues

- **Utilities: 2%**
  Water, electricity, gas, sanitation, phone

- **Services of Debt: 5%**
  Capital improvements, equipment and original loan expense

- **Depreciation: 3%**
  An account established to save for replacement of equipment; creates tax credit

- **Miscellaneous: 1%**
  All other expenses

Total Operating Expense (OE): 88%
Profit: 12%

Expenses and Income

In very basic terms, the financial success, or profitability, of a nail salon is achieved when the income is significantly greater than its total expenses. In even simpler terms, a business makes a profit when it takes in more money than it pays out.

Income refers to all payments received from clients for services performed and home care products purchased. Income is also frequently referred to by accountants as **revenue**.

Operating Expenses (OE) refers to all the costs incurred in the day-to-day running of the salon.

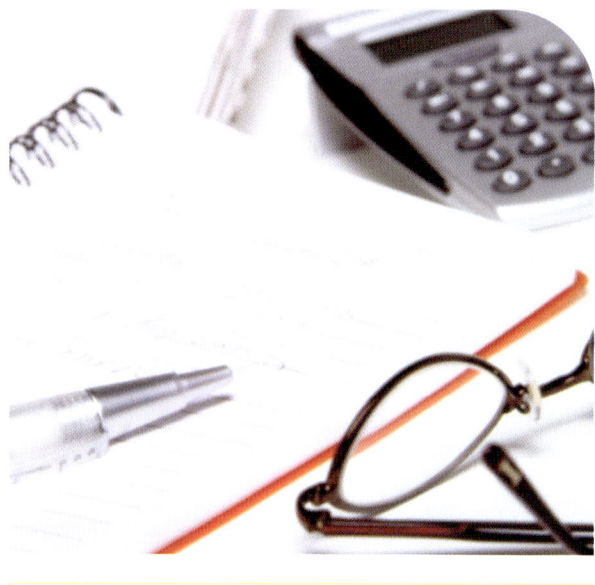

INCOME - EXPENSE = PROFIT

There are two types of operating expenses—fixed and variable. Fixed costs do not change from month to month for at least one year, and would include the rent or mortgage payment, salaries and insurance. Variable costs can change on a monthly basis and would include utilities, supplies, cost of promotions, postage and taxes. A business may operate at a loss while it builds its clientele during the first few weeks, months, and even years after it is open.

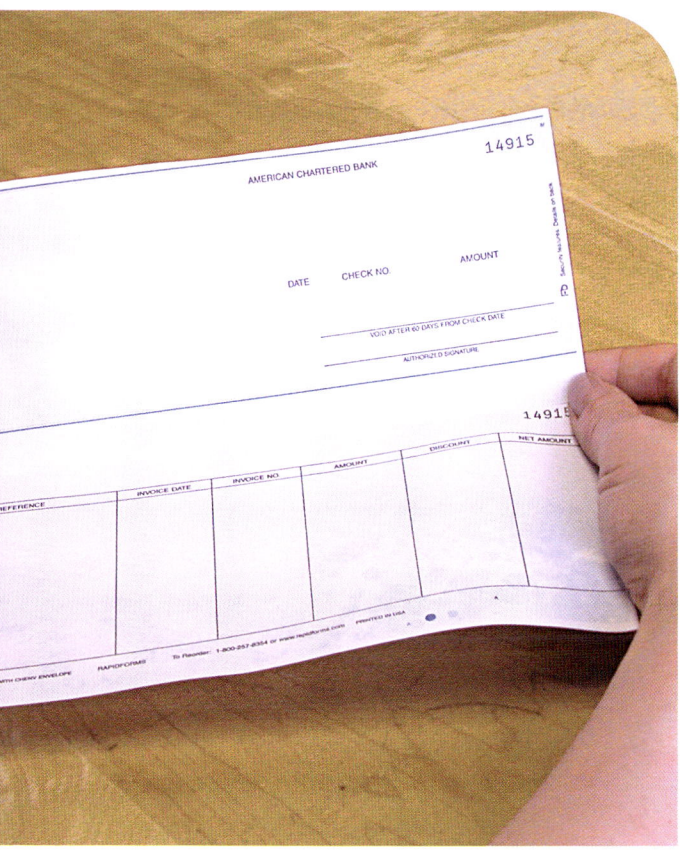

Taxes

A business owner is responsible for paying a wide array of taxes to local and federal governments. It is the owner's responsibility to pay promptly. A bookkeeper can keep track of regular tax payments, but for a full understanding of your tax obligations, seek the advice and expertise of a certified public accountant (CPA).

Withholding Tax

The owner is responsible for withholding, or keeping, a percentage of an employee's income for payment of certain taxes. In the U.S., these include federal, state and local income taxes and Social Security tax. The business owner also has a tax obligation to the employee. For every dollar of Social Security tax paid by the employee, the owner must pay the same amount to the federal government.

Social Security is a planned savings/retirement fund for every worker in the United States. Medicare is part of your Social Security tax and provides medical insurance coverage during retirement. The owner must also provide an annual W-2 form for each employee. The W-2 form indicates all the taxes paid for the past year. In Canada, the business owner is responsible for withholding Federal and Provincial tax, Employment Insurance (EI) and Canadian Pension Tax.

Sales Tax

Most states and some local governments impose sales taxes on products. If there is a tax, business owners are responsible for collecting sales taxes on products and paying these monies to the state on a monthly or quarterly basis. Some states may charge taxes on services, so check with your area's governing agency.

A permit is required to collect taxes, and the payments are a permanent record of the dollar volume of the business. A business owner must apply for a State Sales Tax Permit before collecting taxes on products or services sold. A state sales tax number serves as your "resale number." This means that if you are purchasing items for your salon, such as products or any type of supply that will be re-sold to a client, you are not required to pay sales tax to the seller. You will need to fill out a Resale Certificate and provide your Tax ID number to the seller (the wholesaler) and then you will not be charged sales tax.

This practice prevents clients from essentially having to pay sales tax twice (once to cover the total purchase price from the wholesaler and once at the point-of-sale to the client). Check with an accountant regarding your area's sales tax requirements.

Income Tax

Income tax is paid on the profits (earnings) of a business. In the U.S., the Internal Revenue Service (IRS) establishes criteria for reporting profit and loss. Again, be sure to consult with an accountant on IRS tax compliance. When a business makes a profit, it is required to pay a percentage of that profit to the federal, state and local governments. If a business suffers a loss, it receives a tax credit, which means it pays little or no tax. You can see the importance of careful planning and control of expenses. Careful record keeping is required by law. For your own protection, keep all records of daily sales and service for seven years. If a business is audited by the IRS, these records are proof of income. Failure to keep records is against the law in most areas.

Internal Revenue Service (IRS) rules require you to register a daily log of all your tips, which is income. Keep a copy for yourself and submit a copy to your employer. The salon owner is responsible for reporting employees' tips.

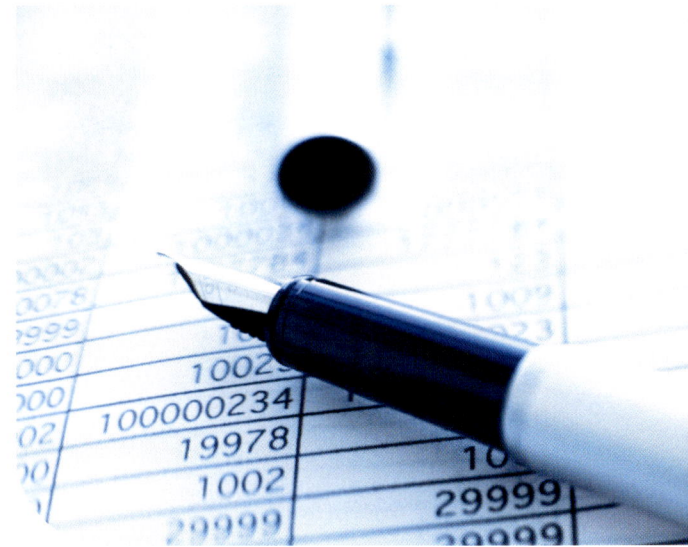

Nail Salon Philosophy, Policies and Procedures

A nail salon should have a professional philosophy or standard of ethics. Creating a Policies and Procedures Handbook is the first step in developing these standards. Such a handbook should thoroughly outline the owner's expectations of employees.

A salon handbook should also inform the employee about what to expect from management. The employer is expected to provide a safe and pleasant working environment, reasonable working hours, equitable salary structure, products and supplies and sanitation services.

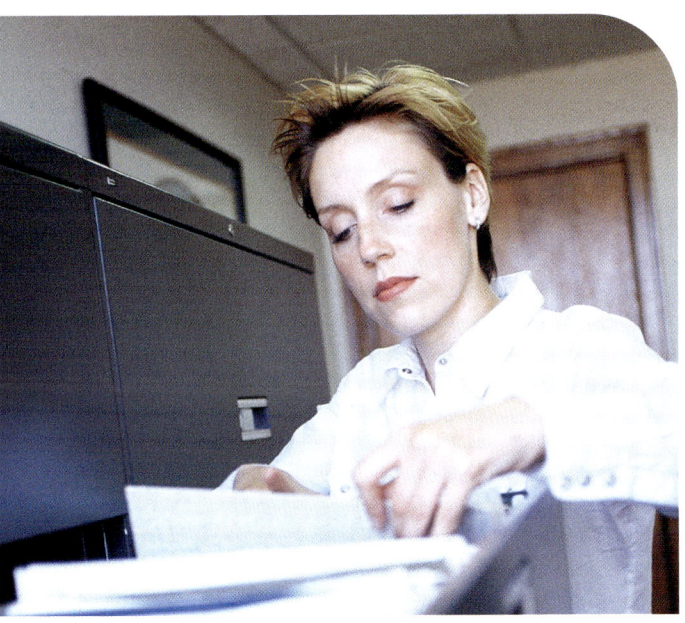

Record Keeping

In addition to keeping accurate records for tax purposes, you must also keep detailed financial records. You may wish to hire a full- or part-time bookkeeper, or accountant, to help you keep track of all income and expenses. A bookkeeper is also responsible for paying bills, making sure all periodic tax payments are made, overseeing payroll, keeping payroll

records, reconciling the checking account, and conducting tasks to maintain the financial health of the business.

Reports required by federal, state and city agencies need financial records that pertain to such issues as worker's compensation, unemployment and disability insurance, income taxes and Social Security payments. Appointment and sales records are extremely important to maintain daily and analyze regularly—either weekly or monthly. By doing so, you will be able to:

- Notice when inventory supplies are running low so that you can re-order.
- Observe what types of services are being requested (or not requested) in order to make adjustments in your service menu.
- Be aware of the kinds of materials that are being used for different types of services.
- Control waste.

Other kinds of records aid business as well. Customer service records track services provided and merchandise purchased by each client. They also improve the personal service the client receives and can help to increase sales.

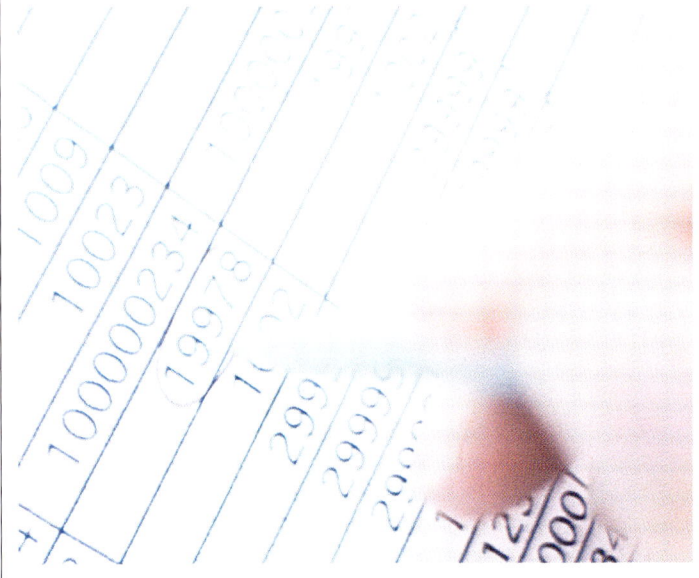

2

Inventory and Product Control

All products purchased by the salon owner for use during client services and for retailing are **inventory**, or stock in quantity. Inventory is generally identified by two categories: professional and retail. A strong inventory system allows close management of these valuable products. Proper inventory practices also require the timely ordering of products.

The term **inventory control** applies to procedures used in the salon to ensure that products are accounted for from the time they are added to the inventory until they are sold or used. Owners or managers usually establish inventory-control guidelines to monitor the sales of a specific product within an assigned timeframe.

A salon owner should expect the nail technicians to recommend products for home care to their clients. Setting sales goals is essential to providing retail income to both the owner and the technician.

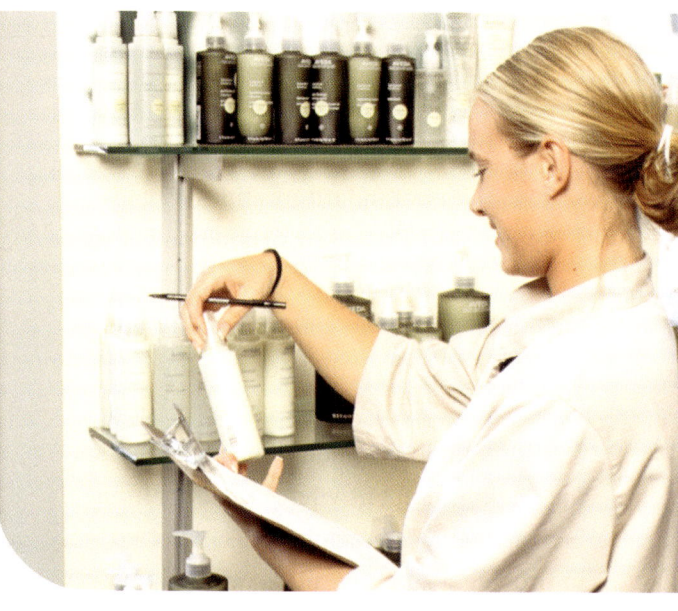

Stock:
The total merchandise kept on hand for future use by a merchant, commercial establishment, warehouse or manufacturer.

Stock inventory:
A detailed itemized list, report or record of items; a periodic survey of all goods and materials in stock.

Pricing

Determine service prices by conducting a market survey before opening the salon. Price the services at a reasonable rate to fit the income range of the clients you want to attract. Determining what other salons are charging can be helpful, but remember, price is not the only reason clients select a particular nail salon.

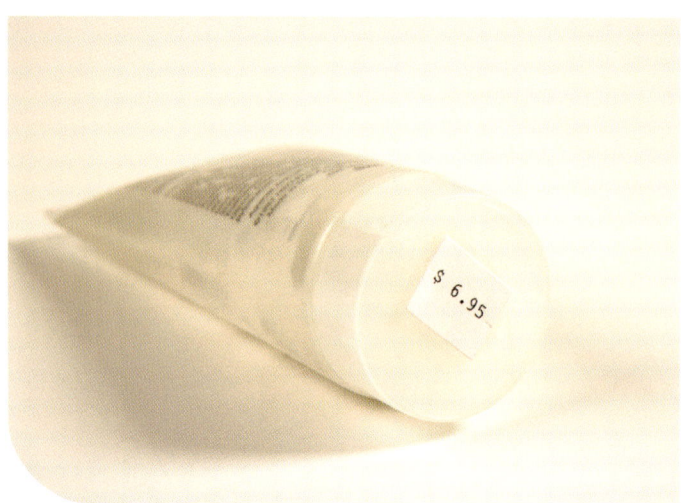

Price products to recapture the cost of what you paid the manufacturer or distributor while building in a profit margin. Profit margins can range anywhere from 50% to 100% and beyond. As a guideline, rely on the manufacturer's suggested retail price. This way you are assured of being competitive with other salons selling the same product.

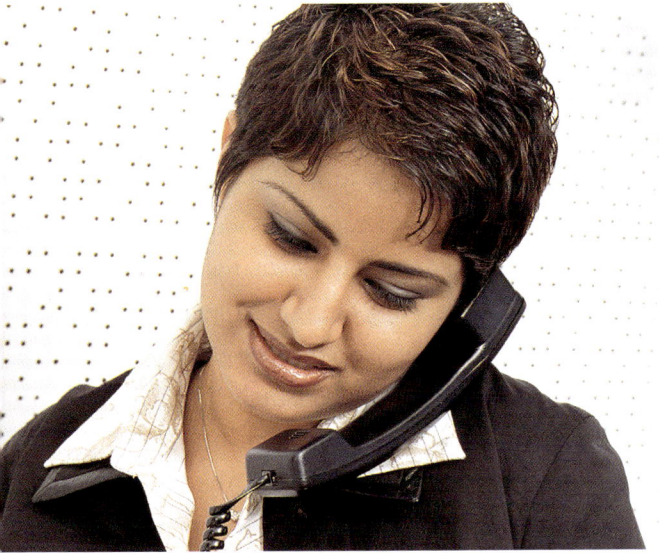

A poorly-trained receptionist can ruin a salon's operations. Clients often judge the salon by how phone calls are handled and how they are treated within the first few minutes after their arrival.

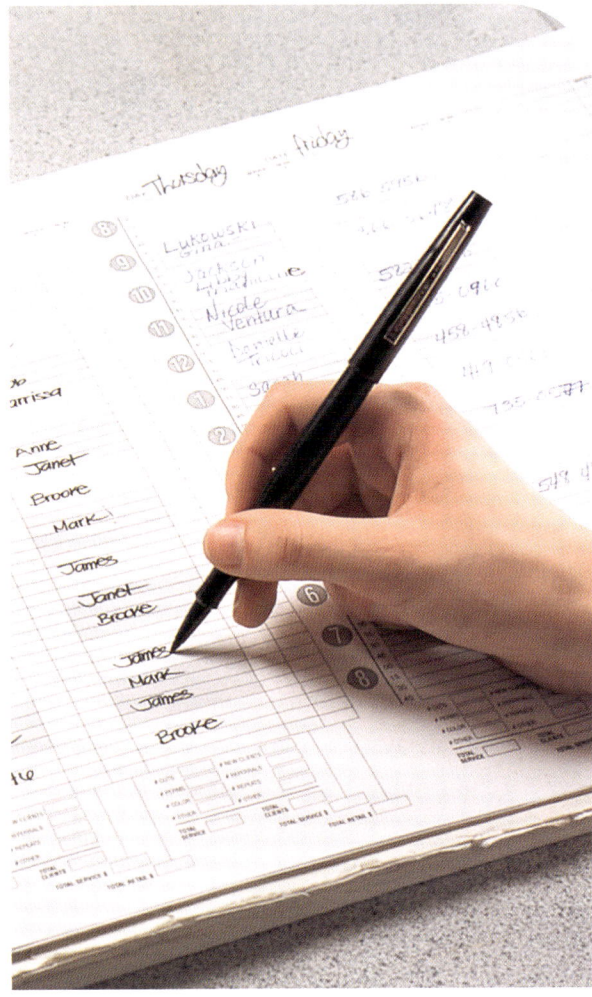

Receptionist Duties

In many cases the receptionist is the first person to greet clients as they arrive. If the salon does not have a full-time receptionist, the owner usually appoints another employee to serve in this capacity as needed. Or, employees can rotate throughout the day to meet the needs of this area. In some cases, the receptionist also acts as the cashier.

The primary duties of this very important position are to:

- Greet each person with a smile.
- Schedule appointments in a fair and efficient way.
- Manage incoming and outgoing calls regarding appointments and other questions.
- Work with the nail technician to ensure that the appropriate amount of time is allowed for each individual service being scheduled.
- Inform technicians of client arrival.
- Supervise the reception and waiting area to ensure organization and efficiency.
- Handle client complaints calmly and efficiently.
- Ensure client services are all paid for and documented.

The process of scheduling appointments is of primary importance within the operation of the salon. Generally, appointments are scheduled according to the type of service and the speed of the nail technician. Important information to be noted in the appointment book includes the following:

- Client name
- Scheduled service
- Appointment time
- Client phone number

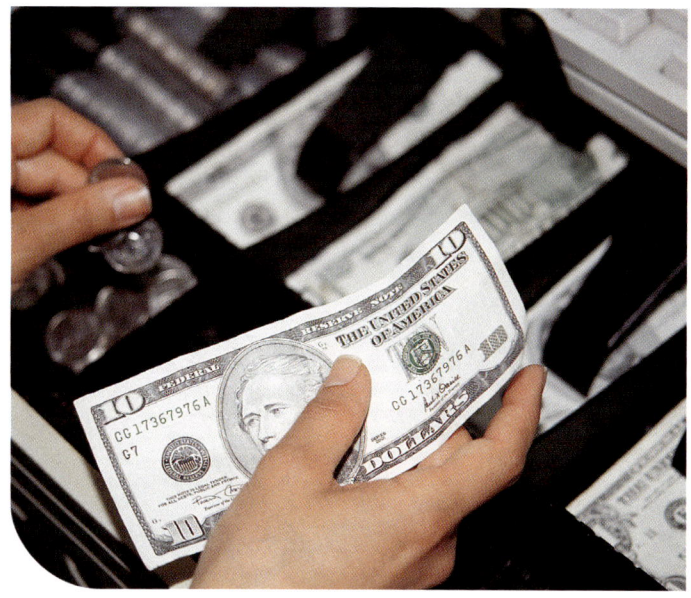

Handling Money

Cash operations are important to every business and the nail salon is no exception. The receptionist or assigned cashier needs to ensure accuracy and efficiency. He or she must also be able to provide the correct denomination of bills and coins for cash transactions and troubleshoot during credit transactions. The most efficient method of offering change is to always give the client the fewest bills necessary to complete the transaction.

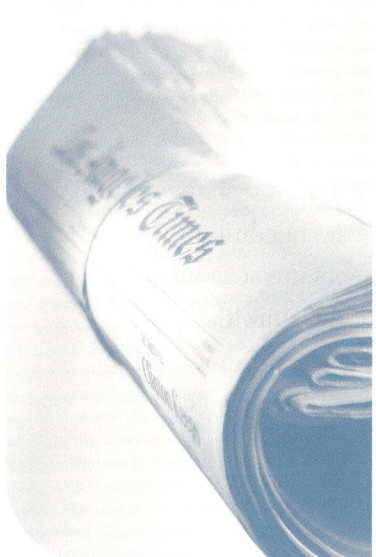

Advertising

Advertising incorporates all activities that attract attention to your salon or spa and create a positive impression. Your advertising image should be consistent and "fresh." The best form of advertising is often word-of-mouth.

Satisfied clients nearly always tell others about your salon. More conventional forms of advertising, such as print media like newspapers or magazines, can be very effective. The most selective and efficient form of advertising for local businesses is direct mail. This method of advertising involves sending postcards or flyers to prospective clients, encouraging them to try a new service. Daily or weekly newspaper ads can create an image in the consumers' minds through the repetition of your name and logo. Magazines or periodicals that reach the types of clientele you are trying to attract can also be effective, as can other types of mass media such as billboards or bus stops.

> Marketing your business is very important. After all, you could have the best nail salon in the world, but if no one knows about it, what good is it? Good marketing can be compared to target practice. Rather than "Ready! Fire! Aim!" you should practice finding your targets, then "Ready! Aim! Fire!"

Remember new media options, too; Advertising on the Internet can be quite affordable, highly effective and relatively easy to do on a limited budget. Simple banner ads can be purchased on smaller Web sites. Consider sites that list city events, restaurants, and so on. Also, it is now quite easy to create your own home page, or with time and money you can hire someone to do an entire Web site that features your product and service menus.

Plan a yearly advertising budget and stick to it. Alternate expensive methods of advertising with inexpensive methods. If one form of advertising works, repeat it. If something fails, drop it. Consider surveying clients once a year for their opinions about services, community image and advertising programs.

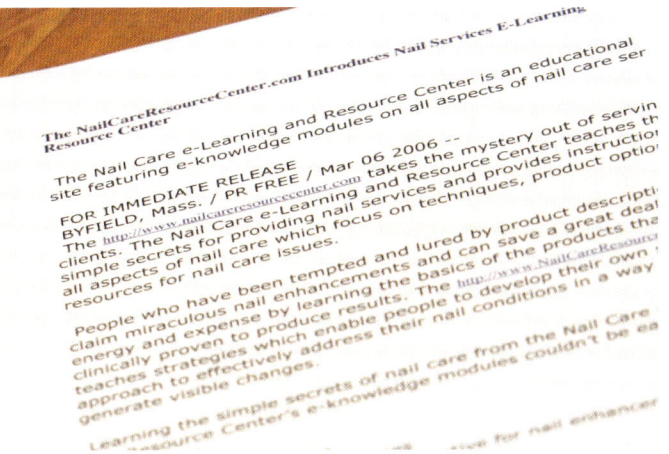

Public Relations

Spreading the word about your business doesn't have to be expensive. In fact, it can even be free! **Public relations (PR)** is an essential component of any advertising plan. The term defines itself: Relating to the public. Public relations involves the shaping of your public image in ways other than advertising. Involvement in community affairs, the chamber of commerce or service organizations can help promote the business' professional image in the area.

2

Another typical public relations strategy is to try to get your salon's name featured in the media— in local newspapers, magazines, television news or entertainment programs. Getting such coverage requires coming up with a story idea, writing it down, and sending it, along with photographs or other support materials, to a host of media contacts.

Promotion Calendar

The best way to ensure an effective advertising and promotion campaign is to create a promotion calendar for an entire year. In this way, you will establish deadlines for yourself and be able to plan promotions around special events or new product or service announcements you have planned for your salon. Also, a calendar helps you plan regular seasonal promotions, which can become a mainstay of your advertising.

Building a career in the nail care industry means learning about the business you are in. Whether you are starting out in the industry, or opening your own salon, there are many ways you can develop yourself into the nail care professional you would like to become. By establishing professional relationships, learning to retail, and becoming familiar with business essentials, you are ensuring that your career will be filled with a lifetime of opportunity.

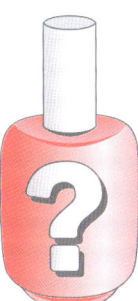

In successful businesses, everyone communicates openly and freely exchanges ideas and information. How would you keep everyone in your salon informed on issues, such as emergency procedures, inventory and product control, telephone techniques and scheduling appointments?

DECISION-MAKING SKILLS

Case Studies

The following situations are designed to help you build your decision-making skills. Using your training to this point, review the following scenarios, then think through and describe how you would handle each challenge.

1. You are interviewing with a company that you hope will hire you. You have been asked many questions about your work experience, education, your view of customer service, and so on. Then, the interviewer turns the tables by asking "Do you have any questions for me?" List the three most important questions you would ask.

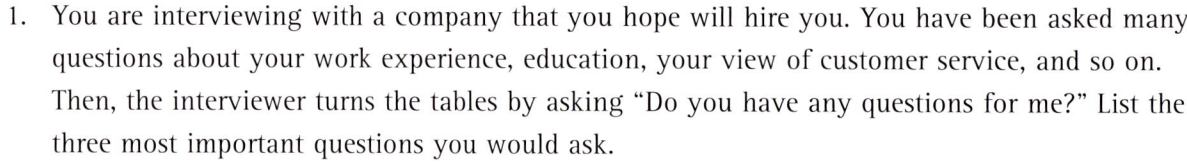

2. The salon manager has just met with you during your first week on the job and has suggested that you establish a goal of developing five new clients in the next two weeks. You have also been challenged to have these five clients be anyone other than your family, since you can already probably count them as clients for nail care services. List your top three plans of action.

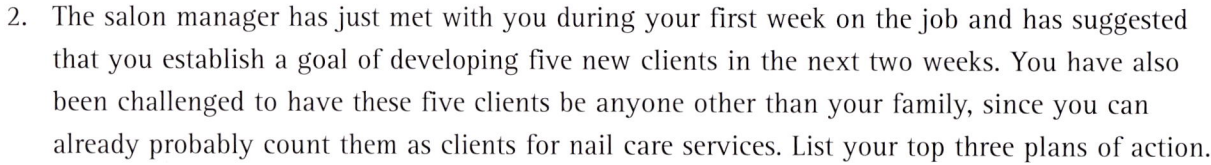

3. You have just completed your very first service on a client in the salon. Your client is very satisfied with the final results and you are just finishing your comments regarding his or her home care plan. As you walk your client to the retail area, you notice that the cuticle conditioner you have recommended is completely sold out. What would you do?

salon FUNDAMENTALS™
NAILS

Unit 2: The Science of Nail Care

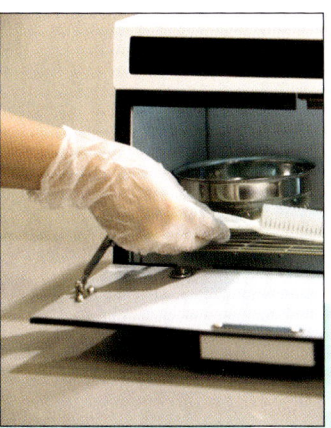 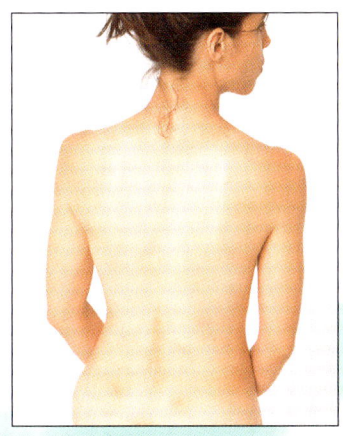 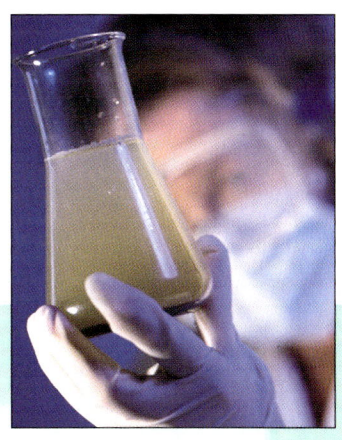 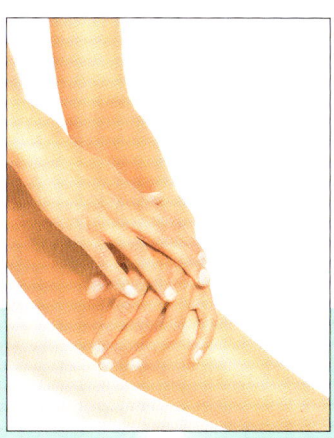

CHAPTER 3, NAIL SALON ECOLOGY

CHAPTER 4, ANATOMY

CHAPTER 5, CHEMISTRY

CHAPTER 6, NAIL AND SKIN PHYSIOLOGY

UNIT 2 THE SCIENCE OF NAIL CARE features the theory behind nail care technology. Nail care is both a science and an art that requires an understanding of the scientific concepts associated with chemistry, anatomy and microbiology. The concepts and guidelines found in these four chapters promote safe and practical methods that will prove invaluable when performing nail services in the salon.

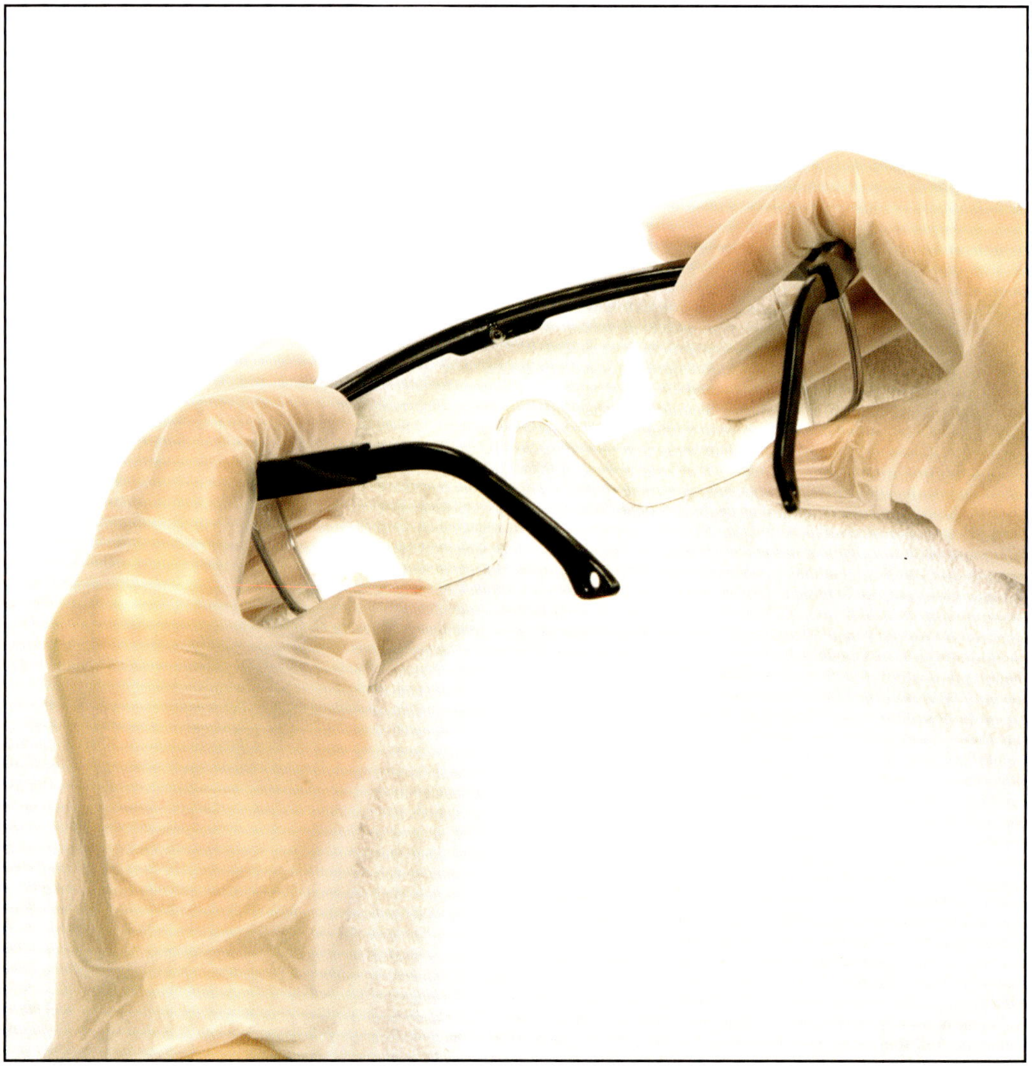

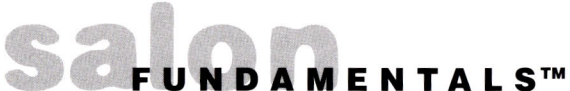

salon FUNDAMENTALS™

Did you know that people are much more relaxed and optimistic when they feel safe and secure? For this reason, most successful businesses place a high priority on maintaining clean, attractive and safe environments. This is especially true for businesses that provide personal services like nail care. Cleanliness and professionalism with regard to infection control are industry standards that translate into higher levels of client satisfaction and repeat business. A healthy environment is a powerful way to assure your clients that their comfort and safety are important to you.

VALUE

A basic understanding of nail salon ecology will enable you to better implement safety procedures that prevent the unnecessary spread of infectious diseases and protect the well-being of clients and co-workers.

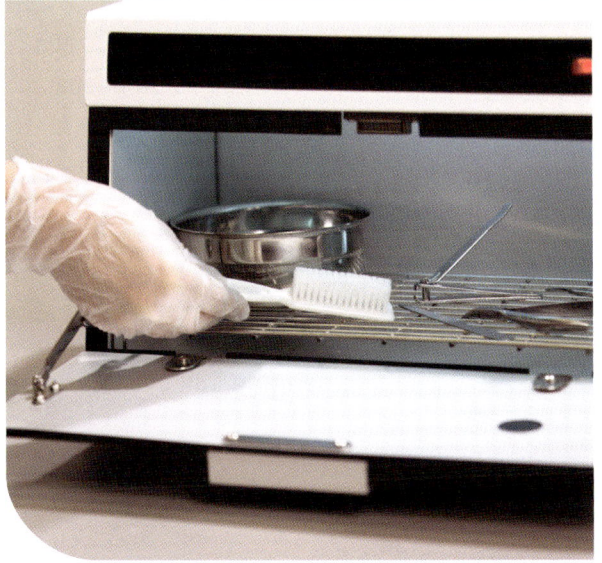

MAIN IDEA

Because services that could result in the transmission of germs and infectious diseases or pose safety hazards are performed in salons or spas, nail technicians must maintain strict infection control and safety standards. These standards, often mandated by law, regulate the ecology of each salon or spa. They guarantee cleanliness, sanitation, hygienic handling of tools and equipment and adherence to first-aid and safety procedures. By tending to these standards, the nail technician can help eliminate the transmission of germs and demonstrate a genuine concern for the health and safety of the clients who visit the salon. This chapter covers microbiology, infection control and first aid as they relate to safety and cleanliness in the nail salon or spa.

PLAN	OBJECTIVES
Microbiology • Bacteria • Growth of Bacteria • Viruses • External Parasites • Infection • Immunity	Recognize the structure and function of bacteria and viruses by the following: • Types • Classifications • Growth and reproduction patterns • Relationship to the spread of infection
Infection Control • Sanitation • Disinfection • Sterilization • Equipment	Describe the three levels of infection control and explain the procedures and precautions for each level. Identify two regulating agencies that enforce safety and health standards in the workplace and describe their specific functions. Explain how infection control equipment works to prevent cross-contamination.
Safety and First Aid • Electrical Safety • Chemical Safety • Allergic Reactions • Bleeding and Wounds • Burns • Choking • Fainting • Eye Injury	Describe basic electrical and chemical safety precautions when working in the nail salon or spa. Identify the symptoms and effects of overexposure. List simple safety and first-aid applications for cuts, minor burns, choking, fainting and eye injury.

MICROBIOLOGY

Microbiology – what a big word to describe the study of extremely small organisms! Yet, that's exactly what microbiology is, the study *(ology)* of small *(micro)* living *(bio)* organisms called microbes. Despite being invisible to the naked eye, microbes are important to nail technicians as they are known to cause infectious diseases via the use of **contaminated** *(dirty)* implements and equipment.

That is why a basic knowledge of microbiology is required of all nail technicians. By adhering to standard infection control procedures, nail technicians can prevent the unnecessary transmission of infectious, disease-spreading microbes.

Bacteria

Bacteria, also called germs, are one-celled microbes. While thousands of different kinds of bacteria exist, they are generally classified into two types:

1. **Nonpathogenic**–Nondisease-producing bacteria
2. **Pathogenic**–Disease-producing bacteria

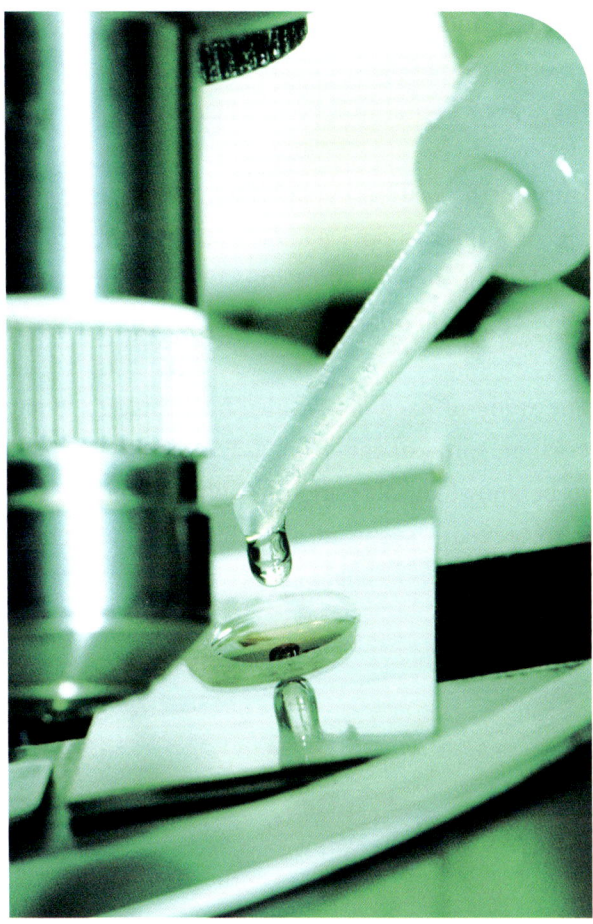

3

There are more than 2,000 different kinds of bacteria, and most are harmless—or even helpful!

Here is an easy way to remember these words. The Greek word *pathos* means suffering. Pathogenic bacteria cause disease = suffering. Nonpathogenic bacteria do not cause disease = nonsuffering.

Nonpathogenic Bacteria

Nonpathogenic bacteria are harmless and can at times be very beneficial. Approximately 70 percent of all bacteria are nonpathogenic, many of which live on the surface of the skin. Some nonpathogenic bacteria have medical applications. Other bacteria, like those found in certain dairy products (such as yogurt), have health-enhancing properties, and still others cause the decay of refuse or vegetation and thereby improve the fertility of soil. **Saprophytes** (SAP-ro-fights) are nonpathogenic bacteria that live on dead matter. Without this type of bacteria, the earth would literally be covered with dead matter!

Pathogenic Bacteria

Pathogenic bacteria live everywhere in your environment and even exist inside your body. Several different types of pathogenic bacteria are harmful because they cause infection and disease, and some produce toxins. A toxin is a poisonous substance produced by living cells or organisms. These infectious bacteria can be easily spread in the nail salon or spa through the use of contaminated implements or via dirty hands.

Only in the last 100 years have scientists discovered these microscopic (seen only with the aid of a microscope) bacteria and invented solutions for destroying many of them, thereby combating the spread of infection. Scientists found that bacteria have distinct shapes that aid in microscopic identification.

The study of bacteria is called **bacteriology**. Bacteria are single cells with one of three basic shapes: circular, spiral or rod-shaped. For effective infection control in the nail salon, nail technicians need to be knowledgeable about all types of microscopic bacteria. The nail technician's main responsibility is to prevent the spread of all bacteria by exercising proper hygiene and cleanliness. The following are more common pathogenic bacteria that can be found in the salon or spa.

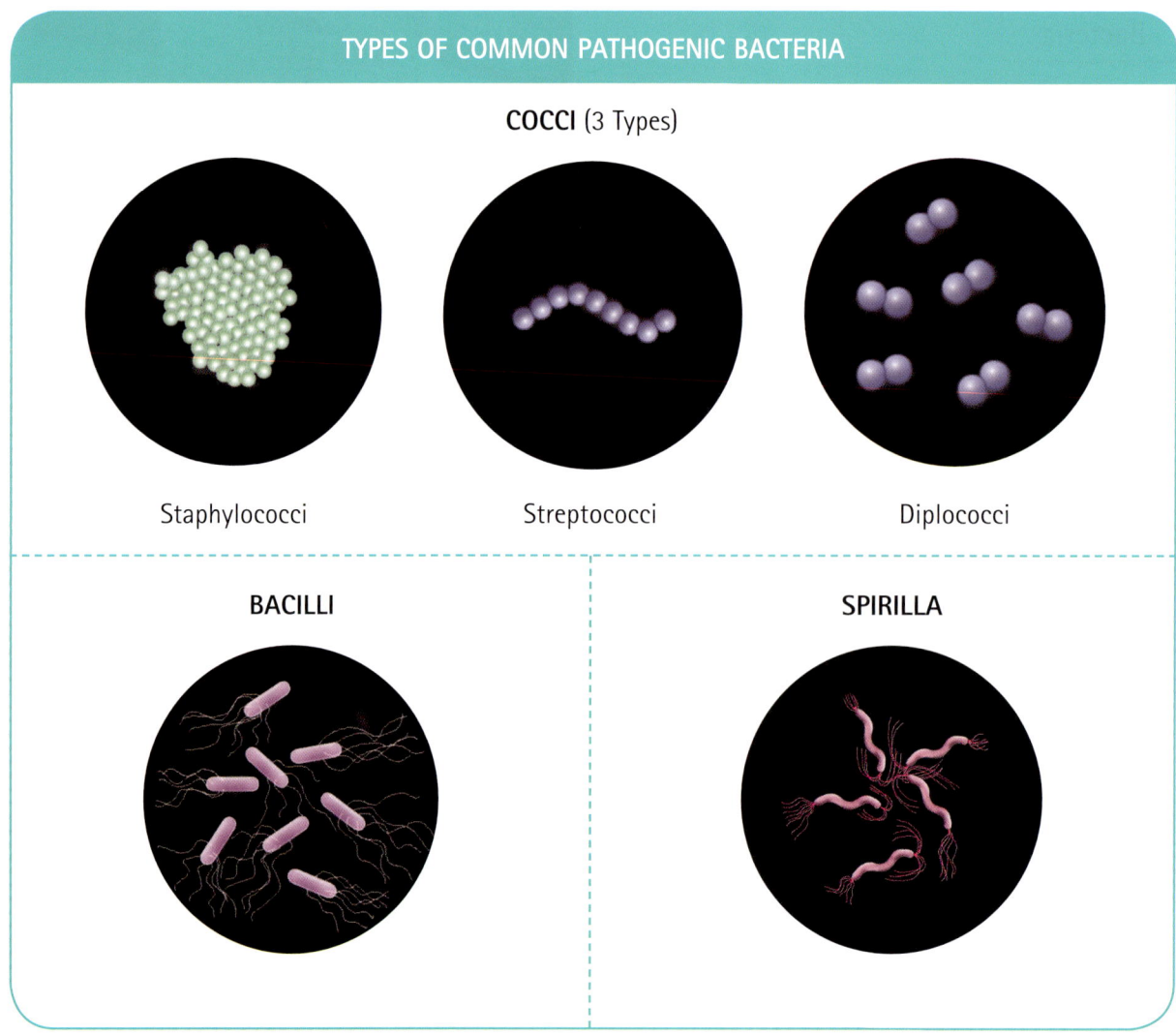

TYPES OF COMMON PATHOGENIC BACTERIA

COCCI (3 Types)

Staphylococci   Streptococci   Diplococci

BACILLI   **SPIRILLA**

Cocci (KOK-sigh) are spherical or round-shaped bacterial cells that appear singularly or in groups. To remember, think c = circle and cocci. There are three groups of cocci:

- **Staphylococci** (staf-i-lo-KOK-sigh) are pus-forming bacterial cells that form grape-like bunches or clusters and are present in abscesses, pustules and boils.

- **Streptococci** (strep-to-KOK-sigh) are also pus-forming bacterial cells that form in long chains and can cause septicemia (sometimes called blood poisoning), strep throat, rheumatic fever and other serious infections.

- **Diplococci** (dip-lo-KOK-sigh) are bacterial cells that grow in pairs and are the cause of certain infections, including pneumonia. To remember, think d = double and diplococci.

Bacilli (ba-SIL-eye) are the most common form of bacterial cells. Bacilli are bar- or rod-shaped cells that can produce a variety of diseases including tetanus, bacterial influenza, typhoid fever, tuberculosis and diphtheria. To remember, think b = bar and bacilli. **Spirilla** (spi-RIL-uh) are spiraled, coiled, corkscrew-shaped bacterial cells that cause highly contagious diseases such as syphilis and cholera. To remember, think s = spiral and spirilla. Keep in mind that this list is never complete. Through research, previously unknown pathogenic bacteria are discovered on an ongoing basis.

Bacteria can cause infections by invading the body through a break in the skin or through any of the body's natural openings (nose, mouth, eyes, etc.). An infection occurs when an insufficient number of antibodies is produced by the body's immune (defense) system to fight harmful bacteria.

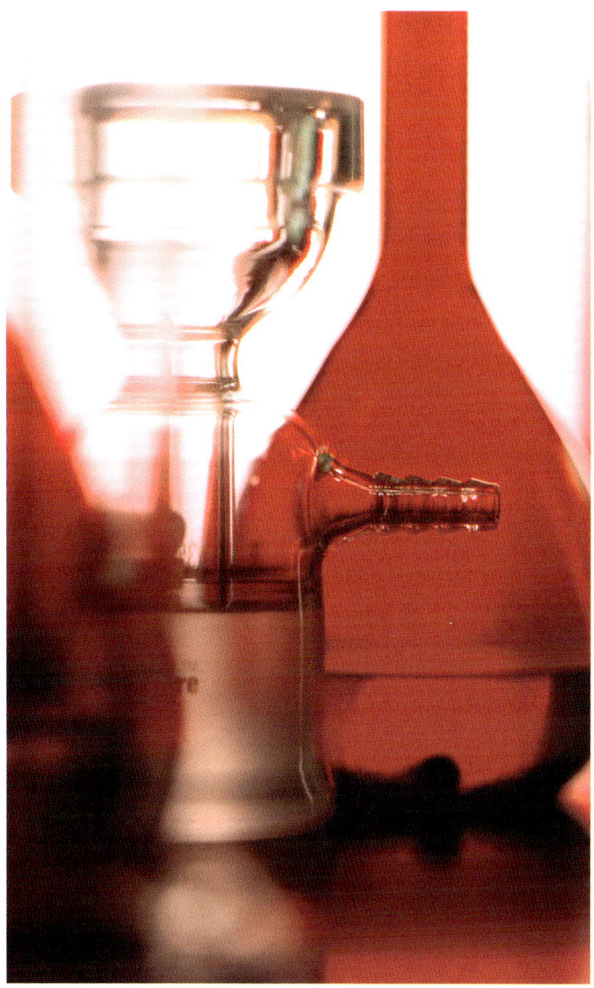

Growth of Bacteria

Bacteria thrive in dark, damp or dirty areas where a food source is available. All bacteria go through a growth cycle that consists of two stages: an active stage and an inactive stage.

Active Stage

During the active stage, also known as the vegetative stage, bacteria reproduce and grow rapidly. As the bacteria absorb food, each cell grows in size. When it is fully grown, it divides to create two cells. This process of cell division in bacteria is called **mitosis**. The process of cell division in bacteria is similar to the budding process in plants. Under favorable conditions, bacteria reproduce quickly, developing as many as 16 million offspring in 12 hours.

Inactive Stage

Bacteria are not always active; in unfavorable conditions, the cells die or become inactive. Some bacteria, such as anthrax and tetanus, also have a normal inactive or dormant stage. When the environment makes the bacteria's survival difficult, some bacteria enter this inactive, spore-forming stage, by creating spherical spores resistant to disinfectants, cold or heat. Spore formation and other means by which bacteria can resist disinfection are factors to be considered when practicing infection-control procedures in the nail salon. Some bacteria can survive for a long time in extreme heat or cold. When conditions again become favorable for the bacteria's growth, the bacteria return to the active stage.

The word *spore* is from the Greek word meaning *seed*. When times are tough for bacterial cells, such as when exposed to extreme temperatures, dehydration or chemical assault, some bacteria form hard protective coatings that encase their key parts to survive. In other words, think of a spore as a peanut that has formed an outer protective layer (the shell) over a thinner membrane (thin leafy inner husk). This outer shell protects the bacterial cell (nut), from the outside environment. Spores can be blown about and become more difficult to kill than active bacteria.

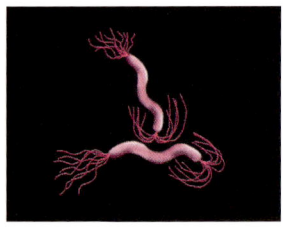

Movement of Bacteria

Because of their tiny size, bacteria can travel easily from place to place through air or water, from you to your client and vice versa. Bacilli and spirilla have the ability to move by themselves, using hair-like projections called **flagella** (flah-JEL-ah) or **cilia** (SIL-ee-a). These projections move the cells using a wave-like motion.

Viruses

The word **virus** comes from the Latin word meaning *poison.* It is defined as a sub-microscopic infectious agent that replicates itself only within cells of living hosts (meaning it "takes over" the cell to survive), and many are pathogenic. Viruses are much smaller than bacteria but cause more serious diseases, such as herpes, influenza and other respiratory and gastrointestinal infections, chickenpox, mumps, measles, smallpox, yellow fever, rabies, Human Immunodeficiency Virus (HIV), hepatitis and polio. Viruses cannot live on their own. They need "host" cells in order to survive.

For computers, the word VIRUS really is an acronym for "vital information resources under siege." Though the names and types have changed over the decades, computer viruses really originated in the 1960s and can cause losses in the billions of dollars for any company. A VIRUS is designed to enter your computer and infect your files by attaching itself to, overwriting or replacing another program—similar to what happens in the body!

Personal Service Workers (PSW), such as nurses, doctors, teachers, cosmetologists, estheticians and nail technicians should take precautions against all viruses, but in particular, two that are life-threatening: **Hepatitis B Virus (HBV)** and **Human Immunodeficiency Virus (HIV)**. HBV is a highly infectious disease that affects the liver. HBV is now preventable through vaccination. Vaccination is usually recommended for professionals such as those previously mentioned whose work may cause them to be exposed to HBV. Check with your local health agency or doctor to determine whether you are a candidate for this vaccination. HIV interferes with the body's natural immune system and causes the immune system to break down. HIV is spread when body fluids from an infected individual are absorbed into the blood stream of an uninfected individual.

Acquired Immunodeficiency Syndrome (AIDS), is a highly infectious disease caused by HIV (or a variant of HIV, called HIV-1), which interferes with the body's natural immune system and causes it to break down. Scientists have gained a great deal of knowledge about HIV, including information about its transmission and prevention. Although HIV is spread through the exchange of fluids between infected and uninfected individuals, the fluids from the infected person must contain sufficient amounts of the virus in order for the disease to be transmitted. Fluids known to contain sufficient amounts of HIV include blood, semen, vaginal fluids and breast milk. Infectious fluids can enter the body through sexual intercourse, childbirth, breastfeeding, cuts, sores or by sharing needles to name a few.

The Centers for Disease Control and Prevention (CDC) assign people in the beauty industry to the category titled "Personal Service Workers" (PSW). Watch for the initials PSW, since information that may pertain to you is released from a local center and mailed to your salon or spa.

External Parasites

External parasites (PAR-ah-sights) are organisms that grow and feed on other living organisms, which are referred to as hosts. They contribute nothing to their host and cause contagious diseases. Two such parasitic animals are head lice (pediculosis capitis) and itch mites (scabies). Clients that have a disease caused by a parasitic animal should not be treated and should be referred to a physician. Parasitic plants, or fungi, are

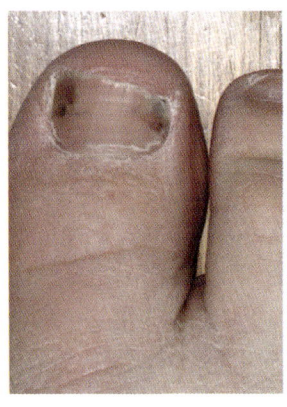

molds and yeast that produce such contagious diseases as ringworm (tinea capitis), honeycomb ringworm (favus) and nail fungus. These can occur on nails and can spread by implements that are not properly disinfected. A nail technician can spread infection to a noninfected area by using the same implements previously used in an infected area. Be aware of this fact when performing nail services.

Infection

An infection occurs when disease-causing (pathogenic) bacteria or viruses enter the body and multiply to the point of interfering with the body's normal state. An **infection** is the growth of a parasitic organism within the body. These microorganisms are referred to as **pathogens**, and include viruses, bacteria and fungi.

An object that contains pathogens is considered contaminated. To prevent cross-contamination, all pathogens need to be removed from the object (decontaminated).

Common means of spreading infection in a salon or spa include:

- Contact with open sores
- Contact with contaminated hands and implements (usually due to improper disinfection between clients)
- Exposure to coughing or sneezing
- Use of common drinking cups and towels
- Exposure to unsanitary conditions
- Use of manicure tables and pedicure tubs that are not properly disinfected

3

Infections can also be prevented by good personal hygiene, public awareness and following infection control procedures in the salon or spa. If you have a contagious or communicable disease, extra caution should be taken in order to prevent the spread of infection. Check with your area's regulating agency for specific guidelines on dealing with contagious diseases.

There are two basic classes of infection:

1. A **local infection** (below) is present in a small, confined area often indicated by a pus-filled boil, pimple or inflammation. To remember, think local = little.

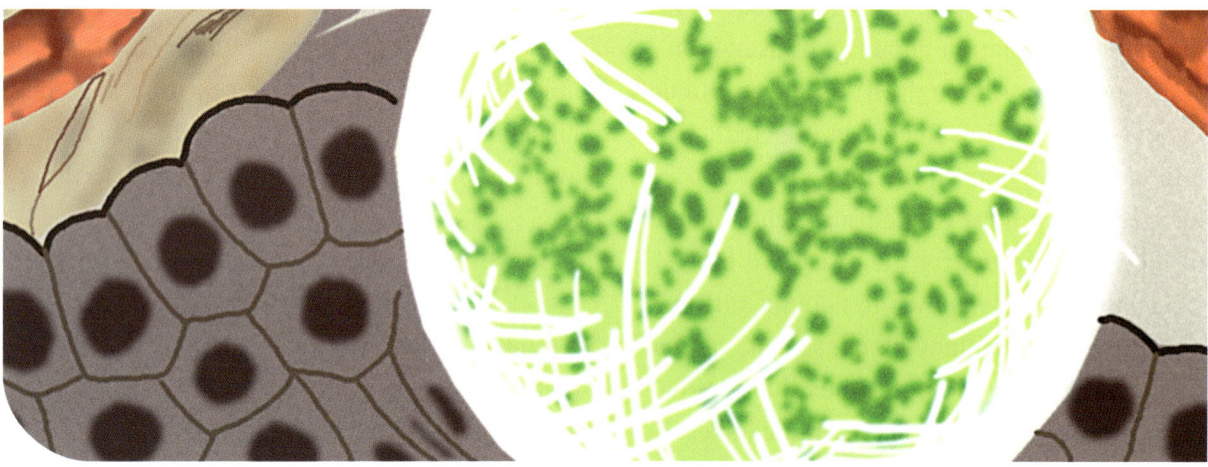

2. A **general** (or **systemic**) **infection** (below) occurs when the circulatory system carries bacteria and their toxins to all parts of the body. To remember, think general = giant.

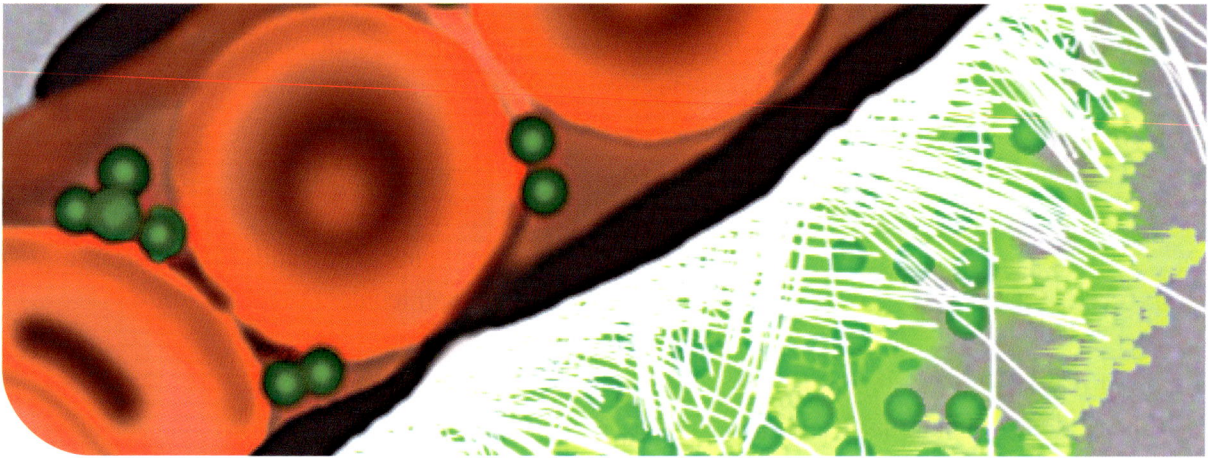

It is possible for a person to carry disease-producing bacteria or viruses with no recognizable symptoms of the disease. Such a person is called an asymptomatic carrier. For this reason, the same infection control procedures should be used with all clients. Using consistent infection-control procedures for all clients is called **universal precautions.**

Immunity

Immunity is the body's ability to destroy infectious agents that enter it. The immune system is a remarkable defense mechanism that fights infections in two basic ways:

1. **Natural immunity** is a partially inherited, natural resistance to disease. A healthy body produces white blood cells and antibodies to fight disease-causing agents. Also, the epidermis (outermost layer of skin) protects the body from microbes. If the skin is punctured, the cut must be treated to prevent microbes from infecting the skin.

2. **Passive (acquired) immunity** occurs through **vaccinations**, or the injection of antigens, which stimulate the body's immune response (i.e., innoculation for polio or flu).

The body's dependence on its immune system inspires most people to protect themselves from coming into contact with potentially harmful bacteria and viruses. Healthy, unbroken skin is the first major defense the body has against infection, since skin is a natural barrier against infection.

Now that you have read about the dangers of microbes, you are ready to learn how you can destroy them and prevent disease from spreading in the salon or spa.

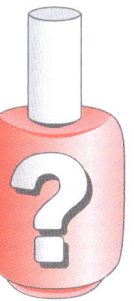

If you were asked to give a presentation in class on how infection spreads, what would you say?

3

INFECTION CONTROL

As you know, microbes are everywhere, including in the air around you; so infection control requires close attention. **Infection control** is the term used to describe efforts to prevent the spread of disease and kill microbes. Prevention is practiced at three varying levels of control, which include sanitation at the lowest level, disinfection at the second level and sterilization at the third, and highest level. General practices used during infection control procedures include handwashing and using personal protective equipment, such as gloves and safety glasses when needed. It also means properly disinfecting all nail implements and surfaces to prevent **cross-contamination**, which means bacteria is spread by contaminated equipment, surfaces or food.

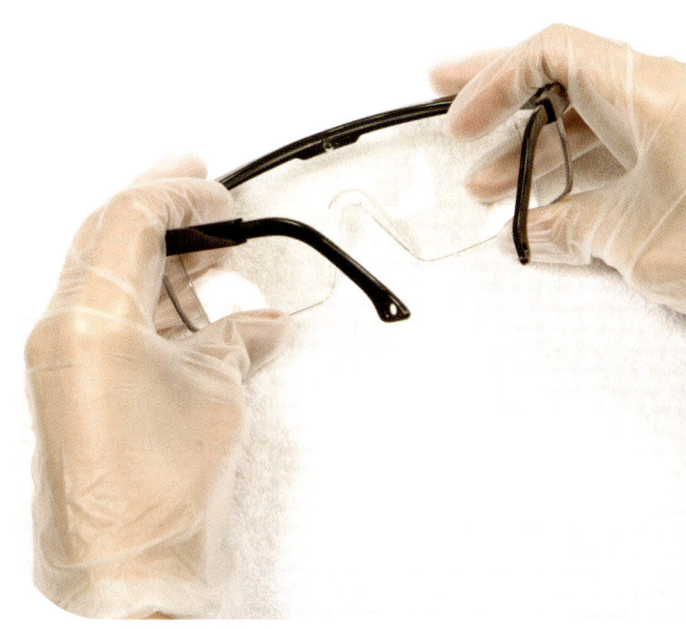

Gloves may be required by some regulating agencies to perform services but must always be worn in the case of a blood spill. Always follow your area's regulatory guidelines for when gloves are required.

Dilution: Mix 2 ozs. per gallon. (16 ml per liter).

Directions for Use: It is a violation of Federal Law to use this product in a manner inconsistent with its labeling. Remove outer cap. While holding bottle by the neck, twist off inner cap and discard. Replace outer cap loosely. Gently squeeze bottle until solution fills upper reservoir to desired level. Use at a dilution of 1:64 (2 ozs. of this product per gallon of water or 16 ml per liter).

Beauty and Barber Shop, Instruments and Tools: Thoroughly pre-clean. Completely immerse brushes, combs, scissors, clipper blades, razors, tweezers, manicure and other shop tools for 10 minutes (or as required by local authorities). Wipe dry before use. Fresh solution should be prepared daily or more often when the solution becomes diluted or soiled.

*Virucidal: For Complete Instructions For Hepatitis B Virus (HBV) and Human Immunodeficiency Virus (HIV-1) DISINFECTION Refer To Enclosed Hang Tag.

Statement of Practical Treatment: In case of contact, immediately flush eyes or skin with plenty of water for at least 15 minutes. For eye contacts, call a physician. If swallowed, drink egg whites, gelatin solution or if these are not available, drink large quantities of water. Avoid alcohol. Call a physician immediately.

Note to Physician: Probable mucosal damage may contra-indicate the use of gastric lavage.

Note: Avoid shipping or storing below freezing. If product freezes, thaw at room temperature and shake gently to remix components.

Manufactured for ULTRONICS 1-800-262-6262
750 Corporate Drive, Mahwah, New Jersey 07430
Made in USA   ©1991   Pat. pending   P/N 81348 M
EPA Reg. No. 61178-1-63562   EPA Est. No. 37365-PA-01

Also important in infection control is the concept of **efficacy**, which means the ability to produce results, or effectiveness. Standards have been established that require efficacy labels, as shown here, on all disinfectants to inform the user about what organisms the product is effective against. An example is a disinfectant label that states "effective against human Hepatitis B Virus and HIV-1." As you gain more information in this chapter, you will notice that you are required to use products based on the efficacy label.

Reading the manufacturer's directions plays a significant role in ensuring proper infection control practices. Methods may vary from product to product. For example, immersion times (length of time for soaking) in a disinfectant, storage and application methods differ for each product. Follow the directions. It cannot be emphasized enough that two steps are necessary for effective infection control, which include reading the label and following the directions.

VOCABULARY OF INFECTION CONTROL

- **Infection control** is the prevention of the spread of infectious agents to you and your clients.

- **Sanitation** is the low-level reduction of surface bacteria.

- **Disinfection** eliminates bacteria, viruses and most organisms on nonliving, nonporous surfaces. This procedure is recommended for all nail implements and surfaces.

- **Sterilization** eliminates all living organisms, including bacterial spores on nonporous surfaces.

- **Decontamination** makes objects and areas safe by eliminating poisonous or otherwise harmful substances.

- **Antiseptics** prevent the growth of microorganisms on the skin.

- **Infection control procedures** include handwashing, using personal protective equipment, such as gloves and safety glasses when necessary, and properly disinfecting all nail service implements and surfaces to prevent cross-contamination.

- **Universal precautions** means using the same infection control practices on all clients. Since we cannot identify clients with infectious diseases, it is safer to handle the blood spills and body fluids of all clients as potentially infectious.

- **Exposure to blood** and other body fluids presents a risk for nail technicians. Exposure can occur during any service when the client may be accidentally cut with a file or nippers.

- **Handwashing** removes microorganisms by lifting them from the surface of the skin. Hands should be washed between each service, before and after a lunch break, after using the restroom, or any time they become contaminated.

- **OSHA's Bloodborne Pathogen Standard**, established by the Occupational Safety and Health Administration (OSHA), should be followed for all tools and implements that come into contact with blood or body fluids. This type of high-level disinfection requires the use of an EPA-registered, broad spectrum (hospital-level) disinfectant that is labeled as effective against HIV-1 and Hepatitis B or tuberculocidal (proven effective against mycobacterium tuberculosis). EPA Standards, provided by the Environmental Protection Agency discussed on page 63, require efficacy labels on all disinfectants to inform the user about what organisms the product is effective against. Reading the label and following the directions ensures that the product will perform according to the efficacy claims on the label.

3

In today's nail salon or spa environment, infection control has become a major focus of attention. Client concerns about safety, along with new standards set by regulatory agencies, have resulted in heightened awareness of the procedures necessary to prevent cross-contamination—particularly involving pedicure services. As mentioned previously, the three levels of infection control are sanitation, disinfection and sterilization, which are used to protect you and the public you serve. Determining the appropriate level of decontamination (free of germs) and infection control depends on how a tool or implement is used as well as requirements set by your area's regulating agency. Since these regulations change from time to time, it is recommended that you frequently review them.

Sanitation

Sanitation is the lowest level of infection control and serves as the foundation of your infection control program. This first level of infection control is the physical removal of debris, which reduces the number of microbes present. Sanitation also removes organic matter, such as blood, nail-filing dust and skin particles, which may interfere with proper disinfection procedures. Infection control practices for sanitation of the spa or salon require shared responsibilities from everyone on the team in order to provide and maintain a healthy environment. The goal of infection control is to minimize the transfer of microorganisms. This goal can be accomplished in many ways, but it begins with cleanliness.

Standards for infection control are developed by your area's regulating agency to protect the general public. Sanitation practices that meet these established rules must be carried out by you to keep the working areas, nail implements and all equipment clean. As the lowest level of infection control practiced in the salon or spa, sanitation is performed on noncritical objects (objects that come into contact with healthy, unbroken skin). Sanitation begins the process of protecting you and your clients from the transmission of diseases. The charts that follow give an overview of steps to take to achieve sanitation.

SANITATION = CLEANING

All visible residues must be removed before implements and equipment can be disinfected properly. If this step is skipped, the disinfection is ineffective and it will contaminate the disinfection solution.

SANITATION GUIDELINES

1. Wash your hands with a liquid soap and water immediately before and after each service. Liquid or foam soap is recommended, since bar soaps can harbor and transmit microbes.
2. Sanitize all surfaces before and after each service.
3. Provide hot and cold running water at all times.
4. Provide clean restrooms, with well-stocked liquid soap, toilet tissue and paper towels. Never use restroom areas for storage of chemicals.
5. Provide disposable drinking cups.
6. Clean all sinks and water fountains regularly.
7. Keep the salon or spa free from insects and rodents.
8. Empty waste receptacles daily or more often if necessary.
9. Wear clean, freshly laundered clothing.
10. Provide freshly laundered towels for each client.
11. Launder all towels on a regular basis.
12. Store soiled towels in a covered receptacle until laundered.
13. Avoid touching your face, mouth or eyes during services.
14. Wear protective gloves if you are exposed to a client's blood or body fluids.
15. Never allow pets or animals in service areas, except for Service Animals as identified in the Americans With Disabilities Act.
16. Dispense all powders with a shaker, dispenser pump, spray-type container, spatula or disposable applicator.
17. Label all chemicals and keep them covered when not in use.
18. Use a fresh spatula or applicator stick for each client every time you dip in for more product. No double-dipping, which means using the same spatula or stick more than one time in any product. This can spread bacteria and contaminate the product.
19. Discard disposable items, porous materials or implements after each service.
20. Wash and dry all reusable implements with soap and water before placing them in disinfecting solution.
21. Maintain a file of Material Safety Data Sheets for all products used in the salon or spa.

PROPER HANDWASHING PROCEDURE

Handwashing is one of the most important sanitation actions you can take to prevent the transfer of microorganisms from one person to another. Washing hands with a liquid or foam soap removes microorganisms from the folds and grooves of the skin by lifting and rinsing them from the skin's surface.

In the salon or spa, wash your hands before and after each service. At the end of the day, wash your hands again thoroughly to prevent carrying microorganisms outside of the salon or spa. This also eliminates any chemicals that you may have come into contact with during the nail service.

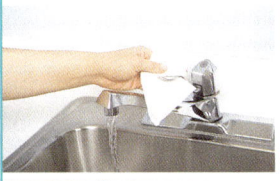

1. Use a paper towel or tissue to turn the water on, if you have a paper towel or tissue dispenser (some facilities only offer hands-free air blowers). Dispense an additional 10" to 12" (25 to 30 cm) and leave hanging in place from the dispenser for later use (#5).

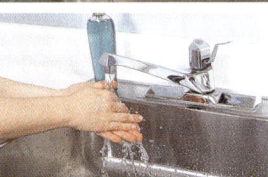

2. Wet hands with warm water.

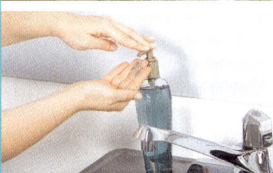

3. Apply soap and clean hands, nails and between fingers.

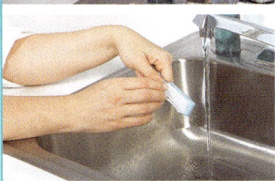

4. Lather and scrub for approximately 15 seconds.

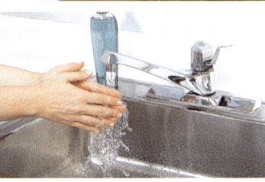

5. Rinse hands; then tear off paper towel and dry.

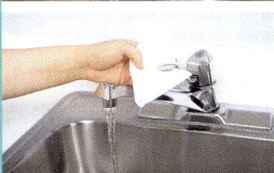

6. Turn off water with paper towel or tissue—not with your clean hands! If more paper is needed, use the paper in your hand on the dispenser handle.

3

Disinfection

Disinfection is the second level of infection control and means using products (or methods) that kill or destroy bacteria and a broad spectrum of viruses. However, chemical disinfectants do not eliminate bacterial spores. This is the main difference between disinfection and sterilization.

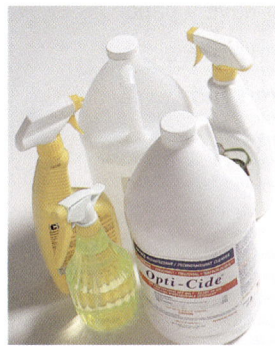

Because disinfection products claim to kill or destroy bacteria, and most of these products are toxic, they are regulated by law through a governing agency such as the **Environmental Protection Agency** (EPA). Standards for disinfection apply to all nonporous surfaces, tools and implements in the salon or spa. For example, nippers and clippers, which can be exposed to blood during service in the salon or spa, as well as all nail implements and surfaces, require pre-cleaning (sanitation) and disinfection after each use. These objects are considered semi-critical objects and require a high level of disinfection since they may come into contact with skin that is unhealthy or broken (not intact).

Implement disinfection and pre-cleaning can be done by hand or with an ultrasonic cleaning machine, which uses high-frequency energy waves. While both methods are acceptable, ultrasonic cleaners have proven to be 16 times more effective than hand scrubbing with a brush. Ultrasonic cleaners also eliminate handling of implements that may be contaminated with blood. (Refer to Disinfection Guidelines, page 65.) The use of an EPA-registered, broad spectrum (hospital-level) disinfectant effective against HIV and HBV, which is also tuberculocidal, is recommended to eliminate or minimize occupational exposure to bloodborne pathogens in the 2001 OSHA Bloodborne Pathogens Standard.

> Regulatory agencies outline very specific rules pertaining to thoroughly pre-cleaning nonporous instruments with soap and hot water before immersing in any disinfectant solution. Pre-cleaning (washing with soap and hot water) implements is the first step to proper disinfection.

> The 2001 OSHA Bloodborne Pathogens Standard requires the use of an EPA-registered, broad spectrum (hospital-level) disinfectant with an efficacy against HIV and HBV or tuberculocidal. This requirement applies to all implements that come into contact with blood or body fluids.

Regulating Agencies

In the United States, the **Occupational Safety and Health Administration** (OSHA) was created in 1971 by the Department of Labor to enforce safety and health standards in the workplace. OSHA standards require that employees be informed of the dangers of the materials used in the workplace and the exposure they might have to toxic substances and that all workplace conditions are sanitary. A **Material Safety Data Sheet** (MSDS) and labeling of products are two important regulations that this agency has instituted to assist in safe operations. An MSDS (sample on next page) provides key information on a specific product regarding ingredients, associated hazards, combustion levels and storage requirements. It is required to keep an MSDS on file for every product used in the salon or spa. Remember that, for your protection and safety, you have a right as an employee to know what is contained in any product being used. OSHA standards significantly impact the industry by helping to ensure general safety, especially in regard to mixing, storing, labeling and disposing of chemicals.

REGULATING AGENCIES

EPA

In the United States, the Environmental Protection Agency (EPA) was created in 1970 to protect human health and to safeguard the natural environment, such as air, water and land. The EPA researches and sets national standards for a variety of environmental programs and delegates the responsibility of issuing permits, and monitoring and enforcing compliance locally. For example, if you have a car, you have most likely taken it in for a "Clean Air Inspection" at an EPA station to ensure that the exhaust emitted from your vehicle is at a safe level for the environment. Prior to the EPA, the national government was not structured to make a coordinated attack on the pollutants that harm human health and the environment.

OSHA

The Occupational Safety and Health Administration (OSHA) was created to ensure health and safety in America's workplaces. The existence of OSHA has reduced workplace fatalities and occupational injury and illness rates by nearly half and plays a vital role in preventing these hazards through outreach, education and compliance assistance. OSHA offers free workplace consultations in every state to small businesses that want on-site help to establish safety and health programs and identify and correct workplace hazards. OSHA classes, literature and information are important to you and your daily work as a nail technician because they set up guidelines for you regarding the use of chemicals.

MATERIAL SAFETY DATA SHEET

An MSDS for every product used in the salon or spa is kept in a file or a binder that is easily accessible to all personnel for reference and in the event of an emergency. The MSDS provides information on the product ingredients, including potential hazards. Such information may prove helpful if an allergic reaction or injury occurs related to the product's usage.

An MSDS is supplied by the manufacturer with each shipment or made available upon request, by the supplier or manufacturer of the product. This standard applies to disinfectants, soaps, lotions, artificial nail products, adhesives, oils and any other products used in the salon or spa.

Section I:
Product Name and Company Name

Section II:
Hazardous Ingredients

Section III:
Physical and Chemical Ingredients

Section IV:
Fire and Explosion Hazard Data

INSPECT THE LABEL

Always follow the manufacturer's instructions, and always wear protective gloves and safety glasses when mixing disinfectants. Read the label on all disinfectant products to determine the specific organisms the product has been proven effective against. EPA-registered, broad spectrum disinfectants, also known as hospital-level disinfectants, will state on the label that they are as follows: Germicidal (jur-mi-SIGH-dahl), Fungicidal (fun-ji-SIGH-dahl), Pseudomonacidal (soo-doh-MON-ah-SIGH-dahl), and Virucidal (vy-ri-SIGH-dahl). If the disinfectant is not proven effective against pseudomonas aeruginosa, or Pseudomonacidal, and if this does not appear on the label along with an EPA Registration Number, the disinfectant is not broad spectrum. The disinfectant must also be effective against HIV and HBV or tuberculocidal. If it is effective against these organisms, it will always be stated on the label as shown below.

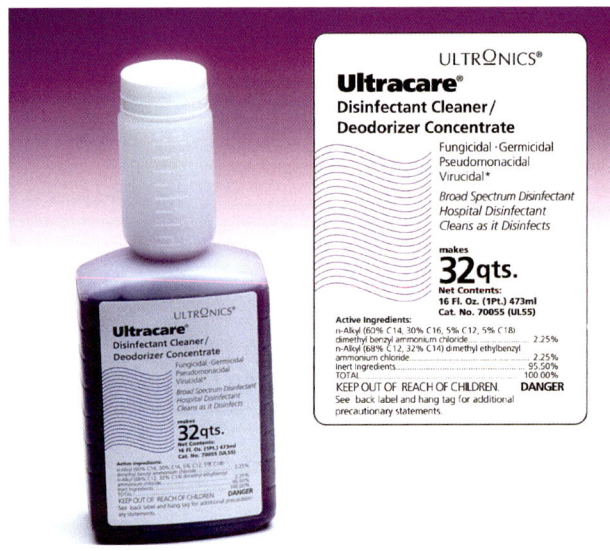

In the United States, the EPA approves the efficacy of products used for infection control. The manufacturer must submit a product to the EPA for verification of effectiveness against the organisms listed on the label. Once verification has been established, the product receives an EPA registration number, along with approval of the efficacy claims on the label, stating what organisms the product is effective against.

Disinfection Considerations

Since the regulatory agency in each area determines efficacy standards, they may vary from place to place. Some areas may recommend disinfecting all tools and implements regardless of whether they have come into contact with blood or body fluids. Others may recommend disinfecting only those that have come into contact with blood or body fluids. A broad spectrum (hospital-level) disinfectant with an efficacy label that reads "effective against HIV and Human Hepatitis B Virus or tuberculocidal" meets both of these requirements.

Chemical disinfecting agents come in varied forms, including liquid, capsule and powder. When choosing one from your supplier, consider the following:

- Is it in compliance with your area's regulating agency or health department?
- Is it economical?
- Is it easy to use?
- Is it an agent that works quickly?
- Is it safe for use with metal and plastic implements?

Porous vs. Nonporous Items

A porous item is anything that is made of a material that can absorb liquid and cannot be disinfected. Some examples of this are orangewood sticks, emery boards or lint-free wipes. Examples of nonporous items are glass files, metal cuticle pushers and metal files. If it is unclear whether an implement is porous or nonporous, a simple way to determine what to do is: "When in doubt, throw it out." Always follow your regulating agency's guidelines for disposing of porous items.

Most files are porous and cannot be properly disinfected. You may wish to offer your clients their personal files as a complimentary gift with their service. To offset the cost, you can include it in the price of your service and delight your clients with this added bonus.

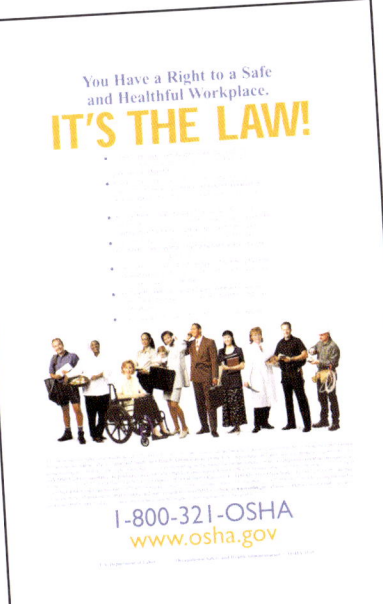

You Have a Right to a Safe and Healthful Workplace.

IT'S THE LAW!

1-800-321-OSHA
www.osha.gov

Read the directions carefully and follow recommended safety precautions! Always note and follow specific immersion times, and always cleanse implements before disinfecting. Remember that disinfection methods do not work instantly but require some time to destroy microbes. Procedures and timing will vary based on the product used to disinfect. Read the label to determine the length of time required for implement and surface disinfection. Sanitation and disinfection practices are the methods most often utilized in the salon or spa. The charts on the following pages present proper disinfection guidelines including how to act in the event of a blood spill.

3

DISINFECTION GUIDELINES

1. Discard or disinfect every implement that comes into contact with the client.

2. Remove all debris from nondisposable implements and pre-clean by washing the implements thoroughly with soap and water by hand or with an ultrasonic cleaner.

3. Rinse thoroughly and pat implements dry prior to immersion to avoid dilution when immersed in disinfectant.

4. Completely submerge all nonporous nail implements in a disinfectant that is EPA-registered, broad spectrum (hospital-level) and designated as effective against HIV and HBV or tuberculocidal. Follow manufacturer's instructions for submersion time—and for dilution, if you are using a concentrated formula.

5. Change disinfection solutions daily, or as recommended by the manufacturer.

6. Remove implements with forceps, tongs or gloved hands, or use a self-draining basket, which is usually included with the soak tray. Rinse disinfection solution off implements. Do not leave implements in solution for extended periods of time, or beyond manufacturer's instructions.

7. Store implements that have been disinfected in a clean, dry, covered container or cabinet until needed.

8. Never use an implement or towel that has been dropped on the floor. Even though your floor may be cleaned daily, always discard or prepare the item for disinfection, then continue services with clean, disinfected materials and implements.

9. If towels are laundered in your facility, use an additive that disinfects and sanitizes wet linens.

10. Keep a first-aid kit on hand.

11. Refer to guidelines on blood spill procedures for cuts or broken skin exposures.

12. Dispose of any material that comes in contact with blood or body fluids, such as discharge from open sores, in a sealable plastic bag. Then, place this sealed bag in a second bag, seal it and discard it in a covered waste can. This process is called "double bagging." You may be required to label this bag with a red or orange marker to indicate that it contains hazardous waste. Check with your area's regulating agency for disposal guidelines.

IMPLEMENT DISINFECTION GUIDELINES

It is important to sanitize and disinfect all implements in order to prevent cross-contamination. Following are guidelines to protect you and your clients:

1. Sanitize (pre-clean) and dry all nonporous implements.
2. Fully immerse the entire implement in an EPA-registered, broad spectrum (hospital-level) disinfection solution, for the manufacturer's recommended time; most require 10 minutes for disinfection.
3. Remove the items with tongs or gloved hands and rinse with water and dry.
4. Store in a clean, dry, covered container or follow your regulatory guidelines.

PEDICURE BASIN DISINFECTION GUIDELINES

To ensure the safety of your pedicure clients, it is especially important to sanitize and disinfect all pedicure basins properly. Following are guidelines to protect your clients:

After Every Client
1. Drain water from pedicure basin or tub.
2. Scrub basin with soap and a disinfected scrub brush. Rinse with water to remove all visible residue.
3. Fill basin with water and the manufacturer's recommended amount of an EPA-registered, broad spectrum (hospital-level) disinfection solution.
4. Allow the solution to circulate through the basin if it has jets. If not, allow the solution to set for the manufacturer's recommended amount of time (generally about 10 minutes).
5. Drain the water and rinse the basin.
6. Dry basin with a clean, disposable towel.

End of the Day
1. Drain water from pedicure basin or tub.
2. Remove all removable parts, such as screens, footplates, impellers (rotating device that forces fluid to move) and scrub with a brush, soap and water. Be sure to also scrub the areas behind the removable components.

3. Replace parts and fill basin with water and chelating detergent (cleansers designed for use in hard water). Allow the chelating detergent to circulate through the spa system for approximately five to 10 minutes or as directed by the manufacturer's instructions. Turn off the jets and let the solution soak for the remainder of the 10 minutes if it generates too much foam.
4. Drain the basin and rinse with water.
5. Fill basin with water and the manufacturer's recommended amount of EPA-registered, broad spectrum (hospital-level) disinfection solution.
6. Allow the solution to circulate through the basin if it has jets. If not, allow the solution to set for the manufacturer's recommended amount of time.
7. Drain the solution and rinse with water.
8. Dry the basin with a clean, disposable towel.

Once a Week
Follow End of the Day guidelines, however, leave the disinfection solution in the basin overnight. In the morning, drain the solution and run clean water through the spa pedicure system.

Precautions for Mixing Chemicals

Since chemical disinfecting agents can be dangerous, remember to take the following precautions to prevent accidents and mistakes:

- Tightly cover and label all disinfecting products and other chemicals for use in the salon or spa.
- Store in a cool, dry area. Air, light and heat can weaken chemicals.
- Purchase chemicals in small quantities.
- Do not inhale (or smell) chemical solutions. Avoid contact with skin and eyes. Wear protective gloves and eyewear. Refer to the MSDS for procedures if contact does occur with the skin or eyes.
- Wash hands after handling all chemicals.
- Avoid spilling chemicals. If a spill does occur, clean it up immediately. Refer to the MSDS for proper handling of specific chemicals.
- Always follow manufacturer's instructions.

3

BLOOD SPILL PROCEDURE

All blood encountered in the workplace should be treated as infectious. Direct contact with blood should be avoided, and protective gloves should be used whenever such contact may occur. If you are exposed to a client's blood during a service, take the following steps:

1. Stop the service and wash your hands.
2. Cover your hands with protective gloves.
3. Supply the injured person with styptic powder or spray, which helps stop the bleeding, and the appropriate dressing to cover the injury.
4. Do not allow containers, brushes, nozzles or the styptic container to touch the skin or come into contact with the wound.
5. Disinfect the station and implements with an EPA-registered, broad spectrum (hospital-level) disinfectant.
6. Double-bag all disposable, blood-soiled (contaminated) articles and discard, making certain that it is sealed to protect anyone from coming into contact with the material.

If you are injured during a service, follow this procedure:
- Stop the service and wash the wound with an antiseptic.
- Cover the wound with a bandage, wear gloves if the wound is on your hand and continue your service.

Sterilization

Sterilization is the third and highest level of infection control. It destroys all living organisms, including bacterial spores, which neither sanitation nor disinfection can kill. Sterilization is used less frequently than disinfection, but is far more effective. However, it is more costly. Certain regulating agencies require sterilization, so check with your area's regulating agency regarding sterilization and its procedures.

> **Calibration** means adjusting the settings on a piece of sterilization equipment so that it operates safely according to the manufacturer's instructions, and within tolerances set forth by your regulating agency law. Each agency has different requirements for sterilizer calibration. Check with your local area regulatory agency to determine calibration settings and requirements for posting proof of calibration in the salon or spa.

Numerous sterilization methods exist, including moist or dry heat (calibrated to various temperatures) and immersion in liquid chemical sterilizers. Specific calibrations and timeframes are normally required for sterilization procedures. In addition, manufacturer representatives or approved technicians must perform periodic checks to ensure proper use of procedures and equipment. Sterilization methods are costly, time-consuming and require a high degree of quality control to ensure results; however, some regulatory agencies require sterilization.

Equipment

Infection control equipment is available to sanitize, disinfect and sterilize, depending on the salon's needs.

UV Light Sterilizer

The **ultraviolet (UV) light sterilizer** is common in most salons or spas, though it is possible to function without one. This machine usually looks like a large toaster oven and utilizes UV light to kill bacteria in a dry setting. Typically, implements are placed in the cabinet after being completely pre-cleaned with warm soap and water and are allowed to sanitize for approximately 20 minutes.

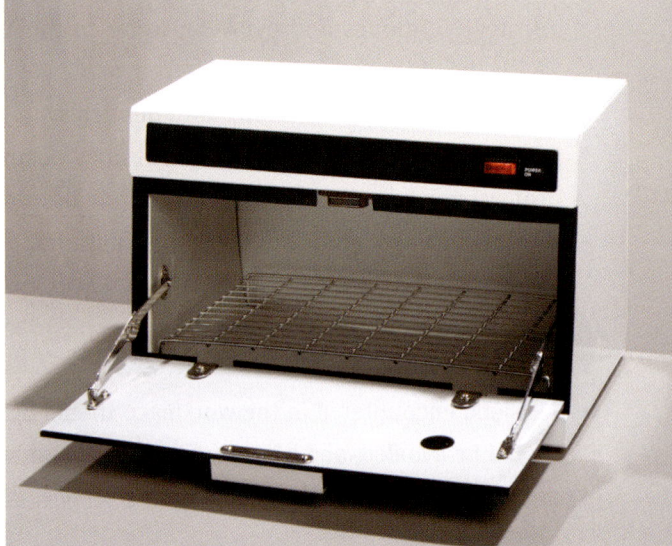

Although this UV light machine is often referred to as a "sterilizer," it is not effective in eliminating all organisms on nail implements and tools. These are usually labeled "UV Sterilizer" on the machine, but since they don't kill all microorganisms, they technically are not sterilizers; they are sanitizers. You may encounter both sanitizers and sterilizers in the salon or spa. The difference between the two is that usually the sanitizer, which utilizes both light and heat, is lower in strength than an actual sterilizer, which is called an autoclave.

The UV light machine can be used as a holding area for implements after they have been properly disinfected. However, a UV light machine is not required for storing implements. Disinfected implements can also be stored in a clean, covered container or drawer. Solutions to consider using for disinfection and sterilization are overviewed on the next page.

DISINFECTION AND STERILIZATION CONSIDERATIONS

There are many different options to consider when applying disinfection or sterilization practices. Listed here are a few of the chemicals you may encounter for both.

Iodophor (eye-OH-duh-for) **Germicidal Detergent Solution**
Iodine solutions or tinctures relieve skin irritation and are antiseptics. They are not suitable disinfectants due to varying concentrations from product to product.

Phenolic (fee-NO-lik) **Germicidal Detergent Solution**
Phenol (carbolic acid) may be used with numerous other additives such as ortho-phenylphenol or ortho-benzyl-para-chlorophenol. Three percent phenolics are not considered high-level disinfectants due to their inability to inactivate bacterial spores, mycobacterium (my-co-bac-TEER-ee-um) tuberculosis and fungi. Phenolic solutions may also have the tendency to destroy plastic containers or implements.

Ethyl – (70%) or **Isopropyl** (eye-suh-PRO-pil) **Alcohol** – (90%)
These alcohols are antibacterial, antifungal and antiviral, but they do not destroy bacterial spores. They are not recommended for high-level disinfection because of their inability to inactivate bacterial spores (and isopropyl's inability to eliminate hydrophilic viruses).

Stabilized Hydrogen Peroxide – (6%)
Properties of hydrogen peroxide include antibacterial, antiviral and antifungal. Commercially available 3% peroxide is a stable and effective disinfectant when used on nonporous surfaces.

Quaternary Ammonium Germicidal Detergent Solution
Quaternaries or "quats" that are sold as disinfectants are antifungal, antibacterial, and antiviral, but are typically not sporicidal or tuberculocidal. They are recommended for use as environmental sanitation of noncritical surfaces such as floors, furniture and walls. The newer quaternary ammonium disinfectant cleaners are proven effective against HIV-1 and Hepatitis B Virus and are recommended for disinfection of all nonporous implements and surfaces.

Glutaraldehyde (gloo-tuh-RAL-duh-hide)- **Based Formulations** – (2%)
Lower levels of glutaraldehyde phenate are no longer considered high-level disinfectants and must be used at 2%. Disinfection time is 20 minutes. Once activated by alkaline solution, it has a shelf life of 14 days. Glutaraldehyde products have a shelf life of 28 days.

Sodium Hypochlorite (hi-puh-KLOR-ight)
Sodium hypochlorite, a liquid chlorine disinfectant found in household bleach, has a wide range of antimicrobial activity, is inexpensive and fast-acting (20 minutes). Its use is limited due to corrosiveness and instability. Chlorine stability is dependent upon pH. As the pH rises with prolonged shelf life, the antimicrobial effects are reduced. Based on this, the product is not recommended for disinfection or sterilization procedures in the salon.

Demand-Release Chlorine Dioxide
This is a relatively new agent that sterilizes after six hours. Refer to the manufacturer's instructions for restrictions and directions.

Heat Sterilization
Dual-purpose autoclaves/sterilizers can be used for steam (moist heat) or dry heat ranging from 320° to 375°. They require distilled water to operate and take approximately 30 minutes to sterilize. They are only for use with hard, nonporous implements that can withstand high temperatures.

Ethylene (ETH-uh-leen) **Oxide Gas**
This sterilization method is ideal for porous or difficult-to-clean, narrow, channeled implements. Sterilization can vary from two to six hours. Follow the manufacturer's instructions for operation and sterilization time.

3

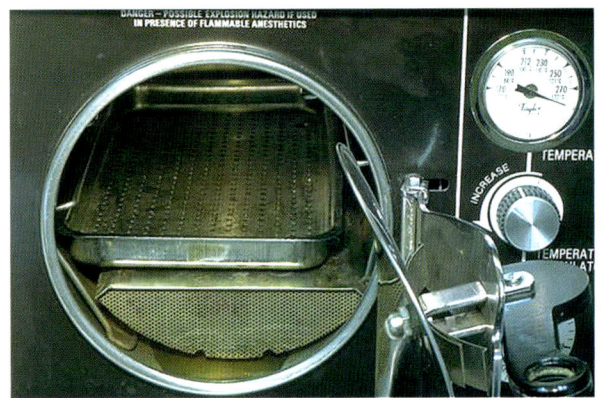

Autoclave

To truly sterilize equipment, an **autoclave** is used. An autoclave is a pressurized, steam-heated vessel that sterilizes objects with high pressure and heat, or pressurized steam, preventing microorganisms from surviving. Autoclave is taken literally from the Greek word *auto*, meaning self, and Latin's *clavis*, meaning key. This is because the vessel can be self-locking, due to pressurization. However, autoclaves are more commonly used in medical or dental offices, where critical instruments such as surgical tools that are designed to puncture body tissue, are used. Autoclaves can be found in some salons or spas as required by local regulating agencies.

Sterilization by a steam autoclave (moist heat under pressure) is very reliable, but must be monitored for effectiveness. For example, on a daily basis, the nail technician may have the responsibility of making certain that the unit is sterilizing by checking readouts as the cycles progress. As with any type of equipment or sterilization process, it is important to follow the manufacturer's instructions to ensure proper sterilization. This applies to instructions for use, proper maintenance and monitoring.

Chemiclave

While an autoclave uses steam to sterilize implements and other objects in the salon or spa, a **chemiclave** uses high-pressure, high-temperature water, alcohol and formaldehyde vapors for sterilization. Unlike the objects in an autoclave, the items sterilized in a chemiclave do not get wet and, in addition, the time it takes for a chemiclave to heat is considerably shorter than with an autoclave.

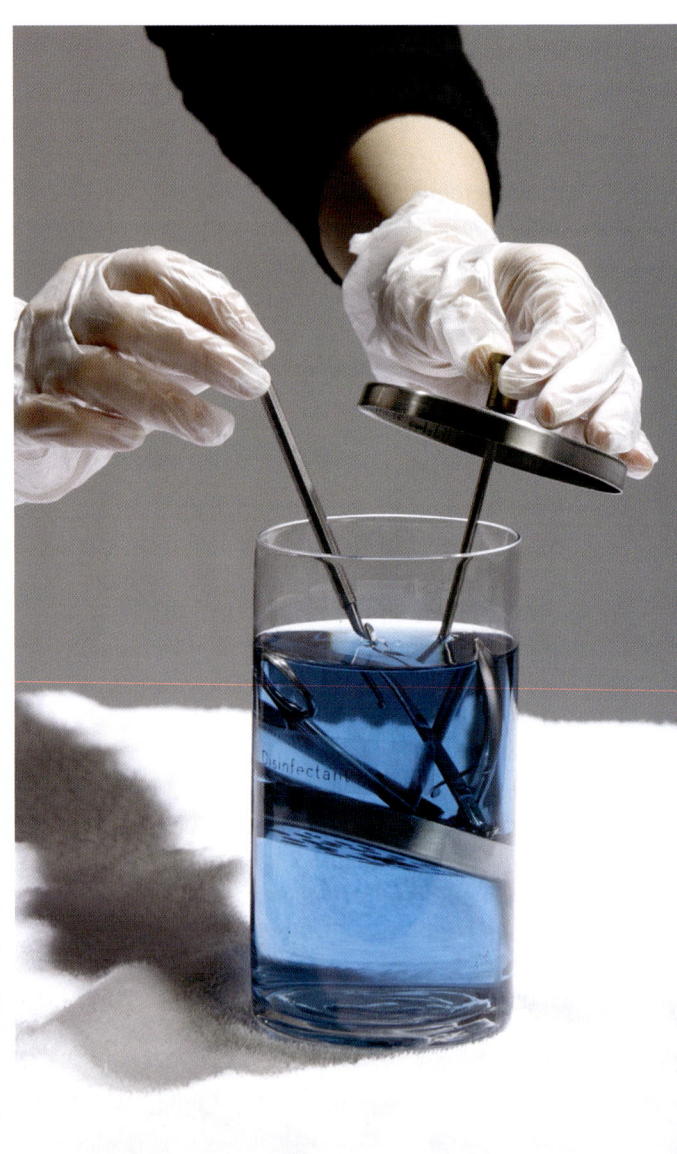

INFECTION CONTROL GUIDELINES

Level of Infection Control	Item	Procedure
SANITATION Items categorized as **noncritical**, meaning they make contact with healthy, unbroken (intact) skin, need to be sanitized.	Countertops, sinks, floors, toilets, towels, linens.	Use appropriate cleaning products. Efficacy label will state "appropriate for floors, countertops, sinks, toilets, towels and/or linens."
	Your hands before each service.	Use liquid soaps. Avoid bar soaps.
	Your hands and client's hands/feet prior to hand or foot service.	Apply antiseptic designed for hands and feet or use a liquid soap.
DISINFECTION Items categorized as **semicritical**, meaning they may make contact with mucous membranes or skin that is unhealthy or broken (not intact), need to be disinfected.	Tools and implements that *have not* come into contact with blood or body fluids.	Use EPA-registered, broad spectrum (hospital-level) bactericidal, viricidal, fungicidal, pseudomonacidal disinfectant mixed according to manufacturer's instructions or as required by your area's regulatory agency.
	Tools and implements that may or *have* come into contact with blood or body fluids.	Use antibacterial, EPA-registered, broad spectrum (hospital-level) disinfectant effective against HIV and HBV or tuberculocidal. Mix and immerse according to manufacturer's instructions or as required by your area's regulating agency.
STERILIZATION Items categorized as **critical**, meaning they are intended to enter the body cavity.	Tools and implements used to puncture or invade the skin.	Use a liquid sterilant or moist or dry heat sterilizer, calibrated to the specified temperatures, to kill all living organisms and bacterial spores.

3

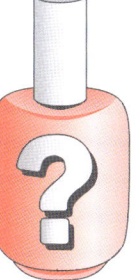

Why is it important to have standardized guidelines for infection-control procedures in the salon or spa?

SAFETY AND FIRST AID

Health and safety considerations for you and your clients are your number one concern when working in a salon or spa. Besides being knowledgeable about protection from harmful bacteria and disease, you also need to be aware of first-aid techniques to help you react properly in an emergency situation. Over the course of your career, you will come into contact with many clients. What if one fainted? What if a chemical gets in your eye? What if you accidentally cut a client? These questions and more are answered in this section.

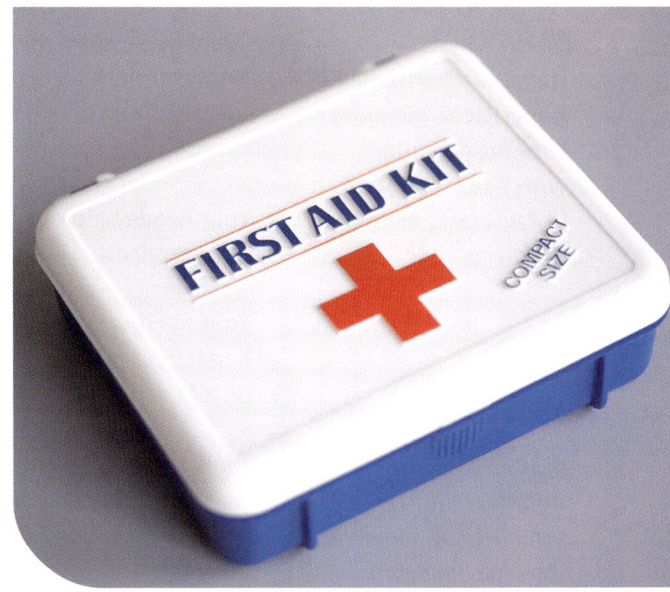

Electrical Safety

You can never take too many precautions when working with electricity. Knowing what precautionary measures must be taken when using electrical devices will help you prevent injuring yourself or your client when providing nail services. The following guidelines are designed to prevent injury while using electrical equipment.

- To avoid overheating, check outlets to make sure there are no loose-fitting plugs. Replace any missing or broken wall plates.
- Cords should be in good condition with no frays or cracks. Do not place cords in high-traffic areas. Do not cover cords with carpet or furniture, and do not staple them to walls or baseboards.
- Make sure the plugs fit the outlet. Never force a plug into an outlet if it does not fit, and never take the third prong off to make a three-prong plug fit into a two-conductor outlet. Adapters are readily available to accomplish this safely.
- If light switches or outlets feel warm, do not use them. Call an electrician to check the wiring.
- If an electrical device falls into water, always unplug it before removing it from the water. Be sure your hands are dry before unplugging the device.
- Always follow manufacturers' instructions carefully.
- Use UL listed equipment to ensure your safety.

Chemical Safety

In the nail salon, you will use and be exposed to numerous chemicals on a daily basis. From cleaning and disinfection solutions to polish remover and artificial nail products, you need to be aware of the proper ways to handle these chemicals. By safely using these chemical products, you will be able to protect your clients, your co-workers and yourself.

Ventilation

With the number and variety of chemicals used in the nail salon, it is important to keep the technicians and the clients safe from overexposure.

Artificial fingernail products are made from many chemicals, but the main one in most of these products is ethyl methacrylate (eth-UHL meth-AK-ruh-late) or EMA. In 1974 the U.S. Food and Drug Administration (FDA) outlawed a similar chemical, methyl methacrylate (MMA), used in fingernail products. MMA was proven harmful to nail technicians and clients. However, both MMA and EMA can cause contact dermatitis, asthma and allergies in the eyes and nose—problems that nail technicians may experience if the salon is not properly ventilated. Both can make the eyes, nose, and other mucous membranes sting, redden, and swell. Clients are at risk, too. It is best to control your exposure to chemicals in the salon before you become sensitized because often it is too difficult to tell which chemical is causing an allergy.

In the nail salon, to eliminate the EMA vapors from the air you breathe, artificial nail products should ideally be used at a ventilated worktable. It is also helpful to keep all bottles of artificial nail products closed or covered when not in use.

Ventilated Manicure Table *

Researchers from the National Institute for Occupational Safety and Health (NIOSH) have found that ventilation tables are best for protecting nail technicians from inhaling EMA. The ventilated table places local exhaust ventilation close to the work area.

Here are some recommendations for the best possible ventilation when working with artificial nail products:

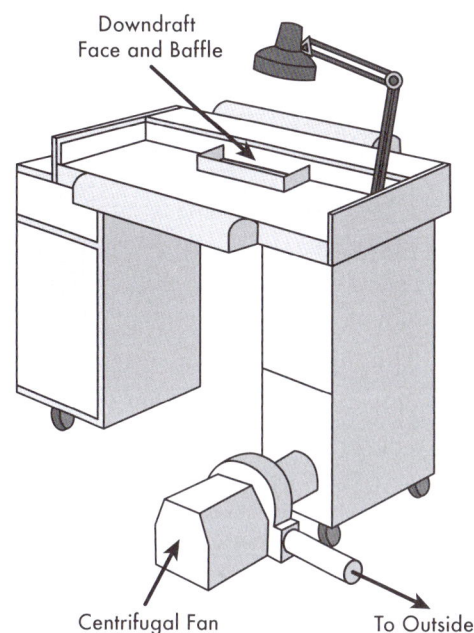

Downdraft
Face and Baffle

Centrifugal Fan   To Outside

- *Place local exhaust ventilation* as close to the EMA source as possible. Exhaust air should be directed out of the building. Charcoal filters are not recommended because they make it difficult to tell when the charcoal is full.

- *Use a ventilated work table.* Ventilated work table sizes will vary from nail salon to nail salon. Choose a wood for your ventilated table that will not soak up the chemicals. A veneer-coated particle board works well for the table material.

- *Make sure enough air blows through the table downdraft* to get rid of the EMA. The downdraft is the hole in the table top for air intake. The amount of air exhausted depends on its speed as it moves through the downdraft face and on the size of the table opening. However, too much air rushing past the fingernails may cause the artificial nail product to cure too fast.

An air speed of 620 feet per minute, directly above the 13" x 4" (33 cm x 10 cm) downdraft face works well. A 22" (55 cm) baffle should surround the downdraft face to pull the moving air closer to the client's hands.

Different drying times are needed for different fingernail products and different application techniques. Although a stronger and larger airflow will collect more dust during filing and dry the color coat faster, a slower and lower airflow gives better results for the artificial fingernail product.

- *Choose an exhaust fan* that can exhaust at least 250 cubic feet per minute of air and has 1/4" (0.63 cm) static pressure. A 1/8 horsepower centrifugal fan should work well. To prevent fan noise from getting in the way of conversation or client comfort, you can do one of three things: 1) buy a quiet fan, 2) put a cover over a noisier fan, or 3) buy an outdoor fan to be placed on an outside wall. The fan should have control settings. Use either a multi-speed or high-volume exhaust fan with a damper.

- *Provide enough make-up air* to replace the exhausted air. If the make-up air is too weak, there will be negative pressure areas and perhaps drafts. The air intake, which pulls outdoor air inside, should not be placed near the building exhaust. If the exhaust and intake vents are too close, dirty air will be pulled back into the room.

- *Avoid allowing comfort fans* to blow directly on the downdraft face because the strong air movement can interfere with the exhaust airflow.

* *Ventilated manicure table information and illustration courtesy of National Institute for Occupational Safety and Health (NIOSH).*

Dispenser Bottles *

Use dispenser bottles that have small openings, only large enough for an application brush to enter. The bottle stoppers should be pressure sensitive. A dispenser bottle with a pressure-sensitive stopper and small opening will result in less evaporation of the fingernail liquid and, thus, will cut down on possible exposures to methacrylates.

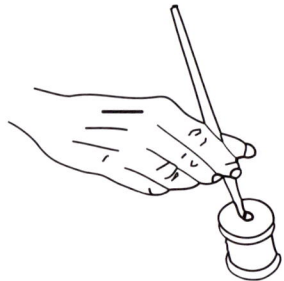

Nail technicians can also lower their exposure to these airborne chemicals by changing some of their work habits:

- EMA-soaked gauze pads should be placed in a sealed bag before being thrown in the trash can.

- Trash can liners should be changed daily.

- No more than the needed amount of product should be poured into the closed dispenser bottle.

- Nail technicians should wear personal protective clothing and glasses. Eye protection can protect technicians from chips of acrylic that sometimes result from removing artificial nails. In addition to safety glasses, technicians also should wear long sleeves and gloves to protect their skin from acrylic dust.

- Technicians should wash their hands, arms and face with mild soap and water several times throughout the day to remove potentially irritating dust.

- Eating and drinking should not be allowed where artificial nails are applied. Methacrylates in nail dust can be carried accidentally to the mouth or face on a cup or other food item. There are many other chemicals used in a salon that could cause health problems if swallowed.

- Smoking should be banned from the salon because many of the chemicals used in a salon or spa, including nail products, are flammable.

* *Dispenser bottles information and illustration courtesy of National Institute for Occupational Safety and Health (NIOSH).*

Overexposure

In the nail industry, technicians are routinely exposed to harmful chemicals throughout their career. This exposure can lead to injury or illness if proper precautions are not taken. **Overexposure** occurs when a safe level of chemical exposure is exceeded, which can happen to any professional who works with chemicals. To prevent overexposure, follow manufacturers' instructions and refer to the MSDS. Overexposure in the salon typically occurs in the following three ways:

1. **Ingestion:** Can occur by not washing hands after a service and eating or keeping food in the same area where chemicals are stored. Avoid eating or drinking while working with chemicals.

2. **Inhalation:** Can occur when there isn't adequate ventilation in areas where chemicals are being used. It's important to have the fumes removed from the salon and to wear a dust mask when filing artificial nails, which is especially important when using an electric file.

3. **Absorption:** Can occur from touching or handling chemicals or items with chemicals on it, such as a file with dust particles on it. Only apply products to the skin if they are intended to be applied to the skin.

Following are guidelines to help prevent overexposure:

- Wash your hands before and after every service.
- Avoid eating or drinking while working with chemicals.
- Avoid storing chemicals and food or drinks in the same area.
- Wash dishes in an area separate from where implements or equipment are sanitized or disinfected.
- Wear protective equipment (gloves, goggles or dust mask) when performing procedures that present the risk of creating an opening in the skin, chemical spills or the inhalation of dust particles.
- Provide adequate ventilation.
- Keep all product containers closed to prevent spills and fumes from escaping.
- Keep all trash in a covered trash can and empty it as frequently as necessary.
- Dispose of all chemicals properly according to your local area regulations.
- Remove any article of clothing that comes into contact with a chemical spill.
- Always follow manufacturers' instructions on use of chemicals.

Signs of Overexposure

- Dizziness
- Insomnia
- Tingling toes
- Fatigue
- Breathing problems
- Watery eyes
- Sore or dry throat
- Runny nose
- Sluggishness
- Lightheadedness

Allergic Reactions

Both clients and nail technicians are susceptible to allergic reactions and skin irritations in the nail salon or spa. Both afflictions trigger inflammation of the skin due to an exposure to an irritant or allergen, a condition known as **contact dermatitis**. Contact dermatitis is characterized by red, itchy skin and certain lesions such as blisters appearing in the area that is in contact with the irritating substance. It may also appear as dry, cracked or scaly skin. There are two common types of contact dermatitis: irritant contact dermatitis (ICD) and allergic contact dermatitis (ACD). Both are usually brought on by an exposure, either high- or low-level, to ingredients or chemicals found in many nail products.

Irritant contact dermatitis occurs when the skin comes into contact with an irritating chemical or substance and a rash or inflammation appears on the surface of the skin. The appearance of ICD is usually immediate or within several hours from the time contact occurred.

In contrast, allergic contact dermatitis is known as a delayed type of contact dermatitis, meaning that in many cases, the development and recognition of the product or chemical as an allergen does not occur immediately. Rather, over a period of time, repeated exposure to products or chemicals can affect the immune system, causing the person exposed to the substance to develop an allergy. This is why it is necessary to take all precautions necessary to avoid an allergic reaction caused by overexposure.

Signs of an Allergic Reaction
- Redness
- Itching
- Burning sensation
- Irritation
- Cracked, dry skin

Here are some general guidelines to follow to avoid prolonged exposure or contact to irritants that would promote contact dermatitis:

- Wash hands and dry thoroughly immediately after services.
- Replace towels used during the service if a product spills.
- Avoid touching the hairs on acrylic or gel brushes.
- Avoid touching any product not intended to be in contact with the skin.
- Use gloves when skin may come into contact with any potentially harmful chemicals.

Clients may have allergic reactions to chemicals used to create artificial nails. To help avoid allergic reactions follow the guidelines listed below:

- Avoid allowing any artificial nail products to come into contact with the skin.
- Use products that are designed by the manufacturer to be used together. Avoid mixing product lines.
- Be sure artificial nail products cure properly by using the correct product consistency, not applying product too thick and making sure UV lights are working properly.
- Avoid smoothing acrylic product with excess monomer (acrylic liquid).
- Avoid using a large brush that holds too much monomer.

If a client has an allergic reaction, discontinue use of the product immediately and inform the client to avoid use of the product in the future. It may take up to four to six months of repeated exposure to the substance for an allergy to a product to develop. For more on artificial nail products, see *Chapter 5, Chemistry*, or *Chapter 9, Artificial Nail Services*.

Bleeding and Wounds

On the rare occasion that a client in your salon or spa becomes cut or wounded and begins to bleed, it is important that you are responsive and prepared to calmly handle the situation.

FIRST AID FOR BLEEDING WOUNDS

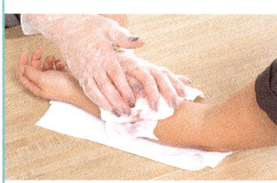
1. Cover wound, apply pressure.

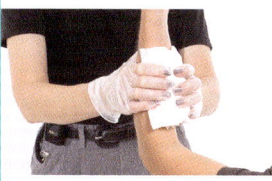
2. Elevate injured limb above heart.

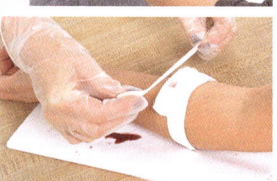
3. When bleeding stops—apply bandage.

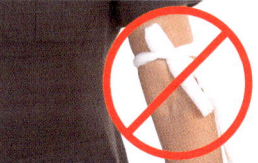
4. **Never use a tourniquet.**

If a client is cut or scraped, wear protective gloves and wash the cut or scrape with soap and water and keep it clean and dry. Avoid using alcohol, hydrogen peroxide or iodine to treat the wound because it can actually cause it to take longer for the wound to heal.

In the event of a more serious wound or injury:
1. Always wear protective gloves when you are exposed to blood.
2. Have the person sit or lie down.
3. Place a gloved hand and a clean cloth or gauze over the wound. Apply firm, steady pressure for at least five minutes.
4. Call 9-1-1 or other emergency personnel if bleeding is severe.

5. Elevate an injured limb above the level of the victim's heart if practical.
6. When bleeding stops, secure the cloth with a bandage. DO NOT try to remove the cloth that is against the open wound as it could disturb the blood clot and restart the bleeding. Be sure the bandage is not too tight. It could restrict circulation.
7. Never use a tourniquet unless you cannot control the bleeding. Tourniquets may result in subsequent medical amputation.
8. Be aware of the symptoms of shock. The victim will feel cold, clammy, lightheaded or dizzy. If this happens, keep the victim warm and seated or lying down.

Burns

In the salon or spa environment, chemical, heat or electrical burns are a possibility, so the first step toward prevention is learning how they can be caused.

The word *burn* is from the Old English word, *beornan*, meaning to be on fire. Burn means to damage or injure by fire, heat, radiation, electricity or a caustic agent such as a chemical.

- **First-degree burns** affect the outer layer of skin (epidermis). These burns are usually minor and may be accompanied by pain, swelling and redness, but they do not produce blisters.

- **Second-degree burns** affect both the epidermis and underlying dermis. They are accompanied by pain, swelling and redness and do cause blisters.

- **Third-degree burns** destroy all layers of the skin and damage underlying tissue, including nerves. In a majority of cases, this means there is no pain.

Chemical Burns

Certain chemicals may cause a burn or a burning sensation to the skin. A chemical burn will cause extreme redness and irritation and possibly mild to severe itching. The skin may also display welts and/or overall puffiness.

If a chemical burn does occur:

1. Remove the product with damp cotton (using either water or a neutralizer).
2. Move any contaminated clothing from the burn area.
3. Apply several cold compresses, or cotton soaked in cold water, to the skin for several minutes at a time.
4. Cover the burn loosely with a clean, lint-free, dry cloth, such as a sheet. Do not use terry cloth towels since they generate lint that can become embedded in the wound.
5. Refer the injured person for medical treatment if necessary.

Performing a patch test and a thorough analysis can help avoid chemical burns caused by products used during services. But it is also important to be cautious when using cleaning and disinfecting chemicals.

Heat Burns

Burns from heat can come from a variety of sources such as electric files, wax or heated towels. Paraffin wax is one of the few heated products you will use in providing nail services in the salon or spa. It is heated up in an electric warmer and if the temperature is too high, it can burn the skin when applied.

Hot towels from towel cabinets are a great addition to a nail service. However, most cabinets can heat up to as high as 110 degrees. Towels can get extremely hot and can cause discomfort, so it is important to cool the towel

prior to applying it to your client's skin. Test the temperature by holding the side of the towel that will not be placed on the client's skin against your own arm to evaluate the heat intensity.

In the event of a heat burn:

1. If the skin is not broken, immerse the burned area in cool (not ice) water or gently apply a cool compress until pain is relieved. Bandage with a clean, dry cloth.
2. Do not break a blister if one forms. Do not apply ointments or creams.
3. If skin is broken or if burns are severe, follow the procedure below:
    - Call 9-1-1 or other emergency personnel.
    - Do not clean the wound or remove embedded clothing.
    - Cover the burn loosely with a clean, dry, lint-free cloth.

Electrical Burns

Electricity is a form of energy that produces light, heat, magnetic and chemical changes. The flow of electricity along a conductor is called **electric current** or **modality**. Materials that transport electricity easily are called **conductors**, and their purpose is to transport current in a circuit to an electrical appliance.

Electrical burns are usually the result of faulty equipment or improper use of equipment. These burns occur when flesh comes into contact with a flow of electrical current, such as when your finger gets caught between the outlet and plug when plugging in an appliance. A burn can also occur when a piece of equipment has a frayed or severed cord that makes contact with the skin. Electrical burns can be prevented by carefully inspecting and handling all equipment used in the salon or spa environment.

Because of the possibility of overloads and short circuits, safety devices are installed in many appliances and buildings. Two of these devices, fuses and circuit breakers, connect directly to the circuits in the power box, the carefully insulated location where the electric current enters a building from a generator or power plant. A **fuse** is a device that contains a fine metal wire that allows current to flow through it. If too much current flows through, known as an overload, the fuse will heat up and the wire will melt, breaking the circuit and cutting the flow of electricity. The fuse will have to be replaced.

A **circuit breaker** is a reusable device that breaks the flow of current when an overload occurs. A heat-sensing device causes the two pieces of metal for a single switch to separate and stop the flow of electricity. The breaker can be reset in two simple steps: 1) Turn off or unplug all appliances connected to the switch. 2) Find the correctly labeled switch and turn it completely to the "off" position first, and then immediately to the "on" position.

Choking

When a person is choking, he or she usually grasps the throat with one hand. The typical choking victim cannot speak and may gasp or wheeze, but is not able to cough. If you are in doubt, ask the person if he or she can talk. If not, no air is entering the windpipe. This person may turn blue and have an expression of panic on his or her face. Properly responding to a person who is choking by using the steps provided could save a life.

1. Determine whether the victim can speak or cough forcibly and is getting sufficient air.
2. Do not interfere with the victim's attempts to cough the obstruction from his or her throat.

3. If the victim cannot speak or is not getting sufficient air, have someone call 9-1-1 while you perform abdominal thrusts, known as the **Heimlich Maneuver**.

This means you should:

1. Stand behind the victim and wrap your arms around his or her stomach to perform abdominal thrusts.
2. Make a thumbless fist with one hand and place that fist just above the navel and well below the ribs, with the thumb and forefinger side toward the victim.
3. Perform an upward thrust by grasping this fist with the other hand and pulling it quickly toward you with an inward and slightly upward movement.
4. Repeat if necessary.

FIRST AID FOR CHOKING–HEIMLICH MANEUVER

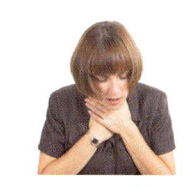
1. Victim begins to choke.

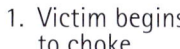
2. Determine if victim can talk or cough.

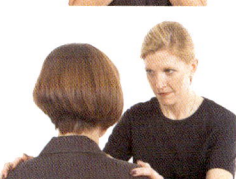
3. Wrap your arms around victim from behind and make a thumbless fist.

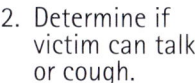

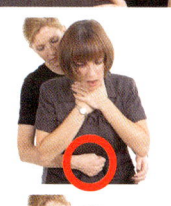
4. Perform an upward thrust.

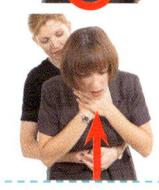

These instructions pertain to choking victims OVER one year of age. Specific guidelines for treatment of infant choking are not outlined in this text.

3

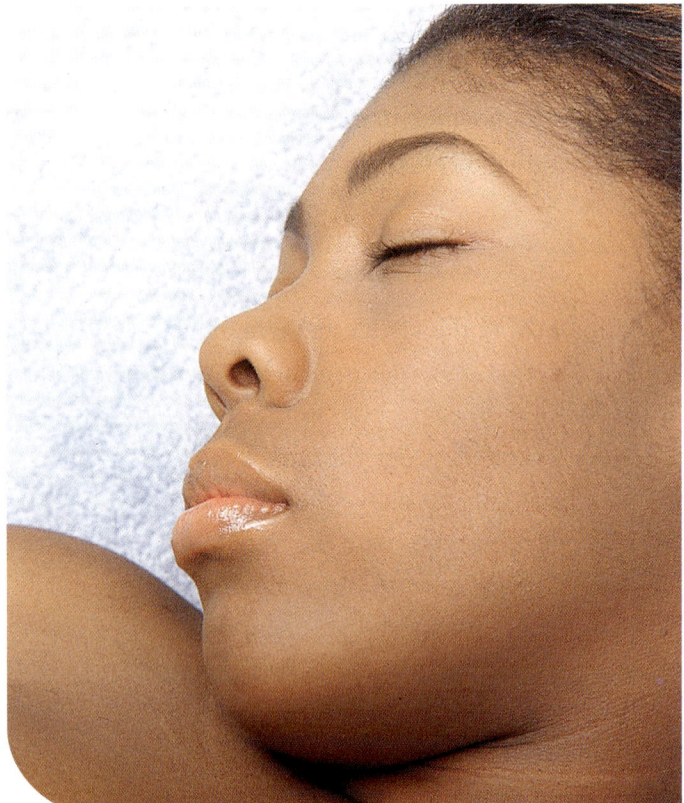

Fainting

A sudden drop in blood pressure can prevent enough oxygen from getting to the brain. This lack of oxygen causes a person to faint, or lose consciousness from a few seconds to a few minutes. Typically the fainting victim collapses suddenly. Listed below are the actions to take if a person becomes unconscious.

1. Turn the victim onto the back and make sure he or she has plenty of fresh air.
2. If vomiting occurs, roll the victim on his or her side and keep the windpipe clear.
3. When the victim regains consciousness, reassure him or her and apply a cold compress to the face.

Fainting victims regain consciousness almost immediately. If this does not happen, the victim could be in serious danger and you should call 9-1-1 immediately.

Eye Injury

In a salon or spa, the possibility for eye injury is a risk. Types of injuries include cuts and scratches or getting an imbedded object or chemical solution in the eyes. Knowing the proper precautions and procedures for dealing with eye injuries can help to avoid serious eye damage.

Cut, Scratch or Embedded Object

1. Place a gauze pad or cloth over both eyes and secure with a bandage.
2. Do not try to remove an embedded object.
3. Get to an eye specialist or emergency room immediately.

Chemical

1. Hold the eyelids apart and flush the eyeball(s) with lukewarm water for at least 15-30 minutes. Be careful not to let runoff water flow into the other eye if only one eye is affected.
2. Place a gauze pad or cloth over both eyes and secure with a bandage.
3. Get to an eye specialist or emergency room immediately.

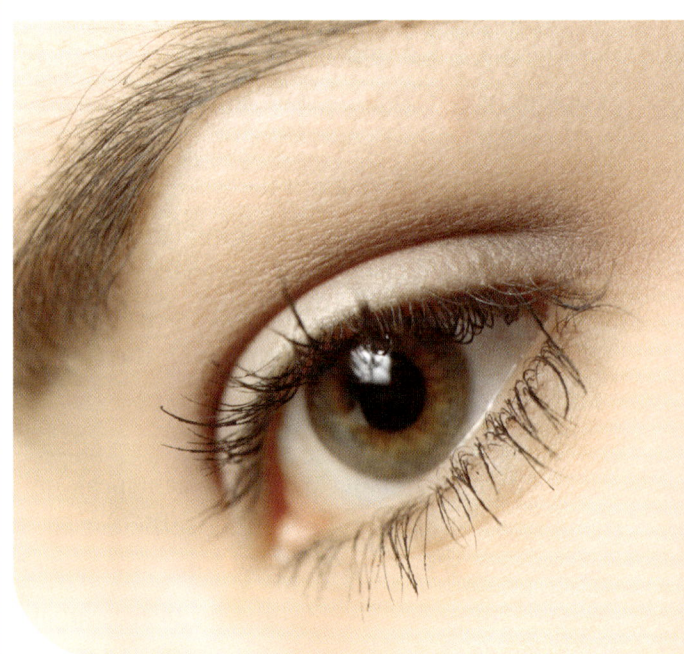

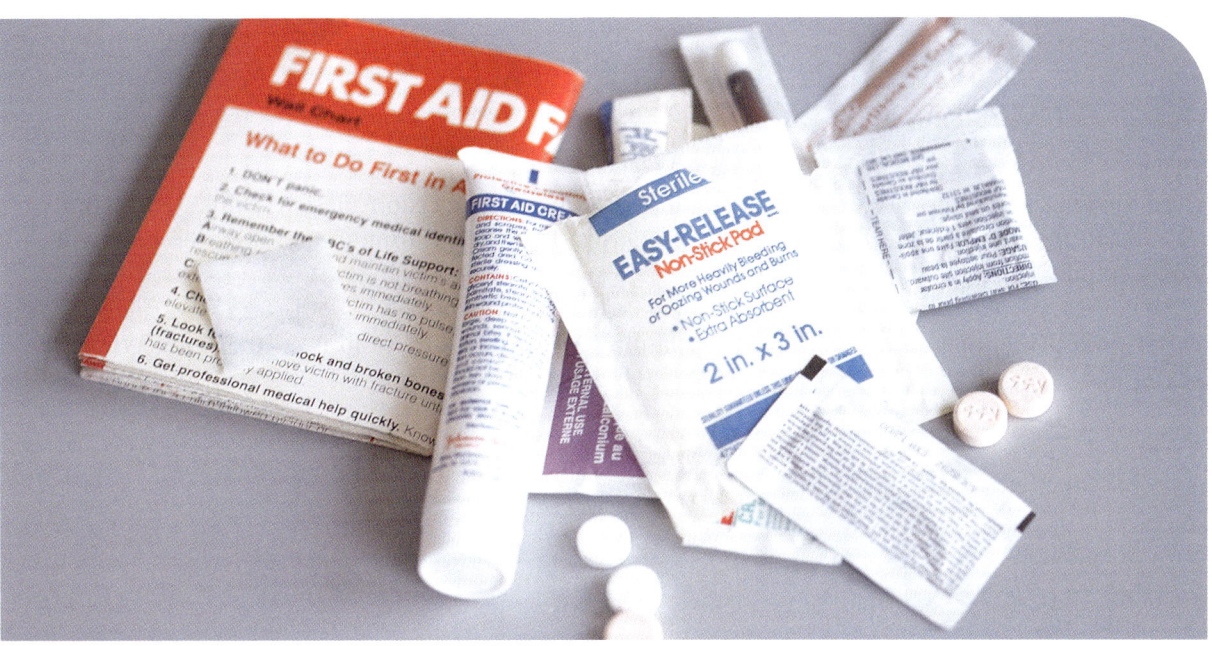

3

The safety, protection and welfare of the clients you serve are among the many reasons you are licensed as a professional. This chapter holds valuable information for you to utilize and practice. Remember that your own health and safety carry significance as well. Make sure you know the procedures necessary to maintain a clean, healthy, safe environment. Your clients will respect your efforts and trust your services.

Microorganisms inhabit bodies at all times—both yours and your clients'. Practicing universal precautions protects everyone and eliminates the spread of infection. By adhering to strict guidelines for hygiene—using the proper procedures, tools and solutions for sanitation, disinfection and sterilization—you exhibit the utmost professionalism. You also demonstrate concern for your clients' health and well-being, putting them at ease and making them feel secure and relaxed in your hands. This is the best peace of mind you can offer them. Protect your clients and yourself by practicing proper infection-control procedures throughout your workplace. Your clients will appreciate your efforts to protect their health, but the true benefactor is you, today's professional nail technician.

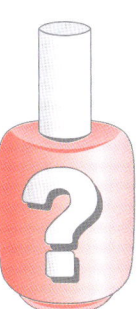

Can you think of any time in your past when knowing first-aid procedures would have come in handy? Give an example.

DECISION-MAKING SKILLS

Case Studies

The following situations are designed to help you build your decision-making skills. Using your training to this point, review the following scenarios, then think through and describe how you would handle each challenge.

1. During a pedicure, you reach for a new spatula and accidentally drop it on the floor. What would you do?

2. You have just finished a manicure and your client has already left the salon. What procedures do you follow to get ready for the next client?

3. What two steps must you always follow to ensure that an infection-control product will do what you want it to do?

4. You are walking your client to the front door after a nail service and she starts to feel faint. What would you do?

Our bodies are often the best source of information about health and personal well-being. For example, studies of human anatomy and physiology reveal that, from birth to old age, our muscles, hearts and nerves respond in healthy ways to a caring touch. Knowing the systems of the body and how they function will help you maintain your personal health as well as your clients'. In this chapter, you will learn about the systems of the human body and how to use this knowledge to perfect the art and science of therapeutic human touch in your work as a nail technician.

VALUE

Only a select group of professionals is licensed to touch people in ways that promote health and well-being. This licensure carries with it an expectation that these professionals understand the human body and its functions. This knowledge is part of your preparation for a career as a nail care specialist.

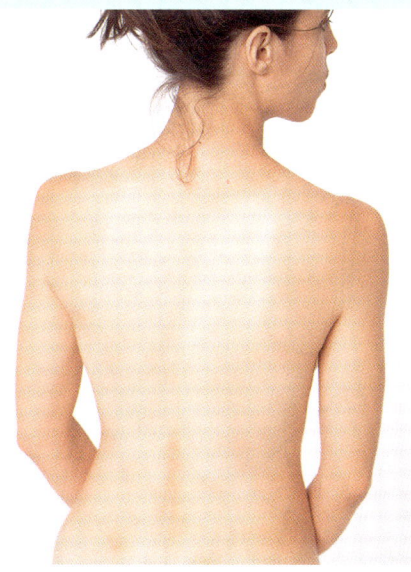

MAIN IDEA

This chapter involves the careful study of the human body, beginning with the simplicity of the single cell, progressing to the wondrous organization of each body system. Of particular importance to the nail technician will be the skeletal, muscular, circulatory and nervous systems. As your understanding of the human body increases, so will your ability to touch your clients in ways that improve their health and well-being.

PLAN	OBJECTIVES

Building Blocks of the Human Body

- Cells
- Tissues
- Organs
- Body Systems

Explain the relationship and function of cells, tissues and primary organs within the human body.

Basic Body Systems

- The Skeletal System
- The Muscular System
- The Circulatory System
- The Nervous System
- The Digestive System
- The Excretory System
- The Respiratory System
- The Endocrine System
- The Reproductive System
- The Integumentary System

Identify the structure and function of the 10 major body systems.

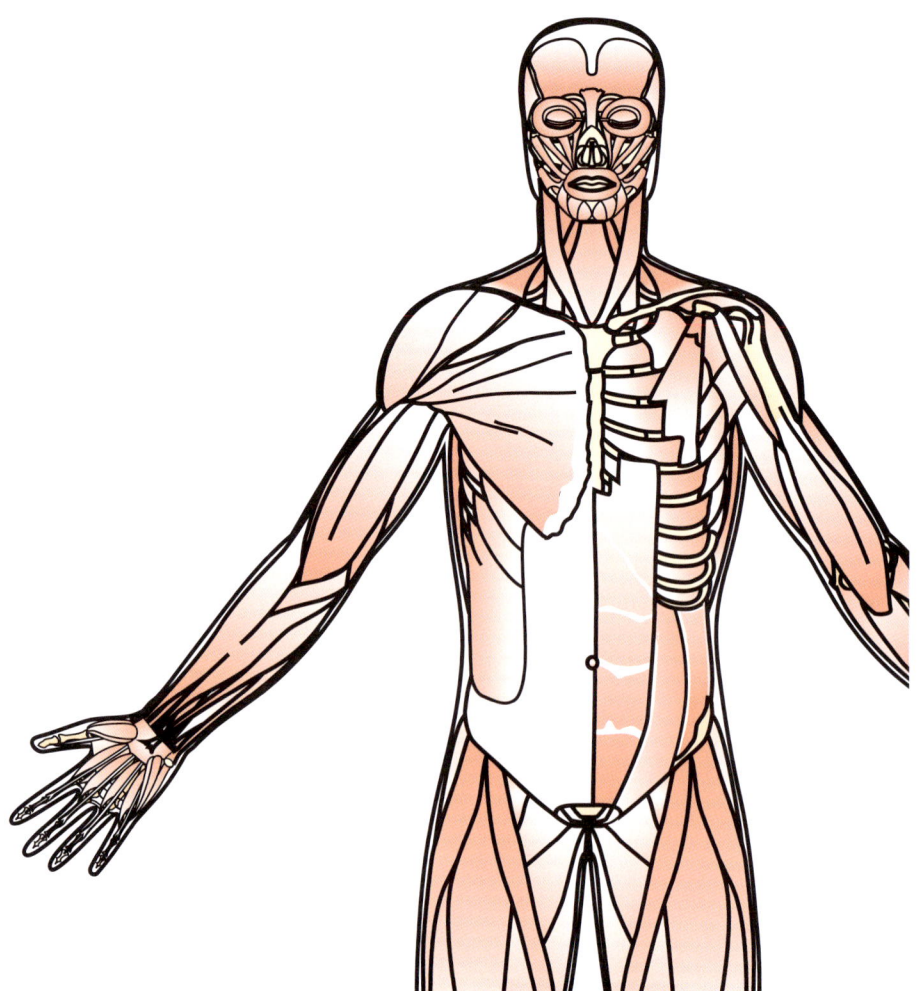

BUILDING BLOCKS OF THE HUMAN BODY

Knowledge of the human body and how the systems work together helps the nail technician provide safe and effective services. Whether you give a manicure, pedicure or a specialized hand or foot treatment, you have the privilege of bringing relaxation and well-being to others.

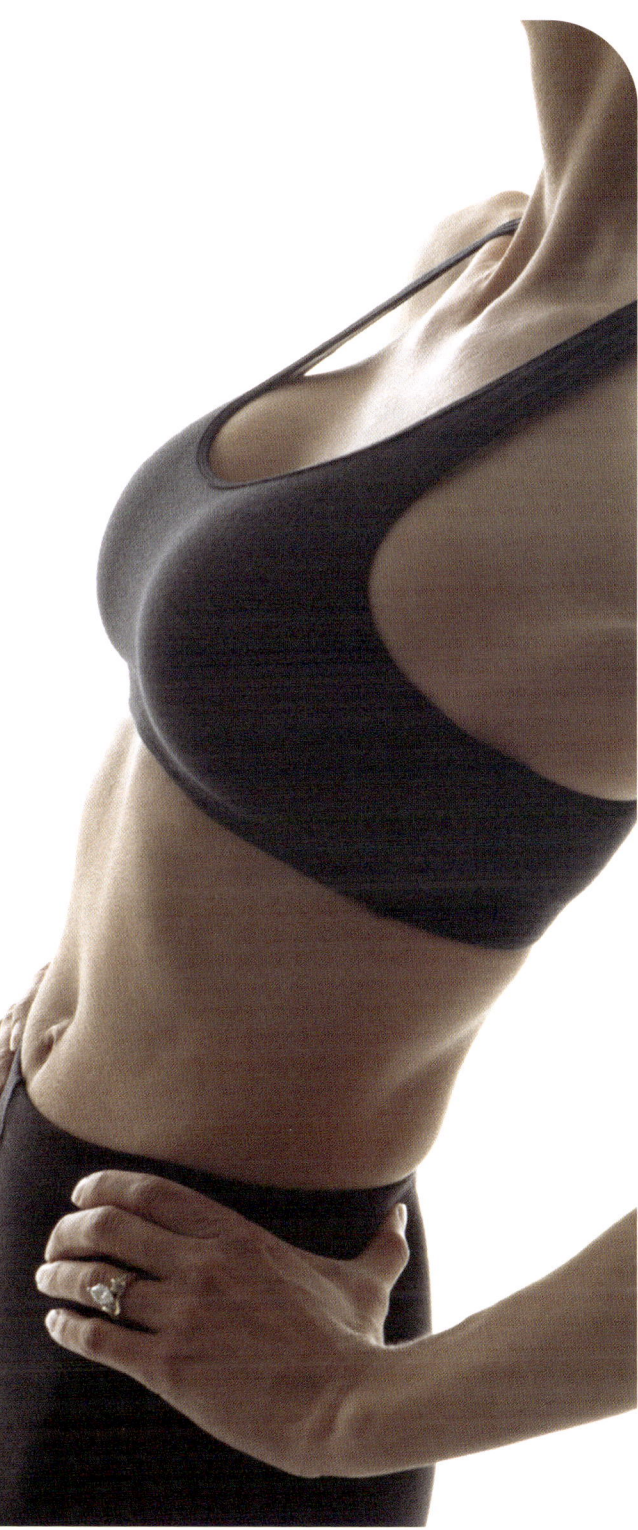

Especially important to the nail technician are the muscular, nervous, circulatory and skeletal systems, specifically focusing on the arms, hands, legs and feet. Knowledge of the human body and its systems provides the foundation for performing beneficial massage techniques and offering quality nail services.

The study of the human body can be divided into two general categories:

- **Anatomy**, the study of the organs and systems of the body.
- **Physiology**, the study of the functions of these organs and systems.

Other subcategories go into greater detail. For example, the study of structures that can be seen with the naked eye is called **gross anatomy**. The study of structures too small to be seen except through a microscope is called **histology**.

To understand anatomy and physiology you must first be aware of the building blocks of the human body, which are:

- Cells
- Tissues
- Organs
- Body Systems

4

STRUCTURE OF A CELL

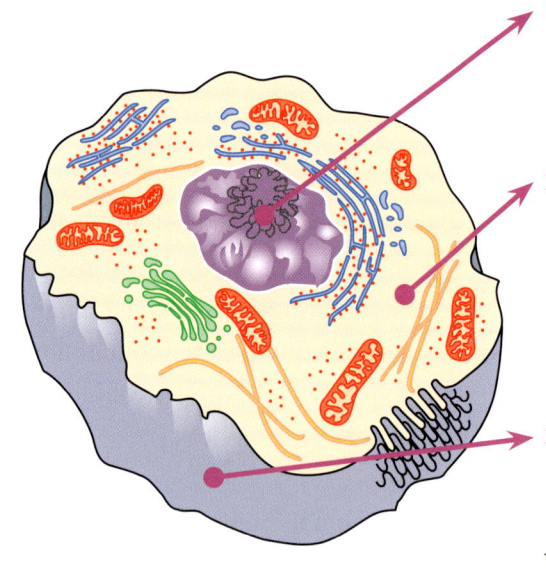

1. NUCLEUS

The control center of the cell. The nucleus controls cell reproduction, growth and metabolism.

2. CYTOPLASM

The production department of the cell. The cytoplasm is the site of most of the chemical activities within the cell. Organelles within the cytoplasm store nutrients. They also repair and restore the cell.

3. CELL MEMBRANE

The outer surface and enclosing structure of the cell.

The word *cell* comes from the Latin word *cella*, which means chamber.

Cells

All muscles, nerves, bones and body systems are made up of cells. **Cells** are the basic units of life. They are composed of **protoplasm** (PRO-to-plazm), a colorless gel-like substance that contains water, salt and nutrients obtained from food. Cells vary in size, shape, structure and function, but they have certain characteristics in common. A cell contains three basic parts:

1. The **nucleus** (NU-kle-us), or control center of cell activities, is vitally important for cell reproduction. The nucleus is located in the cytoplasm, and both are surrounded by the cell membrane.
2. The **cytoplasm** (SI-to-plazm) is the production department of the cell. Small structures called **organelles** perform most of the cell's activities. Organelles store food for growth, as well as repair and restore the cell.
3. The **cell membrane** is the outer surface of the cell.

Cells make up tissues.

Tissues make up organs.

Organs make up systems.

Nucleus is from the Latin word, *nut*, the core around which other parts are gathered or grouped.

In order to grow and remain healthy, cells need enough food, oxygen and water. They also need proper temperature and the ability to eliminate waste products. If these criteria are not met, cell growth is impaired. Human cells reproduce by dividing in half, a process referred to as **mitosis** (my-TOE-sis) or indirect division. Cells receive nutrients for cell growth and reproduction through a chemical process known as **metabolism** (me-TAB-e-lizm).

Metabolism turns nutrients into energy for the body to use or store for later use. A body's metabolic rate is dependent upon heredity, health conditions, medications, exercise, diet and eating habits. Human life depends upon the body's ability to obtain nutrients from foods. In order for nutrients to be used by the body, they must be broken down into smaller components.

Metabolism is from the Greek word *metabole*, meaning, "change." Think of your metabolism as a furnace. Wood burns and is converted into heat, just as food is "burned" and converted into energy.

Different types of nutrients are stored and used differently by the body. For example, carbohydrates are the body's main energy source. However, carbohydrates are converted to glucose (sugar) in the body and excess carbohydrates can result in excess body fat.

Do you know someone who can eat anything and not gain weight? That is because he or she has a high metabolic rate.

A person's metabolic rate can influence his or her energy level and weight. A healthy diet, regular exercise and careful attention to the overall condition of the body can help keep metabolism in check. People with weight problems frequently have metabolic problems. People with low metabolisms take longer to process food, making it hard for them to lose weight. A person with a high metabolism processes food at a faster rate.

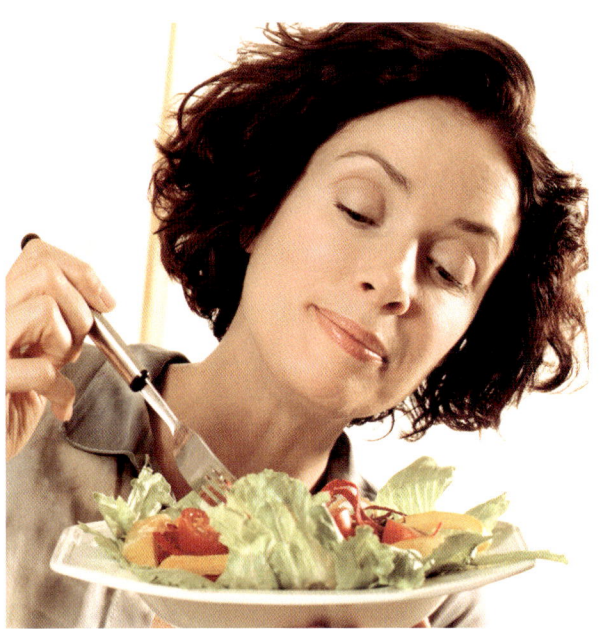

There are two phases of metabolism:

1. **Anabolism** (ah-NAB-oh-lizm), the process of building up larger molecules from smaller ones. During this phase, the body stores water, food and oxygen.
2. **Catabolism** (kah-TAB-oh-lizm), the process of breaking down larger molecules or substances into smaller ones. This releases energy within the cell, which is necessary for the performance of specific body functions, including muscular movements and digestion.

The prefix *ana* is from the Greek word meaning "up." The prefix *cata* is from the Greek word meaning "down." Hence, anabolism implies a building up, or constructive phase; while catabolism is a breaking down, or destructive phase.

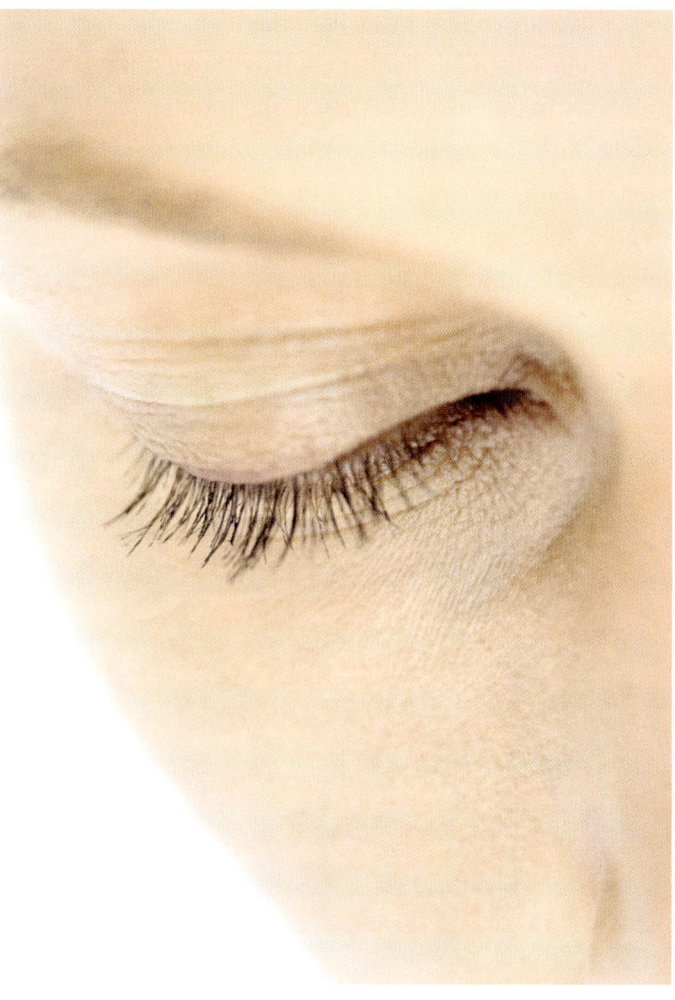

Organs

Organs are separate body structures that perform specific functions. They are composed of two or more different types of tissue. The eight organs of primary importance are:

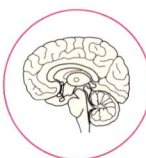 1. The **brain**, which controls all body functions.

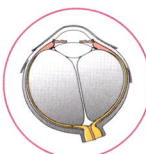 2. The **eyes**, which provide sight.

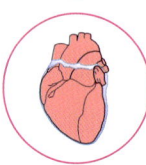 3. The **heart**, which circulates the blood.

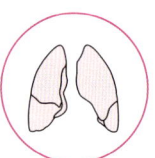 4. The **lungs**, which supply the blood with oxygen.

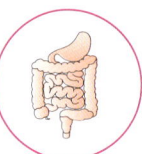 5. The **stomach** and **intestines**, which digest and eliminate food.

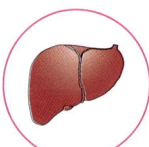 6. The **liver**, which removes the toxic by-products of digestion.

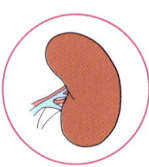 7. The **kidneys**, which eliminate water and waste products.

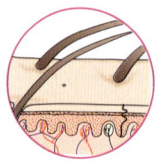 8. The **skin**, the body's largest organ, which forms the external protective layer of the body.

Tissues

Groups of cells of the same kind make up tissues. There are five primary types of tissue in the human body and each differs in structure and function, depending on the type of cells.

1. **Epithelial** (ep-eh-THEE-lee-el) **tissue** covers and protects body surfaces and internal organs.
2. **Connective tissue** supports, protects and holds the body together.
3. **Nerve tissue** carries messages to and from the brain and coordinates body functions.
4. **Muscular tissue** contracts, when stimulated, to produce motion.
5. **Liquid tissue** carries food, waste products and hormones.

Body Systems

A system is a group of organs that, together, perform one or more vital functions for the body. The 10 body systems you will study in this chapter are:

- **Skeletal**
  Provides the framework of the body.
- **Muscular**
  Moves the body.
- **Circulatory**
  Circulates blood through the body.
- **Nervous**
  Sends and receives messages.
- **Digestive**
  Supplies nutrients to the body.
- **Excretory** (ECKS-kre-tohr-ee)
  Eliminates waste from the body.
- **Respiratory**
  Controls breathing.
- **Endocrine**
  Controls growth, health and reproduction.
- **Reproductive**
  Generates new life to carry on the species.
- **Integumentary** (in-TEG-u-men-ter-ee)
  Covers and protects the entire body.

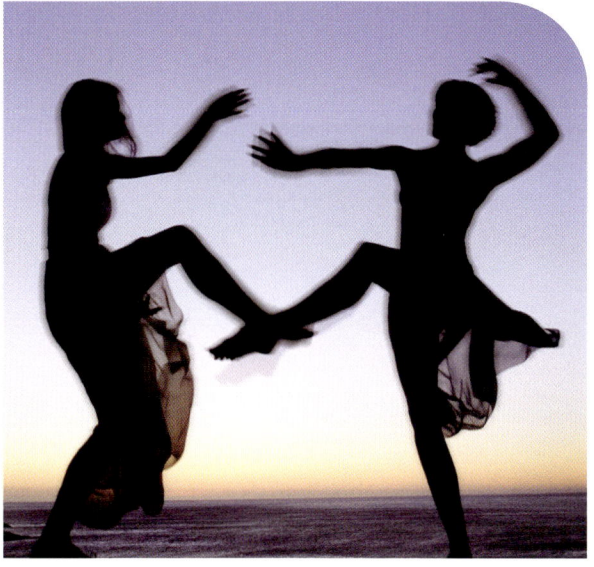

The next section explains how these systems function to provide structure, energy, movement, protection and the ability to regenerate and reproduce.

Some clients may have health concerns or injuries that they reveal to you during the Client Consultation (Client Consultations are discussed in depth in *Chapter 7, Client Care*). Knowing the bones, muscles, organs, nerves and other systems of the body can help you understand your clients' needs as they describe their health concerns.

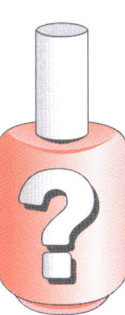

The human body is one of the most complex systems known to humankind. How is the structure of a car like the human body? How is the design of a house like the body?

BASIC BODY SYSTEMS

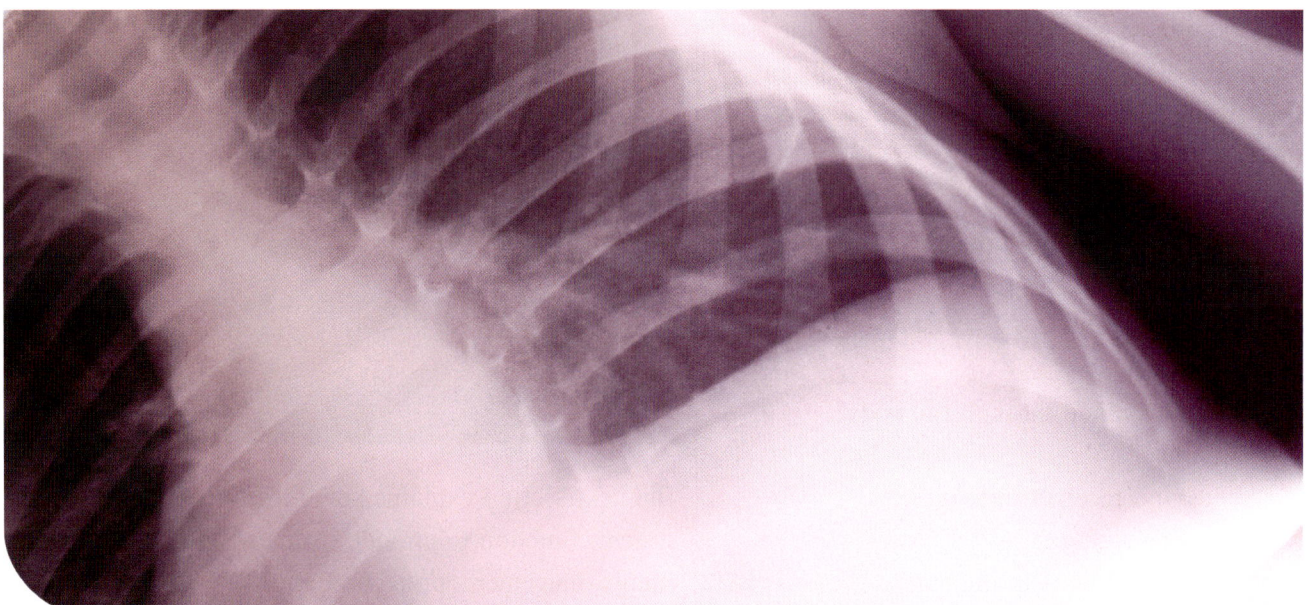

All body systems are dependent on each other to carry out their functions. In fact, many organs are part of more than one system. The lungs, for example, are part of the respiratory system because they bring in oxygen, but they are also part of the excretory system because they exhale carbon dioxide. An explanation of each system and its interrelated functions is important to the work of a nail technician as a foundation for recognizing healthy conditions.

The Skeletal System

The **skeletal system** is the physical foundation of the body. It consists of 206 bones of different shapes and sizes, each attached to others at movable or immovable joints.

Osteology (as-tee-AL-e-jee) is the study of bones. Bones can be long, flat or irregular in shape. Long bones are found in the arms and legs. Flat bones are plate-shaped and include bones located in the skull as well as the scapula, hip bone, sternum, ribs and according to some,

the patella (knee cap). Irregular bones are found in the wrist, ankle and spinal column (the back). Bone is the body's hardest structure, which is made up of two-thirds mineral matter and one-third organic matter.

The functions of the skeletal system are to:
- Support the body by giving it shape and strength.
- Surround and protect internal organs.
- Provide a frame to which muscles attach.
- Allow body movement.
- Produce red and white blood cells.
- Store calcium.

Though nail technicians generally only work with the lower arms, hands, lower legs and feet, it is important to be familiar with the bones of the entire body so you can speak professionally about every area. The illustrations on the next two pages identify the major bones of the skeleton.

SKELETAL SYSTEM – ANTERIOR

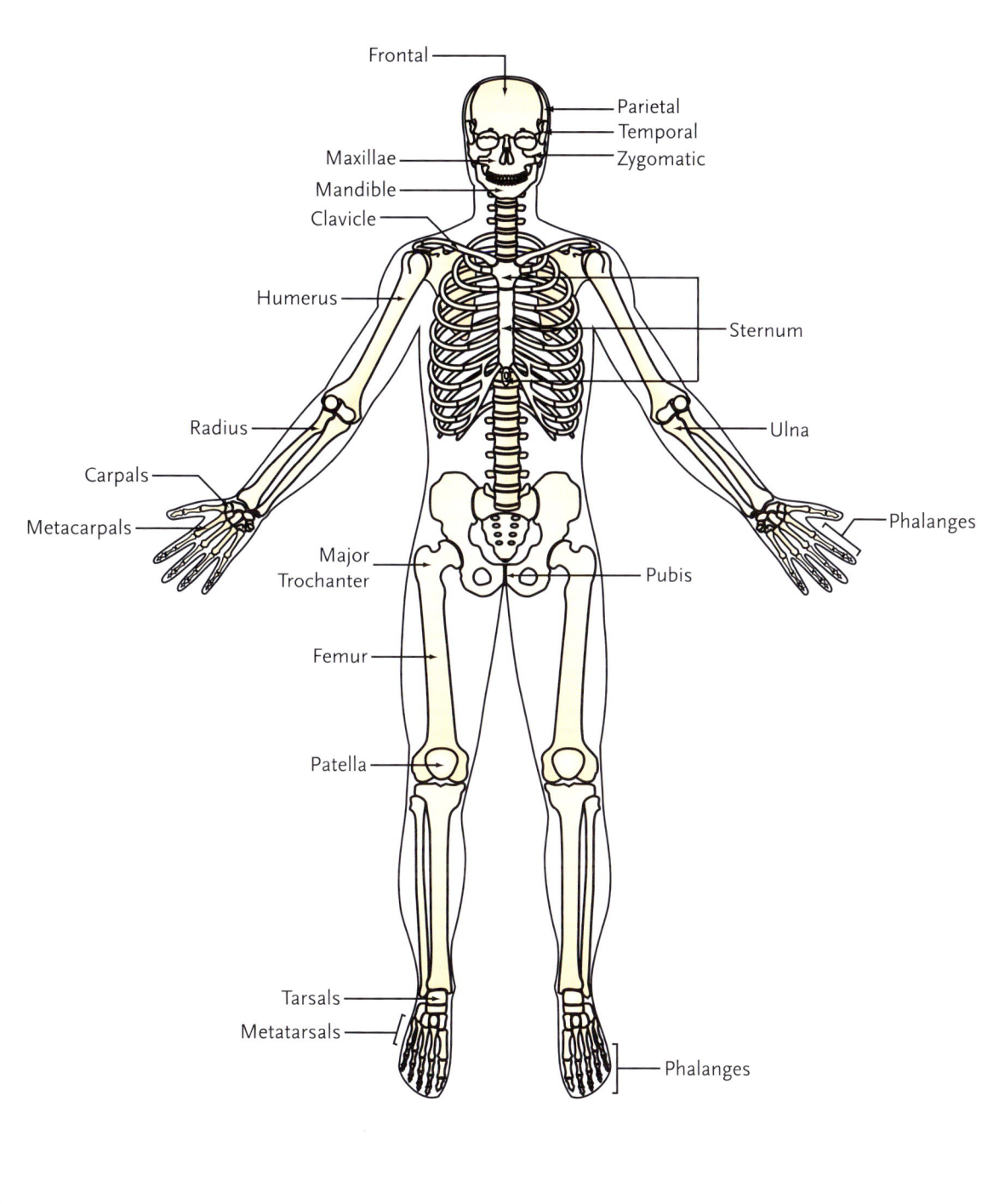

Frontal

Parietal
Temporal
Zygomatic

Maxillae

Mandible

Clavicle

Humerus

Sternum

Radius

Ulna

Carpals

Metacarpals

Phalanges

Major
Trochanter

Pubis

Femur

Patella

Tarsals

Metatarsals

Phalanges

4

SKELETAL SYSTEM – POSTERIOR

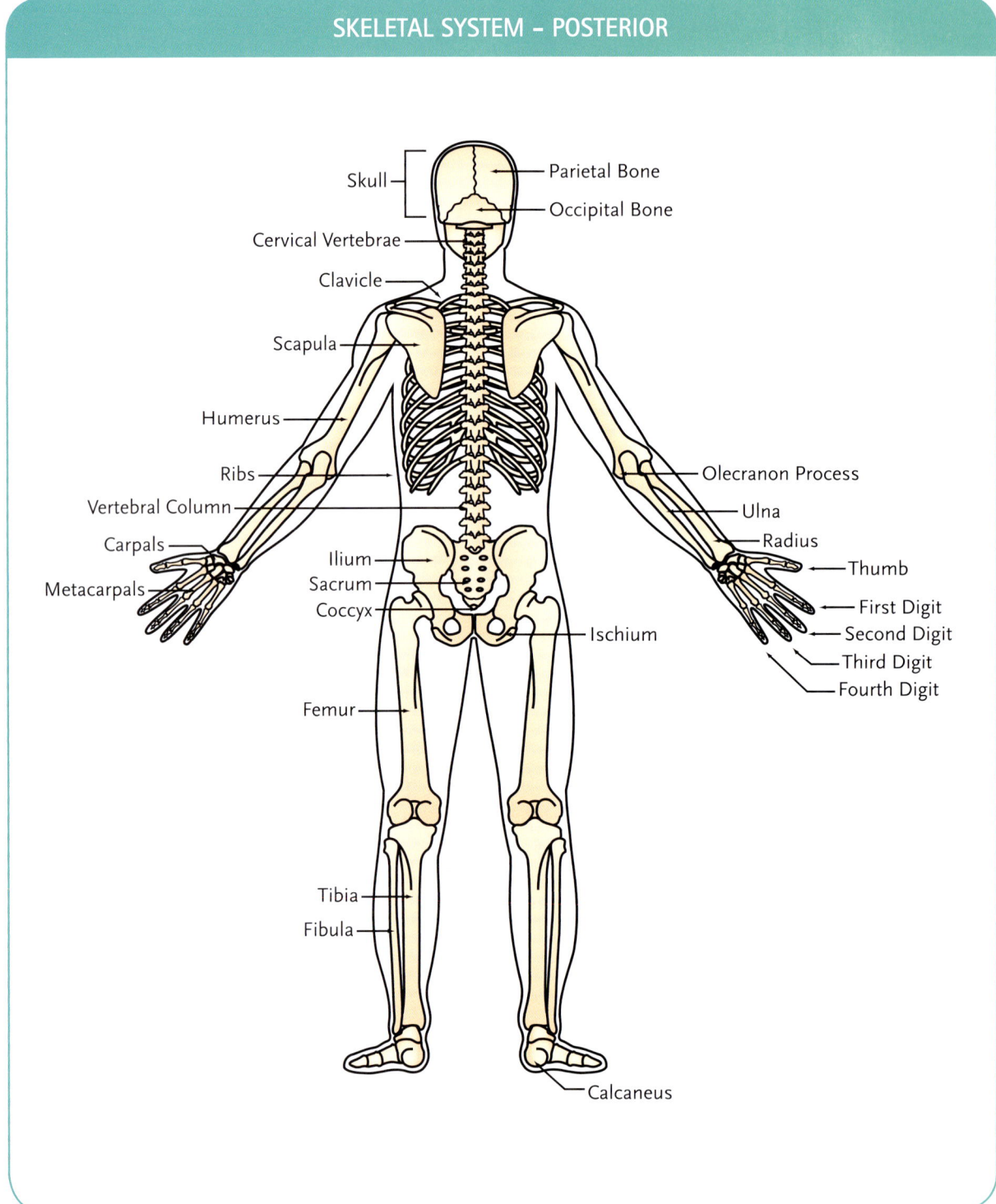

Skull

Parietal Bone

Occipital Bone

Cervical Vertebrae

Clavicle

Scapula

Humerus

Ribs

Vertebral Column

Carpals

Metacarpals

Ilium

Sacrum

Coccyx

Olecranon Process

Ulna

Radius

Thumb

First Digit

Second Digit

Third Digit

Fourth Digit

Ischium

Femur

Tibia

Fibula

Calcaneus

Knowing the names and the positions of the bones in the arms, hands, legs and feet helps nail technicians better understand what they feel as they perform a service. Quite often knowing the location of a bone makes it easier for the nail technician to locate a particular muscle. The illustrations on the following pages identify the bones of the shoulders, arms, wrists, hands, legs, ankles and feet.

SHOULDER BONES

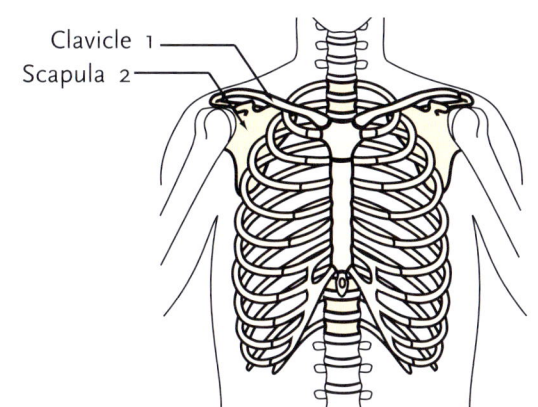

Clavicle 1
Scapula 2

1. The **clavicle** (KLAV-i-kel) or collar bone.
2. The **scapula** (SKAP-yu-lah) or shoulder blade.

4

ARM BONES

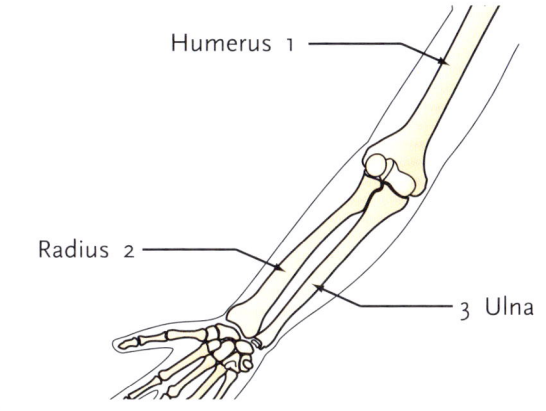

Humerus 1

Radius 2

3 Ulna

1. The **humerus** (HU-mur-us), the largest bone of the upper arm, extends from the elbow to the shoulder.
2. The **radius** (RAD-ee-us) is the smaller bone on the thumb side of the lower arm or forearm.
3. The **ulna** (UL-nah) is the bone located on the little finger side of the lower arm.

WRIST AND HAND BONES

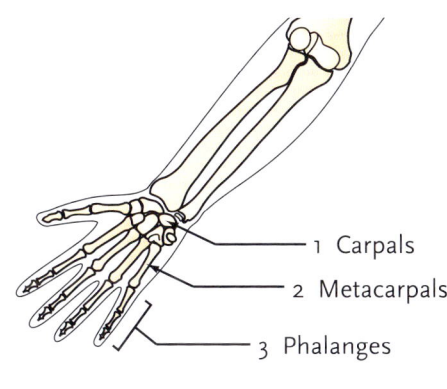

1 Carpals
2 Metacarpals
3 Phalanges

1. The **carpals** (KAR-pels) are the eight small bones held together by ligaments to form the wrist or carpus.
2. The **metacarpals** (met-ah-KAR-pels) are the five long, thin bones that form the palm of the hand.
3. The **phalanges** (fah-LAN-jees) are the 14 bones that form the digits or fingers. Each finger has three phalanges, while the thumb has only two.

LEG BONES

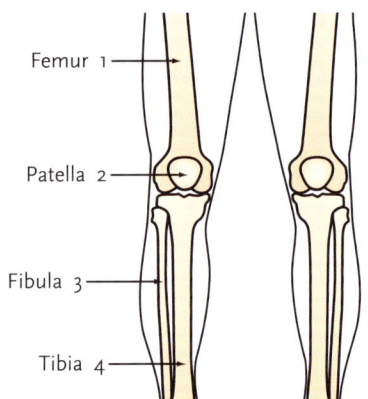

Femur 1
Patella 2
Fibula 3
Tibia 4

1. The **femur** (FEE-mur), the largest bone of the leg, extends from the hip to the knee.
2. The **patella** (pah-TEL-lah) or accessory bone is commonly known as the knee cap.
3. The **fibula** (FIB-ya-lah) is the smaller bone on the little toe side of the lower leg.
4. The **tibia** (TIB-ee-ah) is the larger bone on the big toe side of the lower leg.

ANKLE AND FOOT BONES

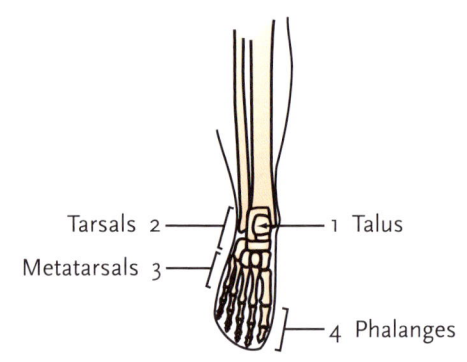

Tarsals 2
Metatarsals 3
1 Talus
4 Phalanges

1. The **talus** (TA-lus) bone is the ankle bone.
2. The **tarsal** (TAHR-sul) bones consist of seven bones in the foot composing the ankle joint including the talus.
3. The **metatarsal** (met-ah-TAHR-sul) bones consist of five bones in the foot between the ankle and toes similar to the metacarpal bones of the hand.
4. The **phalanges** (fah-LAN-jees) are the 14 bones that form the toes. Each toe has three phalanges, while the big toe has only two.

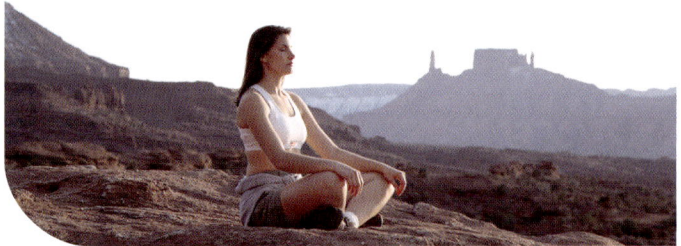

Bone appears to be non-living. In fact, the word skeleton is derived from a Greek word meaning dried up. However, bone is actually a dynamic structure composed of both living tissues, such as bone cells, fat cells, and blood vessels, and non-living material, including water and minerals.

The Muscular System

Nail technicians perform services to benefit the nails and skin. Often these services involve relaxing or stimulating the muscles that lie between the skin and bones.

Myology (mi-OL-o-jee) is the study of the structure, function and diseases of the muscles. There are more than 500 large and small muscles in the body, which account for approximately 40% of the body's weight. Muscles are fibrous tissues that contract or relax to produce movement.

To understand the functions of the muscular system, remember MAPS:

- Movement
- Attachment
- Protection
- Shape

There are three types of muscle tissues:

1. The **voluntary** or **striated** (STRI-at-ed) muscles respond to conscious commands.

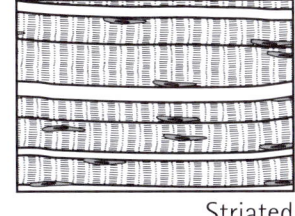
Striated

2. The **involuntary** or **non-striated** muscles respond automatically to control various body functions, including the internal organs.

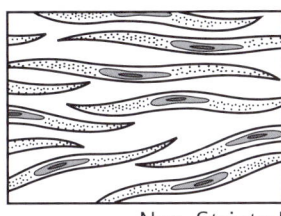
Non-Striated

3. The **cardiac** (heart) muscle is the muscle of the heart itself and the only muscle of its type in the human body. This muscle functions involuntarily or automatically.

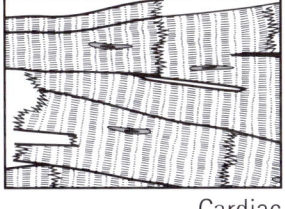
Cardiac

Some muscles function both voluntarily and involuntarily. For example, eye muscles respond to a conscious command to blink, but they also blink automatically to maintain eye moisture. The nail technician is primarily concerned with the voluntary muscles of the arms, hands, legs and feet.

Each muscle has three parts, as shown in the following illustration.

THREE PARTS OF A MUSCLE

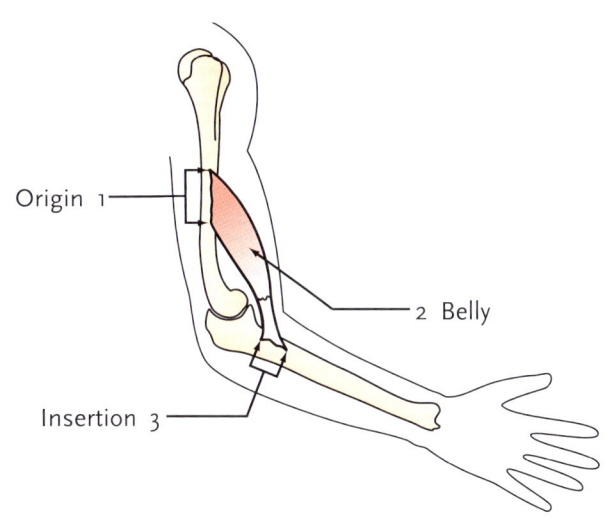

Origin 1
2 Belly
Insertion 3

1. The **origin** is the nonmoving (fixed) portion of the muscle attached to bones or other fixed muscle. The term "skeletal muscles" refers to the part of the muscle attached to the bone.
2. The **belly** is the term applied to the midsection of the muscle, between the two attached sections.
3. The **insertion** is the portion of the muscle joined to movable attachments: bones, movable muscles or skin.

When contraction occurs, the insertion of the muscle moves. The origin of the muscle remains fixed.

Muscles produce movement through contraction (tightening) and expansion (relaxing). When a contraction occurs, one of the muscle attachments moves at the insertion point, while the other remains fixed at the muscle's origin. All muscles are attached at both ends to either a bone or another muscle. **Tendons** are the bands of fibrous tissue that attach muscles to bones. This is what allows bones to move when muscles contract and expand. **Ligaments** are dense, strong bands of fibrous tissue that connect bones to other bones at the joints.

4

Stimulation of muscular tissue can be achieved by using the following methods:

- Massage
- Light rays (infrared rays and ultraviolet rays)
- Heat rays (heating lamps)
- Moist heat (warm steam towels, warm water)
- Nerve impulses (through nervous system)
- Chemicals (certain acids and salts)

The arms, hands, legs and feet muscles are of primary concern to the nail technician when performing services. Muscles affected by massage are generally manipulated from the insertion to the origin attachment.

The charts that follow illustrate and define the muscles of the shoulders, arms, hands, legs and feet.

Abductor and adductor muscles have opposite functions and are found in several places in the body such as the fingers, arms and toes. An easy way to remember this is: An abductor takes away, as in a kidnapper. The adductor draws toward.

SHOULDER AND ARM MUSCLES

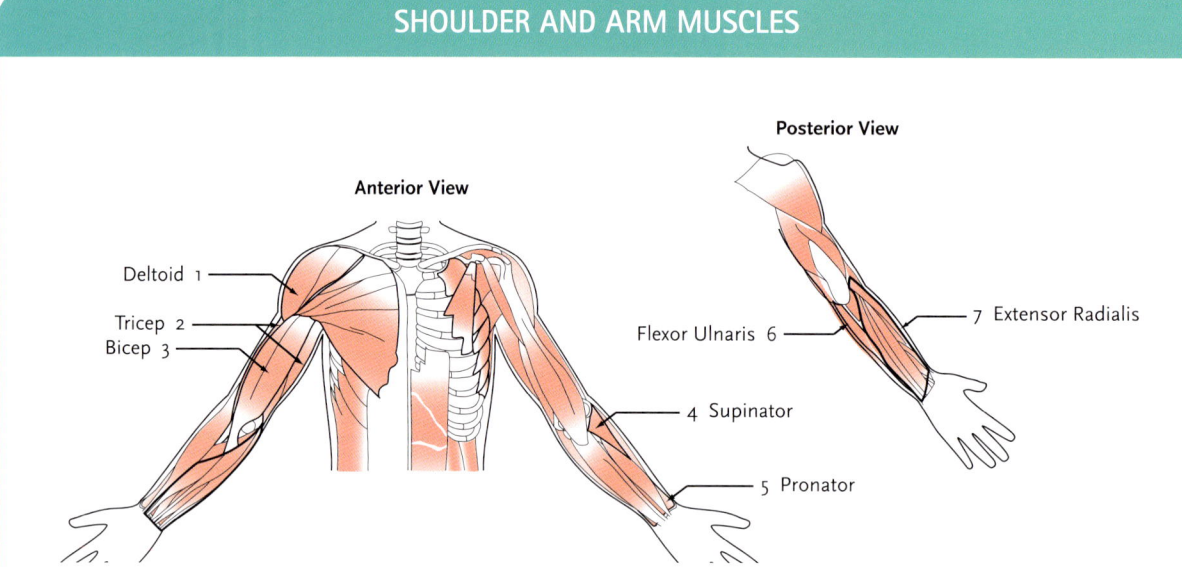

Anterior View

Deltoid 1
Tricep 2
Bicep 3

Posterior View

Flexor Ulnaris 6
7 Extensor Radialis
4 Supinator
5 Pronator

Shoulder Muscles

1. The **deltoid** (DEL-toid) covers the shoulder. This triangular-shaped muscle lifts the arm or turns it.
2. The **tricep** (TRI-sep) extends the length of the back of the upper arm. This muscle pulls the forearm down.
3. The **bicep** (BI-sep) is the primary muscle in the front of the upper arm. This muscle raises the forearm, bends the elbow and turns the palm of the hand down.

Forearm Muscles

4. The **supinator** (SU-pi-nat-or) runs parallel to the ulna and it turns the palm of the hand up.
5. The **pronator** (PRO-nat-or) runs across the front of the lower part of the radius and the ulna. This muscle turns the palm of the hand downward and inward.
6. The **flexor ulnaris** (FLEX-er uhl-NAR-is) is located mid-forearm, on the inside of the arm and it bends the wrist and closes the fingers.
7. The **extensor radialis** (eks-TEN-sor ray-dee-AHL-is) is located mid-forearm, on the outside of the arm. This muscle straightens the fingers and wrist.

HAND MUSCLES

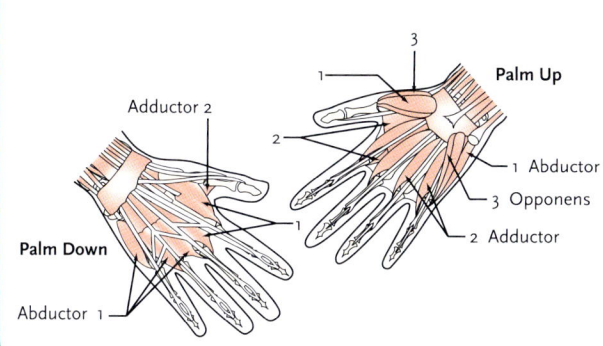

Palm Up

Adductor 2

1 Abductor

3 Opponens

2 Adductor

Palm Down

Abductor 1

A number of small muscles stretch over the fingers, connect the joints and provide dexterity. **Abductor** (ab-DUK-tor) muscles (1) separate the fingers while **adductor** (ah-DUK-tor) muscles (2) draw them together. The **opponens** (uh-POHN-nenz) muscles (3) are located in the palm of the hand and cause the thumb to move toward the fingers, giving the ability to grasp or make a fist.

4

LOWER LEG MUSCLES

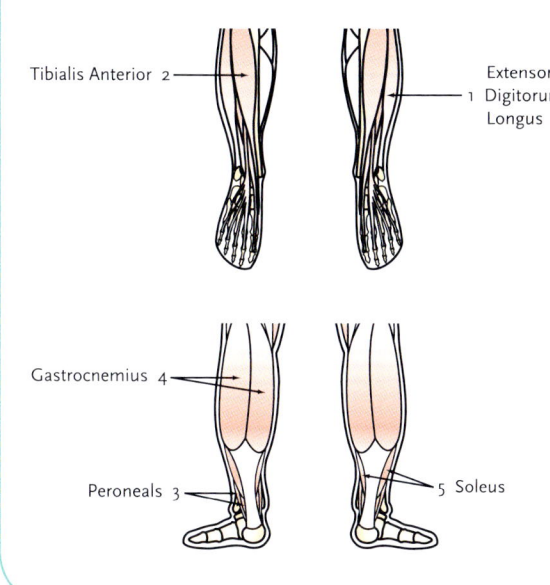

Tibialis Anterior 2

Extensor 1 Digitorum Longus

Gastrocnemius 4

Peroneals 3

5 Soleus

1. The **extensor digitorum longus** (eck-STEN-sur dij-it-TOHR-um LONG-us) extends the toes.
2. The **tibialis anterior** (tib-ee-AHL-is an-TEHR-ee-ohr) covers the front of the lower leg and pulls the foot upward.
3. The **peroneals** (per-oh-NEE-als) (peroneus longus and peroneus brevis) are located on the outsides of the legs and point the toes.
4. The **gastrocnemius** (gas-truc-NEEM-e-us) runs from the back of the knee to the heel of the foot and pulls the foot downward. Also known as the "calf muscle."
5. The **soleus** (SO-lee-us) runs from the mid-calf to the heel of the foot and pulls the foot upward.

FOOT MUSCLES

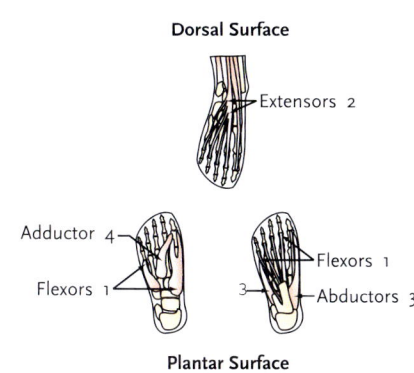

Dorsal Surface

Extensors 2

Adductor 4

Flexors 1

Flexors 1

Abductors 3

Plantar Surface

As with the hands, there are a number of small muscles located in the foot, which work together to produce movement of the toes and feet as well as provide cushion and balance when walking. The **flexor** (FLEX-er) muscles in the foot (1) when contracted bend the joints of the foot, while the **extensor** (eck-STEN-sur) muscles (2) extend or straighten the joint. The **abductor** muscles in the foot (3) draw the toes apart or away from a middle point while the **adductor** muscles (4) draw them together.

The Circulatory System

The **circulatory** or **vascular system** controls the circulation of blood and lymph through the body. As a professional nail technician, you may use massage techniques or perform services that will directly influence or stimulate this important body system. The circulatory system is made up of two interrelated subsystems:

1. The **cardiovascular** or **blood vascular** system, including the heart, arteries, veins and capillaries, circulates the blood.
2. The **lymph vascular** system circulates lymph (described on page 101) through lymph glands, lymph nodes and vessels.

The illustration below shows the muscles of the heart.

THE HEART

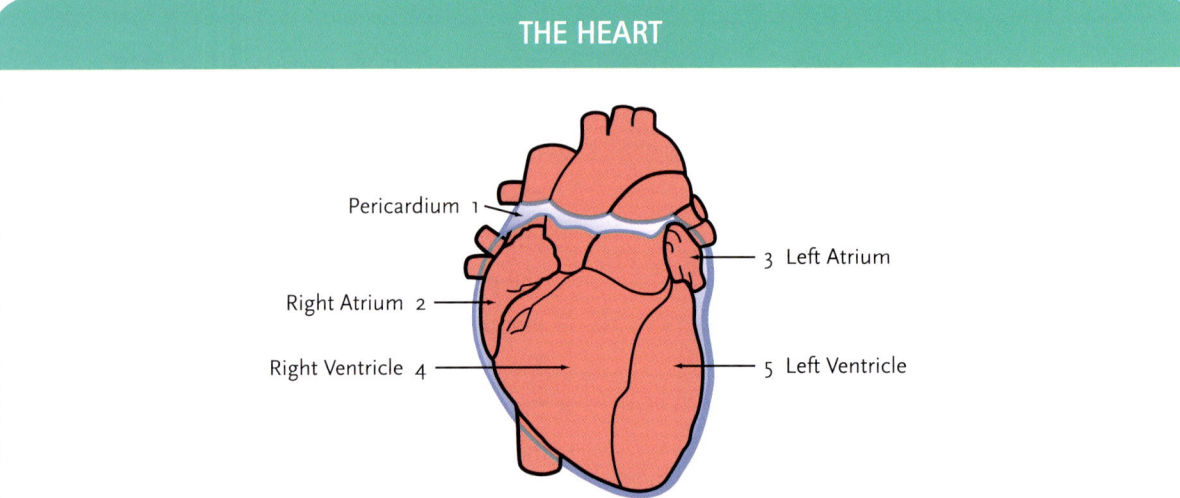

The heart is a fist-sized, cone-shaped, muscular organ located in the chest cavity. It is entirely encased in a membrane called the **pericardium**. The heart contracts and relaxes to force blood through the circulatory system. The interior of the heart contains four chambers: the upper chambers consist of the **right atrium** and the **left atrium**. The right and the left atrium are commonly referred to as the right and left auricles. The lower chambers consist of the **right ventricle** and the **left ventricle**.

A normal heart beats 60 to 80 times per minute. The heartbeat is regulated by the sympathetic nervous system and the **vagus** (tenth cranial nerve).

1. **Pericardium** (per-i-KAR-dee-um) is the membrane that encloses the heart.
2. **Right atrium** (AY-tree-um) is the right upper chamber and is commonly referred to as the right auricle.
3. **Left atrium** is the left upper chamber and is commonly referred to as the left auricle.
4. **Right ventricle** (VEN-tri-kel) is the lower right chamber of the heart.
5. **Left ventricle** is the lower left chamber of the heart.

The Cardiovascular System

The cardiovascular system transports blood through **arteries**, **veins** and **capillaries**, and combines with the lymph system to maintain steady circulation of the blood.

By the time you turn 70, your heart will have beaten approximately two-and-a-half billion times (based on an average of 70 beats per minute).

Blood is the sticky, salty fluid that circulates through the body, bringing nourishment and oxygen to all body parts and carrying toxins and waste products to the liver and kidneys to be eliminated. An average adult has 8 to 10 pints of blood flowing through the circulatory system. Blood is made up of red and white corpuscles, platelets and plasma. These components are called blood cells and make up the semi-solid part of the blood.

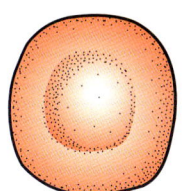 **Red blood cells** (RBC) are also called **erythrocytes** (e-RITH-ro-sites) or red corpuscles. They carry oxygen and contain a protein called hemoglobin. **Hemoglobin** (HEE-mo-glo-bin) attracts oxygen molecules through a process known as **oxygenation** (ok-si-je-NAY-shun). The blood appears bright red in color when oxygen is being carried. As red blood cells move through the body, they release oxygen molecules and collect molecules of carbon dioxide. When oxygen is low, the blood appears darker, nearly blue.

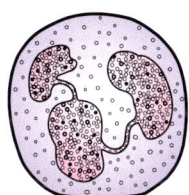 **White blood cells** (WBC) are also called **leucocytes** (LOO-ko-sites) or white corpuscles. They help protect the body by fighting bacteria and other foreign substances, and they increase in number when infection invades the body.

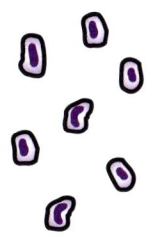 **Blood platelets** (PLATE-letz) or **thrombocytes** (THROM-bo-sites) begin the process of coagulation, or clotting, when exposed to air or trauma in the skin tissue, such as bruising.

Plasma is the fluid part of the blood in which red and white blood cells and blood platelets are suspended. Plasma is about 90% water.

Blood vessels are any vessels through which blood circulates in the body. There are three types of blood vessels:

- **Arteries** are tubular, elastic, thick-walled branching vessels that carry oxygenated blood away from the heart through the body. Oxygenated blood is bright red.
- **Veins** are tubular, elastic, thin-walled branching vessels that carry oxygen-depleted blood from the capillaries to the heart. Veins contain cup-like valves to prevent backward flow. Veins are closer to the outer surface of the body than arteries.
- **Capillaries** are small vessels that take nutrients and oxygen from the arteries to the cells and take waste products from the cells to the veins.

Did you know there is a difference between a heart attack and cardiac arrest? A heart attack is an event that results in permanent damage or death to part of the heart muscle. With cardiac arrest, however, the heart stops beating altogether, resulting in sudden cardiac death in the absence of immediate medical attention. Cardiopulmonary resuscitation (CPR) restores breathing and circulation to help keep the victim alive until further medical attention is found. CPR should only be performed by a person who is certified in it.

4

Arteries transport blood away from the heart and veins return blood to the heart.

The process of blood traveling from the heart throughout the body and back to the heart is referred to as **systemic** or **general circulation**. Blood travels through the pulmonary artery to the lungs where it is oxygenated (combined with oxygen). This phase of the circulation of blood is referred to as **pulmonary circulation**.

Varicose (VAR-ih-kose) veins are veins that are permanently dilated, meaning widened or expanded, most commonly occurring in the legs. They usually appear as reddish-purple or blue-green bulges that form if veins stretch and lose their elasticity. Varicose veins can be brought on by long periods of standing or by limiting circulation when sitting with legs crossed. Preventive measures include wearing support hose and correctly sized shoes.

As a professional nail technician, you will be working with the hands, arms, legs and feet. The following charts show you how blood is supplied to these appendages.

HAND AND ARM BLOOD SUPPLY

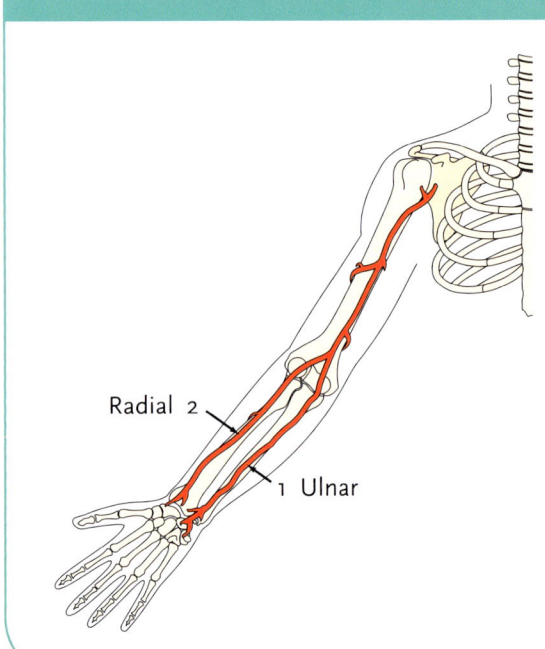

Radial 2
1 Ulnar

There are two main arteries in each arm and hand. Each of these arteries branches out to supply blood to the entire area. The main veins of the arms lie alongside the arteries and are located closer to the surface of the skin. It's important to remember that the veins and arteries of the arms share the same name.

1. The **ulnar** (UL-ner) **artery** supplies blood to the little finger side of the arm and the palm of the hand.
2. The **radial** (RAY-dee-ul) **artery** supplies blood to the thumb side of the arm and the back of the hand.

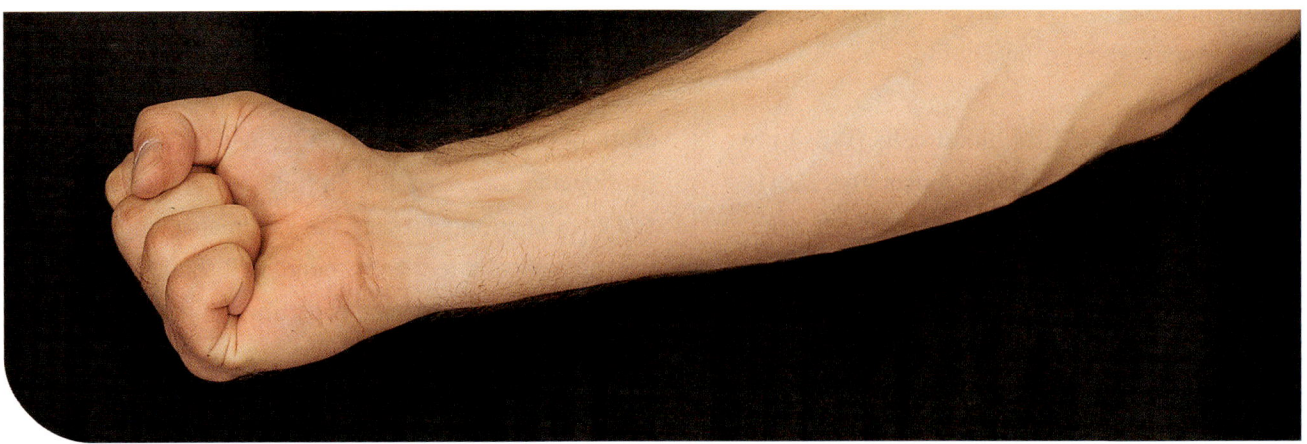

LEG AND FOOT BLOOD SUPPLY

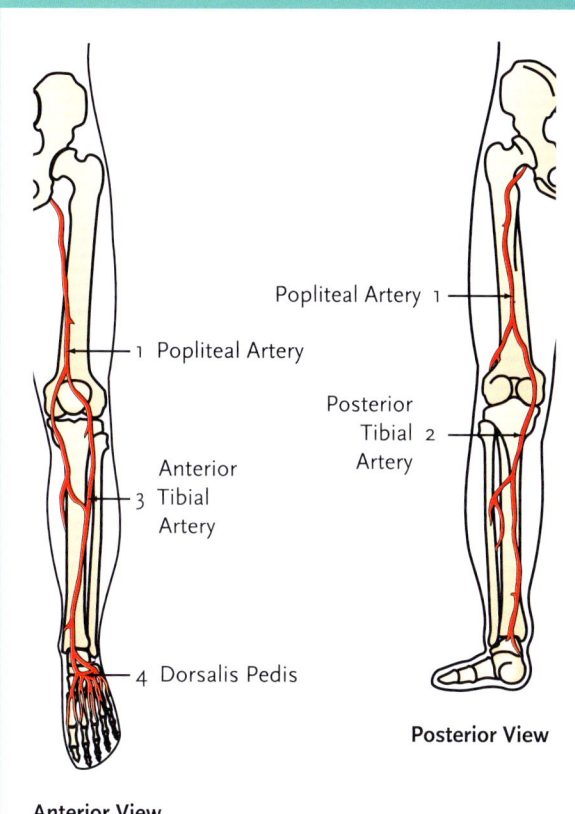

Popliteal Artery 1

1 Popliteal Artery

Posterior
Tibial 2
Artery

Anterior
3 Tibial
Artery

4 Dorsalis Pedis

Posterior View

Anterior View

There are four main arteries of the leg and foot. These arteries have many branches to allow blood to reach the entire area. The main veins of the leg and foot lie alongside the arteries and are located closer to the surface of the skin. Just like the veins and arteries of the arms, the veins and arteries of the legs share the same name.

1. The **popliteal** (pop-lih-TEE-ul) **artery** is located in the upper leg and branches off into the two main arteries of the lower leg.
2. The **posterior tibial** (TIB-ee-al) **artery** is located in the back of the lower leg and supplies the lower leg with blood.
3. The **anterior tibial artery** is located in the front of the lower leg and also supplies the lower leg with blood.
4. The **dorsalis** (dor-SAL-es) **pedis** supplies blood to the foot.

4

The Lymph Vascular System

The **lymph vascular system** (also referred to as the **lymphatic system**) is the second subsystem of circulation. **Lymph** is a colorless liquid produced as a by-product of plasma, passing nourishment to capillaries and cells. It is a product of the blood system and, after traveling through the lymph glands and vessels, moves back into the bloodstream. Lymph filters the blood by removing toxins (poisons) and it contains white blood cells to defend the body against infection. Lymph also nourishes the parts of the body not reached by blood, such as the far extremities.

There are more than 100 lymph nodes in the body that act as barriers to infection from one part of the body to another. As the lymph nodes take on this protective task, they may swell and cause pain. Swollen or tender lymph nodes indicate infection in the body. The lymph nodes most often affected in this way are in the neck and under the arms. Many other circumstances may cause such swelling, so a doctor should be consulted at the first sign of any swelling in these areas.

In Latin, *lympha* means "water nymph." Lymph is a fluid that coagulates like blood, only it contains white blood cells called lymphocytes. You may have noticed your lymph nodes (or glands) if they have ever become swollen and painful in your neck. This is a sign that your lymph nodes are filtering and fighting infection with activated lymphocytes.

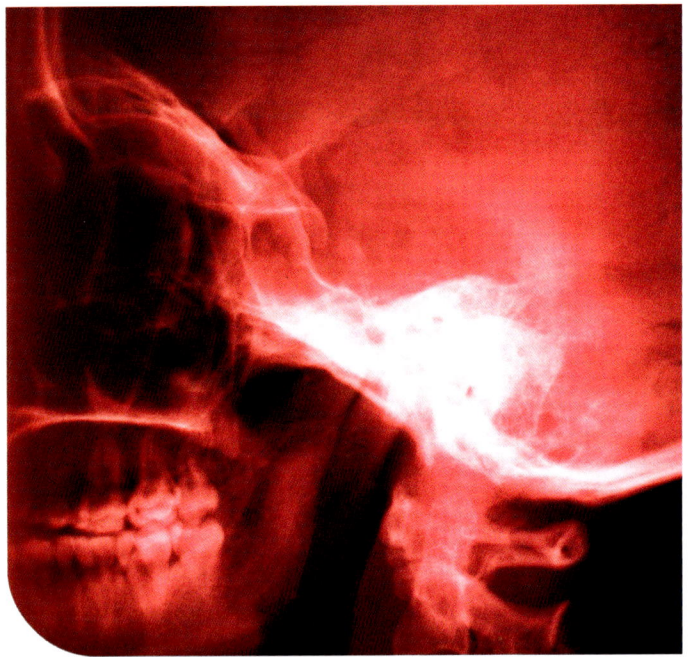

The Nervous System

The **nervous system** coordinates and controls the overall operation of the human body by responding to both internal and external stimuli. The study of the nervous system is called **neurology**.

The nervous system is made up of three subsystems:

1. The **central** or **cerebrospinal** (sa-REE-bro-spy-nel) **nervous system**
2. The **peripheral** (pe-RIF-ur-al) **nervous system**
3. The **autonomic nervous system**

The primary components of the nervous system are the brain, spinal cord and nerves. These components operate together to receive and interpret stimuli (anything that activates the brain) and sends signals to tissues, muscles and organs. The illustration on the opposite page identifies the components of the brain.

The Central Nervous System

The **central** or **cerebrospinal nervous system** is composed of the brain and spinal cord. The central nervous system controls all voluntary and involuntary body action.

The **spinal cord** is made of long nerve fibers that originate in the base of the brain and extend to the base of the spine. The spinal cord holds 31 pairs of spinal nerves that branch out to muscles, internal organs and skin.

The Peripheral Nervous System

The **peripheral nervous system** is composed of sensory and motor nerves that extend from the brain and spinal cord to the voluntary muscles of the body and to the surface of the skin. The peripheral nervous system also carries sensory information to the brain from the ears, eyes, nose and tongue. This information travels to and from the brain through a network of nerve cells. This network also carries messages to and from the central nervous system.

The Autonomic Nervous System

The **autonomic nervous system** is physically part of the central nervous system, and controls the respiratory, digestive, circulatory, excretory, endocrine and reproductive systems. It governs all involuntary body functions such as breathing, blinking, sweating and digesting.

The autonomic system consists of two subsystems:

- The **sympathetic** nervous system, which speeds up the heart rate, constricts blood vessels and raises blood pressure.
- The **parasympathetic** nervous system, which slows the heart rate, dilates blood vessels and lowers blood pressure.

The same nerve tissues are involved in both the sympathetic and parasympathetic nervous systems, but they perform different functions. Sympathetic nerves respond to the body's physiological status. For example, in stressful situations, blood pressure increases. In contrast, when the body is relaxed, the parasympathetic nerves respond by lowering blood pressure. Their opposing functions help keep the body balanced, or in a state of **homeostasis** (ho-mee-oh-STAY-sis).

An adult body has 46 miles of nerves, and nerve impulses travel as fast as 200 miles an hour. The human brain generates more electrical impulses daily than all the telephones in the world.

THE BRAIN

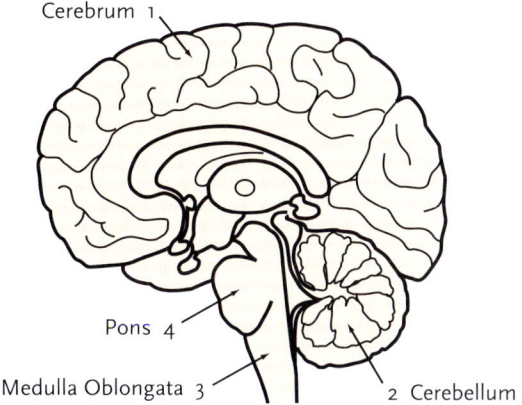

Cerebrum 1

Pons 4

Medulla Oblongata 3

2 Cerebellum

The brain controls all three subsystems of the nervous system. Composed of nerves and tissue, the average human brain weighs between 44 and 48 ounces. The brain has four major parts:

1. The **cerebrum** (se-REE-brum) is the large, rounded structure of the brain that occupies the upper, front part of the cranial cavity. The cerebrum is the center of higher mental functions, such as thought, emotion and memory.

2. The **cerebellum** (ser-e-BEL-um) regulates motor function, muscle movement and balance. Because the cerebellum is located in the occipital area directly below the cerebrum it is also known as the "little brain" or "hind brain."

3. The **medulla oblongata** (me-DOOL-ah ob-long-GA-ta) governs respiration, circulation, swallowing and certain other body functions. Located just below the pons, the medulla is said to be the most vital part of the brain because it controls breathing and heart function. It is also called the "bulb" of the spinal cord because it connects parts of the brain to the spinal column.

4. The **pons** (PONZ) is a prominent band of nerve tissue that connects other parts of the brain to the medulla oblongata. It is located below the cerebrum and directly in front of the cerebellum. Pons is from the Latin word *ponz*, which means bridge.

4

Nerve Cells

Like other cells, the **nerve cell**, or **neuron** (NU-ron), has a nucleus, cytoplasm and membrane. Nerve cells, however, differ in appearance from other cells due to the branches around them called **dendrites** (DEN-dritz), the Greek word for *tree*. Dendrites receive impulses from adjacent neurons and transmit them along long fibers called **axons** (AK-sonz), the Greek word for *axis*. At the end of each axon is a nerve terminal, or **synapse** (SIN-aps). These terminals may connect the neuron to muscles, organs or other nerve cells. They send messages in the form of electrical nerve impulses. These structures receive the messages and relay them to neighboring cells, as shown in the chart to the right.

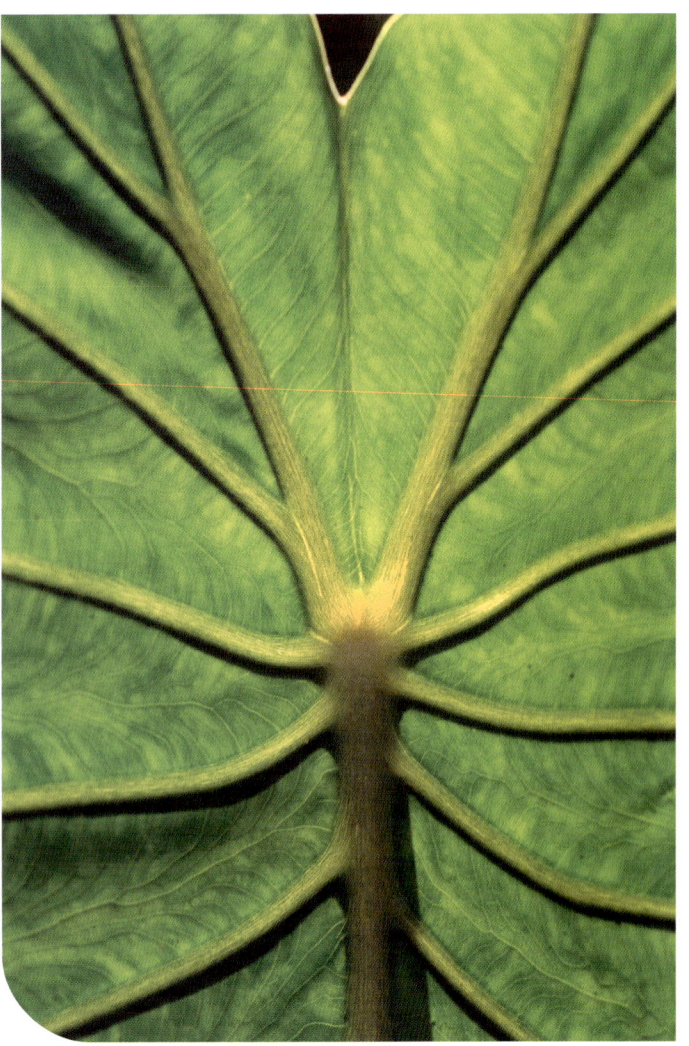

NERVE CELL

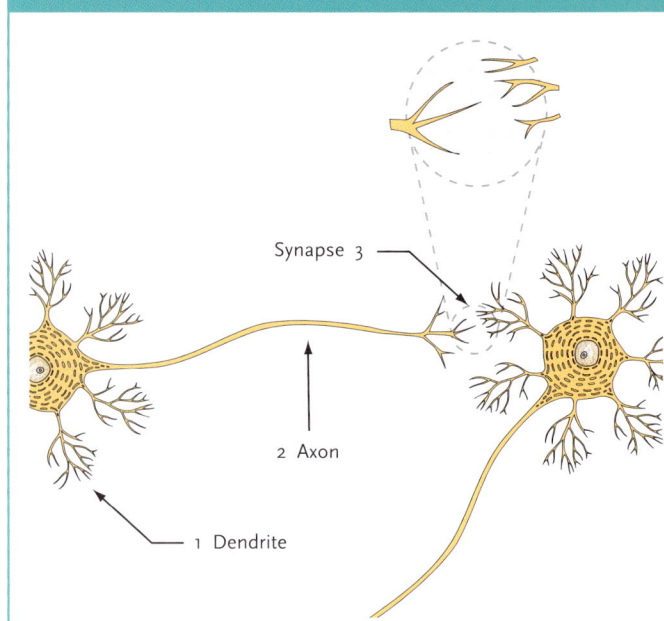

Synapse 3

2 Axon

1 Dendrite

1. **Dendrites** (DEN-dritz) are short fibers extending from the nerve cell.
2. **Axons** (AK-sonz), or **processes**, are the threadlike fibers extending from the cell.
3. **Synapses** (SI-nap-ses) are the bridges across which nerve impulses pass.

The dendrite system is interconnected, like a vast network of highways. Impulses travel back and forth between nerve cells over this network of paths. Certain activities, such as the use of harmful narcotic drugs or a prolonged lack of oxygen, can close the highways down, never to open again. But more commonly, lack of adequate food, rest and exercise causes nerve fatigue. Maintaining a well-balanced diet, sleep schedule, regular exercise routine and relaxation time can alleviate nerve fatigue. Massage also often helps restore nerve energy by stimulating nerves and causing muscles to release built-up toxins.

The three different types of nerves are explained on the next page.

TYPES OF NERVES

Nerves or nerve tissues carry information to and from the brain. Nerves are classified according to the direction in which they carry this information. Sensory and motor nerves can work together or independently. For example, when you chose to open this book, your brain sent a message to the *motor* nerves of your hand. This is a conscious decision. You are in control of your hand movement. But remember the last time you accidentally touched a hot stove? Your *sensory* nerves sent a rapid message to your brain transmitting the sensation you experienced. Your brain immediately responded by sensing pain and by sending impulses back to motor nerves to move your hand away. This interaction of sensory and motor nerves is called a **reflex action**.

4

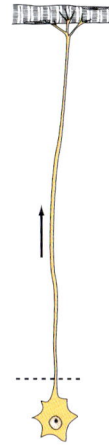

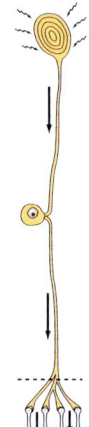

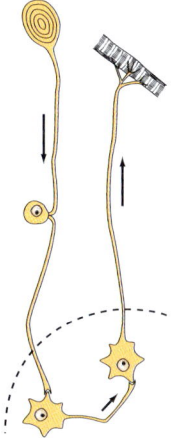

Sensory, or **afferent nerves**, carry messages to the brain and spinal cord. These are the nerves that provide our sense of smell, sight, touch, hearing and taste. Sensory nerves have nerve cells called receptors that are located in the skin. These cells react to outside stimulation by sending a sensory message to the brain.

Motor, or **efferent nerves**, carry messages to the muscles. When the brain sends a message, motor nerves receive the message and cause the muscles to react so movement can occur.

Many large nerves perform both sensory and motor functions. These are called **mixed** or **sensory–motor nerves**. Large nerves have many branches.

Nerves and Massage

The nerves of the arms, hands, legs and feet may be stimulated or soothed during nail services, which include massage. During massage of the arms, hands, legs and feet manipulations can stimulate sensitive nerve tissues, resulting in nerve impulses that expand and contract corresponding muscles.

The same methods used to stimulate muscular tissue are used to stimulate nerve tissues:

- Massage
- Light rays (infrared rays and ultraviolet rays)
- Heat rays (heating lamps)
- Moist heat (warm steam towels and warm water)

- Nerve impulses (through nervous system)
- Chemicals (certain acids and salts)

Through this process, fatigued muscles can be soothed and tense muscles relaxed. Muscle relaxation is also achieved by stimulating nerves using heat to expand muscles and cold to make muscles contract.

As a nail technician your hands are your most valuable tool. Knowing the nerves of the hands, arms, legs and feet and their function will help you deliver excellent nail services. More important, this knowledge will help you in protecting and caring for your own greatest professional assets—your hands.

ARM AND HAND NERVES

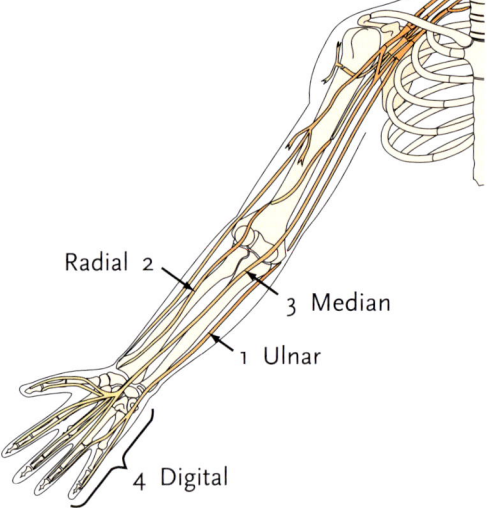

Radial 2
3 Median
1 Ulnar
4 Digital

All four of the primary nerves of the arms and/or hands are mixed nerves; they transmit sensations to the brain and carry impulses from the brain to the muscles.

1. The **ulnar** nerve extends down the little finger side of the arm into the palm of the hand.
2. The **radial** nerve extends down the thumb side of the arm into the back of the hand.
3. The **median** nerve extends down the inside of the mid-forearm into the hand.
4. The **digital** nerve extends into the fingers of the hand.

LEG AND FOOT NERVES

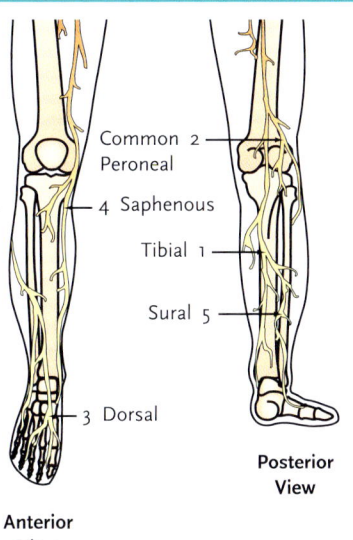

Common Peroneal 2
4 Saphenous
Tibial 1
Sural 5
3 Dorsal

Posterior View

Anterior View

All five of the primary nerves of the lower legs and feet are mixed nerves; they transmit sensations to the brain and carry impulses from the brain to the muscles.

1. The **tibial** (TIB-ee-al) nerve extends behind the knee down the back of the lower leg. This nerve supplies impulses to the knee, muscles of the calf, skin of the leg and the sole of the foot, heel and the bottom of the toes.
2. The **common peroneal** (per-oh-NEE-al) nerve extends from behind the knee to the front of the leg. Its branches (deep peroneal nerve and the superficial peroneal nerve) supply impulses to the muscles in the front of the lower leg and the skin of the lower leg.
3. The **dorsal** (DOOR-sal) nerve extends along the top of the foot and supplies impulses to the skin on top of the foot and toes.
4. The **saphenous** (sa-FEEN-us) nerve extends along the inside of the leg and supplies impulses to the skin on the inside of the leg and foot.
5. The **sural** (SOO-ral) nerve extends down the back and outside of the lower leg and supplies impulses to the skin on the outside and back of the foot and lower leg.

The **digestive system** breaks down food into simpler chemical compounds that can be easily absorbed by cells or eliminated from the body as waste. The digestive process begins as soon as food is ingested, when **enzymes** (EN-zimz) secreted by the **salivary** (SAL-i-ver-ee) **glands** start breaking down the food. Food travels down the **pharynx** (FAR-ingks) and through the **esophagus** (e-SOF-ah-gus) into the stomach, propelled by a twisting and turning motion of the esophagus called **peristalsis** (per-i-STAL-sis). In the stomach, **hydrochloric** (hi-dro-KLO-rik) **acid** and several other enzymes further break down food. One of these other enzymes, called **pepsin**, is responsible for the breakdown of protein into **polypeptide** (pol-ee-PEP-tide) **molecules** and free amino acids, which are of particular importance to the production of hair, skin and nails.

As partially digested food passes from the stomach into the **small intestine**, the breakdown of nutrients begins. Nutrients are absorbed by the **villi** (VIL-i), which are finger-like projections of the intestine walls, and transported through the circulatory system to the tissues and cells of the body.

It is recommended to drink eight, eight-ounce glasses of water a day, since the average adult loses two to three quarts of water a day. Other tips include drinking twice as much as it takes to quench your thirst and drinking frequently throughout the day to avoid dehydration. Drinking water helps keep your skin fresh, and has also been shown to lower the risk of heart attacks.

4

Undigested food passes into the **large intestine**, or **colon**, which stores the waste for eventual elimination through the anal canal. The entire process of digestion takes about nine hours. The illustration below identifies the organs of the digestive system.

DIGESTIVE SYSTEM

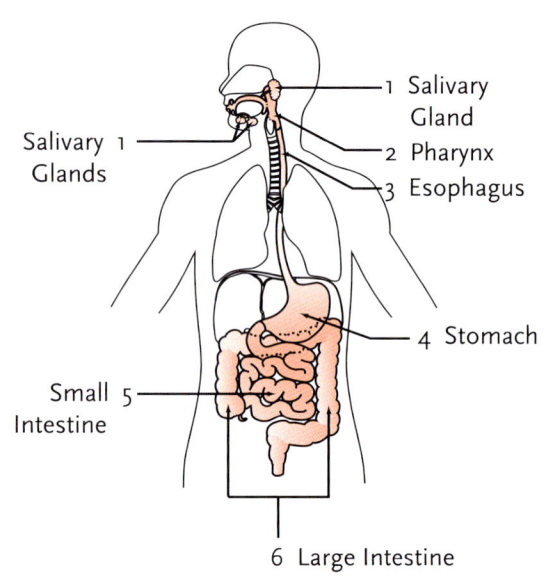

Salivary Glands 1
1 Salivary Gland
2 Pharynx
3 Esophagus
4 Stomach
Small Intestine 5
6 Large Intestine

The digestive system processes nutrients and eliminates waste.

1. **Salivary glands** break down food.
2. **Pharynx** is the passage to the stomach and lungs.
3. **Esophagus** is the passage between the pharynx and the stomach.
4. **Stomach** is the organ where digestion occurs.
5. **Small intestine** begins the breakdown of nutrients.
6. **Large intestine** or **colon** stores the waste for eventual elimination through the anal canal.

The Excretory System

The **excretory system** eliminates solid, liquid and gaseous waste products from the body. Organs of the excretory system include the skin, liver and kidneys.

1. The **skin** is the body's largest organ. The skin releases water, carbon dioxide and other waste through the sweat glands. Sweat glands are a type of excretory gland, since they open onto the surface of the skin outside the body.
2. The **liver** secretes bile and converts and neutralizes ammonia from the circulatory system to **urea** (u-REE-ah). Urea is then carried, through the bloodstream, to the kidneys for excretion.
3. The **kidneys** receive urea from the liver and then pass the urea through small tubelike structures known as **nephrons** (NEF-ronz) as shown in the illustration that follows. The urea is then excreted from the body as urine.

KIDNEY

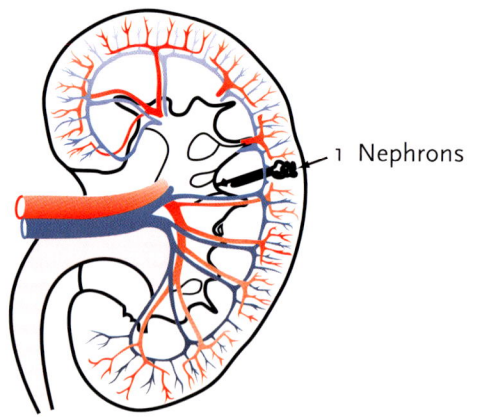

1 Nephrons

1. **Nephrons** filter out waste products and water, allowing usable nutrients to be reabsorbed into the blood. Excreted waste products travel through the **ureters** (U-re-turz) and bladder and are eliminated from the body in urine.

The Respiratory System

The **respiratory system** consists of the upper and lower respiratory tracts, the lungs and the thoracic (THO-rah-sic) cavity, which protects and supports the lungs. This system maintains the exchange of oxygen and carbon dioxide in the lungs and body tissues.

The primary functions of the respiratory system are:

1. **Inhalation**, or the intake of oxygen to be absorbed into the blood.
2. **Exhalation**, or the elimination of oxygen's toxic by-product, carbon dioxide, by breathing out.

Both of these functions take place every time you breathe.

While it is possible to breathe through both the mouth and the nose, breathing through the nose is healthier. The mucus membranes in the nose, called **vibrissae** (vi-BRIS-see), filter out dust and dirt. **Conchae** (KONG-kee) warm the inhaled air as it travels through the nasal passages.

The **upper respiratory tract** consists of the nose, mouth, pharynx and larynx. Air enters the body through the nostrils, and passes through the pharynx. The **larynx** (LAR-ngks), which contains the vocal cords, connects the pharynx to the trachea.

RESPIRATORY SYSTEM

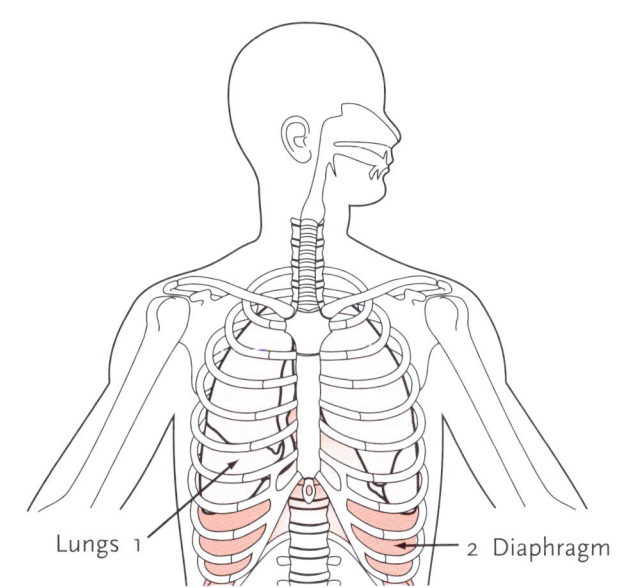

Lungs 1   2 Diaphragm

The primary respiratory system organs are:

1. The **lungs** are spongy muscles composed of cells into which air enters when you inhale. These cells process oxygen for absorption into the blood and release carbon dioxide as you exhale.
2. The **diaphragm** (DIE-ah-fram) is a muscular organ that separates the chest cavity from the abdomen. The diaphragm expands and contracts automatically, assisting in forcing air into and out of the lungs.

A newborn baby breathes 40 times a minute, and up until the age of six or seven months, a child can breathe and swallow at the same time. An adult cannot. On average, an adult breathes almost seven quarts of air every minute. And, during 24 hours, the average person breathes 23,000 times.

The **lower respiratory tract** consists of the trachea, bronchi and the lungs. The **trachea** (TRAY-kee-ah) is a conducting pathway through which air flows. The **bronchi**, (bron-KEE) sometimes called the bronchial tree because of its branched shape, delivers air directly to the lungs.

The Endocrine System

The **endocrine system** is composed of a group of specialized ductless glands that regulate and control the growth, reproduction and health of the body. These glands manufacture chemical substances called **hormones** and release them directly into the bloodstream.

The endocrine system is a carefully balanced mechanism that directly affects hair growth, skin conditions and energy levels. Nutrition plays a key role in the proper regulation of this system. Signs of fatigue, changes in hair growth or in skin condition may signal the need for medical attention.

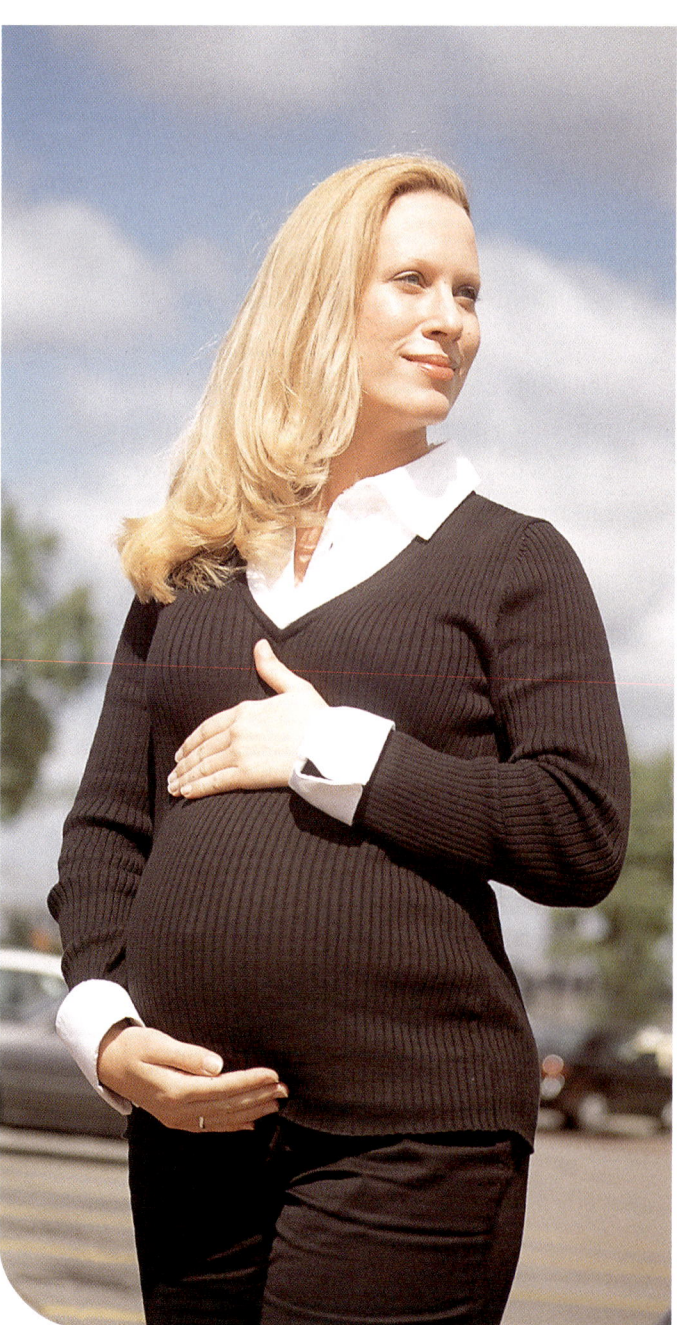

The Reproductive System

The **reproductive system** allows a living organism to procreate. With an understanding of the reproductive system, nail technicians can anticipate the ways hormones may influence changes in the nails.

In pregnancy, hormonal imbalances, or fluctuations in hormone levels, often cause the nails to become soft and brittle. It is important to hydrate the nails with lotions and cuticle conditioners. Lines may appear on the nails, which usually fade after giving birth. Most women will also experience an increased growth rate of their nails due to these hormonal changes.

Often during pregnancy, women experience increased sensitivity to heat, exfoliants and active ingredients, such as Vitamin C. Be aware of a pregnant client's comfort during a service.

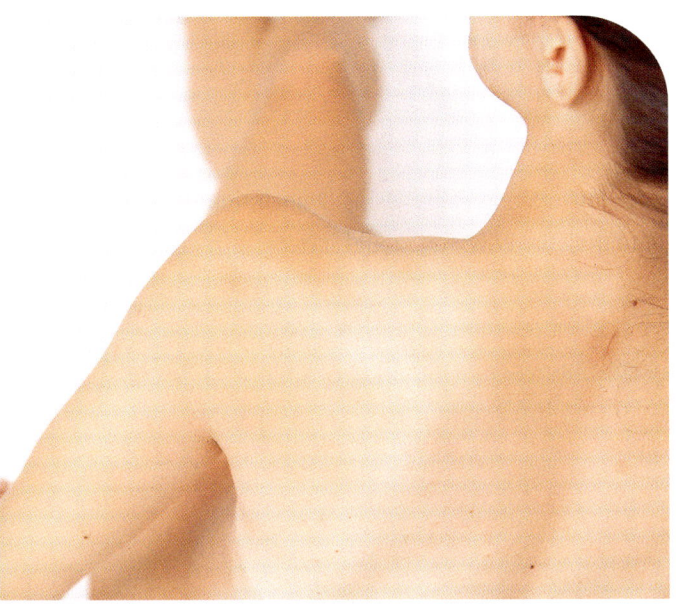

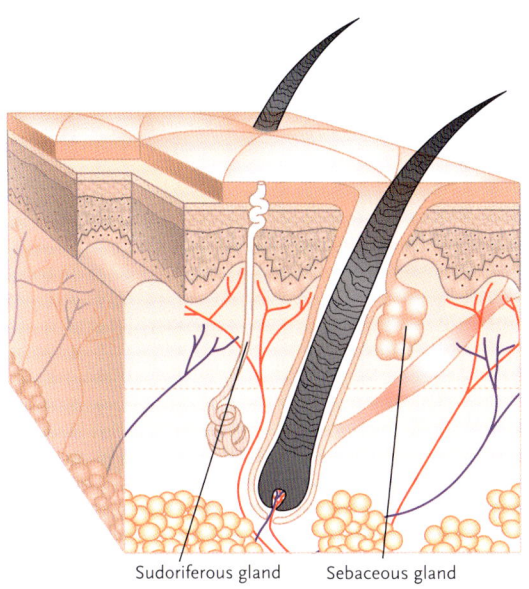

Sudoriferous gland   Sebaceous gland

4

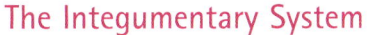
The Integumentary System

The layers of the skin make up the **integumentary** (in-TEG-u-men-ter-ee) **system**. The two primary glands of the integumentary system are the **sebaceous** (si-BAY-shus), or **oil glands**, and the **sudoriferous** (soo-dohr-IF-er-us), or **sweat glands**. These glands are referred to as duct glands because both release their contents into canal-like structures, or ducts, that open onto the surface of the skin.

This introduction to the integumentary system demonstrates its relationship to the other body systems and their functions. *Chapter 6, Nail and Skin Physiology* provides an in-depth look at the skin—both inside and out!

Understanding the human body will help you make decisions that will enhance your client's appearance, health and well-being. In addition, reviewing the fundamental structures and systems of the body prepares you to learn massage techniques used in nail care services. Your mastery of the important aspects of physiology and anatomy is essential as you develop your skills as a nail technician.

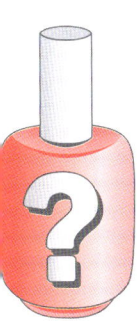

We have all learned about the basic body systems, whether in school or on a visit to the doctor. Having read this section on body systems, which are you most interested in learning more about?

DECISION-MAKING SKILLS

Case Studies

The following situations are designed to help you build decision-making skills. Using your training to this point, review the following scenarios, then think through and describe how you would handle each challenge.

1. A fellow student has been unenthusiastic about her studies on the chapter on anatomy. She wonders why she needs to know about nerves, muscles, bones, and the like. She says: "I'm not studying to be a doctor or anything. What good is all this information to me?" You value this friend and study partner. What would you say to her?

2. A client has just received her first pedicure and says she would like to discuss setting up a regular schedule of pedicure appointments. The client has a friend who has told her how enjoyable foot and leg massage are as part of a pedicure service. Describe the results that could be achieved from this added service using some of the terminology you have learned in this chapter.

3. A client you have known for a year has lost an excessive amount of weight, maintained a very hectic schedule and has suffered the loss of an immediate family member. You are concerned because you can see a noticeable difference in her skin and nails. How could you professionally bring up the importance of a proper diet and good digestion in an effort to help correct this situation?

In your career as a nail technician, you will be in daily contact with products containing powerful chemicals. This means that it is important to have a basic understanding of them, especially the chemicals found in nail and skin products. In addition, knowing how these chemicals interact with one another and what precautions to take helps keep you and your clients safe. Whether you are removing polish or explaining the curing process for gel nails, a working understanding of the fundamental principles of chemistry adds considerable value to the quality of your service.

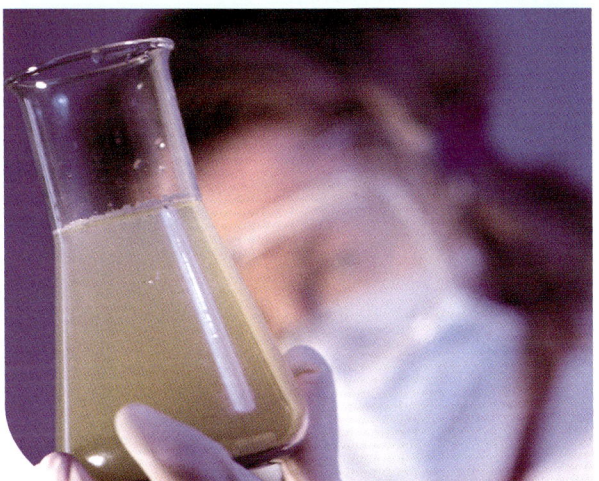

PLAN		OBJECTIVES
Fundamentals of Chemistry	• Classifications of Matter • Chemical Reactions	Describe the three basic forms of matter and the differences between elements, atoms, molecules and compounds. Explain how initiators and catalysts cause polymerization.
Chemistry of Nail Products	• Nail Product Removers • Nail Polish Ingredients • Adhesives and Priming Agents • Monomers and Polymers	Name the common uses of solvents in the nail industry. List the different ingredients that make up nail polish. Explain how a nail plate and a nail product are able to adhere to each other. Describe how monomers and polymers relate to each other.
Chemistry of Artificial Nail Systems	• Nail Wrap Systems • Liquid and Powder Acrylic Systems • Light-Cured Gel Systems	Compare the differences of the three artificial nail systems.

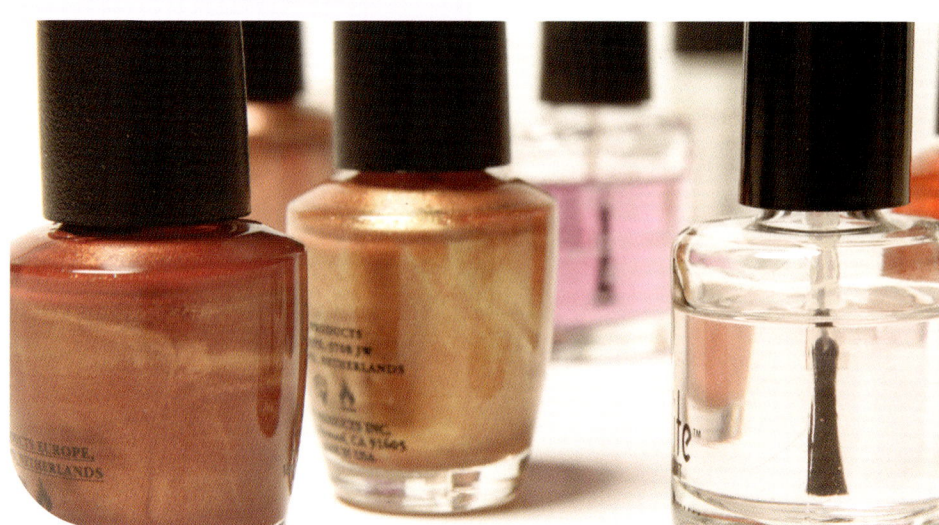

FUNDAMENTALS OF CHEMISTRY

Chemistry is the scientific study of **matter**, which is anything that occupies space. It is also the scientific study of the physical and chemical changes of matter. In addition, chemistry deals with the transformation of substances and the interaction of these substances with energy. For example, plastics, rubber, paint and detergents are all inventions that were made possible through the application of modern chemistry. Nearly every industry in the world—including the nail industry—involves an application of the principles of chemistry in some way. Now, as you read on, you will learn more about how these principles apply to your profession.

Classifications of Matter

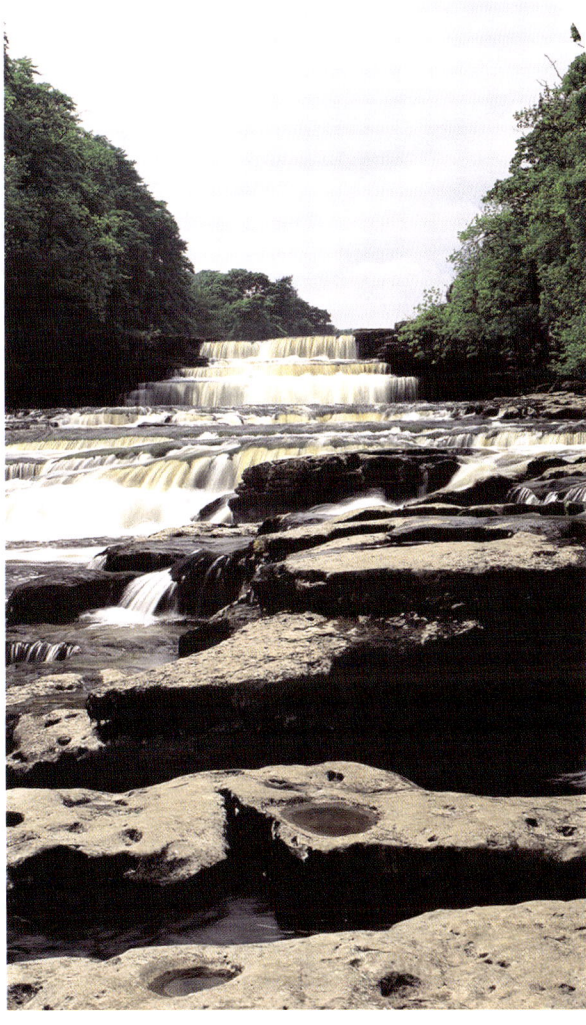

Matter is all around you. From the air you breathe to your own physical body, almost everything you can see or detect under a microscope is made of matter because it takes up physical space. Light and electricity are the only two things in this universe that are not matter, and are categorized as energy.

In chemistry, there are three basic forms of matter:

- **Solids**—Matter with definite weight, volume and shape.
- **Liquids**—Matter with definite weight and volume, but no shape.
- **Gases**—Matter with definite weight, but indefinite volume and shape.

A fingernail is a solid because it has a definite weight, volume and shape. Nail polish is a liquid because polish has a definite weight and volume, but no shape. Oxygen is a gas because it has a definite weight—even though it might not seem like it—but no volume or shape.

Vapor is the gaseous state of a substance that is liquid or solid under normal conditions. Although vapors in the air *can* produce odors, not *all* vapors can be detected by smell. Since vapors cannot always be detected by an odor, it is necessary to have proper ventilation when working with any chemical products. For more information on proper ventilation, refer to *Chapter 3, Nail Salon Ecology*, page 73.

Matter can be changed from one of these forms (solid, liquid or gas) to another in two ways:

- **Physical change** is a change in the physical form of a substance without creating a new substance possessing a distinct material composition. An example of this is the freezing of water. Although the water has changed from a liquid form to a solid form, the substance is still water; only the way it looks has changed.

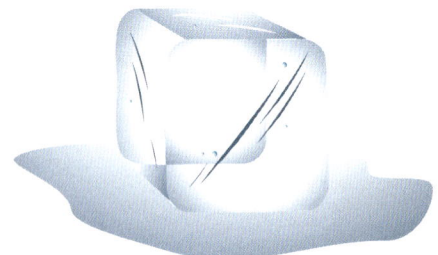

- **Chemical change** is a change in a substance that creates a new substance with different material characteristics from those of the original substance. For example, when you chemically react the two gases, hydrogen and oxygen, the new substance created is water.

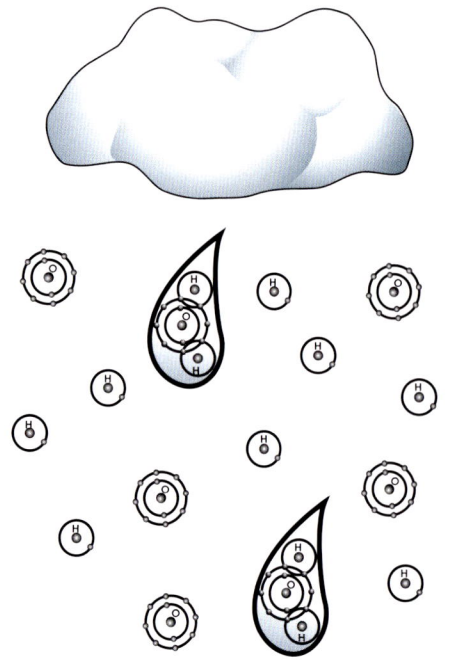

Elements

All matter, whether solid, liquid or gas, is made up of elements. **Elements** are fundamental substances that cannot be broken down into simpler substances (except by nuclear reactions). One example would be an element of iron. **Atoms** are the smallest possible unit of an element that possesses the characteristics of that element. There are 92 naturally occurring elements, but only five of these elements form the primary basis of the protein found in nails known as keratin. These elements are carbon, oxygen, hydrogen, nitrogen and sulfur.

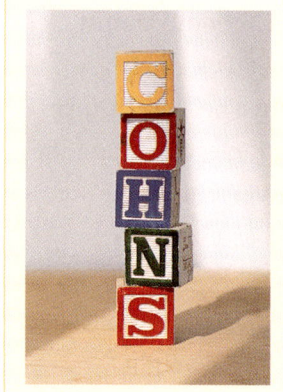

One easy way to remember the elements that make up nails is the acronym: COHNS (carbon, oxygen, hydrogen, nitrogen and sulfur).

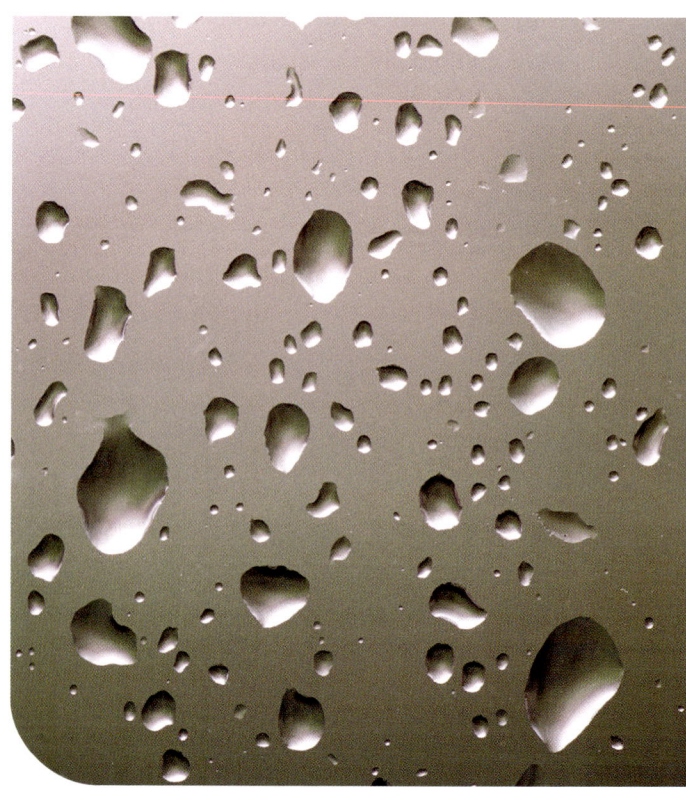

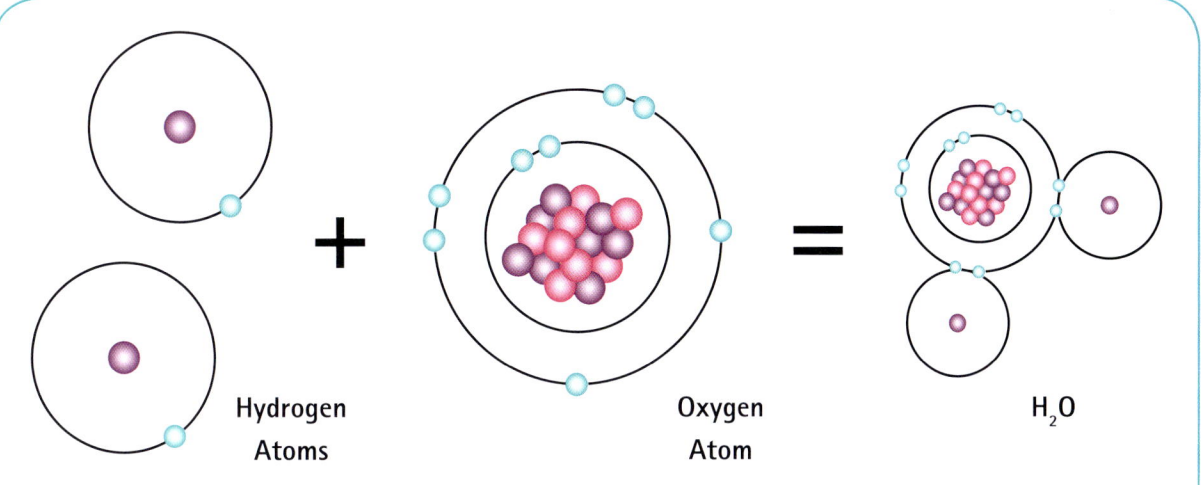

Hydrogen
Atoms

Oxygen
Atom

H_2O

5

When two hydrogen atoms combine with one oxygen atom, the result is the compound H_2O, which is a water molecule. This diagram shows two gases—hydrogen and oxygen—uniting and becoming a liquid.

Molecules and Compounds

Molecules are two or more atoms joined together by a chemical bond. For example, if you keep tearing a sheet of paper into shreds down to the smallest piece, that smallest piece of paper is your molecule of cellulose, the agent that is used to make up paper. Although it's smaller, that shred of paper is still paper. Meanwhile, a **compound** is a molecule composed of two or more different kinds of atoms joined together. When that happens, the original elements lose their physical and chemical characteristics. The perfect example occurs when two hydrogen atoms and one oxygen atom, both of which are gases, join to form a liquid compound of water.

Remember the five primary elements that make up nails? Through chemical bonds, carbon, oxygen, hydrogen, nitrogen and sulfur combine to create a compound that eventually creates the protein of nails. Also, amino acids are the building blocks of protein, which form the most important chemical bonds. Amino acids link together in a chainlink configuration to create different types of protein. For example, keratin is the type of protein found in nails, hair and the top layers of the skin.

Chemical Reactions

A **chemical reaction** occurs when the substances of two or more molecules interact and undergo a chemical change. A simple way to see a chemical reaction right before your eyes is to cut open an apple and leave it exposed to the air. When the chemicals within the apple combine with the

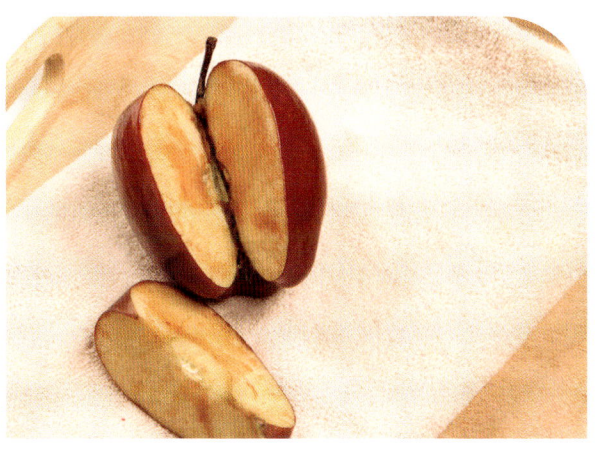

oxygen, a chemical reaction occurs, which causes the apple to turn brown. Because the surface of the apple cannot return to its original state, you know it has undergone a chemical change rather than a physical change.

Polymerization

A majority of the chemical reactions nail technicians commonly experience take place when using artificial nail enhancement products. The chemical reaction that takes place when creating artificial nails is called polymerization. **Polymerization** is the process that occurs when a certain type of molecule, called a monomer molecule, comes together with other monomer molecules in a chemical reaction to form three-dimensional networks, or **polymer chains**. This is more commonly referred to as the curing or hardening process in the nail industry. Two important components of a chemical reaction are an initiator and a catalyst.

Initiator

For a chemical reaction to occur an **initiator** is necessary to begin the process. An initiator is a chemical compound that causes the chemical reaction to start. Without an initiator, the chemical reaction will not occur.

Another way to initiate a chemical reaction is through the use of photo initiators. **Photo initiators**, which are used in light-cured products, are ingredients that absorb light to create the energy needed to begin the curing process. Remember that a photo initiator alone will not start the chemical reaction. A light source must hit the photo initiator in the product to start the chemical reaction.

Catalyst

Sometimes chemical reactions can take a while to occur. This is why there is often a **catalyst**, which is a substance that controls the speed at which the chemical reaction occurs. For instance, when applying a nail wrap, an accelerator is applied over the resin to reduce the curing time. The resin will cure without the use of an accelerator, but the process would take much longer. Keep in mind that when it takes less time to perform the service, you will have additional time for more clients.

> An easy way to understand polymerization, initiators and catalysts is to think of the initiator (in the acrylic powder) as a match and the catalyst (in the acrylic liquid) as the striking board. When the powder and the liquid are mixed, the catalyst and initiator together spark the curing reaction, just as if a match and a striking board were brought together to produce a flame.
>
> *- Courtesy of Paul Bryson, Ph.D., OPI Products Inc.*

Many products also contain **inhibitors**, which are chemicals that prevent the product from polymerizing, or hardening, too soon. This helps to increase the shelf life of the products. Inhibitors work to reduce the reaction caused by the catalyst. It stunts or reduces effectiveness but does not eliminate it.

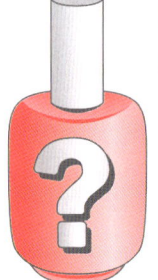

How can an understanding of the basic principles of chemistry relate to your career as a nail technician?

CHEMISTRY OF NAIL PRODUCTS

From acrylic monomers to nail polish, clients need to be assured that the chemical substances contained in nail products will accomplish the desired results and are safe to use. As mentioned previously, knowing the basics of how different chemicals work and interact with one another is an important part of your training as a nail technician. In this section, we will discuss common chemical ingredients found in nail products, as well as principles of adhesion.

HEATING NAIL PRODUCT REMOVER

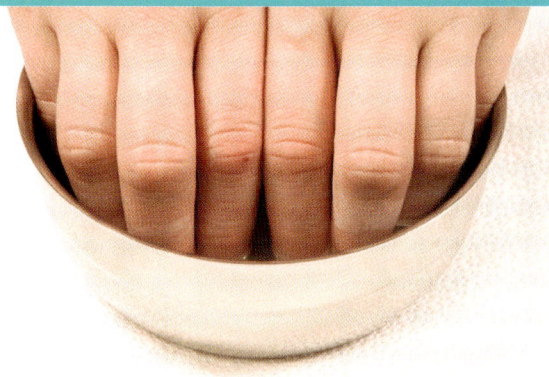

Product remover can be heated to speed up the process of removing artificial nails. A note of caution: Acetone and non-acetone removers are highly flammable liquids and should never be heated in a microwave, on a stove or over an open flame. The only safe methods for heating any solvent are to:

- Loosen the lid and run hot water over the bottle.
- Saturate a cotton ball, place it on the finger and wrap with foil. Body heat will warm the solvent.
- Place a small bowl of solvent into a larger bowl of warm water. Do not allow water to mix with the solvent. Place the client's fingers in the bowl of solvent.

To help contain the odor, place a damp towel over the client's hands while in the bowl.

Nail Product Removers

There are several types of nail product removers. Some are used to remove nail polish and others are used to remove artificial nail products, such as nail wraps and acrylic nails, which are discussed in *Chapter 9, Artificial Nail Services*. The main ingredient in nail product removers that dissolves or chemically breaks down the product is referred to as a solvent, which will be covered later in this chapter.

Acetone

The most widely used solvent in the nail industry is acetone. Acetone is a clear, highly flammable liquid solvent, which is used in both nail polish removers and artificial nail product removers. Although acetone is an effective solvent, it can dissolve the skin's

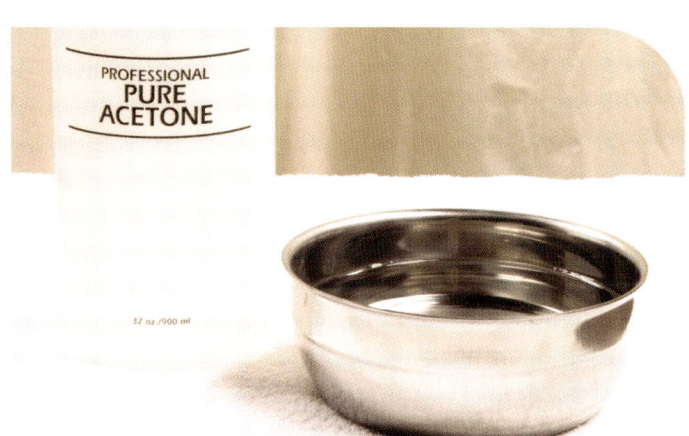

natural oils and dry out the skin. However, there are specific product removers on the market that contain other ingredients along with the acetone to counteract the drying effects. Also, adding a small amount of water to pure acetone can significantly reduce the drying effects while it remains an excellent solvent. Knowing this, you can assure the client who is concerned about the damage caused by acetone that there are other chemicals working that prevent the skin from drying out.

Non-Acetone Polish Remover

For the removal of nail polish, acetone is highly effective. However, when using an acetone polish remover on artificial nails, the acetone can soften the artificial nail product. Non-acetone polish removers are available to prevent this from occurring due to a solvent called ethyl acetate, which is an effective polish remover, even though it works slower.

Nail Polish Ingredients

Nail polish contains six main ingredients: resins, solvents, plasticizers, UV stabilizers, pigments and dispersants. It is the exact proportions of these ingredients that make each type of polish unique.

Resin

Resin is the tough material that holds polish together. Resins are a type of polymer, which means they are composed of giant molecules that were made by linking smaller molecules into long chains and networks. Be aware that different resins have different properties. For example, nitrocellulose resin is a film former that gives the polish strength and a shiny surface. A top coat may contain more of this resin in order to achieve the high shine, but

too much of this ingredient may make the nail polish too strong, reducing flexibility and causing it to become brittle. Some polishes contain tosylamide/formaldehyde resin, which is NOT the same chemical as formaldehyde. This resin makes the polish adhere better and adds some flexibility, preventing it from becoming like glass and breaking or chipping easily. Other polymers that may be used include polyvinyl butyral (for adhesion), cellulose acetate butyrate and acrylates copolymer (for hardness).

FORMALDEHYDE VS. FORMALDEHYDE RESIN

Formaldehyde is a small, reactive molecule that is used at a very low level in nail hardeners to cross-link nail proteins. **Cross-linking** causes the creation of additional chemical bonds between different protein strands in the nail, which works well for many clients. However, some clients' nails can become over-cross-linked and brittle as a result. In such a case, it's better to alternate every few weeks between a hardener and a regular clear coat, rather than only using hardener.

Many other products contain a resin called tosylamide/formaldehyde resin. As the name suggests, formaldehyde is one of the building blocks of this resin. However, since the formaldehyde is bound up in long molecular chains (polymers), it is far less active and will not cross-link the nail protein as does free formaldehyde.

Solvents in Nail Polish

Solvents are liquids that dissolve a solid, liquid or gas. The most common solvent is water. The substance dissolved by the solvent is called a solute. Solvents usually evaporate easily leaving the dissolved substance behind. When a solvent can no longer dissolve a substance, it is considered saturated. For example, when a cotton ball is wet with polish remover, and you've already removed some polish it will no longer remove any more because it is saturated.

Solvents work differently when used in nail polish. They act as the ingredients responsible for the "workability" by dissolving the pigments and other ingredients and drying the polish by evaporating and leaving the pigments and resin behind. Evaporation is the act of liquids leaving a substance, with only the solids remaining. There is no curing involved in nail polish drying; it all happens by evaporation of the solvents.

The solvent must be compatible with the resin in the polish so that it can be spread on the nail. After the polish has been applied, the solvent must evaporate evenly, leaving behind a smooth, hard coat. Because solvents that evaporate too slowly or too quickly can ruin the coat of polish, the right solvent combination must be used. A fast-drying top coat may contain different types or amounts of solvents in order to achieve the fast-drying action. Some common solvents are butyl acetate, toluene, ethyl acetate and isopropyl alcohol.

As the solvents evaporate, nail polish in the bottle becomes thicker. It is not recommended that polish remover or acetone be used to thin old polish because these solvents may not be compatible with the resin in the polish. Always follow the manufacturer's instructions.

Plasticizers

Plasticizers are additives that keep the polish flexible after it is dry. Think of plasticizers as sort of a lubricant in between the polymer chains, which allows them to move around without breaking. This makes the polish stronger and less likely to chip. Some common plasticizers

are dibutyl phthalate, camphor, trimethyl pentanyl diisobutyrate and triphenyl phosphate. Plasticizers can also be used in artificial nail products to keep polymer chains flexible.

UV Stabilizers

UV stabilizers are additives that help keep the polish from changing color when it is exposed to too much UV light from the sun. Some UV stabilizers are the same chemicals used in sun-protection lotions applied to the skin. Benzophenone-1 is an example of a UV stabilizer found in nail polishes. UV stabilizers can also be additives found in artificial nail products.

Pigments

Pigments or colors are the essence of polish. A variety of drug and cosmetic-approved dyes are used. Most polish colors require a combination of different pigments, which have been ground into very fine powders and mixed in the right proportions to create the desired color. Frost and shimmer polishes are created by adding sparkling, reflective particles, such as mica. The size of the particles helps determine the way the polish sparkles. Pigments are not just used in nail polish, since they can also be found in acrylic monomer liquids, acrylic polymers and gels to give them a colored effect.

Dispersants

Dispersants are additives that help the pigments mix with the resin and solvent. Sometimes pigments have a tendency to settle or separate from the solvent/resin mixture. Dispersants partially prevent this. However, even with the best dispersants some settling of the pigments may eventually happen. This is why it's important to mix the polish before using it.

All information on Nail Polish Ingredients courtesy of Paul Bryson, Ph.D., OPI Products Inc.

5

Adhesives and Priming Agents

Adhesion is a type of molecular attraction that causes two different surfaces to stick together by an interaction between molecules. It's important to understand adhesion in order to know how and why nail products adhere to the nail plate. Adhesives and priming agents make two incompatible surfaces adhere to one another. For example, a nail tip won't stick to the nail plate by itself. Adhesive allows the materials in the nail tip to adhere with the keratin in the nail. Two of the most common products used in the nail industry for adhesion are adhesives and priming agents, or primers.

Have you ever painted a wall that has cobwebs, crayon marks or dirt on it? The paint will chip or peel. Remember to remove all oils and debris from the nail plate before applying any product. That is why a clean, oil-free surface is key in the adhesion process. Without a clean surface, adhesion cannot take place even when using a primer.

Adhesives

Adhesives are products that create a bond between two incompatible surfaces, such as a nail tip and the nail plate. In order for an adhesive to work effectively it must be compatible with the two surfaces it bonds together. For example, ordinary school glue is made to bond porous surfaces like paper, cloth and wood. But if this same adhesive is used to bond two pieces of plastic, the bond can be broken with little force because it is not porous. However, when used on paper the bond is very strong and the paper will tear before the bond is broken. Nail adhesives are created to be compatible with the keratin in the nail and common materials found in nail enhancement products.

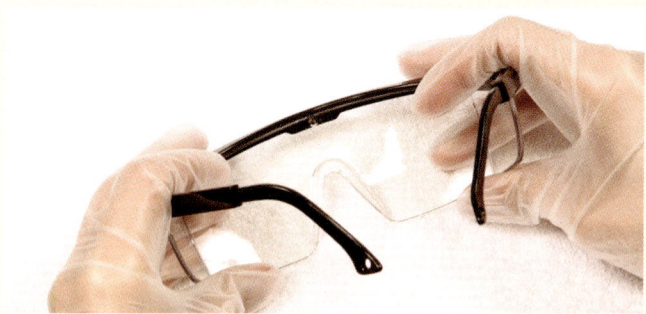

When using primers, it's recommended to use safety goggles and gloves to avoid contact with skin during application. This is especially important when applying a primer containing methacrylic acid.

Priming Agents

Priming agents, or primers, are products that help create the adhesion needed between the nail plate and a nail enhancement product such as acrylic artificial nail product. Primers are used in most acrylic liquid and powder systems and some gel systems. Since the nail plate and an acrylic product are incompatible surfaces, adhesion would be very weak without the use of a primer. Typically, the ingredient in the primer that helps with adhesion is a corrosive acid called methacrylic acid. Methacrylic acid works to rid the nail plate of any remaining oils in order to create a strong bond between the nail product and the nail plate. However, in general, primers are not meant to eliminate bacteria or dissolve any oils, so it is important to properly prepare the nails first.

Although "non-acid" or "acid-free" primers may be found in the marketplace, keep in mind that these typically contain some type of acid, even though it may be less corrosive.

Don't be afraid of the word acid. Acid doesn't necessarily mean harmful. For example, there is a big difference between corrosive car-battery acid, and common salad vinegar, also known as acetic acid.

- *Courtesy of Paul Bryson, Ph.D., OPI Products Inc.*

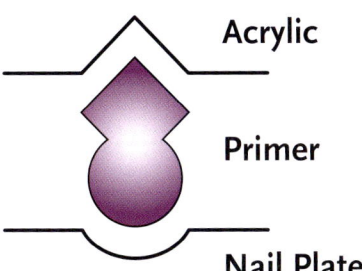

Acrylic

Primer

Nail Plate

Methacrylic acid and the milder acid primers work in the same way: the molecules have an "acid group" at one end and an "acrylic group" at the other. The acid group bonds to the nail protein and the acrylic group bonds to the acrylic enhancement as it cures. The difference is the size and configuration of the acid molecules. The methacrylic molecules are much smaller, which allows them to penetrate the skin and can cause burning or irritation.

5

Monomers and Polymers

As a nail technician you will hear and use the words monomers and polymers when talking about artificial nail products. All artificial nail products contain monomers and polymers, and most often you will hear these terms referred to in acrylic liquid and powder systems. However, remember that all artificial nail enhancement products contain monomers and polymers.

A **monomer** is a small, single molecule that may become chemically bonded to other monomer molecules to form a polymer when it comes into contact with an initiator.

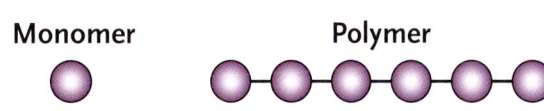

Monomer   **Polymer**

A **polymer** is made up of many monomers that are chemically bonded to form chains or networks. Polymers are formed by monomers that undergo polymerization, a chemical reaction that links the molecules together from end to end.

Monomers are typically in free-flowing liquid form, which is combined with powder polymer to form an acrylic nail. However, monomers are also found in wrap resins and gels, which are pre-mixed with polymers.

Mono is from the Greek prefix meaning one. **Poly** is from the Greek prefix meaning many. One polymer chain can contain thousands or even millions of monomers, and one small granule of acrylic powder contains thousands of polymer chains.

Cross-Linking Monomers

Simple polymer chains are formed when monomers link together end-to-end in a single-file line. However, cross-linking monomers create a web effect by linking one monomer to four or sometimes six monomers

Simple Polymer   **Cross-Linked Polymer**

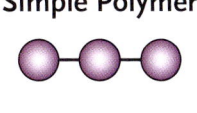

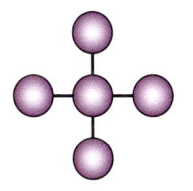

to create a cross-linked polymer. Basically, the cross-linking monomers allow polymer chains to link with other polymer chains. These form an even stronger bond that imparts strength to the nail or artificial nail.

While the advantage of a cross-linked polymer is additional strength, the drawback is that the excessive cross-linking makes it more difficult for solvents to break down the product for removal. For example, wrap resins are simple polymer chains and can be easily removed with acetone. However, gels are highly cross-linked polymers and are more difficult for a solvent to break down. Too much cross-linking can also make the nails too brittle. Knowing this, as well as the information you just learned on removers and polish ingredients, will aid you in your abilities to make the right choices when applying and removing nail products.

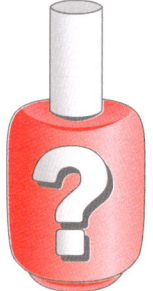

When a client expresses concern about the chemicals in products such as polish remover or product remover, what would you say to put her at ease?

CHEMISTRY OF ARTIFICIAL NAIL SYSTEMS

Have you ever wondered why sometimes creating an artificial nail requires the mixture of a powder and a liquid and others require you to place your hands under a light? Well, an understanding of chemistry answers these questions and provides you with the knowledge of how artificial nail products work. Since there are several types of artificial nail systems, it is important to know the chemical differences between them. Not only does good product knowledge help you answer questions your clients ask, it also helps you gain confidence in your ability to provide artificial nail services. Let's look at the main types of artificial nail systems: nail wraps, acrylic nails and gel nails.

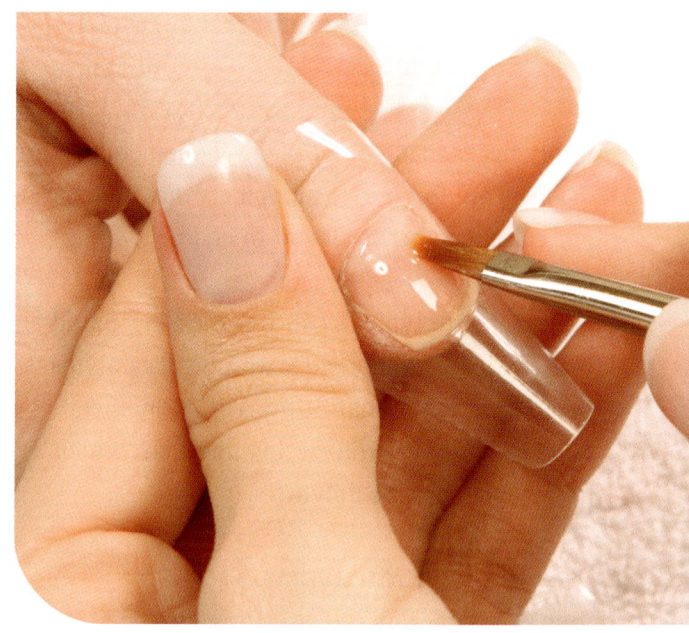

Nail Wrap Systems

Nail wrap systems involve the application of a thick resin over a piece of fabric. Most nail wrap systems contain three key products: wrap resin, accelerator and fabric. In *Chapter 9, Artificial Nail Services*, you will learn more about the various products and how to apply them, but first you need an understanding of their chemical makeup.

Wrap Resin

Wrap resin is an adhesive used to create layers over the nail when using a wrap system. Wrap resin primarily contains a monomer from the acrylic family called cyanoacrylates, as well as a polymer that acts as a thickener and inhibitor to prevent the resin from curing too fast.

Cyanoacrylates are known as instant adhesives because they rapidly polymerize in the presence of water, forming long, strong chains that join bonded surfaces together. Another feature is that cyanoacrylates set or dry fast, often in less than a minute. A normal bond reaches full strength in two hours and is waterproof.

Because the presence of moisture causes the adhesive to set, exposure to moisture in the air can cause a tube or bottle of resin or adhesive to become unusable over time. Therefore, it is important to always make sure your bottles are sealed tightly.

Be aware that cyanoacrylates usually have a shorter shelf life—approximately six months. This is why you may have a brand new bottle of adhesive that is completely dried up!

Cyanoacrylates or resins are used in other types of systems commonly called no-light gels or dip systems.

Accelerator

Accelerators are ingredients used to set wrap resins in just a few seconds. Accelerators are known as catalysts, since they help control the speed of the chemical reaction, which in this case, is the curing process. Wrap resins will cure without using an accelerator but will do so much more slowly. Since the accelerator speeds up the chemical reaction, your client may experience a warm feeling on the nails. Because of this, take caution during your application of the wrap resin and catalyst.

Heat Reaction

Sometimes chemical reactions cause heat to be released. If your client experiences this, it means that too much product is undergoing the chemical reaction too quickly. For this reason, some products are applied in several layers instead of in one thick layer.

To prevent your client from experiencing an uncomfortable heat reaction, be sure to keep the layers of resin thin and apply all products according to the manufacturer's instructions.

Fabric

Different types of fabrics are used with nail wrap systems. These include fiberglass, silk, linen and nylon. Fabric is used with a nail wrap system to add strength since wrap resins are usually not cross-linked. Since fabrics do not undergo a chemical reaction, fabrics can also be added to a gel service to add more strength to the nail.

Liquid and Powder Acrylic Systems

Liquid and powder acrylic systems are another option when creating an artificial nail. Unlike nail wraps, the nail is created by combining a liquid and a powder, placing them onto the nail and letting the product cure, or dry. An acrylic system typically contains two key ingredients: a liquid monomer and powder polymer.

Liquid Monomer

Most liquid monomers, also known as acrylic liquids, contain acrylic monomers, cross-linking monomers, catalysts and inhibitors. Typically, ethyl methacrylate is used as the primary monomer in acrylic liquid. However, other monomers are added to give different properties. Cross-linking monomers are added to create a strong network. Commonly used cross-linking monomers are dimethacrylate or trimethacrylate.

Catalysts are also added to speed up the chemical reaction as previously discussed.

Methyl Methacrylate Monomer
In the early 1970s, the Food and Drug Administration (FDA) received a number of complaints of personal injury associated with the use of acrylic monomers containing methyl methacrylate. On the basis of its investigations of the injuries and discussions with medical experts in the field of dermatology, the FDA concluded that liquid methyl methacrylate is a poisonous substance that should not be used in acrylic monomers. However, methyl methacrylate is safe to use in acrylic polymers.

Inhibitors are used as preservatives that keep the monomers from "setting up" or curing on their own. Properly inhibited liquids will last one to two years before the inhibitor runs out. This will also happen if it becomes contaminated or is exposed to heat or sunlight.

Traditional Monomer vs. Odorless Monomer
The sizes of the molecules in different liquid monomer products play a role in determining whether there is an odor associated with the product and the evaporation of the product. The smaller the molecule size, the faster it evaporates, producing more odor. Generally, odorless acrylic monomers have larger molecules, which is why an odorless acrylic system has little or no odor compared to a traditional acrylic system. Also, odorless acrylic liquid doesn't evaporate as quickly.

EMA – Ethyl Methacrylate
- Commonly used traditional acrylic monomer
- High evaporation

MEM – Methoxyethoxy Ethyl Methacrylate
- Commonly used odorless acrylic monomer
- Low evaporation

Other additives that may be contained within the liquid monomer are dyes, plasticizers and UV-protective color stabilizers.

A light-cured powder and liquid acrylic system is similar to a traditional powder and liquid system. However, the initiator and catalyst are removed from the liquid and powder so that the product will not polymerize by simply mixing the two together. Instead, a photo initiator is added to the liquid and polymerization begins when it is exposed to a light source. This begins the curing process.

Powder Polymer
Most powder polymers, also referred to as acrylic powders, contain polymers and initiators while others also contain pigments to give color and silica to keep them free-flowing. Initiators are necessary for the liquid monomer to begin its chemical reaction. This is why acrylic monomer does not begin polymerization until it is mixed with the powder polymer.

Light-Cured Gel Systems

Gel systems are different from acrylics in two ways. First, the product comes in gel form, which doesn't require the combining of a liquid and a powder. Second, the product doesn't cure without exposure to a light source. Most often gel systems are referred to as UV gels. This is because UV gel products must be exposed to ultraviolet (UV) light to cure. However, there are also other gel systems that use other light sources, such as halogen light, to cure.

Gel
Gels are mainly made of acrylic **oligomers**. An oligomer is a short chain version of a polymer. Whereas a polymer may have thousands or millions of monomer links, an oligomer consists of a limited number of monomer links—anywhere from five to 500.

All light-cured gels use photo initiators to begin the curing process. Gels can also contain a wide variety of other ingredients depending on their usage. Base gels, also referred to as gel primers, contain priming molecules. Some gels may have monomers for thinning and speeding up the curing process. For example, for a smooth finish, a sealer, also called a finishing gel, is applied on top of the gel nail causing it to self-level, or spread evenly on its own. A building, or sculpting gel, used to create the artificial nails, may contain silica or polymers for thickening so they will hold their shape. Some gels may contain cross-linking monomers; however, most oligomers used in gels are diacrylates or dimethacrylates, which act as their own cross-linkers. Some also contain pigments to give color.

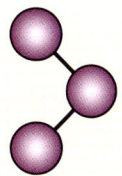

UAO – Urethane Acrylate Oligomers
- Commonly used oligomer for light-cured gels
- No evaporation

As you can see, gels are also odorless due to the size of their molecules in comparison to acrylic monomers. This molecule size is much larger because of the multiple monomers. This means there is no evaporation, and the product does not produce an odor.

5

Frequently Asked Questions About Gels

Q. Why do different gels cure at different speeds?

A. Heat is released during the curing process and may need to be slowed down to prevent burning. Also, in colored gels, pigments partially block the curing light, which slows down the curing process.

Q. Why is it so important to use the same brand of gel and lamp?

A. Different lamps operate at different intensities and manufacturers make their products to be compatible only with their lamps. If you use a mismatched lamp, the cure may happen too quickly and create too much heat, or it may happen too slowly and never cure at all.

– Courtesy of Paul Bryson, Ph.D., OPI Products Inc.

Remember that many of the clients you will encounter in your professional career will express concerns over the chemicals related to the nail products and services you will be providing them. It is your responsibility to put their minds at ease through your knowledge of how nail chemicals work and react. If you're able to do that with confidence, they will trust and rely on you for years to come.

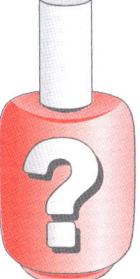

Can you explain why some artificial nail services require the use of a light, while others do not?

DECISION-MAKING SKILLS

Case Studies

The following situations are designed to help you build decision-making skills. Using your training to this point, review the following scenarios, then think through and describe how you would handle each challenge.

1. A new client for artificial nails can't decide which type she would like: wraps, acrylic or gel. How would you explain the products' differences to her so she understands and can decide among them?

2. A client comes in with a broken nail. When you ask if she wants it repaired with a wrap, she states "Oh, no, I don't want any chemicals on my nails." What would you say?

3. A client is concerned when she looks at the ingredients on the nail polish and sees the words "tosylamide/formaldehyde resin" because she's heard that you should never use a polish with formaldehyde in it. How would you explain to her that it is safe to use?

Did you know that nails and skin can tell us a lot about the overall health and condition of the body? It's true. As a nail technician, your primary concern will be taking care of nails by providing services that promote and preserve their healthy condition. Knowing how the services you provide will benefit your clients begins with an understanding of the structure and functions of the nails and the skin that surrounds them. Equally important when providing nail services is to protect you and your clients from the spread of infection. In this chapter, you will also discover how to identify nail and skin diseases and disorders to help you determine when it is safe to proceed with a service.

VALUE

The ability to identify—not diagnose—nail and skin diseases and disorders and know their causes adds value to the services you provide your clients.

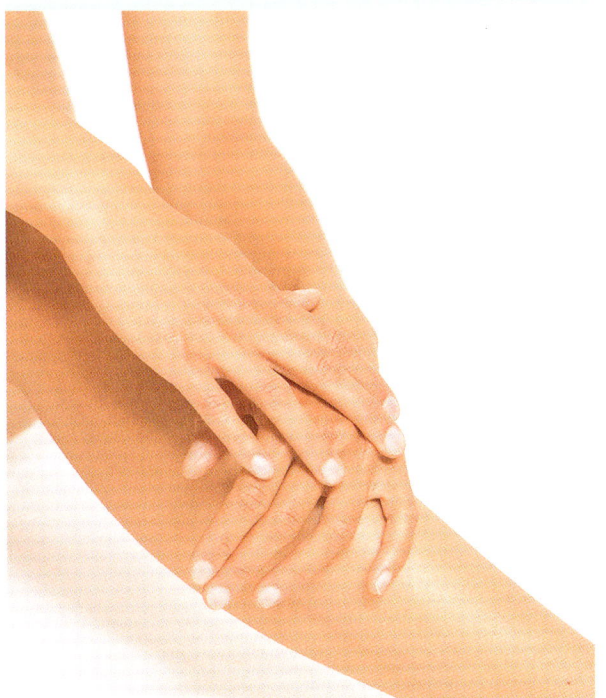

MAIN IDEA

All successful nail technicians need an understanding of the nail from the inside out. This chapter focuses on the structure and growth of nails as well as the diseases and disorders that you may encounter. As a professional nail technician, you will be working with the skin on the hands and feet as well. This chapter provides information on the functions and composition of the skin, as well as the diseases and disorders that nail technicians need to be aware of in order to provide safe and effective services.

PLAN	OBJECTIVES
Nail Physiology • Composition of the Nail • Nail Growth • Nail Diseases and Disorders	Describe the structure of the nail. Explain the growth process of the nail. Identify and describe common nail diseases and disorders.
Skin Physiology • Functions of the Skin • Composition of the Skin • Skin Diseases and Disorders	List the six primary functions of the skin. Describe the basic physiology of the skin. Recognize common diseases and disorders of the skin.

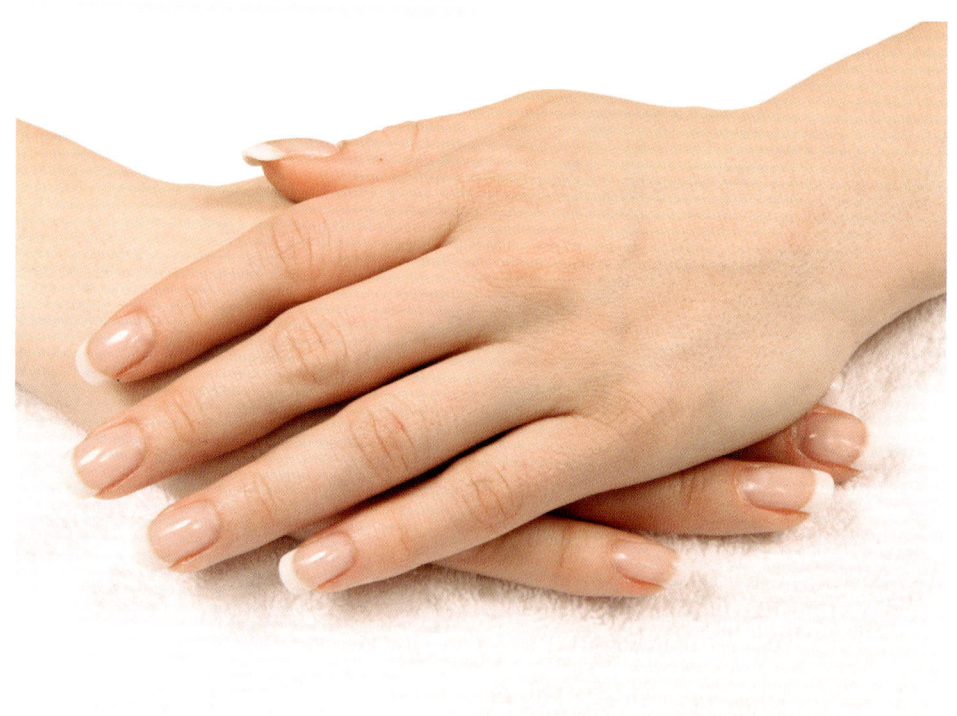

Composition of the Nail

To understand the growth of healthy nails, you must become familiar with the structure, or composition, of the nail. The best way to begin your study is to familiarize yourself with the location and function of essential parts of the nail structure.

1. The **free edge** is the part of the nail plate that extends beyond the end of the finger or toe and protects the tip of the finger or toe.

2   The **onychodermal** (ON-ih-koh-DER-mal) **band** appears as a glassy, grayish band at the point where the nail plate meets the hyponichium.

3. The **nail plate**, sometimes referred to as the nail body, is the visible nail area from the nail root to the free edge. It is made up of several transparent layers of hardened cells, which do not contain any nerves or blood vessels.

4. The **nail wall** consists of the folds of skin on either side of the nail groove.

5. The **lunula** (LOON-oo-la) is the white, half-moon shape at the base of the nail.

> The lunula, from the Latin word meaning *moon*, appears white due to a reflection of light at the point where the nail matrix and nail bed meet.

6. The **eponychium** (ep-o-NIK-ee-um) is the area that overlies the matrix at the base of the nail. It also serves as a watertight seal that protects the matrix against infection.

7. The **cuticle** is the loose and pliable overlapping skin, which forms a watertight seal around the nail. It is a thin layer of skin that, as it sheds, attaches to the top layer of the nail plate.

Hyponychium 15
1 Free Edge
2 Onychodermal Band
Bed Epithelium 14
3 Nail Plate (Nail Body)
Perionychium 13
4 Nail Wall
Nail Folds 12 (Nail Grooves)
5 Lunula
Nail Bed 11
6 Eponychium
7 Cuticle
8 Nail Matrix
9 Nail Root
10 Mantle

2 Onychodermal Band
14 Bed Epithelium
8 Nail Matrix

8. The **nail matrix** is the active tissue that generates cells, which harden as they move outward from the nail root to the nail plate.

9. The **nail root** is attached to the nail matrix at the base of the nail, under the skin and inside the mantle.

10. The **mantle** is the pocket-like structure that holds the nail root and nail matrix.

11. The **nail bed** is the area of the nail on which the nail plate rests. Nerves and blood vessels found here supply nourishment to the entire nail unit.

> **Specialized ligaments,** also called **nail body ligaments**, attach the nail bed to the bone.

12. The **nail folds**, sometimes referred to as **grooves**, are the tracks on either side of the nail that the nail moves on as it grows.

13. The **perionychium** (PER-i-o-nik-ee-um) is the skin that touches, overlaps and surrounds the side of the nail.

14. The **bed epithelium** (ep-i-THEE-lee-um) is a thin, sticky layer of the epidermis (uppermost layer of skin) that attaches the nail plate to the nail bed.

15. The **hyponychium** (hy-poh-NIK-ee-um) is the skin under the free edge, which acts as a watertight seal to prevent bacteria from entering the nail bed.

Now that you know where each of the parts of the nail is located, it will be easier to understand the way the nail grows.

NAIL PHYSIOLOGY

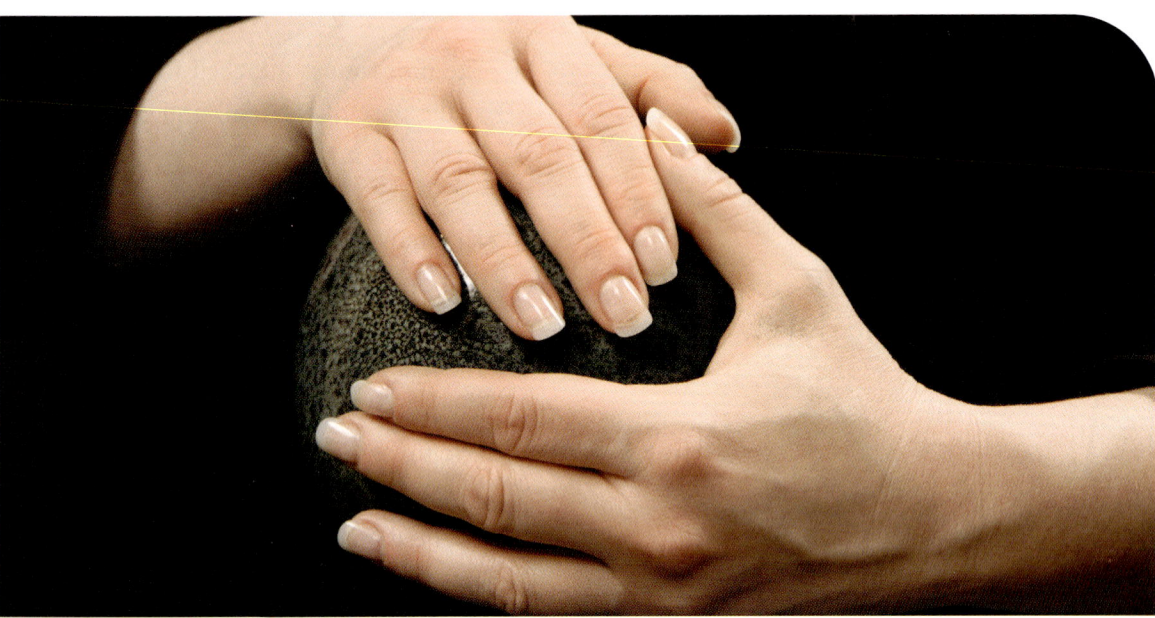

Nail Growth

Nails, skin and hair are all formed by a protein substance called **keratin**. While skin and hair are made up of soft keratin, nails are composed of hard keratin that helps protect the tips of the fingers and toes. Nails are appendages of the skin, which means that they are a part of the skin, the largest organ of the body.

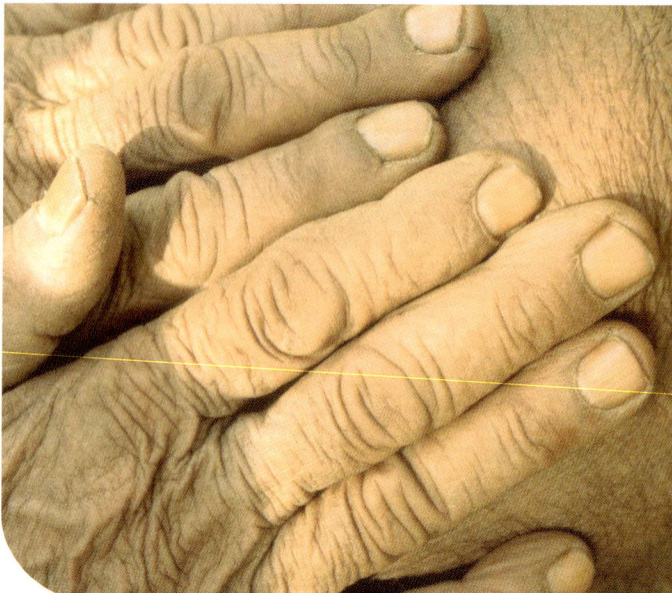

Aging and the Nail
As a person ages, nail growth tends to slow and nails are likely to be more brittle. Prominent ridges may also appear on the nail plate.

6

Throughout history nails have been used for various purposes: as weapons for self defense, for prying open objects, hunting, digging and eating. In addition to being useful, nails have evolved as physical features that can be beautified to express personal style. What many people forget, though, is that nails are also a valuable indicator of a person's health. It is important that, as a nail technician, you are able to recognize any abnormalities that indicate the presence of a disease or disorder of the nail. This way, you will be able to identify when it is safe to perform a service on a client and when it is necessary to refer a client to a physician.

The technical name for the nail is **onyx** (ON-iks) just like the gemstone of the same name. The study of the structure and growth of the nails is called **onychology** (on-ih-KOL-o-gee).

You already know from *Chapter 4, Anatomy,* that -ology means the study of something. If you add onyx + ology, you get onychology.

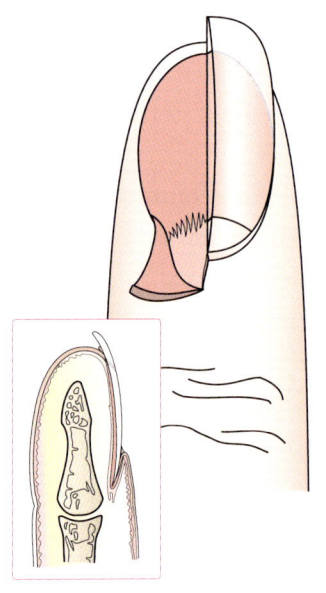

Turn the page to view the **"Composition of the Nail"** fold-out.

Nail growth originates from active tissue known as the nail matrix, located in the mantle. The nail matrix contains lymph, blood vessels and nerves that create cells, which are pushed outward from the nail root. These cells **keratinize**, or harden, as they grow toward the nail plate and become fully hardened by the time they reach the eponychium. These hardened cells form the visible nail plate that grows along tracks on either side of the nail called nail folds. The nail plate can be thin, normal or thick, depending on the rate of production of cells in the nail matrix. The nail bed on which the nail plate rests contains many nerves, as well as blood vessels for continuous nourishment.

Nails grow at an average rate of 1/8" (.375 cm) per month in adults. Under normal circumstances, growth of a new fingernail takes about four to six months. Toenails, which are harder and thicker than fingernails, grow at a slower rate and take about 10-12 months to grow a new nail plate. Nails grow more rapidly in younger people because general cell reproduction is occurring at a faster rate. Thus, as one ages, the growth of nails slows down.

Nail growth is faster in summer than in winter, and can be affected by nutrition, health or disease. The longer the nail matrix, the faster the nail grows. This fact explains why each nail grows at a different rate. For example, the thumbnail grows slowest, while the nail on the middle finger grows the fastest.

Injuries to the nail can result in shape distortions or nail discoloration. Most nail injuries are minor and resulting distortions and/or discoloration are temporary. Permanent distortions can occur when:

- A nail is lost due to injury and, without the protection of the nail plate, the nail bed or nail matrix is injured.
- A nail is lost through disease or infection. The regrown nail, in these circumstances, is often distorted in shape.

Nail Diseases and Disorders

It is important that a nail technician be able to tell the difference between a diseased or damaged nail and a healthy one since certain precautions are required when servicing them. A disease is a pathological condition that results from causes associated with genetic ailments, environmental factors or infections. Infectious diseases can stem from bacteria, viruses or fungi. A disorder is an ailment from injury or imbalance that affects the functions of the mind and/or body.

Any disease or disorder of the nail is called an **onychosis** (on-i-KO-sis). A study of onychosis considers four factors:

1. Identification of the disease or disorder.
2. **Etiology** (e-te-OL-o-je) or the study of the cause of a disease or disorder.
   a) Systemic causes are internal and occur throughout the system. They are related to illness, disease, nutrition or heredity.
   b) Environmental causes include injury to the nail or nail services or products (chemicals) that have adversely altered the skin or nail.
   c) Disease-related causes are often invasion of the skin or nail tissues by an agent like bacteria or fungi. These agents are contagious and spread by contact.
3. Indications of an onychosis include the symptoms and appearance of the nail and surrounding skin.
4. Services:
   a) Products used and recommended for home care.
   b) Techniques used and taught to the client.

In order to determine whether it is safe to perform a service on a client, it is helpful to refer to these guidelines:

- If a disease is present, nail services may not be performed on affected nails or, in some cases, on any nails at all; the client must be referred to a physician.
- If a disorder is present, nail services may be performed with care; the client may want to consult a physician for help treating it.

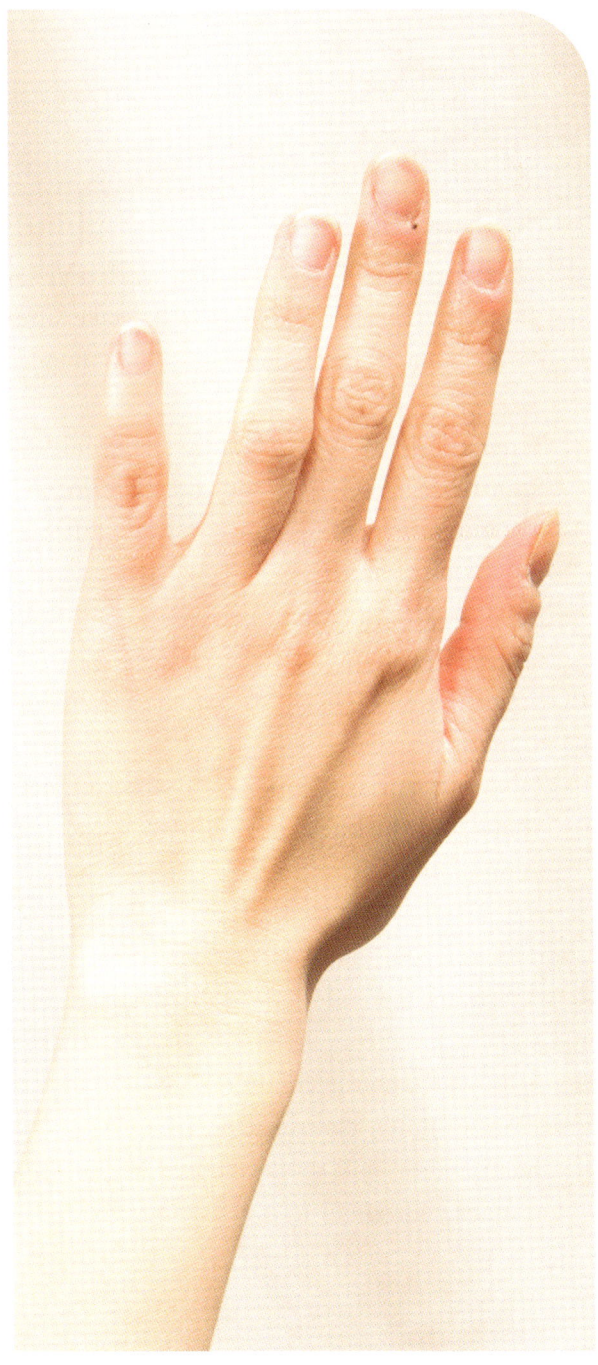

6

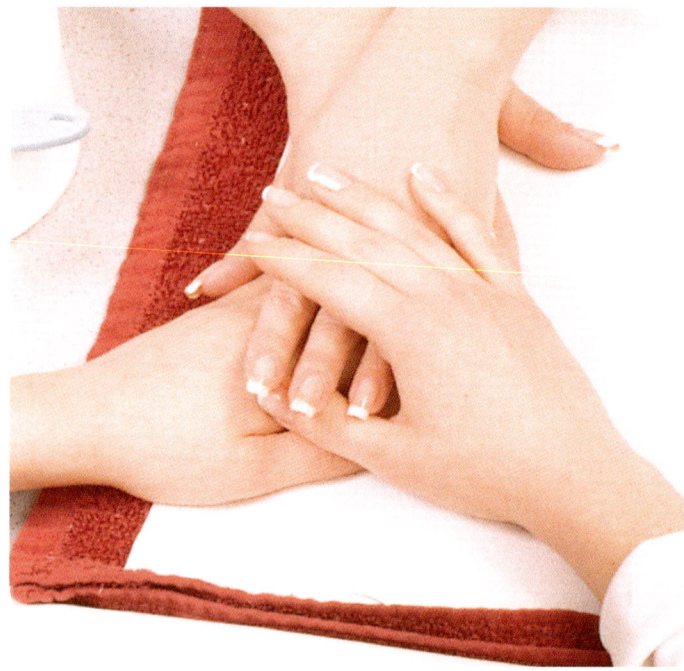

Hand and Nail Examination

To discover problems associated with the hands, nails or growth of nails, begin with a hand and nail examination. During a medical exam, a physician may look at a patient's hands, since they can indicate the health of the body. As a nail technician, you observe the hands and nails to determine the types of services that should be performed to improve their condition and appearance. There are six signs of infection that can be found on the hand or nail: pain, swelling, redness, local fever, throbbing and pus. If an infection is present, no service should be performed. A healthy nail is smooth, curved and without hollows or wavy ridges. It is flexible, translucent and pinkish in color.

Before performing an examination, wash and sanitize your hands and require that the client wash and sanitize his or her hands as well. Make sure to put on protective gloves if required by your regulating agency. Then, hold the client's hands and look at both front and back while observing:

- **Temperature of skin**—Coldness may indicate poor circulation; heat may indicate infection.
- **Skin texture/feel**—May indicate need for moisture.
- **Inflammation/redness on hand or nail**—May indicate need for moisture or possible disease or disorder.
- **Color/condition of nail bed**—May identify visible injuries, disease and/or indication of poor circulation.
- **Condition and length of free edge**—May identify nail biter or "picker;" may indicate dry, brittle nails.
- **Tenderness or stiff joints**—May indicate need to alter massage to ensure client comfort.
- **Shape and thickness of nail plate**—May indicate a disease or disorder and how to properly file.

Upon recognizing that a special condition exists, explain the condition to the client and suggest products and care techniques that can help overcome the condition. Certain nail irregularities (often disease-related), however, must be referred to a physician for diagnosis or treatment and no nail service should be performed until the condition is alleviated. When in doubt, refer your client to a physician.

> Avoid changing polish more than once a week. The use of polish remover when changing polish tends to strip the nails of natural oils causing dryness.

Nail Diseases

As a professional nail technician, you will encounter clients with nail diseases. Of diseases and disorders, diseases are more serious. Clients with nail diseases must be referred to their physician for treatment before nail services can be provided, so it is beneficial for you to familiarize yourself with signs that can indicate a disease. Nail diseases can be caused by bacteria, fungi, viruses or illnesses. Identification of the nail diseases that follow is important to protect the health of you and your client.

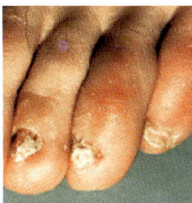

Onychomycosis (o-ni-ko-mi-KO-sis) or **tinea unguium** (TIN-ee-ah UN-gwee-um) or **unguis** (UN-gwees) is ringworm of the nail.
Cause: Fungal infection; disease-related; can result from a nail injury invaded by fungus.
Indications: Nail becomes thick and discolors from black to brown or beige to white; can develop white scaly patches with yellow streaks under nail plate; deformed nail may fall off.
Service: No service may be performed. Refer client to a physician.

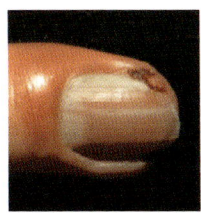

Paronychia (par-o-NIK-e-a), or **felon**, is inflammation of skin around the nail.
Cause: Bacterial infection; disease-related condition of the tissue surrounding the nail; can occur if a hangnail becomes infected. Prolonged exposure of hands to water can create conditions favorable for paronychia to develop.
Indications: Red, swollen, sore, warm to touch, can lose the nail; nail can grow out deformed but can recover shape.
Service: No service may be performed. Refer client to a physician.

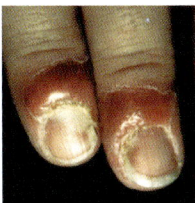

Onychia (o-NIK-e-a) is inflammation of the nail matrix.
Cause: Bacterial infection; disease-related.
Indications: Inflammation of the nail matrix, pus formation; red, swollen and tender; nail may stop growing and plate may detach; nail may grow back deformed or not at all.
Service: No service may be performed. Refer client to a physician.

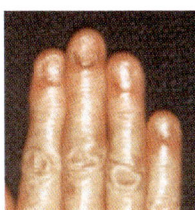

Onychoptosis (o-ni-kop-TO-sis) refers to shedding or falling off of nails.
Cause: Disease-related or injury to nail.
Indications: If the disease causing the problem is cured, the nail will regrow; may occur on only one or two nails; nail bed will be sensitive and should be protected while nail regrows.
Service: No service may be performed on affected nails. Refer client to a physician.

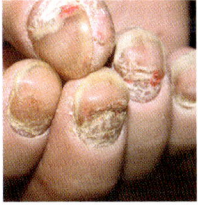

Onychomadesis (on-i-ko-MAH-de-sis) refers to loss of the nail plate with separation occurring at the nail matrix.
Cause: Disease-related or injury to nail.
Indications: A new nail will grow and push the previous nail off. It may occur on only a few nails.
Service: No service may be performed on the affected nails. Refer client to a physician.

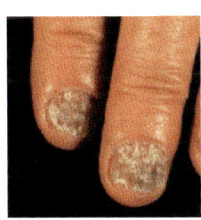

Onychatrophia (o-ni-ka-TRO-fe-a) is atrophy of the nail or wasting away of the nail.
Cause: Injury to nail; systemic; disease-related.

Indications: Nail shrinks in size and may separate from nail bed; may not improve if matrix is damaged.
Service: No service may be performed on affected nails. Refer client to a physician.

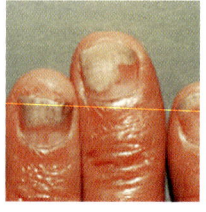

Onycholysis (o-ni-KOL-i-sis) refers to a loosening or separation of the nail.
Cause: Infection or drug treatment; systemic; disease-related; injury to nail.

Indications: Loosening of the nail plate starting at the free edge and progressing to the lunula; stays attached at root area.
Service: No service may be performed on affected nails. Refer client to a physician.

Discoloration of the nail can be due to numerous causes, both internal and external. These include: drugs, dyes, damage, disease, injury, illness, medication reactions, infections and vitamin deficiencies. Some chemicals can stain the nail plate. Base coats not only help colored polish adhere to the nail, they also help prevent staining from pigmented polish. In general, all changes of nail color should be referred to a physician unless they can be removed by a cleansing agent like soap.

NAIL DISEASES

Name	Description	Service
Onychomycosis	Ringworm of the nail	No service
Paronychia or felon	Inflammation of the skin around the nail	No service
Onychia	Inflammation of the nail matrix	No service
Onychoptosis	Shedding or falling off of the nail	No service on affected nails
Onychomadesis	Separation of the nail plate from the nail matrix	No service on affected nails
Onychatrophia	Wasting away of the nail	No service on affected nails
Onycholysis	Loosening of the nail	No service on affected nails

Nail Disorders

Nail disorders can be the physical result of an injury or nail disease. Clients with nail disorders may receive modified services if no infection is present. The following is a list of nail disorders with service modifications.

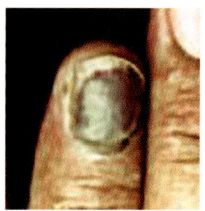

Blue nails appear bluish in color.
Cause: Systemic problems of the heart; poor circulation; injury to nail.
Indications: "Blue" color in skin under nails; common in older people.
Service: Make client aware of problem; refer client to a physician; perform services with caution using light pressure.

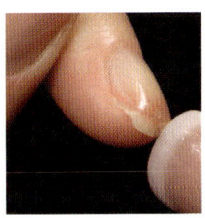

Eggshell nails are very thin, soft nails and sometimes curve over the free edge.
Cause: Heredity; nerve disorder.
Indications: Thin nails; almost see-through or transparent.
Service: Regular application of top coat, nail strengtheners or artificial nails.

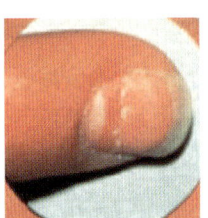

Corrugations (kor-u-GA-shuns) are horizontal wavy ridges across the nail.
Cause: Injury to nail; systemic; uneven growth.
Indications: Easily recognizable; if injury-related, it may grow out; if systemic, may cause permanent ridges.
Service: Lightly buff to level the nail surface without overbuffing; apply a base coat or ridge filler to protect and even out surface.

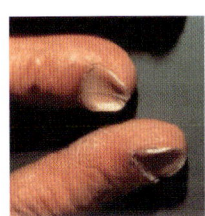

Koilonychia (kol-e-o-NIK-e-a) or **spoon nails** are nails with a concave shape.
Cause: Systemic; long-term illness; nerve disorder.
Indications: Unusual nail shapes; unlikely to disappear.
Service: File carefully; apply no pressure to nail plate; use polish to harden and protect nails.

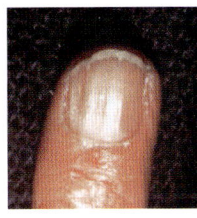

Furrows (FUR-ohs) are indented vertical lines down the nail plate.
Cause: Injury to matrix that causes cells to reproduce unevenly; nutritional deficiency; illness-related; using too much force when pushing back cuticles; exposure to harsh chemicals.
Indications: Easily recognizable; may grow out; may be permanent.

Service: Lightly buff; apply base coat or ridge filler to protect and even out surface; perform nail service as usual.

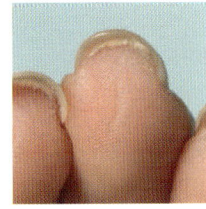

Pterygium (te-RIJ-ee-uhm) refers to living skin that becomes attached to the nail plate either at the eponychium (dorsal pterygium) or the hyponychium (inverse pterygium).
Cause: Severe injury to the eponychium or hyponychium.
Indications: Excess living skin that can remain attached to the nail plate and disrupt normal nail growth.
Service: No service may be performed on affected nails. If severe, refer the client to a physician.

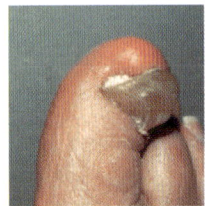

Onychogryposis (o-ni-ko-GRI-po-sis) also called "claw nails" represent an increased curvature of the nails.
Cause: Systemic.
Indications: Increased thickness and curving of the nail that may occur with age or injury to nail; most often occurring on the big toe; physician may remove nail if severely deformed or difficult to keep clean.
Service: Look for signs of infection; clean well under free edge; file with emery board and keep nails short; only a podiatrist (foot doctor) or physician should trim affected toenails.

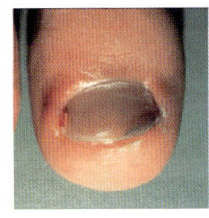

Onychocryptosis (o-ni-ko-KRIP-to-sis) are ingrown nails.
Cause: Poor nail trimming practices; trauma; heredity; can become infected; may also occur on toes if shoes are too tight, or if the toenails are filed too deeply on sides.
Indications: If the nail grows into the edge of the nail fold and becomes infected, refer client to a physician.

6

Service: Thoroughly soften skin; trim nail straight across to prevent pressure on the nail fold. Do not perform service if infection is present or the area is tender. Refer client to a physician.

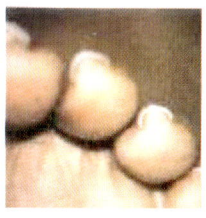

Tile-shaped nails have an exaggerated or deep "C" curve. **Cause:** Heredity. **Indications:** Appears to curve deeply into the nail folds; causes no discomfort. **Service:** Follow the curve of the nail when clipping; avoid cutting the nail too short; use caution not to cut into the skin under the nail.

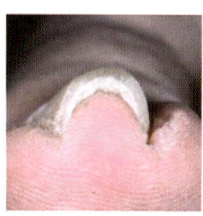

Pincer nails, also referred to as **trumpet nails,** have a nail plate that appears to narrow toward the free edge as the corners fold inward at the tip of the finger or toe. **Cause:** Heredity; bone spur beneath the nail; injury caused by wearing shoes too tight. **Indications:** Corners curve inward toward the free edge of the nail; may cause discomfort or pain. **Service:** Follow the curve of the nail when clipping; avoid cutting the nail too short; use caution not to cut into the skin under the nail; refer client to a physician if severe.

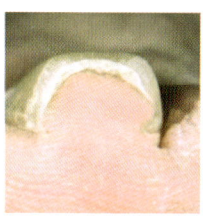

Plicatured nails appear to have a 90° or greater fold that begins at the matrix and extends the length of the nail plate to the free edge. **Cause:** Heredity; injury to nail; injury caused by wearing shoes too tight. **Indications:** Nail begins folding inward at a sharp angle into the surrounding skin; more predominant in toenails than fingernails.

Service: Follow the curve or angle of the nail when clipping; avoid cutting the nail too short; use caution not to cut into the skin under the nail.

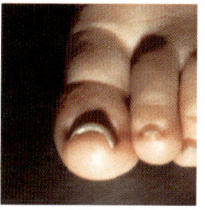

Onychauxis (o-ni-KOK-sis) or **hypertrophy** is a thickening of the nail plate or an abnormal outgrowth of the nail. **Cause:** Injury to nail; systemic. **Indications:** Easily recognizable; likely to disappear. **Service:** Can be lightly buffed to even out the nail plate.

Onychophyma (on-ih-ko-FEE-ma) is the swelling of the nail and is often associated with onychauxis.

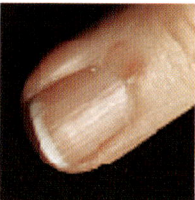

Agnails (hangnails) are split cuticles; loose skin partially separated from the cuticle. **Cause:** Cuticle is overly dry and splits; environmental. **Indications:** Skin breaks at corners of nails; can be trimmed with cuticle nippers if permitted by regulating agency; can be recurring. **Service:** Trim only separated hangnail skin completely; moisturize and avoid massaging the area; recommend that the client use cuticle conditioner daily. Hangnails may become infected if not properly treated.

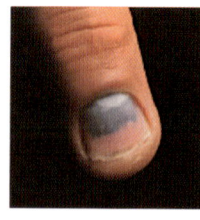

Bruised nails (also called splinter hemorrhages) show dark purplish discoloration under the nail. **Cause:** Injury to nail; environmental; blood trapped under nails or small capillaries that have hemorrhaged. **Indications:** Discoloration under nail; normal nail growth can continue; bruised area can grow out. **Service:** Use no pressure on nail plate.

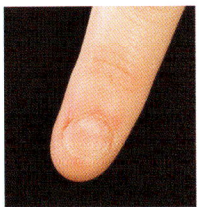

Onychophagy (o-ni-KOF-a-je) refers to bitten nails. **Cause:** Nervous habit; stress-related. **Indications:** Easily recognizable; if biting stops, the nails can regrow; may be sensitive to touch; nail plate will appear flat and may be deformed until an entire nail has regrown from the matrix. **Service:** Perform nail service weekly; apply polish to nails.

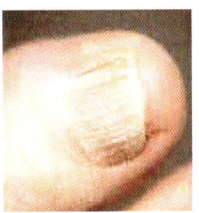

Onychorrhexis (o-ni-ko-REK-sis) are split or brittle nails. **Cause:** Injury to nail; improper filing; harsh chemical contact; aging. **Indications:** Easily recognizable; may be a permanent condition. **Service:** Soften nails well before trimming; file carefully with emery board; perform hot oil manicure; advise client to perform moisturizing treatments daily at home and to wear rubber gloves when hands come into contact with water or chemicals.

Brittle nails are the result of an imbalance of moisture and oil on the nail plate. Common causes of brittle nails include:
- Overuse of cuticle solvents containing AHA or glycolic acid
- Overexposure to water or other solvents
- Frequent nail polish changes

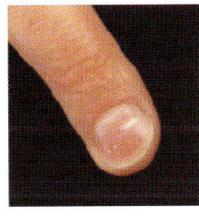

Leuconychia (loo-ko-NIK-e-a) are white spots appearing in the nail. **Cause:** Injury to nail; heredity; systemic; nutritional deficiency. **Indications:** Small separation from the nail bed; grows out. **Service:** Make client aware of possible cause; perform nail service as usual.

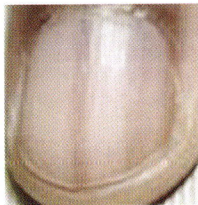

Melanonychia (mel-an-oh-NIK-e-a) generally appears as a tan, brown or black pigmented stripe down the length of the nail. **Cause:** Heredity. **Indications:** This tends to be more common in people with darker skin and is harmless. **Service:** Perform nail service as usual.

Melanonychia is more common in dark-skinned people than their light-skinned counterparts. If it is present in a light-skinned client, recommend that he or she see a physician to rule out a more serious health condition.

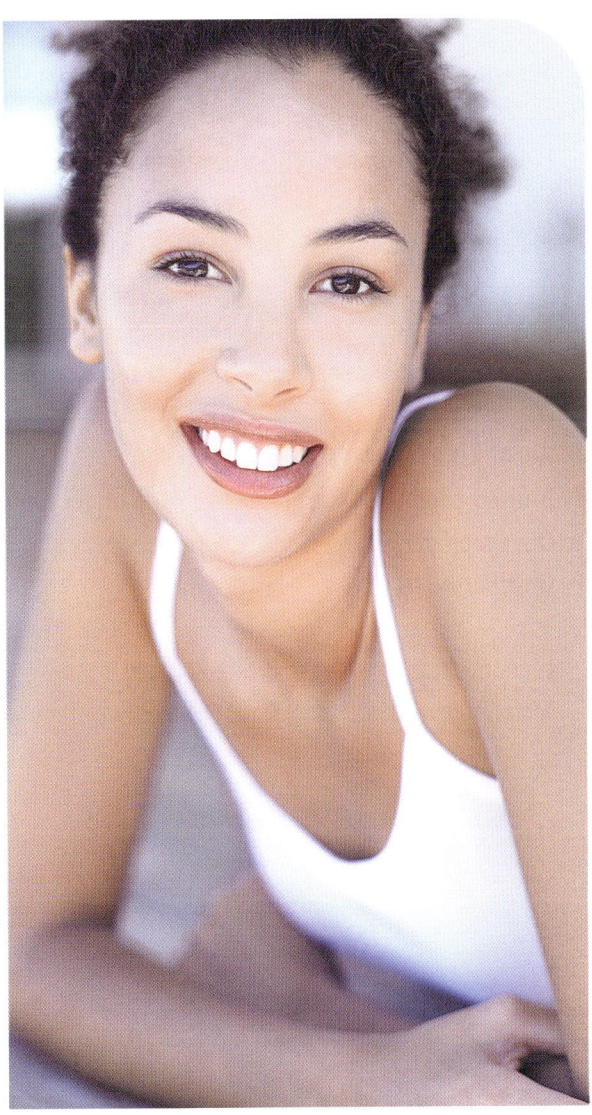

6

NAIL DISORDERS

Name	Description	Service
Blue nails	Appear bluish in color	Service; use light pressure
Eggshell nails	Thin, soft nails	Service; use light pressure and nail strengthener
Corrugations	Horizontal ridges across the nail plate	Service; lightly buff the surface
Koilonychia	Nails with a concave shape	Service; use light pressure and nail strengthener
Furrows	Indented vertical lines down the nail plate	Service; lightly buff the surface
Pterygium	Living skin attached to the nail plate	No service on affected nails
Onychogryposis	Claw nail; increased curvature	Service if there is no sign of infection; do not trim the nail; file to shorten
Onychocryptosis	Ingrown nail	Service if there is no sign of infection or tenderness; trim straight across
Tile-shaped nails	Exaggerated or deep c-curve	Service; use care when trimming; avoid trimming too short
Pincer nails (trumpet)	Corners fold inward at the tip of the finger or toe	Service; use care when trimming; avoid trimming too short
Plicatured nails	90° or greater fold	Service; use care when trimming; avoid trimming too short
Onychauxis hypertrophy	Thickening of the nail plate or an abnormal outgrowth of the nail	Service; use caution
Onychophyma	Swelling of the nail	Service; use caution
Agnails (hangnails)	Split cuticles	Service; use cuticle conditioner
Bruised nails	Discoloration under the nail plate	Service; no pressure on the nail
Onychophagy	Bitten nails	Service
Onychorrhexis	Brittle nails	Service; use cuticle conditioner and lotion
Leuconychia	White spots	Service
Melanonychia	Dark stripe down the nail	Service

BACTERIAL VS. FUNGAL INFECTIONS

Nail infections, bacterial or fungal, can occur:

- on the nail plate
- in the nail plate
- under the nail plate

Bacterial infections commonly occur either on the surface of the nail or underneath the nail, between the nail plate and the nail bed. They are most often seen as a green discoloration on the nail plate caused by the waste products of the bacteria. They are also most commonly caused by improper nail preparation before applying artificial nails.

Fungal infections generally occur inside the nail plate and on the nail bed causing it to swell and separate in layers. Early stages of nail fungus are indicated by a yellow-green spot that eventually becomes black. The area will look as though it is spreading toward the cuticle the larger it becomes.

Despite a commonly held belief, bacterial infections are much more common than fungal infections, but you will see both in the salon setting.

6

Diseases and infections are not spread simply by performing salon services; they are spread as a result of contact with an infected client and improper sanitation and disinfection procedures. It is critical to protect your clients and yourself by practicing proper infection control procedures.

The nail diseases and disorders you have learned in this section are typical of those that you may encounter every day in the salon. It is up to you to know how to identify and handle the service when you do recognize a nail disease or disorder. This knowledge will contribute to your success as a nail technician.

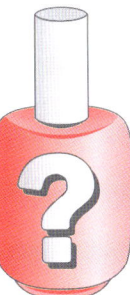

Why is it important to be able to recognize the characteristics of nail diseases and disorders?

SKIN PHYSIOLOGY

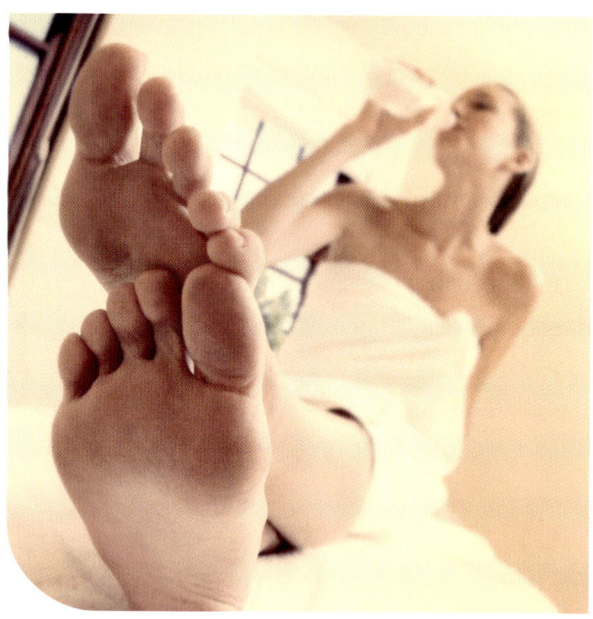

The skin is the largest organ of the body, and other than the brain, it is the most complex. Sensitive and durable, the skin requires special attention and care to maintain its health, elasticity, color and vibrancy. It acts as a shield between your body and your environment and performs many functions. The skin and its layers make up the **integumentary** (in-TEG-u-men-tary) **system**.

> As you learned in *Chapter 4, Anatomy*, the major systems of the body are the integumentary (skin), skeletal, circulatory, muscular, nervous, endocrine, excretory, digestive, respiratory and reproductive systems.

Functions of the Skin

The study of the skin's functions is referred to as **skin physiology**. The skin performs six primary functions. These include protection, absorption, secretion, excretion, regulation and sensation. The skin contains thousands of pores, which are tiny openings or "passageways," that allow sweat or **sebum**, a complex mixture of fatty substances also known as oil, to pass through the surface of the skin. A pore can contain a hair follicle, an opening that contains the root of a hair. Pores assist the skin in performing its six functions.

Protection
The skin shields internal tissues from toxins such as pollutants, smoke, ultraviolet radiation and other harmful chemicals and substances. It also acts as a barrier to infectious bacteria and extreme heat and cold.

Absorption
The skin permits certain substances like water and oxygen to pass through its tissues. Certain types of ingredients, such as vitamins and acids, are absorbed by thousands of pores on the surface of the skin to provide necessary moisture, nourishment and protection.

Secretion
The skin secretes sweat and sebum (oil) to keep it soft, supple and pliable. These two substances mix together to maintain the skin's moisture balance, which serves as a protective barrier to prevent bacteria from invading the skin.

Excretion

The skin is the body's largest waste removal system. The skin eliminates toxins and waste material, such as carbon dioxide, which are released through the sweat glands and pores. Sweat is water mixed with salt and other chemicals that have built up in the body.

Regulation

The body maintains an internal temperature of 98.6° Fahrenheit (37° Celsius). Skin regulates the body's temperature through mechanisms such as shivering and goosebumps. The contraction of a muscle called the arrector pili causes goosebumps, while shivering releases energy that warms the body. The skin also changes blood flow to regulate body temperature. For example, when the body temperature drops, blood flow increases. When body temperature increases, sweat on the skin cools the body.

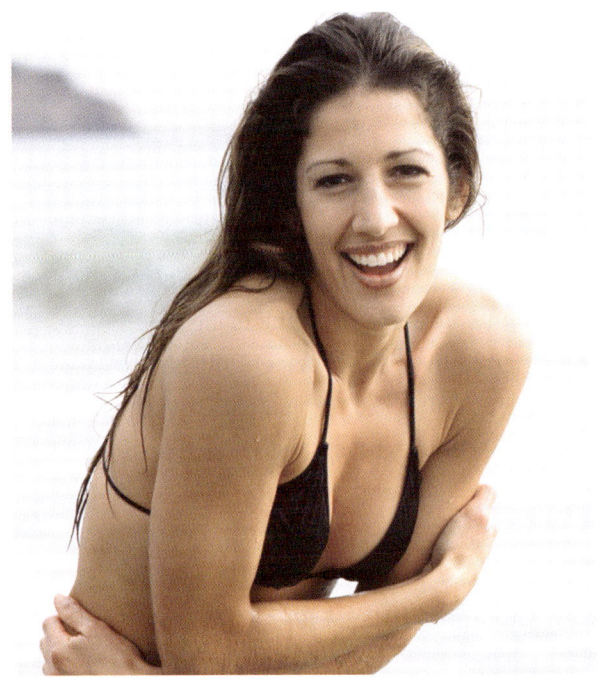

6

Amazingly, 1,250 pain receptors, 155 pressure receptors and 12 cold and heat receptors can be found in only one square inch (2.5 cm) of skin.

Sensation

The surface of the skin contains millions of nerve end fibers that send messages from the brain to corresponding parts of the body. These nerve end fibers allow humans to feel heat, cold, touch, pain and pressure.

Composition of the Skin

Skin histology is the microscopic study of the skin's tissue. There are three main layers of the skin:

1. **Epidermis,** which is the outermost layer of skin (also referred to as cuticle or scarf skin);
2. **Dermis,** which is the underlying, or inner, second layer of the skin (also called derma, corium, cutis or true skin);
3. **Subcutaneous layer,** which is located below the dermis and is composed primarily of **adipose** (fatty) tissue (also called subcutis or subdermis).

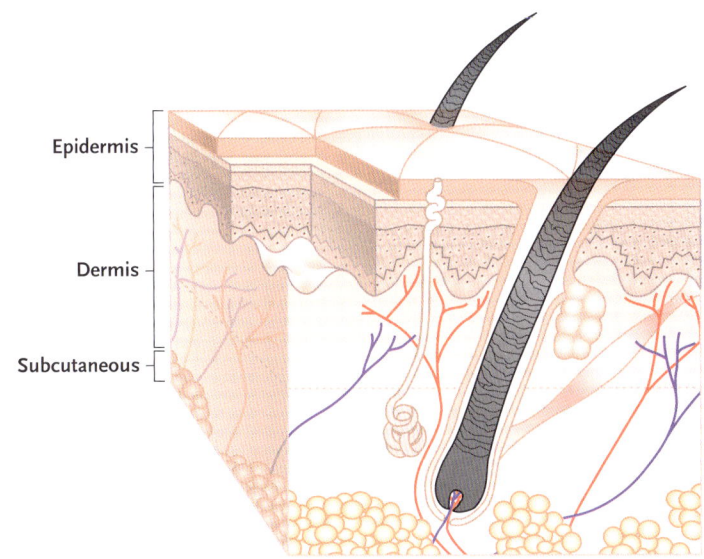

These layers are made up of a variety of cells, each serving a specific function. The primary component of skin cells is a protein substance called keratin. There are two forms of keratin. Hard keratin makes up nails, while soft keratin makes up the hair and skin.

When looking through a microscope, the epidermis and dermis are easy to identify. You can think of the epidermis as shingles on a roof, while the dermal layer below is like the plywood under the shingles. The epidermis attaches to the dermis just as the shingles attach to the plywood of the roof. A layer of "felt" material goes between the shingles and the plywood. This would be the lowest layer of the epidermis, sometimes referred to as the basement membrane (the skin's "felt"), which attaches the epidermis to the dermis. You can also think of the subcutaneous layer as the space between the floor and the roof.

Epidermis

The **epidermis** is the outermost layer of the skin, visible to the eye. Known as the protective layer, its primary function is "to keep the insides in and the outside out." There are no blood vessels found in the epidermis, which receives nourishment from the layer below it, the dermis.

The epidermis has five different layers of cells. These five layers are: stratum corneum, stratum lucidum, stratum granulosum, stratum spinosum and stratum germinativum.

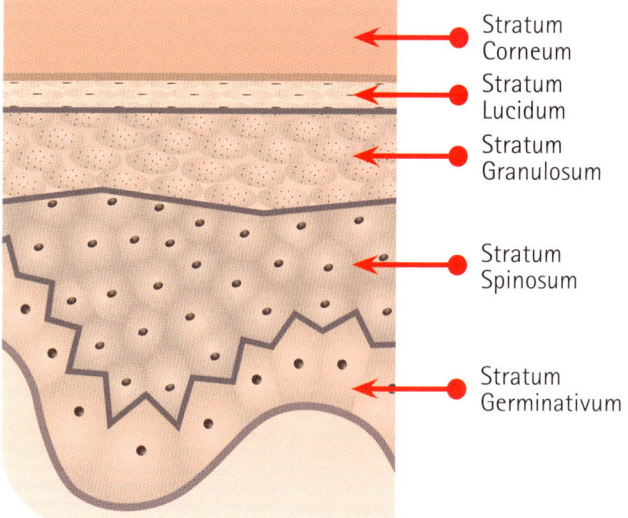

Stratum Corneum
Stratum Lucidum
Stratum Granulosum
Stratum Spinosum
Stratum Germinativum

Stratum Corneum

The uppermost layer, the **stratum corneum** (KOHR-nee-um), sometimes called the horny layer, is the toughest layer of the epidermis and is composed of keratin protein cells that are constantly shed and replaced with cells from below. Unlike the hard keratin found in nails, the keratin produced by the skin remains soft throughout the keratinization and shedding process. **Keratinization** is the chemical process in which living cells turn into dead protein cells.

The stratum corneum acts as a protective layer for the layers below it. It protects the skin's moisture balance by acting as a barrier to moisture loss. It, in turn, is protected by an **acid mantle**, which is a mixture of sweat and sebum.

Keratinization takes place on all exposed skin surfaces except the cornea of the eye.

Stratum Lucidum

The **stratum lucidum** (LOO-sid-um) is a transparent layer that lies between the stratum corneum and stratum granulosum. Although it is spread throughout the body, this layer is thickest on the palms of the hands and soles of the feet. These thick skin areas have ridges that provide your palms and soles with traction. You can grasp things with your hands more easily because of these ridges, and they cause friction so you don't slip while walking barefoot.

The ridges on your fingertips form fingerprints, which have been used for more than a century in crime detection. Your fingerprints are unique and consistent—they do not change with age.

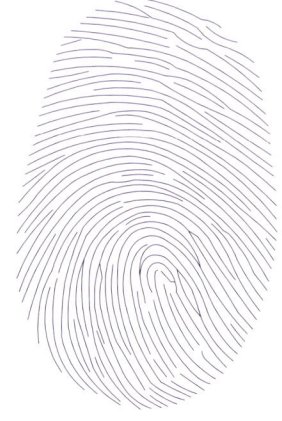

Stratum Granulosum

The next layer, the **stratum granulosum** (gran-yoo-LOH-sum), contains cells that are more regularly shaped and resemble many tiny granules. These granules (dying cells) are on their way to the skin's surface to replace cells that are shed from the stratum corneum. The process of keratinization is completed in this layer.

Keratinization, the chemical change of living cells into dead protein cells, begins when the newly produced cells are pushed toward the surface. As newly produced cells move toward the surface and farther away from the stratum germinativum, they flatten out, lose most of their water, die and, as keratinized cells, are finally shed. This process takes from 25 to 28 days, depending mostly on the area of the body, as well as the age and/or health of the individual.

Stratum Spinosum

The **stratum spinosum** (spin-OH-sum) is often called the spiny layer because the connections between the cells appear like "spines." These spines provide strength and support between the cells. The cells in this layer also help protect the body from infection by identifying them as harmful foreign substances, known as **antigens**.

An easy way to remember that the stratum spinosum protects is to think of "SPINES," as in the spines of a porcupine.

Stratum Germinativum

The lowest layer of the epidermis is the **stratum germinativum** (jur-mih-nah-TIV-um), also called the **basal layer**. This layer contains basal cells that continually divide through a process called **mitosis**, to replace the cells that are lost from the hardened (keratinized) outermost layer, the stratum corneum.

Melanocytes are also found in the stratum germinativum. These cells produce the **melanosomes**, or pigment granules containing **melanin**, that give color to the skin. The number, size and distribution of melanocytes determine skin color.

Melanocytes increase the production of melanosomes in response to the UV rays of the sun, which explains how skin tans or burns. This increase protects the keratinocytes from the destructive UV rays and allows them to continue producing healthy skin. However, excessive exposure to UV rays can eventually destroy protective melanocytes.

Dermis

The **dermis**, or **dermal layer**, is often referred to as the "true skin" or corium. This layer nourishes the lower epidermis and is the skin's main support structure, since it is comprised of many connective tissues and is rich in capillaries and blood vessels. Connective tissues are composed of a semi-fluid substance containing collagen protein and elastin fibers, both of which lend support to the epidermis and give the skin its elastic quality. **Collagen** protein fibers are strong and flexible while the **elastin** fibers are soft and pliable. It is in this layer that the collagen and elastin fibers deteriorate, causing the skin to wrinkle during the aging process. Also found in the dermis are the sweat glands called **sudoriferous** (soo-dohr-IF-erus) **glands**, oil glands called **sebaceous** (sih-BAY-shus) **glands**, sensory nerve endings and receptors, blood vessels, arrector pili muscles and a major portion of each hair follicle. Remember that hair is an appendage of the skin just as nails and the sweat and oil glands are.

6

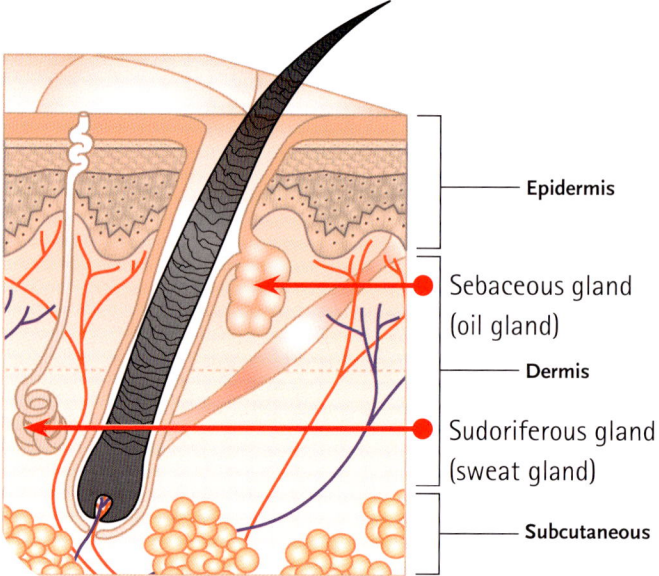

- Epidermis
- Sebaceous gland (oil gland)
- Dermis
- Sudoriferous gland (sweat gland)
- Subcutaneous

> The dermis is called the "true skin" because it is the layer of skin that is completely alive. The epidermis, on the other hand, is composed mostly of dead cells.

The dermis has two layers: the papillary dermis and the reticular dermis, which contain a variety of glands. These layers nourish the epidermis and connect the dermis to the layer below it, the subcutaneous layer.

Subcutaneous Layer

The **subcutaneous layer**, also called the subcutis or subdermis, is located beneath the dermis and is composed of primarily adipose (fatty) tissue. This layer is the body's cushioning that acts as a shock absorber and insulator to protect the bones and help support other delicate structures, such as blood vessels and nerve endings. This layer gives contour and shape to the body and serves as an emergency source of food and water.

Skin Pigmentation

As previously mentioned, melanin-producing cells (melanocytes) are located in the basal layer of the epidermis. These cells, loaded with melanin, move toward the surface at a faster

rate than other cells. Melanin is distributed throughout all epidermal cells and forms an effective barrier from the penetration of ultraviolet rays to deeper layers of the skin.

Melanin tans the skin to protect it from the burning rays of the sun. Dark skin contains more melanin, which serves as a more effective barrier to the damaging rays of the sun than is seen in light skin. Skin with little melanin present is light, pale or may appear slightly pink. The "pink" tone visible in pale skin is the reflection of red blood through the epidermis. No matter what color, all skin needs protection from the sun.

> Studies show that 90% of wrinkles are caused by excessive exposure to the sun, and only 10% by the natural aging process. It is said that the hands give away a person's age. Remind your clients that wearing sunscreen on their hands can help prevent damage caused by the sun and keep them looking younger.

Skin Diseases and Disorders

Dermatology is the study of the skin, its structure, functions, diseases and treatment. A **dermatologist** is a physician who specializes in diagnosing and treating diseases of the skin, hair and nails. As a nail care professional, you will need to be familiar with the indications of skin diseases and disorders so that you can recognize any problems that would prevent you from performing a nail care service. The following section covers common indications of diseases and disorders that includes lesions, infections, rashes, hyperkeratoses and pigmentation disorders. Keep in mind that only a dermatologist or physician should diagnose and treat them.

The symptoms or signs of a disease or disorder are divided into two classifications:

• Subjective—Those you feel
• Objective—Those you see

In other words, signs of a disease or disorder may be felt but nothing may be visible. Itching, burning, pain or symptoms that are felt are examples of subjective symptoms. Blisters or inflammation are objective symptoms because they are visible. In some cases, both objective and subjective symptoms may be present. Avoid direct contact with open skin.

There are six signs of infection: pain, swelling, redness, local fever (heat), throbbing and pus. Always avoid performing services on skin that displays any of these symptoms.

Lesions

Diseases and disorders are often accompanied by skin lesions. Being familiar with skin lesions will lead you to recognize skin diseases and disorders because lesions indicate any abnormal changes in the structure of an organ or tissue. There are three categories of lesions: primary, secondary and tertiary. As a nail care professional, it is helpful to recognize primary and secondary lesions.

Primary Skin Lesions

Primary skin lesions are changes in the structure of the skin during the early stages of change and development and include the following:

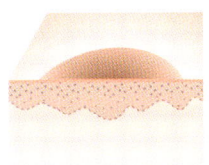 A **macule** is a discoloration appearing on the skin's surface. Macules are flat areas and, although they are usually rounded and distinct, they may be oval, irregular or have an outline that gradually fades into surrounding tissues. They may vary in size but are generally less than one centimeter (1 cm) in diameter. A large freckle is an example of a macule. The technical name for freckle is lentigines (len-tih-JEE-nees).

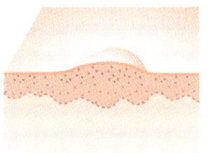 A **papule** is a hardened red elevation of the skin in which no fluid is present. These lesions normally vary in size from that of a pinhead to that of a pea. The actual shape and coloration of the lesions may vary. Consistency may vary from hard to soft. Papules may persist unchanged but they can, sometimes, proceed to other types of primary lesions. A large papule is known as a tubercle. A pimple is an example of a papule.

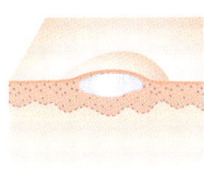 A **vesicle** is a fluid-filled elevation in the skin caused by localized accumulation of fluids or blood just below the epidermis. Vesicles may develop from poison oak or poison ivy and are generally short-lived.

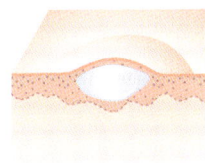 A **bulla** is a lesion, like a vesicle, but larger. Found above and below the skin, bullae contain a clear, watery fluid. A friction blister is an example of a bulla.

A friction blister is a small bulla filled with a semi-clear fluid, and it is usually caused by friction or rubbing on hands or feet. Friction blisters may be surrounded by redness.

No service may be performed until the blister is healed.

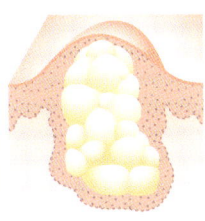 A **pustule** is a small elevation of the skin similar to a vesicle in size and shape, but containing pus. Pustules appear whitish or yellowish in color and may be surrounded by a reddish inflammatory border. They may develop from vesicles or papules. A pimple with pus is an example of a pustule.

6

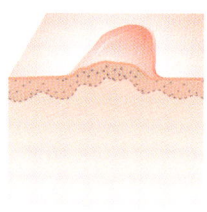

A **wheal** is a solid formation above the skin, often caused by an insect bite or allergic reaction. Wheals are sharply defined and solid, rising above the skin (i.e., a mosquito bite). These lesions usually develop rapidly, disappear slowly and are accompanied by itching or tingling.

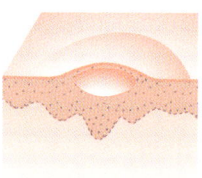

A **tumor** or **nodule** is a solid mass in the skin. These lesions are usually more than one centimeter (1 cm) in diameter. They may be hard or soft, depending on their makeup, and may be fixed or freely movable. This classification often includes any new skin growths and any localized swelling, which may be elevated or deep. Skin tumors generally have a rounded shape.

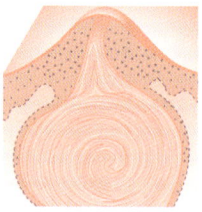

A **cyst** (sist) is an abnormal membranous sac containing a gaseous, liquid or semi-solid substance.

Secondary Skin Lesions

Secondary skin lesions appear as a disease or disorder that progresses into the later stages of development and needs to be treated by a dermatologist or physician.

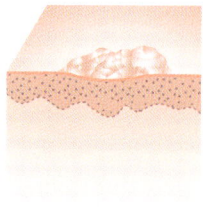

A **scale** is a shedding of a dead cell from the uppermost layer of the epidermis. The epidermis normally undergoes constant exfoliation (removal) of small, barely perceptible flakes of skin. When the formation of epithelial cells speeds up or the normal process of keratinization changes, an abnormal exfoliation of the epidermis occurs, which results

in scales. They may be dry, such as psoriasis, or oily, such as dandruff.

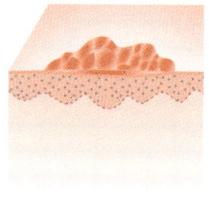

A **crust** is a dried mass that is the remains of an oozing sore. A scab is an example of a crust.

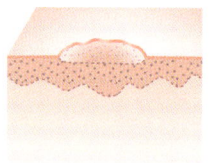

An **excoriation** is a mechanical abrasion to the epidermis (or an injury to the epidermis). It appears bright to dark red, because of dried blood, and can occur when an insect bite or scab is scratched. A scratch to the surface of the skin is considered an excoriation.

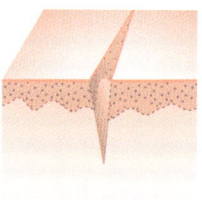

A **fissure** is a crack in the skin. These lesions usually appear as cracks or lines that may go as deep as the underlying dermis. They may be dry or moist. These lesions often occur when skin loses its flexibility due to exposure to wind, cold, water and other elements. Chapped lips are an example of fissures.

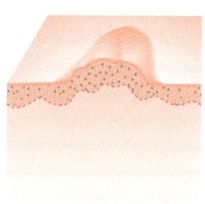

A **scar** is a formation resulting from a lesion, which extends into the dermis or deeper, as part of the normal healing process. Scars are permanent; however, they generally become less noticeable with time. The size and shape of a scar are dependent upon the extent of the original injury. Keloids (KEY-loyds) are thick scars.

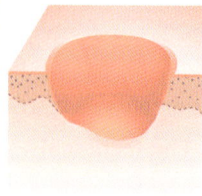

An **ulcer** is an open lesion visible on the surface that may result in the loss of portions of the dermis and may be accompanied by pus.

Skin Infections

As a nail technician it is important to be able to recognize skin infections in order to perform safe services for you and your clients. Skin infections cannot be worked on and need to be referred to a physician.

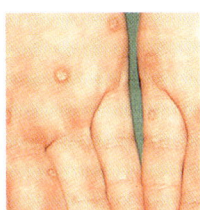

Verruca is the name given to a variety of warts. Plantar warts are very common. They are located at the bottom of the foot. They look like calluses on the outside, and the warts (characterized by little black dots) are on the inside. A dermatologist or physician should be consulted for removal of warts.
Cause: Human papilloma virus (HPV); can be contagious; can be spread to other areas of the body if contact is made with an opening in the skin.
Indications: Small area that resembles cauliflower; may have little black dots.
Service: Avoid servicing the area; never cause a wart to bleed.

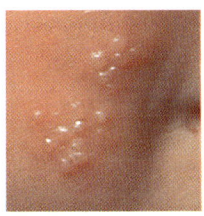

Herpes Simplex is a highly contagious viral infection that causes eruptive, blister-like clusters that are typically found on skin around the mouth, nose or genital area. They can also appear inside the mouth. Outbreaks of the blisters do not always appear on the skin at all times. The blisters and lesions associated with herpes must be completely dry and healed before the client is no longer contagious.
Cause: Herpes Simplex Virus Type-1; contagious through skin-to-skin contact or sexual transmission.
Indications: Blisters or sores on the lips, around or inside the mouth.
Service: Service may not be performed on affected area.

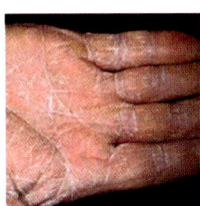

Tinea manus (TIN-e-ah MAN-es) is ringworm of the hand.
Cause: Fungal infection; disease-related.
Indications: Appears as rings containing tiny blisters, dark pink to reddish in color; can have dry flakes; can be confused with eczema or contact dermatitis; can spread to nails, scalp, feet or body.
Service: No service may be performed. Refer client to a physician.

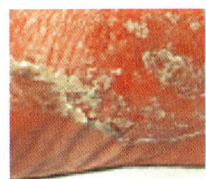

Tinea pedis (TIN-e-ah PED-is) is "athlete's foot" or ringworm of the feet.
Cause: Fungal infection; disease-related; thrives in dark, moist places.
Indications: Itching and peeling of the skin on feet; may look like dry skin; blisters containing colorless fluid form in groups or singly on sores and between toes, leaving sore or itchy skin on one or both feet.
Service: No service may be performed. Refer client to a physician.

SKIN INFECTIONS		
Name	**Description**	**Service**
Verruca	Variety of warts	No service in the area of the warts
Herpes Simplex	Blisters or sores around and on the mouth	Service after proper handwashing
Tinea manus	Ringworm of the hand	No service
Tinea pedis	Athlete's foot or ringworm of the feet	No service

Skin Rashes

As a nail technician it is important to be able to recognize when a skin rash is present to protect the client and yourself. Remember never work on a client with open skin, and refer the client to a physician.

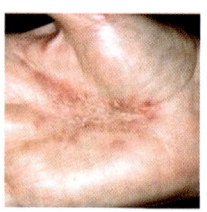

Contact dermatitis (dur-mah-TEYE-tis) is a rash. **Cause:** Allergic reaction from contact with substances such as dyes, detergents, nickel, fabrics or plants or a non-allergic irritation from contact with these substances.

Indications: Red, itchy, irritated eruption in the specific area of contact with the substance. The longer the skin is in contact with the irritating agent, or the more concentrated the substance, the more severe the reaction.

Service: No service may be performed if the skin is inflamed or broken in the area to be serviced.

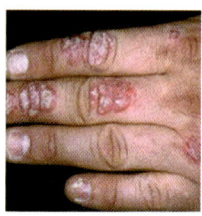

Psoriasis is characterized by the production of an excess of thick, scaly, silvery skin patches surrounded by a red area. It is not contagious and cannot be cured, but symptoms can be temporarily relieved with treatment.

Cause: Heredity; can be triggered by environmental factors if a person is genetically predisposed to the disease.

Indications: Often seen on the elbows, knees, back and scalp, and is an increased growth of skin cells from the lower dermis that appear as patches on the surface of the skin.

Service: Use caution and no service may be performed if the skin is inflamed or broken in the area to be serviced. Refer client to a physician.

> Psoriasis of the nail may appear as pitting on the surface of the nail. In other cases, lines may develop across the nail plate or the skin under the nail may thicken and cause the nail to loosen.

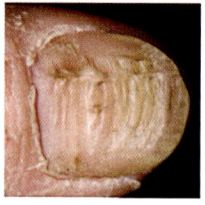

Eczema (EK-see-mah) is characterized by dry or moist lesions, an eruption of small vesicles and watery discharge. It is generally accompanied by an inflammatory redness and itching. The vesicles usually dry up, leaving the skin covered with crusts. Eczema is not contagious but requires medical attention. Eczema of the nail may be characterized by irregularly pitted nails with ridging and thickening of the nail plate. It may be chronic (lasting three months or more, or recurring frequently) or acute (a severe outbreak lasting less than six weeks).

Cause: Heredity; can be triggered by irritants if predisposed to the disease.

Indications: Dry, itchy and inflamed areas; can cause the skin to become broken or raw.

Service: Use caution and no service may be performed if the skin is inflamed or broken in the area to be serviced. Refer client to a physician.

SKIN RASHES

Name	Description	Service
Contact dermatitis	Rash	No service
Psoriasis	Thick, scaly, silvery skin patches surrounded by a red area	Service unless skin is inflamed or broken in the area to be serviced
Eczema	Dry or moist lesions, an eruption of small vesicles	Service unless skin is inflamed or broken in the area to be serviced

Hyperkeratoses

A **hyperkeratosis** is a thickening of the epidermis to protect the hands and feet due to friction or pressure. The excessive growth of keratin in the epidermis causes the skin to develop corns or calluses.

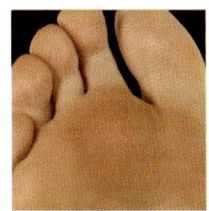

A **callus** is a thickening of the epidermis. The technical term for callus is tyloma.
Cause: Pressure and friction applied to the skin.
Indications: Rough, hardened patch of skin, usually found on the palms of the hands or soles of the feet.
Service: Smooth and soften the area using a file or foot file. It is not recommended to cut the callus.

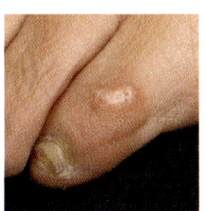

A **corn** is hard or soft tissue growth due to inflammation.
Cause: Friction or pressure applied to the skin.
Indications: Small, inflamed bump, usually found on the top or between toes.
Service: Gently file the outer layer of the corn using caution. No service may be performed if the skin is inflamed or broken in the area to be serviced. If painful, refer client to a physician.

HYPERKERATOSES		
Name	**Description**	**Service**
Callus	Thickening of the epidermis	Service
Corn	Excessive tissue growth	Service; use caution around affected area

Pigmentation Disorders

Pigmentation disorders are a result of abnormal production of melanin in the skin. An excess production of melanin causes the skin to appear darker in certain areas and is referred to as **hyperpigmentation**. A lack of the production of melanin causes the skin to appear lighter in spots and is referred to as **hypopigmentation**. If infection is present, no service should be performed on clients with pigmentation disorders.

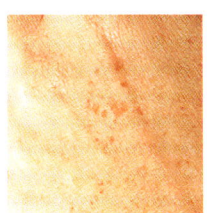

Melanoderma is the term used to describe any hyperpigmentation caused by overactivity of the melanocytes in the epidermis. It can be triggered by overexposure to sunlight, overactivity of the pituitary gland, circulation of hormones, disease and drugs. Some examples of melanoderma are chloasma and lentigines (freckles).

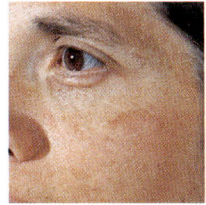

Chloasma (kloh-AZ-mah) is a group of brownish macules (nonelevated spots) occurring in one place. Chloasma is commonly referred to as liver spots and often occurs on the hands and face.

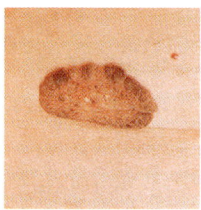

A **mole** is a small, brown pigmented spot that may be raised. Hair often grows through a mole, but should not be removed, unless advised by a physician. If there is any change in appearance of a mole, seek medical advice. Melanotic sarcoma, or melanoma, is a skin cancer that begins with a mole.

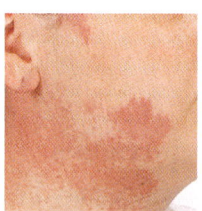

A **naevus** (NEE-vus) is a birthmark or a congenital mole. A birthmark may look like a stain on the face or other part of the body and is generally a reddish purple flat mark. The stain is caused by dilation of the small blood vessels in the skin.

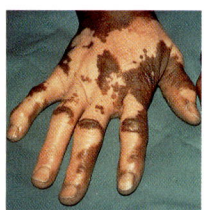

Leukoderma (loo-ko-DUR-mah) describes hypopigmentation (lack of pigmentation) of the skin caused by a decrease in activity of the melanocytes. Leukoderma is occasionally the result of a congenital defect such as albinism. However, hypopigmentation can be acquired, as in vitiligo.

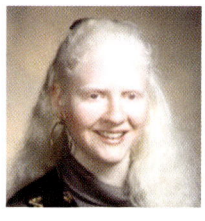

Albinism (AL-bin-izm) (oculocutaneous) is a group of hereditary conditions that results in the failure of the skin to produce melanin. Persons with albinism usually have pale skin, light blond hair and light blue eyes. They have a strong hypersensitivity to light and sun and their skin ages faster than the average person. This skin must be protected from exposure to sunlight or ultraviolet rays.

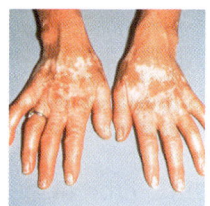

Vitiligo (vit-I-LEYE-goh) is characterized by oval or irregular patches of white skin that do not have normal pigment. Vitiligo is usually seen on the face, hands and neck as patches of hypopigmentation that may enlarge slowly. These patches of skin must be protected from exposure to sunlight or ultraviolet lamps.

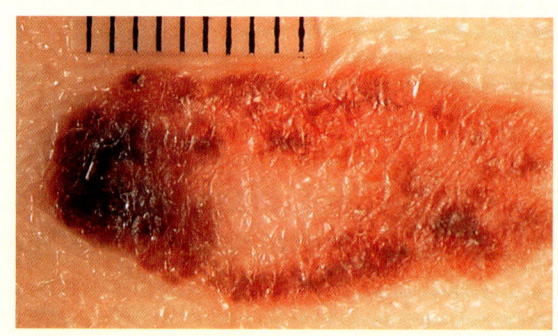

Melanoma is a serious form of skin cancer that causes the most skin cancer-related deaths. Melanomas originate as flat or raised pigmented lesions or moles. It is important to know what melanoma looks like to help determine whether to refer your client to a physician. The following are the **ABC's** of melanoma:

A — Asymmetry: If the mole is not symmetrical...

B — Border: If the border is irregular...

C — Color: If the mole contains multiple colors or has variation in color...

D — Diameter: If the mole is more than 6 mm in diameter...

...Refer your client to a physician. Remember to never diagnose a client.

The ability to identify the characteristics of nail and skin diseases and disorders helps ensure that the services you provide are safe for both you and your clients.

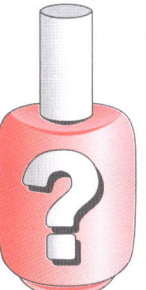

Why is it important to be familiar with the characteristics of common skin diseases and disorders?

6

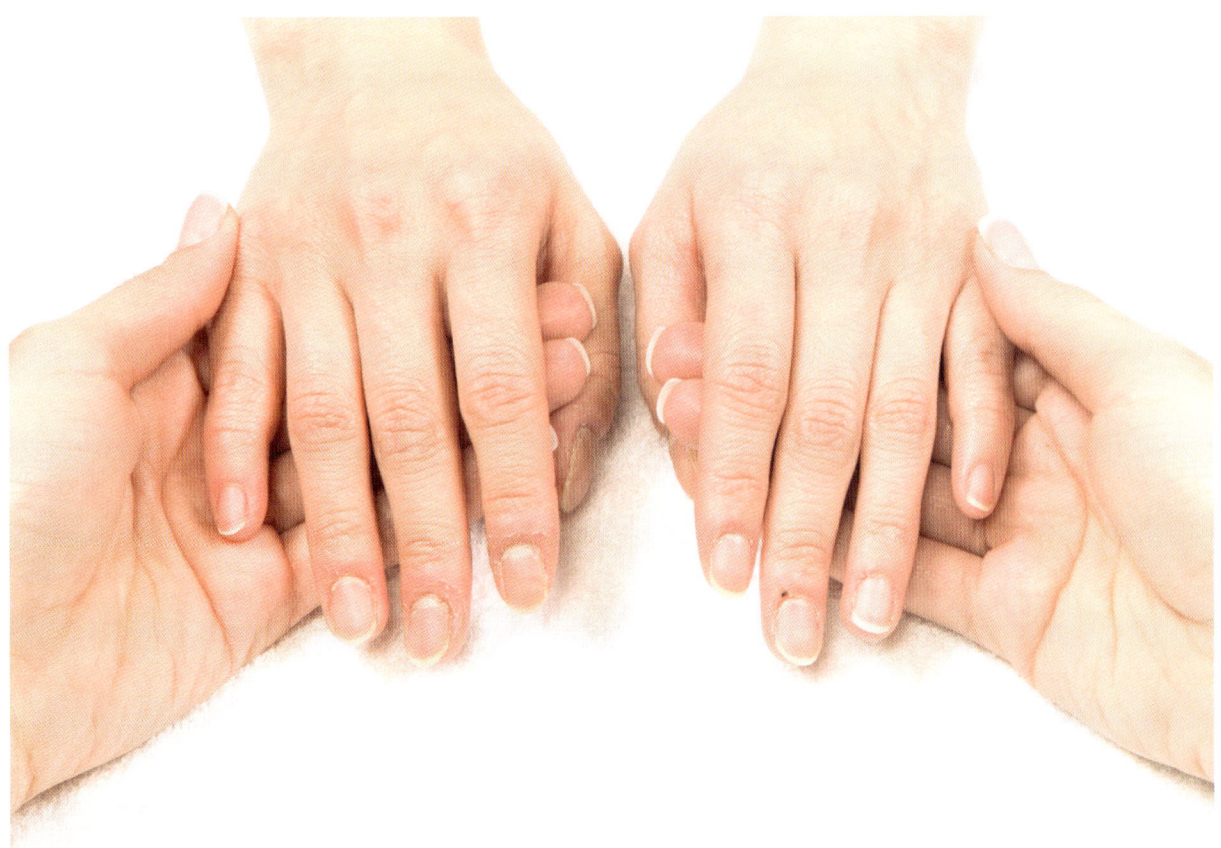

DECISION-MAKING SKILLS

Case Studies

The following situations are designed to help you build your decision-making skills. Using your training to this point, review the following scenarios, then think through and describe how you would handle each challenge.

1. A new client arrives for a pedicure and has a few warts on the bottom of his feet. Would you perform the procedure? Why or why not? If not, how would you explain your decision to your client?

2. Susan is a relatively new client. She has been in before for manicures. You notice that she has more hangnails than normal and it looks as though she has been tearing them. How would you explain to Susan how important it is not to tear the hangnails and why you would recommend a hot oil manicure?

3. A new client arrives for a pedicure and you notice a few areas that are irritated and red between her toes. She is also complaining of itching. You suspect that she has athlete's foot (tinea pedis). How would you explain to her that you cannot perform a service?

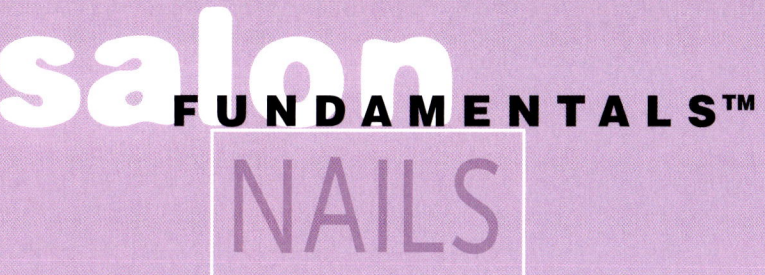

Unit 3: Nail Services

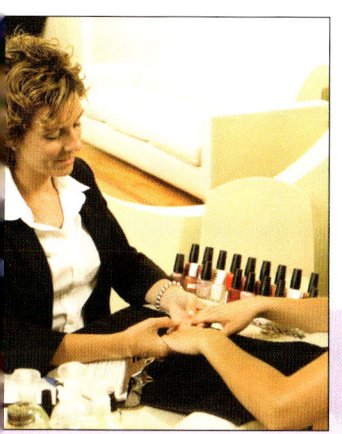 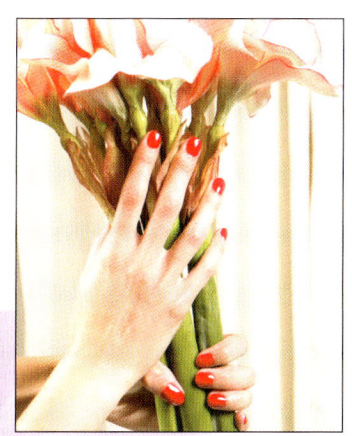 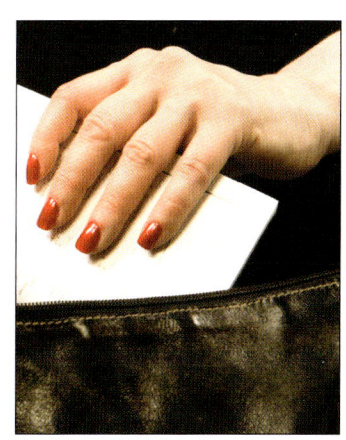 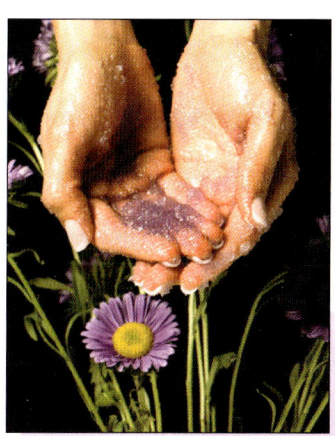

UNIT 3 NAIL SERVICES focuses on the abilities and skills required by every successful nail technician. This unit offers sound lessons in exceptional client service in addition to hands-on step-by-step procedures that are essential for any nail technician looking to perform with confidence and capability.

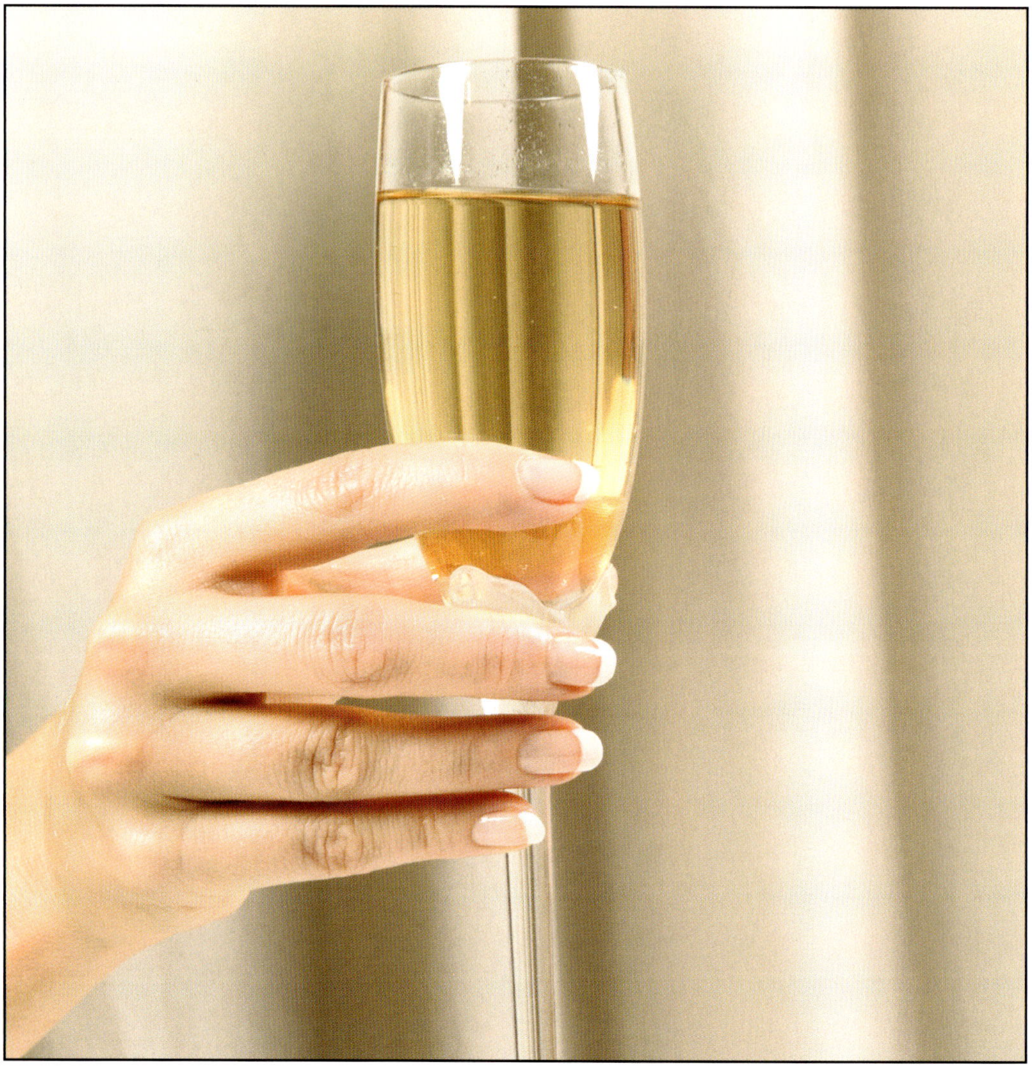

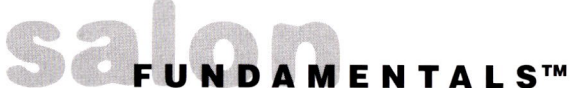

salon FUNDAMENTALS™

Most people are very selective when it comes to choosing someone to care for their personal needs. They expect this professional to treat them with respect, advise them honestly and provide appropriate professional services in a safe and supportive environment. In the nail care industry, personal care, also known as client care, is a business essential. When clients are well cared for, everyone benefits.

VALUE

Professional nail technicians who develop strong interpersonal and consultation skills can expect more repeat business and word-of-mouth referrals.

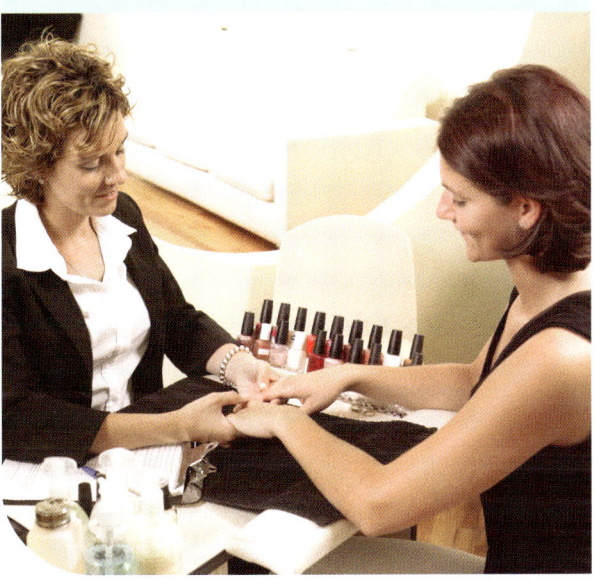

MAIN IDEA

The phases of client service are designed specifically to guarantee client comfort and safety with all nail care services. Skillfully completing each phase in the service process will help you build lasting relationships with clients. The quality of these relationships will play a big role in your success as a nail technician. This chapter defines the essentials of client care before, during and after the service.

PLAN	OBJECTIVES
Before the Service • Greeting • Ask, Analyze and Assess • Agreement	Describe the personal impressions that play a key role during the Greeting Phase of service. Identify the purpose of obtaining a medical history on the Client Consultation Form. Explain the Agreement Phase of service.
During and After the Service • Delivery • Completion	Describe the elements of client education used in the Delivery Phase of service. Identify the importance of soliciting feedback, retail sales, rebooking and follow-up care used in the Completion Phase of service. State the various types of follow-up care.

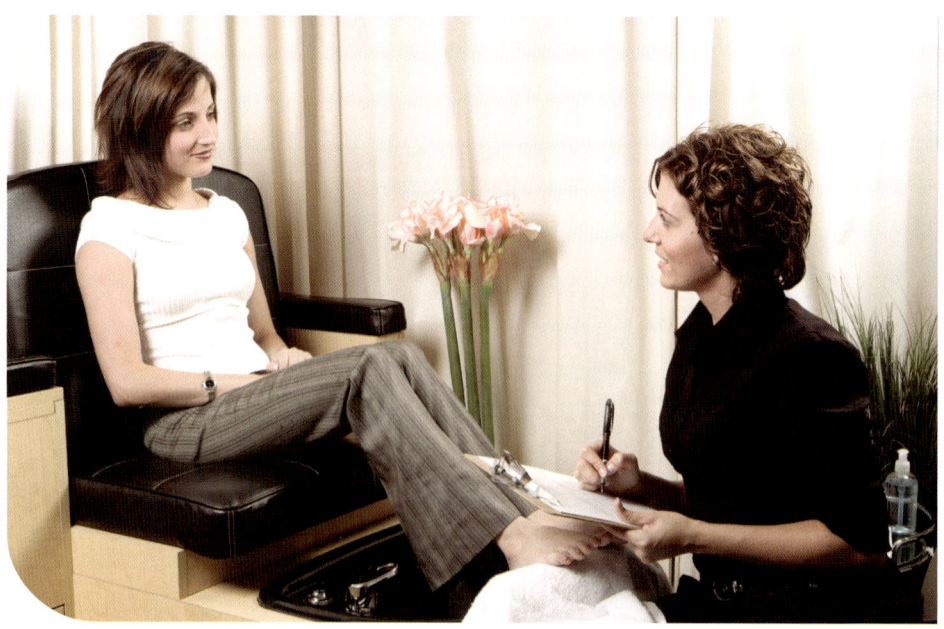

BEFORE THE SERVICE

The goal of client care is to help guarantee client satisfaction. There are five phases of service that help the nail technician achieve this goal, and each of the phases has a different objective in the service process. For example, exchanging greetings, establishing rapport and building trust are the goals of the Greeting Phase. In the Ask, Analyze and Assess Phase, the focus shifts from relating personally to offering professional advice. The Agreement Phase is performed to clarify client expectations and desired results with an agreement between the client and the technician. In the Delivery Phase, the service shifts from consultation to action and the service is actually performed. The Completion Phase occurs when the service is concluded, and the technician makes recommendations for a home care regimen, rebooks the next service and gives the client the opportunity to express an opinion about the experience.

5. Completion **1. Greeting** **2. Ask, Analyze, Assess** **3. Agreement** **4. Delivery**

7

These phases are designed to keep the lines of communication open while allowing clients to be actively involved before, during and after the professional service. This section focuses on the first three phases of service, which occur before the actual delivery.

The phases help you build rapport with your clients and allow you to learn your clients' needs and desires so that you can put your professional skills into action. The first three phases are:

- Greeting—establish rapport
- Ask, Analyze and Assess—offer professional advice
- Agreement—clarify expectations

Gaining clients' trust, understanding their nail care needs and establishing agreement in regard to the services they will receive allows you to deliver the necessary and appropriate services. These first three phases are extremely important in helping to ensure client safety, comfort and satisfaction.

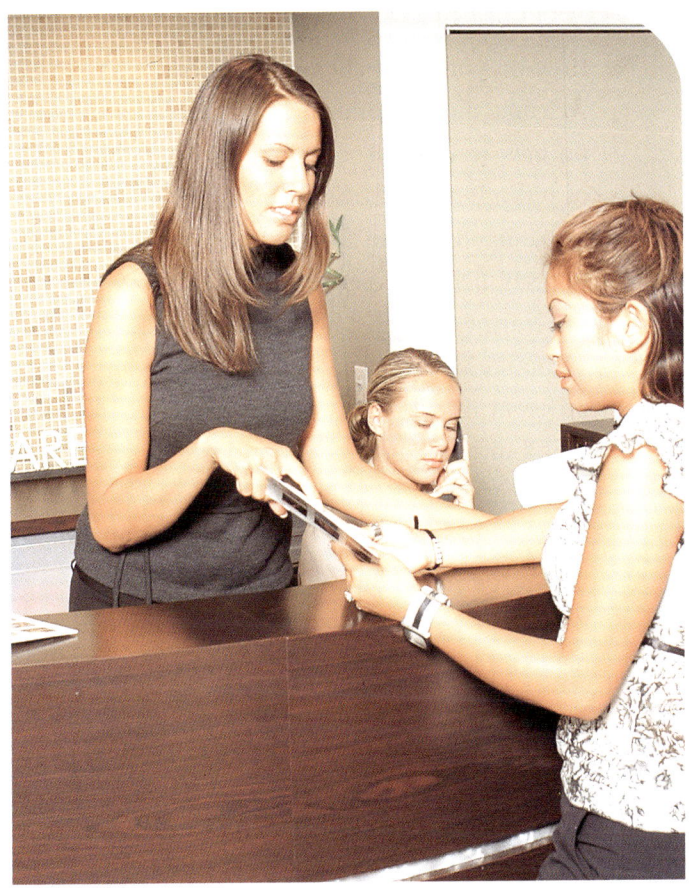

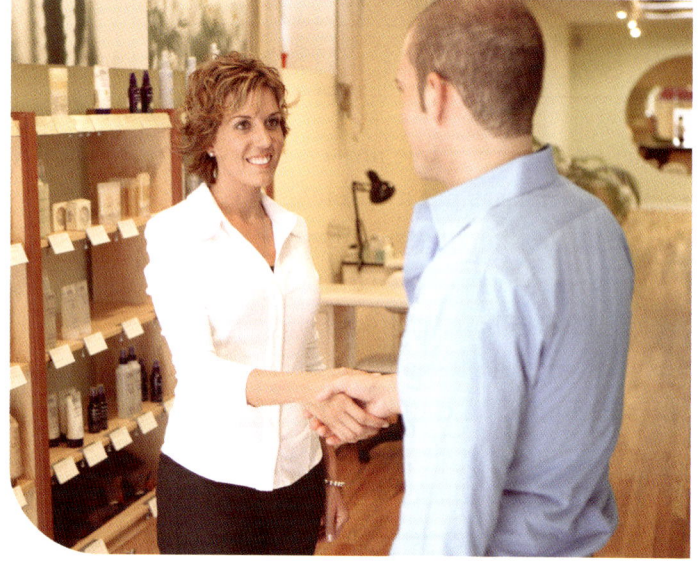

Greeting

Have you ever noticed how different professionals greet clients? Some greet clients with a shower of attention and recognition, while others are more reserved. Most clients prefer a greeting somewhere in the middle—a polite and genuine greeting is always appropriate.

How do you greet clients to help them feel welcome and important? Most likely it depends on how well you know them or if they are new or returning clients. Some people are inclined to shake hands, some kiss and hug, while others just say hello. These exchanges are common in the Northern Hemisphere (Canada, U.S., Puerto Rico and Mexico) and Europe, but are quite different in parts of Asia. For example, in China, a nod or bow is the common form of greeting. In Hong Kong, the older Chinese clasp their hands together at throat level and nod. In India, the palms of the hands are placed together, then followed with a slight bend or nod. Indonesians greet each other by saying "selamat," which means "peace." People in Japan greet each other by bowing from the waist, palms on thighs and heels together. In Thailand, palms are placed together, elbows down, and the head

is bowed slightly, called "wai." In Northern Europe, three kisses, alternating from cheek to cheek, is a common greeting. In Southern Europe, Central and South America, it is customary to shake hands warmly and for a longer period of time. Each handshake differs slightly, but the traditional American handshake is very similar.

In the U.S., the most common greeting is to shake hands firmly and make direct eye contact. Historians have found that the handshake has several origins, the most interesting being the medieval custom of extending the hand, palm up, as a friendly gesture that demonstrated there was not a weapon in hand. If the other person also extended a hand, hands were clasped as a sign of friendship. The common factor in all greetings is a gesture of respect.

Throughout your career, you may meet many different people from all around the world. In the Greeting Phase, you can win your clients' respect by greeting them professionally and respectfully:

- Offer a friendly smile
- Make direct eye contact
- Extend your hand and shake hands firmly
- Welcome them warmly

The telephone is often the first contact a client has with you or your place of business. Telephone contact in the salon or spa can help create an impression that is just as powerful and important as the first physical impression. (See *Chapter 2, Business Basics*, for more on telephone answering techniques.) Although telephone contact usually happens first, meeting clients in person gives you a chance to make a positive personal impression as a professional. In person, impressions are formed based on professional atmosphere, eye contact, touch and tone of voice.

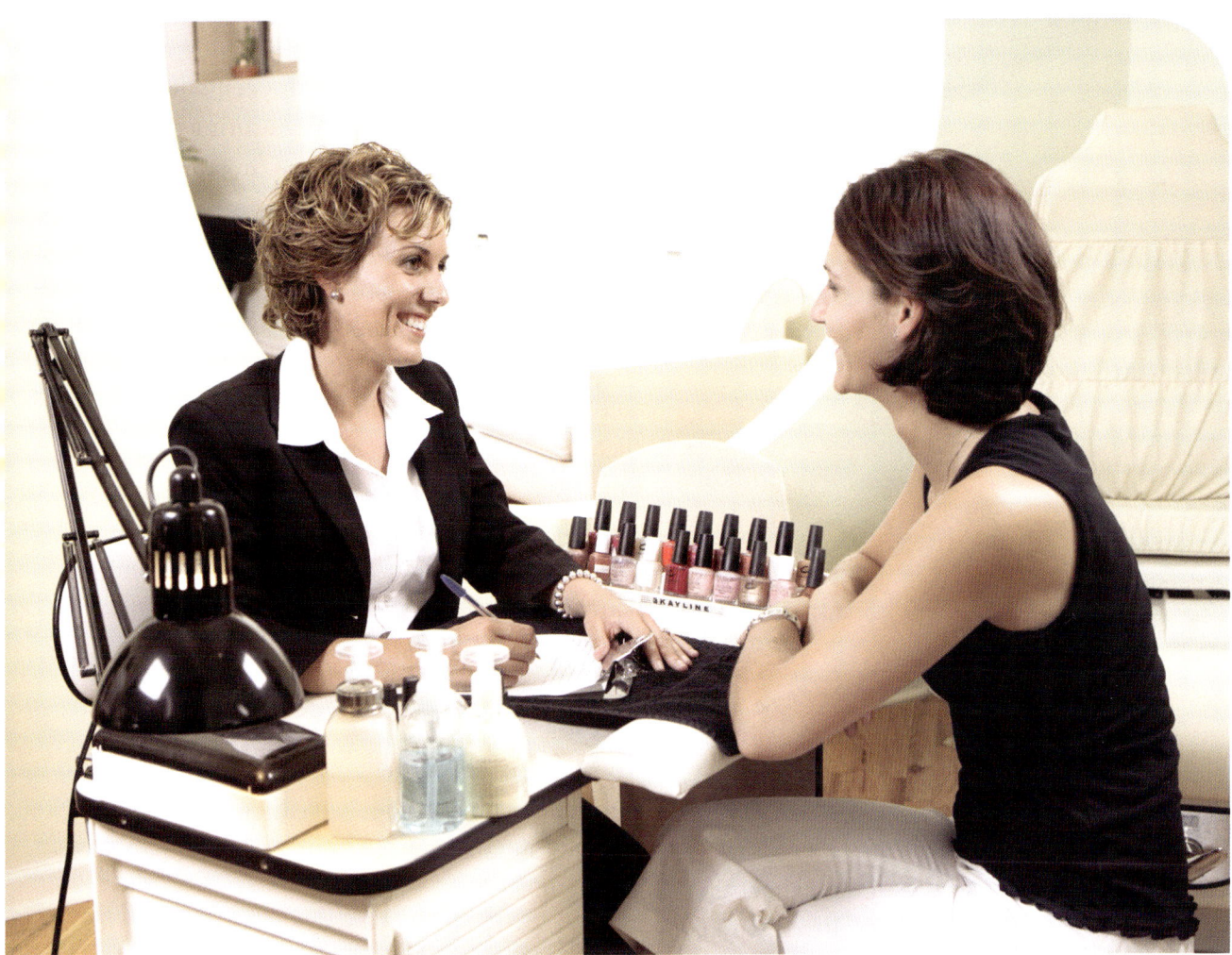

7

Professional Atmosphere

The atmosphere and physical arrangement of the salon or spa in which you work will significantly influence a client's impression of you. Every aspect of your workplace is a representation of you and your commitment to excellence. The service area, as well as the salon or spa, conveys powerful impressions about your dedication to cleanliness and professionalism. In addition, prominently displayed licenses, certificates and awards let your clients know that you are dedicated to excellence.

Is it easier to smile or frown? It is easier to smile because it takes only 17 muscles to create a smile, but it takes 43 muscles to make a frown. So smile—it's much easier—and friendlier!

Eye Contact

Eye contact is a nonverbal gesture that conveys an impactful message. It says, "You have my undivided attention." Looking a person in the eyes when talking and listening also demonstrates personal confidence. For example, when a client tells you about a concern and you listen attentively and look at him or her, without saying one word, you have communicated that you are interested in what is being said. By contrast, looking around the room during a client consultation sends a clear signal that you are distracted or unsure of yourself. To create a positive lasting impression on a client, try giving him or her your undivided attention. It works!

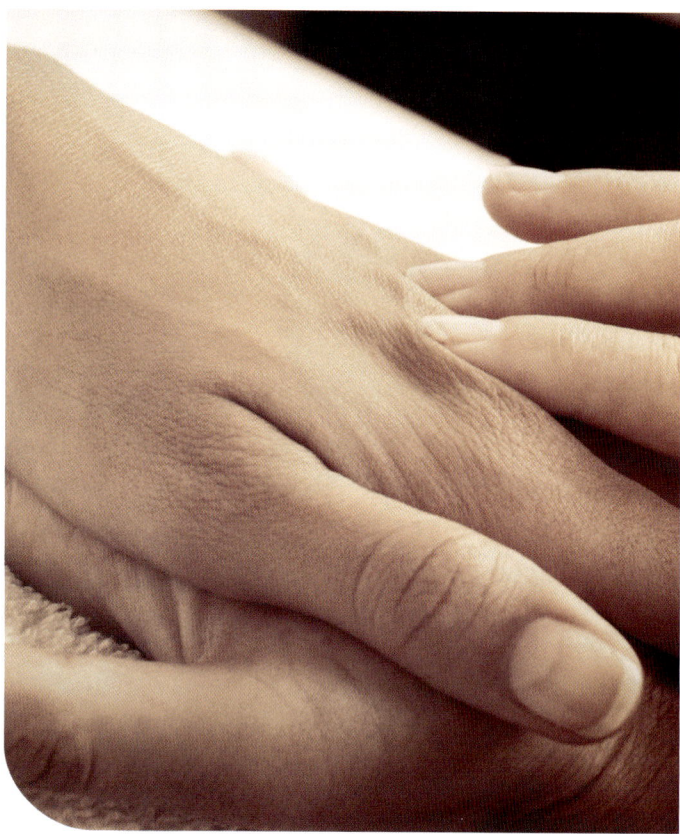

Touch

Therapeutic touch has been used throughout the ages and now, in this technology-driven world, it is even more valuable. Touch is considered the most personal of the five senses. It can lower blood pressure, relieve stress, stimulate circulation and promote feelings of security and comfort. The healing effects of touch are also well-established. For example, in pediatric hospitals, touch is used to stimulate growth and improve the health of premature babies.

Therapeutic touch is an essential skill in the nail care service industry. The initial physical contact with a client is usually through touch when shaking hands. To create a positive first impression, approach your new client, make eye contact, introduce yourself and firmly grasp his or her hand. Once you develop a relationship with your client, you may find other ways to communicate welcome and confidence, such as a gentle hand on the shoulder.

Tone of Voice

When it comes to relating with clients, what you say and how you say it can turn a first-time customer into a return client. In professional settings, a firm and low-key tone of voice is preferred over a loud or high-pitched voice. Words that describe a professional tone of voice include the following: confident, calm, respectful and non-judgmental. It is important to be honest and sincere when explaining your services to clients. It is to a technician's advantage to select words that apply directly to the client's needs or concerns and describe products and services in terms that are accurate and easy to understand. Your first opportunity to begin this dialogue is in greeting the client.

For example:
"Hi Madison. My name is Sarah and I'll be your nail technician today. Please have a seat and we can talk about the services you'll be getting today."

As opposed to:
"Madison, go ahead and choose a nail polish color and let's get started."

As you can see, the Greeting Phase is more complex than a simple "Hello." However, it can be easy, and now that you understand what it takes to make positive personal impressions when greeting clients, you are ready to shift into the next phase of service.

Most people do not know what their tone of voice sounds like to others. Do you? Find out by recording yourself while you role-play a service or consultation. The results might be surprising!

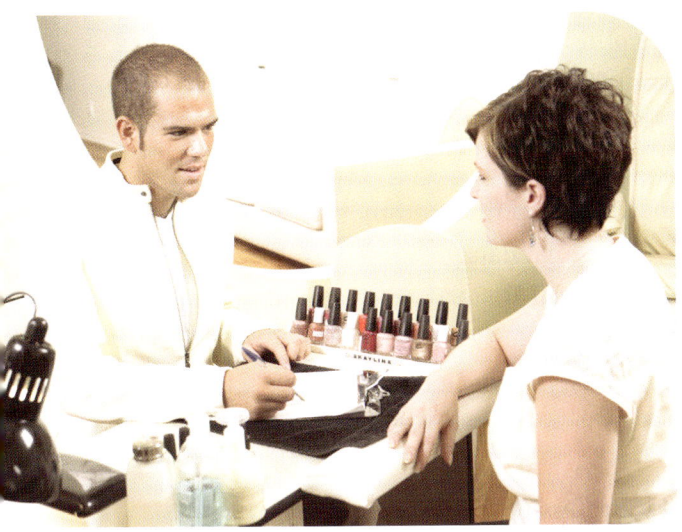

Ask, Analyze and Assess

The Ask, Analyze and Assess Phase is more than a question-and-answer exchange between client and technician. It is a guided conversation that invites clients to share their expectations as well as their reasons for requesting services. A typical conversation might start like this:

Technician: "What would you like to accomplish today?"

Client: "I am in a wedding this weekend so I need my nails to look nice."

Once the general reason for the service is established, then the dialogue can shift to personal nail care concerns.

Learning to uncover a client's motive for requesting a specific service is an essential part of nail care training. These interpersonal skills develop over time as you learn to be more sensitive to client requests, ask the most effective questions and listen intently to their responses. Having a new client fill out a Client Consultation Form allows you to retain valuable information gained from asking, analyzing and assessing before the service.

Client Consultation Form

The Client Consultation Form helps the technician obtain information relating to the client and allows for good record keeping. The policies on how much information is documented and how much is gained during a client consultation varies from salon to salon. All information discussed here will allow you to offer a professional service.

Consultation forms are provided to clients at the beginning of the first visit. The nail technician should give a brief overview of each section and explain why it is important to thoroughly complete the form. These forms are updated with all future visits.

7

CLIENT CONSULTATION FORM
PERSONAL INFORMATION

Date

Name
Address
City
Home Telephone
Email Address
Recommended by

State
Zip
Work Telephone

Optional Information
Significant Other's Name
Birthday
Anniversary
Are you interested in receiving emails on our special offers?
Yes   No

MEDICAL HISTORY

Allergies?   Yes   No
(If yes, explain)
Recent Surgery(ies)

Health conditions: Please check all that apply.
Pregnancy   Diabetes   Heart Conditions   Varicose Veins
High Blood Pressure   Arthritis   Stroke   Skin Disease
Fungal Infection (on hands or feet)   Other

List any other medical conditions, which we need to be aware:

Medications and Treatments: Please check all that apply.
Blood Thinners   Antibiotics   Steroids   Radiation Treatment
Chemotherapy   Other

LIFESTYLE

Occupation
What type of work do you perform using your hands each day?

Are your hands submerged frequently in water? Yes   No

Do you participate in sports? Yes   No
If yes, what type of sports do you enjoy?

What other types of activities or hobbies do you take part in?

CLIENT CONSULTATION FORM
PERSONAL INFORMATION

Date

Name
Address   State   Zip
City   Work Telephone
Home Telephone
E-mail Address
Recommended by

Optional Information
Significant Other's Name   Anniversary
Birthday
Are you interested in receiving e-mails on our special offers?
Yes   No

MEDICAL HISTORY

Health conditions: Please check all that apply.
Pregnancy   Diabetes   Heart Conditions   Varicose Veins
High Blood Pressure   Arthritis   Stroke   Skin Disease
Fungal Infection (on hands or feet)   Other

Allergies?   Yes   No
(If yes, explain)
Recent Surgery(ies)

CLIENT CONSULTATION FORM
LIFESTYLE EVALUATION

Occupation
What type of work do you perform using your hands each day?

Are your hands submerged frequently in water? Yes   No

Do you participate in sports? Yes   No
If yes, what type of sports do you enjoy?

What other types of activities or hobbies do you take part in?

Do you do household cleaning, gardening or dish washing by hand?
Yes   No
If yes, do you wear gloves? Yes   No

Do you take steps at home to care for your hands? Yes   No
If yes, what steps do you take and what products do you use?

Do you take steps at home to care for your feet? Yes   No
If yes, what steps do you take and what products do you use?

CLIENT CONSULTATION FORM
PROFESSIONAL EVALUATION

...stand that withholding
...or irritation to the
..., and I release this
...ereof.

...te

Observations:
Nails:

Cuticles:

Skin:

Goals:

Course of action:

SERVICE RECORD

TECHNICIAN

PRODUCT USED

SERVICE

DATE
1
2
3
4
5

REMARKS
1.
2.
3.
4.
5.

Keep in mind that Client Consultation Forms vary from salon to salon. However, most will incorporate the five sections listed below:

1. **Personal Information,** which includes personal data.
2. **Medical History,** which includes the client's medical history.
3. **Lifestyle,** which includes daily activity to help determine the best service for the client.
4. **Professional Evaluation,** which allows the technician to note and record professional observations.
5. **Service Record,** which allows the technician to document specifics such as services received, products used and purchased, and to track changes or improvements in the client's nails.

The Client Consultation Form is an important element in demonstrating your professionalism, the effectiveness of your nail care services and the achievement of the best results. Each section asks questions that provide a wealth of information about the condition of the client's nails and skin. Although some of the questions asked may seem odd or even intrusive, they can help to properly determine and document the client's needs.

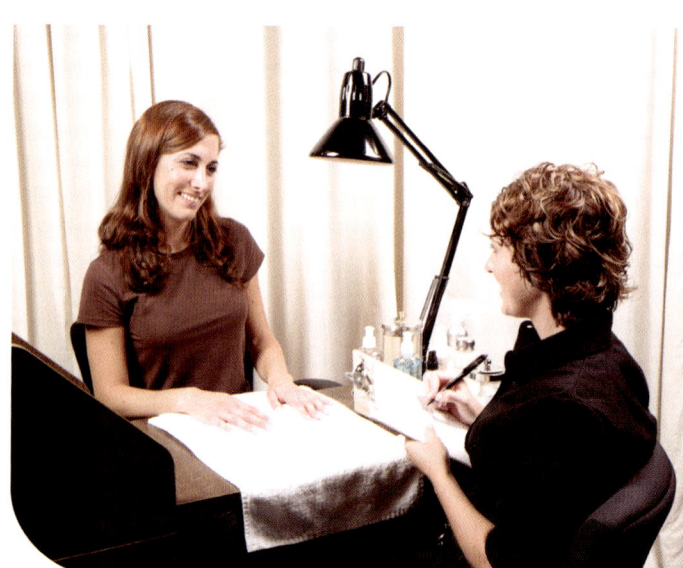

Personal Information

The first part of the Client Consultation Form, titled "Personal Information," asks for basic data necessary for good record keeping. This includes information such as the client's full name, address, phone numbers (home, work and mobile, if applicable), e-mail address and how the client was referred. For marketing purposes, salons or spas can give clients the option of listing their anniversary, birthday, and the name of a significant other. Clients may appreciate reminders to purchase gift certificates for special occasions or anniversaries. Make sure the questions regarding personal information, such as age, are marked "optional" on the form, as shown above.

CLIENT CONSULTATION FORM
PROFESSIONAL EVALUATION

Name _____ Date _____
Address _____
City _____ State _____ Zip _____
Home Telephone _____ Work Telephone _____
E-mail Address _____
Recommended by _____

Optional information:
Significant Other's Name _____
Birthday _____ Anniversary _____
Are you interested in receiving e-mails on our special offers? Yes ____ No ____

Medical History

The second part of the Client Consultation Form, "Medical History," deals with the client's personal health and medical history. This information provides important facts about the client that will be necessary to help determine what products and equipment to use and what services to offer. Most importantly, this information will help you identify factors, or existing conditions that make it inadvisable for particular products, equipment or services to be used or performed.

This section includes questions about allergies, medications and recent surgeries. Additional questions concerning health conditions such as heart conditions, high blood pressure, diabetes, pregnancy and arthritis will help you avoid services that could cause adverse reactions or cause the client discomfort during the service. These questions are vital in providing safe and effective services. For example, when giving a pedicure to a client with diabetes it is important to use lukewarm water. Clients with diabetes may experience a loss of sensitivity in the extremities, which could prevent them from feeling that the water is too hot. Client safety is of the utmost importance when providing any type of service.

MEDICAL HISTORY

Health conditions: Please check all that apply.
___ Pregnancy ___ Diabetes ___ Heart Conditions ___ Varicose Veins
___ High Blood Pressure ___ Arthritis ___ Stroke ___ Skin Disease
___ Fungal Infection (on hands or feet) ___ Other _____

Allergies? ___ Yes ___ No
(If yes, explain) _____

List any other medical conditions of which we need to be aware of such as recent surgeries:
_____

Medications and Treatments: Please check all that apply.
___ Blood Thinners ___ Antibiotics ___ Steroids ___ Radiation Treatment
___ Chemotherapy ___ Other _____

Health Conditions

The state of a client's health may influence the way services are performed. In fact, some conditions may indicate that a service should not be performed at all. Listed here are some health conditions you may encounter during the Ask, Analyze and Assess phase of the service, along with some characteristics, recommendations or cautions.

HEALTH CONDITIONS

Condition	Characteristics	Recommendation/Caution
Pregnancy	• Heightened skin sensitivity • Stimulation of pressure points located on the hands and feet may cause contractions	• Avoid massage or only use light effleurage movements • Check for client comfort
Heart Conditions/High Blood Pressure	• Over-stimulation may harm the client by raising the blood pressure • Light-headedness	• Avoid massage unless given permission by physician • Use less heat and stimulation (water temperature and jets in pedicure basin) • Check for client comfort
Diabetes	• Slower rate of healing • Increased risk of infection • Decreased sensitivity in hands and feet	• Use extra care not to cause an opening in the skin • Check temperature of water, paraffin wax or other items that may use heat • Get permission from physician before performing a service
Varicose Veins	• Bulging, prominent veins • Increased risk of forming a blood clot	• Avoid massage over varicose veins • Use caution when massaging around varicose veins
Arthritis	• Painful movements • Joint pain	• Use care when massaging client • Check for client comfort
Stroke	• Over-stimulation may harm the client by dislodging plaque found within the arteries	• Avoid massage unless given permission by physician • Use less heat and stimulation with water temperature and jets in pedicure basin • Check for client comfort

HEALTH CONDITIONS

Condition	Characteristics	Recommendation/Caution
Skin Disease/Disorder	• Irritation such as redness or cracked/peeling skin • Open sores	• Analyze client carefully • Check for any signs of redness, open sores, rash, irritation or infection • Do not perform a service if any of these characteristics are present
Fungal Infection	• Spread easily • Nail plate thickens • Nail plate becomes discolored and appears black to brown or beige to white • Nail plate may loosen from the nail bed	• Analyze client carefully • Check for thickening of the nail plate, discoloration or loosening of the nail plate • Do not perform a service if any of these characteristics are present • Refer client to a physician
Edema (swelling)	• Sign of another disease or disorder the client may not know about • Sign of injury	• Avoid massage unless given permission by physician

7

Allergens

An **allergen** is a substance or ingredient likely to cause an allergic reaction. An allergic reaction to a particular product and/or ingredient may make it inadvisable to proceed with the service, or to use a product. It is important that the technician is able to recognize some of the most common allergens. Following is a list of allergens that you might encounter.

• **Cosmetic ingredient allergens:** Colors and fragrances are ingredients found or contained in products that commonly cause allergic reactions.

• **Hydroxy acid allergens:** Both alpha and beta hydroxy acids promote cell turnover and exfoliation. These ingredients can be found in some cuticle treatments. Allergies to these ingredients can cause irritation, redness and increased sensitivity in the area to which they are applied.

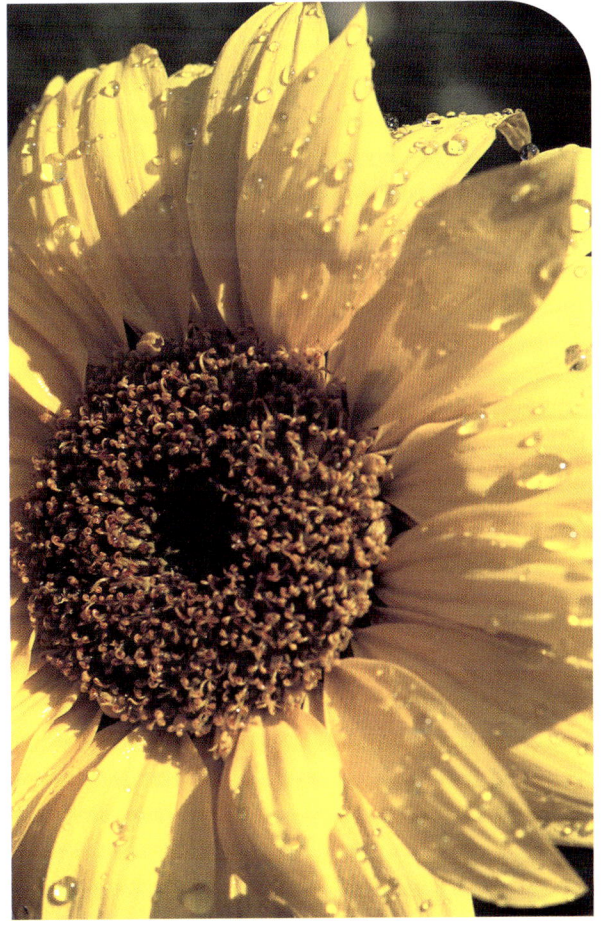

• **Environmental allergens**: Clients with allergies to pollen, mold, animal dander and saliva, food and other environmental substances often show increased sensitivity to some products and to stimulation of the skin. Some products may contain seaweed or algae, which could trigger an allergic reaction in someone who has an iodine or shellfish allergy.

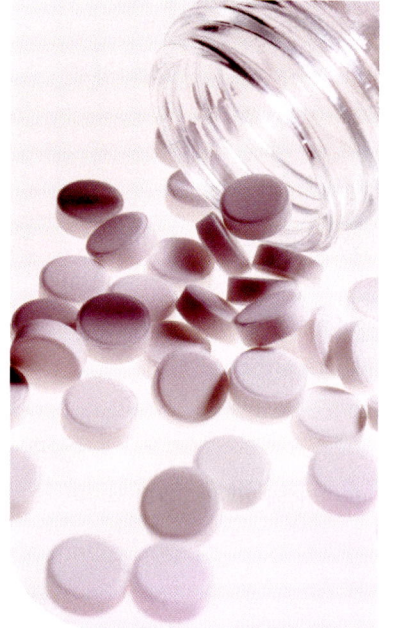

Medications and Treatments

Certain medications can also give reason to avoid specific services, treatments or products. What clients put into their bodies has an influence on the condition and appearance of the skin and nails. Knowing the types of medication that a client is taking is important to the results of professional services.

• **Oral antibiotics**: The use of oral antibiotics can create dryness, increase sensitivity and cause the blood to thin.

• **Steroids and blood thinners**: The use of steroid medications and blood thinner medications can cause the blood to thin.

• **Chemotherapy/radiation treatment**: Chemotherapy or radiation treatments heighten a client's sensitivity and may cause thinning of the skin.

If a client is taking any of these medications or treatments, take caution not to create an opening in the skin. Also avoid aggressive massage because it can cause bruising.

Lifestyle Evaluation

The third section of the Client Consultation Form, titled "Lifestyle Evaluation," allows clients to offer information based on their daily routines and how they treat their hands and feet. Do they work with their hands for extended periods of time during the day? Do they garden? If so, do they wear gloves? There is also space for clients to write what their home care regimen is, including products used and how much time they spend caring for their hands and feet.

CLIENT CONSULTATION FORM
LIFESTYLE EVALUATION

Occupation _____
What type of work do you perform using your hands each day?
_____

Are your hands submerged frequently in water? ___ Yes ___ No

Do you participate in sports? ___ Yes ___ No
If yes, what type of sports do you enjoy? _____

What other types of activities or hobbies do you take part in?
_____

Do you do household cleaning, gardening or dish washing by hand? ___ Yes ___ No
If yes, do you wear gloves? ___ Yes ___ No

Do you take steps at home to care for your hands? ___ Yes ___ No
If yes, what steps do you take and what products do you use?
_____

Do you take steps at home to care for your feet? ___ Yes ___ No
If yes, what steps do you take and what products do you use?
_____

Knowing a client's lifestyle helps you, as a professional, determine the best service for him or her. The following information provides a brief overview of typical lifestyle considerations that may help you determine the best services as well as the appropriate nail shape and length.

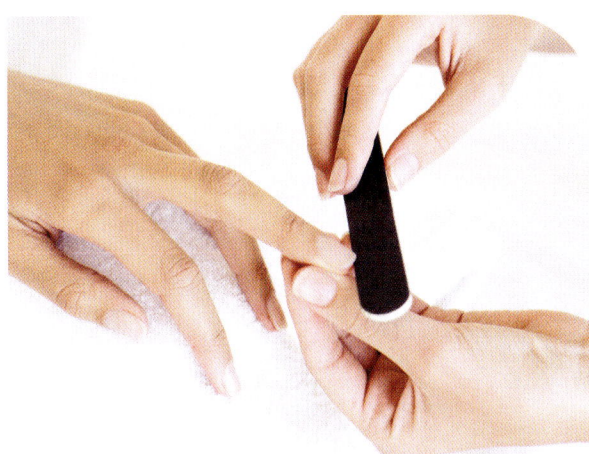

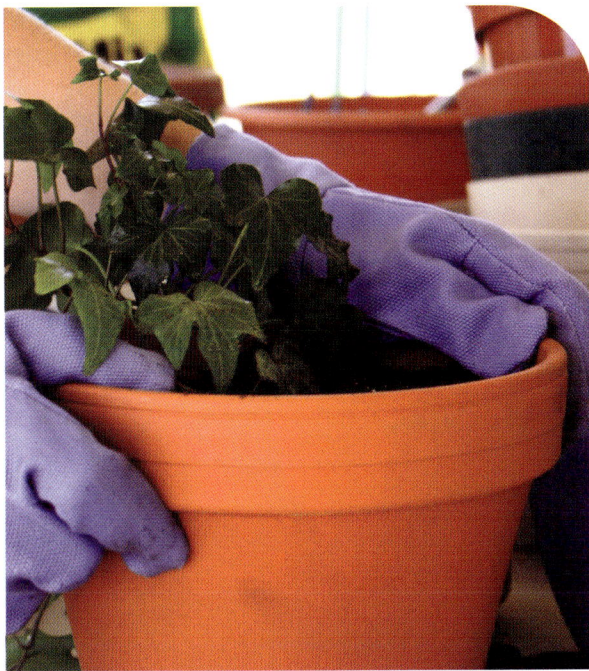

recommend a hot oil manicure with a paraffin dip. You would also recognize that a florist's nails would most likely need to be short.

- **At home nail care:** Knowing what products your clients use and what they do to their nails on a daily, weekly, or monthly basis can help you determine if they need a service that is fairly low maintenance, or if they are willing to spend some time at home to maintain the services they receive. It will also help you to determine if they are willing to work with you to achieve their desired results.

- **Hobbies:** Certain hobbies can be hard on the hands, feet and nails. Knowing what your client does on a daily basis will help you to determine the best course of services to reach your client's goals and expectations. For example, someone who does gardening or ceramics may have different needs than someone who does needlework.

- **Occupation:** Knowing a client's occupation will help you to determine what the best choice of service is and also what shape and length the nail should be. For example, if her occupation requires that she has her hands in water throughout the day, nail enhancements might not be the best choice because of an increased risk of a bacterial infection. Many florists have very rough, dry hands. Knowing this, you can

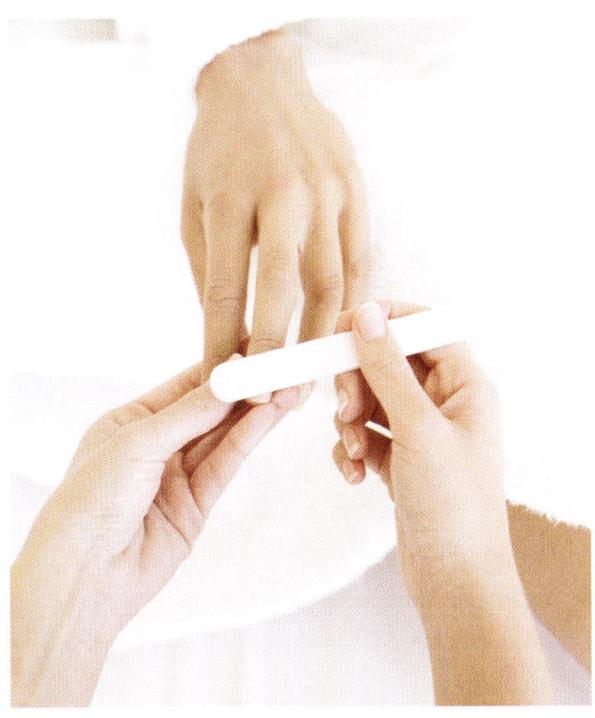

7

At the bottom of the Client Consultation Form is a "Client Release Statement," which gives you permission to service your clients based on the information they have provided on the form and during your consultation.

CLIENT RELEASE STATEMENT

I have read, understand and completed this questionnaire truthfully. I understand that withholding information or providing misinformation may result in undesired results and/or irritation to the skin or nails from services received. The services I receive here are voluntary, and I release this business and/or nail technician from liability and assume full responsibility thereof.

Signature _____ *Date* _____

Professional Evaluation

After clients have filled out their section of the form and shared their concerns, it is time for the technician to objectively review and evaluate the nails and skin. It is up to the technician to determine the best service to help the client reach his or her goals based on observations made and information obtained from the client.

During the professional evaluation, you will observe the nail plate and note any of the following:

- Split nails
- Ridges in the nails
- Discolored nails
- Evidence of nail biting
- Dry, brittle nails
- Strong nails

This is also where you would note the client's goals, such as to grow out damage from previous services or to quit biting his or her nails. Look at the cuticles—are they dry and cracked? Does the client bite his or her nails or pull on hangnails? Observe the overall skin condition of the hands and/or feet. Is the skin dry? Are there callused areas? The more observant you are as a technician, the better you can help your clients work toward their goals.

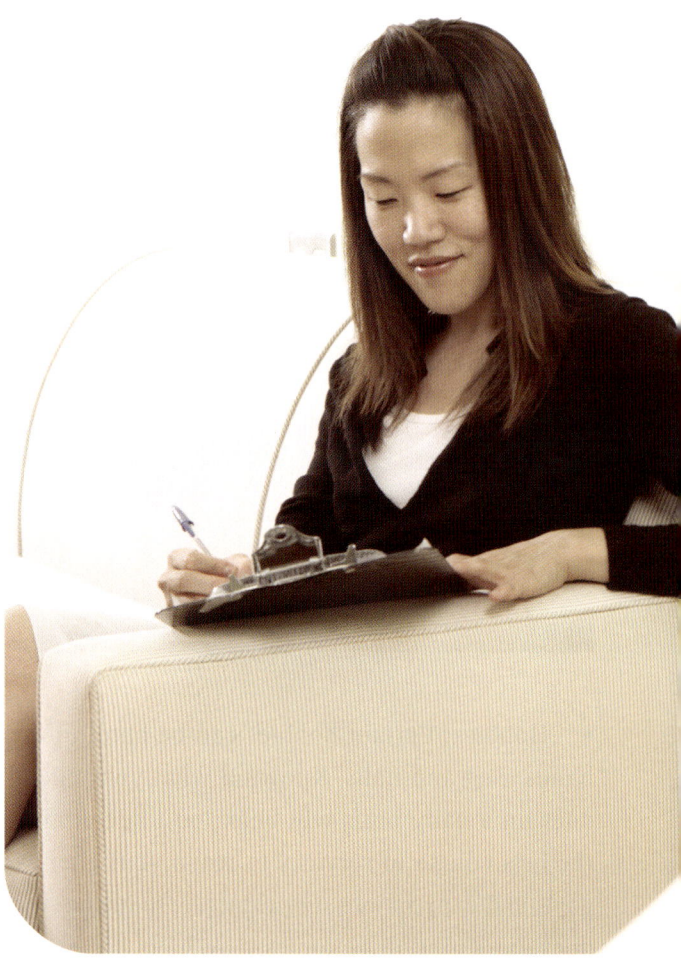

CLIENT CONSULTATION FORM
PROFESSIONAL EVALUATION

Observations:
Nails: _____
_____

Skin: _____

Goals: _____

Course of action: _____
_____

SERVICE RECORD

	DATE	SERVICE	PRODUCT USED	TECHNICIAN
1				
2				
3				
4				
5				

REMARKS

1
2
3
4
5

Service Record

The last section of the Client Consultation Form is to be filled out by the technician and used as a reference at the time of each future appointment. Each visit should be documented with the date of the visit, specific products that were used, any notes and the technician's initials. This allows the technician to remember the details of a client's previous visit. It is also important in the event that more than one technician sees the same client. Assessing changes in the nail condition is an important part of the nail care service. Noting the current condition of the client's nails and keeping records of any changes from visit to visit can help track the effectiveness of services and products that have been used.

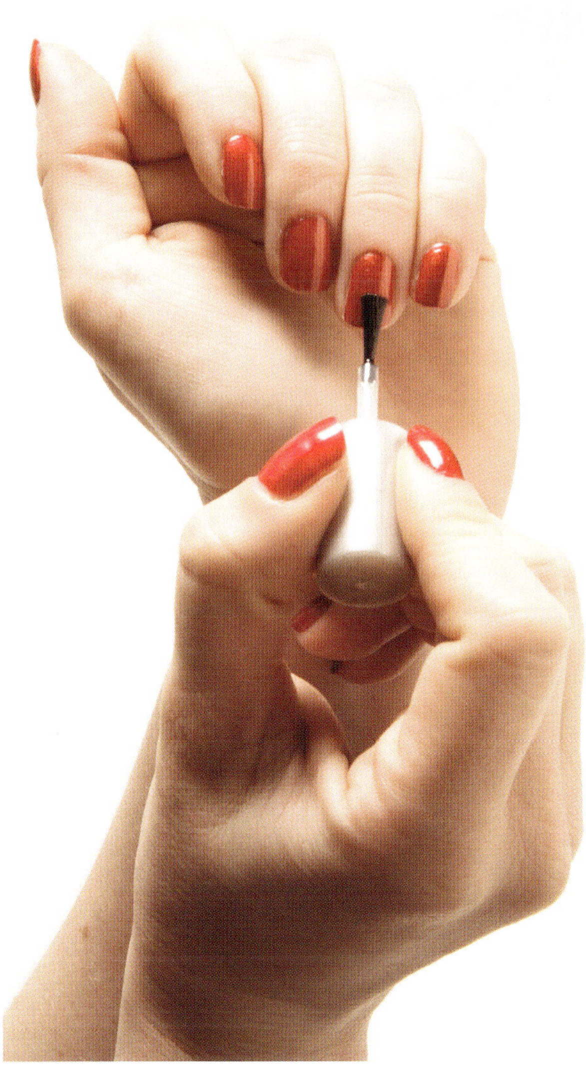

This information ensures consistency for future visits and allows you to follow up with specific questions from the previous visit such as, "How did you like the new polish color?" or "Are you noticing an improvement in the condition of your cuticles since using cuticle oil?"

Asking the right questions and analyzing client feedback will help you make the proper assessment and help guarantee the best possible service for your clients. Noting the relevant data and any special considerations on the Client Consultation Form provides a source for future reference and also helps maximize your efficiency. Once you have determined the needs of an individual client, you are ready to discuss recommendations for meeting these needs and achieving the desired results.

7

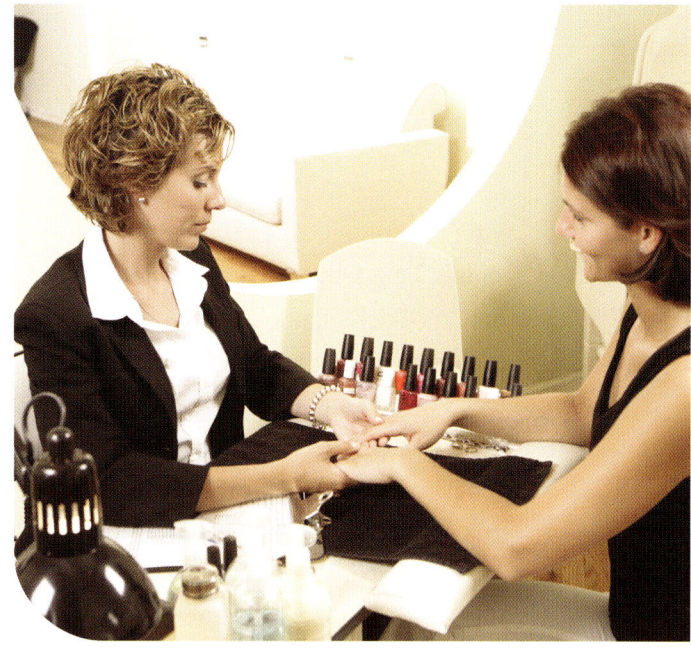

Agreement

Following the first two phases of service is the Agreement Phase. During this phase of the service, the technician summarizes and makes sure that the client agrees on the recommended services. Generally, clients have an easier time understanding when the technician avoids using professional "lingo," or technical terms. Using technical terms may intimidate clients and cause them to hesitate rather than move forward. The technician should try to use everyday language and reassure clients that the service is safe, comfortable and effective.

During the Agreement Phase:
- Summarize and explain the recommended service(s).
- State the cost of today's service, future services and home care products.
- Gain feedback from the client on your suggestions.
- Ensure that you and the client are in agreement before beginning the service.

To reach an agreement on the type of service that is going to be performed, it is important for the clients to understand what is going to be done and why. By explaining to the clients how a particular service is going to address their nail concerns, they will be more confident with the service.

In order to reach a mutual agreement, inform the client of the cost of the recommended service, along with the costs for projected future services and home care products. Providing the client with accurate information about the cost prior to the delivery can help build trust throughout all of the phases of service.

Open communication is important in being able to answer your client's questions regarding the service or your recommendations. Making sure the client understands what it is you are going to do is instrumental in helping gain and retain clients. Use visual support whenever possible by showing the equipment or products you will be using as you make recommendations.

Next, ask the client if he or she is ready to continue to the delivery of the service (agreement). If the client hesitates or has additional questions, keep communication open and do your best to alleviate any concerns.

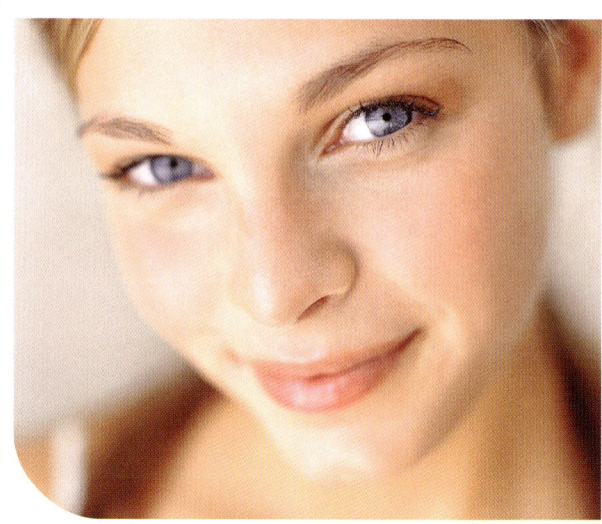

FIRST THREE PHASES OF SERVICE

Phase One
Greeting

How
Welcome client; introduce yourself with a firm handshake; make direct eye contact.

Why
Break the ice; learn the client's name; learn clues about personality; begin building rapport with client.

What
Good appearance for positive first impression; friendly smile; good posture; firm handshake.

7

Phase Two
Ask, Analyze, Assess

How
Escort client to seating area and ask him or her to complete a Client Consultation Form. Then, at the service station, perform a more thorough consultation: Ask about client's nail concerns; observe the nails and skin; review "Medical History" section of Client Consultation Form to make sure all medical and health-related conditions are listed. Finally, discuss nail care objectives with the client.

Why
Begin a record for each client; establish key contact information so that you can easily reach your client; learn about your client's nail conditions, concerns and any health conditions that could prevent you from proceeding with the service.

What
Client Consultation Form; good lighting; consultation and listening skills.

Phase Three
Agreement

How
Communicate your observations to your client including the condition you believe his or her nails are in and what services you recommend. Explain in detail the methods, equipment and products you will use.

Why
Educate your client about nail needs and how various products and services can help; reassure your client that he or she is in the hands of a professional.

What
Client Consultation Form; consultation and listening skills; knowledge of services and recommended products; skill in explaining product features and benefits.

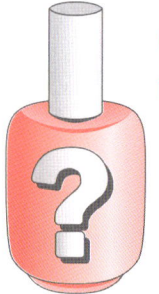

Which of the three phases that occurs before the service will be easiest for you to master? Which phase before the service will be the most difficult? Why?

DURING AND AFTER THE SERVICE

Now that you've successfully completed the first three phases of service, you are ready to move to the last two phases:

- Delivery–perform the service
- Completion–confirm satisfaction, recommend and rebook

You may think that the communication ends after reaching an agreement with the client regarding the service about to be performed. After all, it's time to perform the service. However, it is very important to continue the dialogue during and after the service to ensure that the client is comfortable and expectations are met. It also provides the opportunity to recommend a proper home care regimen and follow-up after the service.

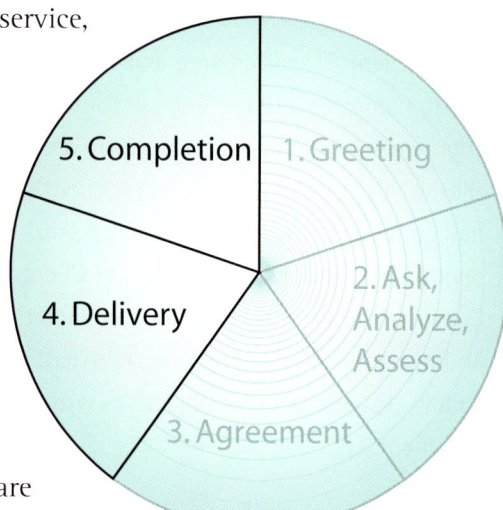

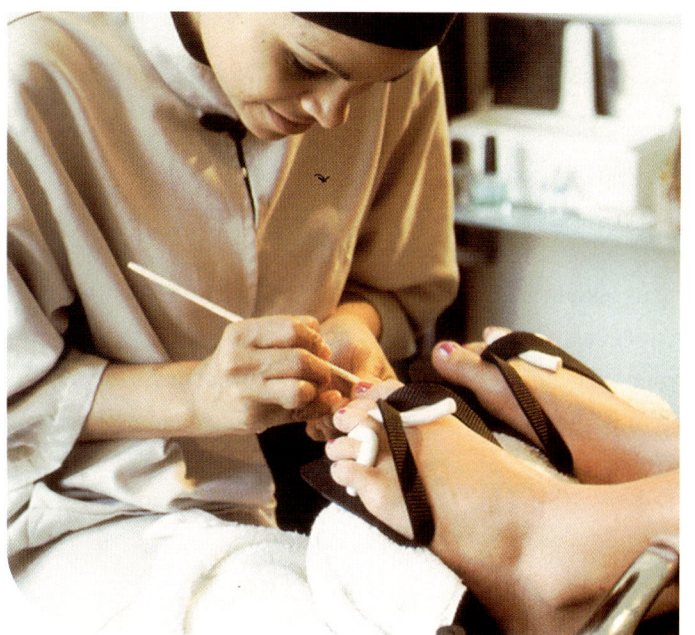

Delivery

Following agreement with the client, you are ready to provide the recommended service. During the Delivery Phase, you can continue to build trust and a sense of confidence. The goals of this phase are to ensure client comfort during the service; to educate the client and explain what is taking place; and to attain results that satisfy the client's needs and expectations.

Client comfort can be approached in many different ways. Never assume that the client is comfortable. Approach each and every client with a desire to make the session as comfortable as possible. For example, you can ask the client if you are using too much pressure at certain points or if he or she would like a glass of water. You can also ask whether the client likes the color of the polish chosen once the first nail is polished. Paying attention to small details during the service will help create a positive, memorable experience. When it comes to client care, little things can make all the difference.

Educating clients is an important step in helping them achieve the results they desire. It is important that clients understand why their nails are in the condition they are, what can be done to improve them and what results can be expected. A thorough educational process, led by the technician, can help achieve this.

In order to achieve desired results with nail care services, it is often best to recommend that the client commits to a series of services, such as regular monthly pedicures. Recommending services in a series is a perfect way to gain commitment from clients as well as provide them with an opportunity to maintain their nails more economically. Packages or sales of a series of services are usually offered at a slight discount.

Always tell clients what to expect during the service and what products will be used so that they understand what steps will be performed and why. The **feature** of a particular product is the key ingredient it contains that makes it effective. The **benefit** is the result that the ingredient delivers to the nails or skin. Each time a product—any product—is applied to the client's nails or skin, tell him or her what you are using, why you are using it and what benefits to expect from its use.

For example:

Technician: "I am going to apply a cuticle remover that contains alpha hydroxy acids. The alpha hydroxy acids will help to exfoliate the cuticles while allowing moisture to penetrate. This will help treat the hangnails which you mentioned during our consultation."

What you tell your client about the feature/benefit of a product is called a **product statement**. The product statement should be unique to you. Develop your own special way of describing the features and benefits of a product so that you express your belief in the product and the effectiveness of the results.

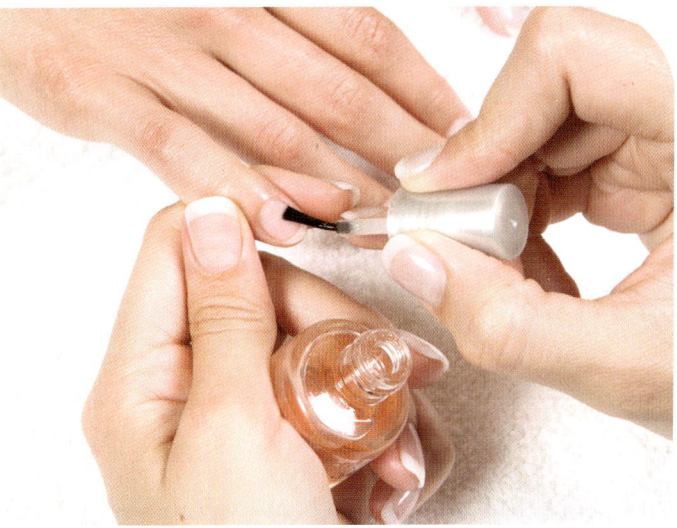

It is advisable to recommend the products that were used throughout the service for use at home. You have already described the importance of each product, the features and benefits, and how the products are to be used. This final step completes the professional "selling" process. If you have already provided your clients with knowledge of what the products will do for their nails and skin and the visible benefits they will receive without making unrealistic claims or guarantees, there is no need to "sell" them on the products—your clients will already be convinced of the benefits and want to purchase the products.

7

A thorough educational process ensures that clients are fully informed about the service and aware of the importance of home care. Your descriptions of the products will help the client be realistic about the expected results from nail care products. A well-informed client can translate into increased retail sales for you, so you can satisfy clients and be financially rewarded at the same time. This is what happens in the Completion Phase.

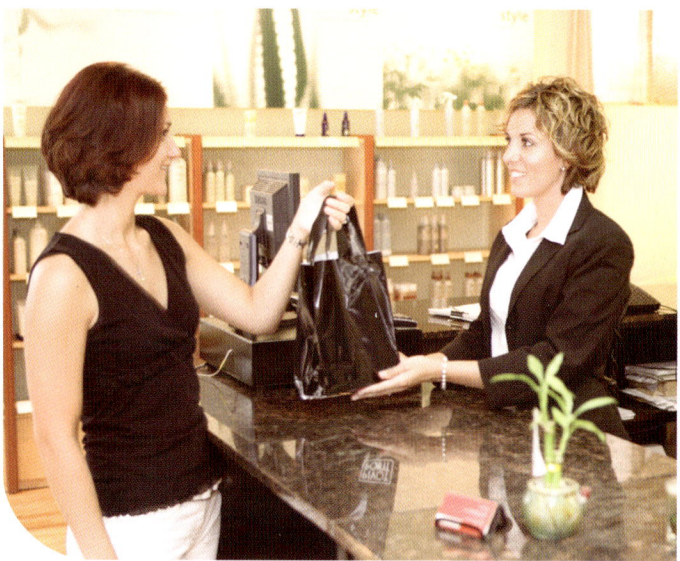

Completion

The final step of the client's visit is the Completion Phase. During this phase you are soliciting feedback, recommending a home care regimen and retail products, scheduling the client's next appointment and expressing appreciation as you say goodbye. The Completion Phase also includes following up with clients to help ensure satisfaction with the service.

Soliciting Feedback

Making a client feel like a guest during a visit to a salon or spa is more likely to result in a client who will rebook the service. Of course, you hope every client has been treated well, has enjoyed the experience and is eager to return. But the truth is, not all clients are,

nor will they be completely honest about this. In cases when the client is noncommittal or responds indifferently when asked, it's best to use intuition. Encourage the client to communicate freely, even if it is a complaint. It is true that you cannot satisfy all of the people all of the time, but your goal will be to satisfy the majority of your clients. Be sure to stick to the policies of the salon or spa. If you have any concern regarding a difficult situation, consult with a manager, owner or supervisor to help resolve the situation so you can ensure the client leaves satisfied. Typically, unhappy clients do not return, and very few call after the visit to express their feelings.

In general, when communication is kept open and clients are encouraged to give feedback, unexpected negative complaints are reduced significantly. Keep in mind that even an angry client can be turned into a happy, loyal client simply by feeling that his or her input is not only heard, but is valued. After you gain feedback from the client, use this time to thank the client for selecting your salon or spa and, more specifically, your services.

Home Care Regimen and Retail Sales

It is best to recommend that clients use nail care products that are suited to their particular needs. Appropriate products, selected for clients based upon consultation and analysis, further personalize your service. These products will need to be used during the service so clients can gain an understanding of the product that you will recommend for use at home.

Upon completion of the service, guide clients toward the retail and/or front desk area. This is the time to review with them the products used during the service, and recommend that they continue using these products at home.

As mentioned earlier, properly teaching clients about the products used during the service is the first step in recommending a home care regimen and establishing a strong retail sales business. By teaching clients about each product during

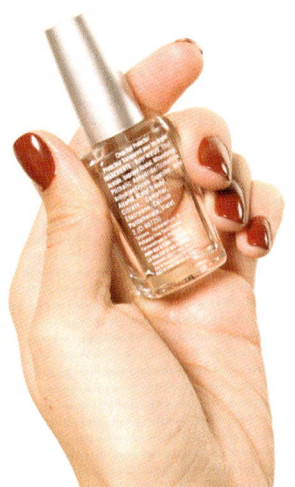

the service, your recommendation or selling process is almost complete. You can end your service by saying, "The products that I just used are those that I recommend for you to use at home in order to continue achieving the benefits that we have started today. I have selected a cuticle oil that you can use every day. This will help keep your cuticles moisturized and your nails more flexible so they are less likely to break."

It is important never to discredit products that clients are currently using, but rather to stress the features and benefits of your recommended products. You can also address how the product selection can help meet the client's nail care concerns.

Before clients leave, explain how to use each recommended product. It will be virtually identical to the procedure that you used during the service. For example, inform clients that they need to use a cuticle oil in the morning

and at night to have healthier cuticles and nails. When clients believe in your professional knowledge and that you care for their nails, your sales in products and services increase. Be ready to explain how to use all products and why some products are more expensive than others.

By following the client education guidelines described here, technicians are able to make home care recommendations with ease. When recommending products for home use, it is important to speak with knowledge and confidence. Clients must believe that the professionals have faith in the products they recommend. Technicians who personally use the products they sell can impact their clients' trust in the products as well.

Referrals

Word-of-mouth, which means news that is spread by verbal communication, is the best form of advertising in any customer service business. This is particularly true in the beauty business. Clients trust the care and health of their nails to proven professionals. So, clients themselves are a very important part of an advertising campaign. If they are happy with your services, they will be eager to pass along a recommendation to friends, family members and co-workers. Generally, a new client who has been referred by an existing client is quite likely to become a regular.

Many businesses offer incentives or discounts for regular clients who refer a new client, such as one free manicure for every five clients referred. One idea is to give clients five business cards each, ask them to write their name on the back, and give them to interested prospects. Each new client can bring the card in with him or her so the original client can get credit for the referral.

7

Rebooking the Next Appointment

An important part of the Completion Phase is scheduling the client's next appointment, also referred to as **rebooking** or **pre-booking**. This helps to ensure repeat business. Building a strong client base can take several years or more, and repeat business is one of the keys to creating this base. It is much easier to utilize the base you have rather than constantly seeking out new clients. A good practical guideline is that once you have established a client base, you should still strive to acquire new clients each week.

New clients are a necessity, but repeat clients ensure that appointment books are full from week to week and month to month. Offer clients a suggested date for a future appointment, then offer alternative appointment times that allow the client to select morning, afternoon or evening. Suggesting that the client rebook is always advisable. Many salon and spa owners and/or managers establish a goal number or percentage of all clients who should be rebooking appointments. This provides a way to measure success and can sometimes be an incentive for an additional financial reward.

> You can help guarantee repeat business by satisfying clients while they are in your care. By using the techniques discussed in this chapter, you can meet the needs of each client and deliver individual client satisfaction. Satisfied clients are likely to return and become regular clients. It is easier to retain a client than it is to find a new client. This is why client care is so important!

Follow-Up

Following up with clients after a service is necessary in order to help guarantee client satisfaction. There are three primary reasons to follow up with clients:

1. To check on the condition of the client's nails and skin following the service. This lets the technician know whether a client is satisfied with the service results and that there were no adverse reactions.

2. To check on the client's satisfaction with any products purchased. Often a client will forget what a particular product may be for or when and how to use it. Follow-up calls provide the client with an opportunity to ask questions.

3. To build a good working relationship and rapport with your clients. This will open the lines of communication between you and your clients. They will feel more comfortable discussing their nail care needs and services with you.

There may be times when a client is not completely satisfied with either the service or the products purchased. Some clients call

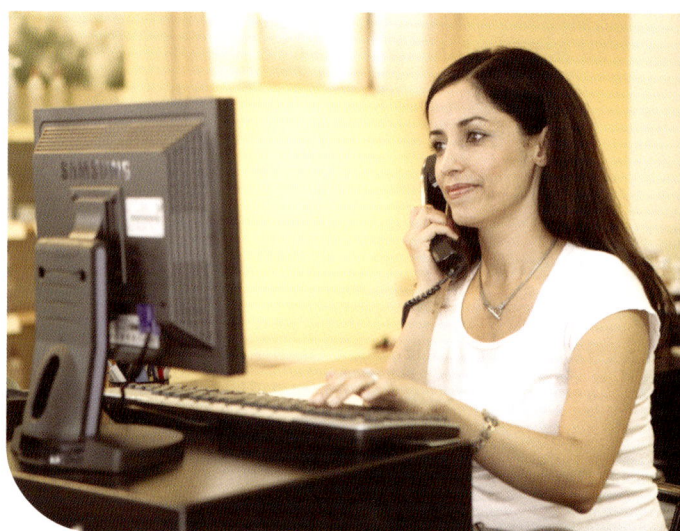

to complain, but the majority never return. Following up within 72 hours of a service invites clients to freely express dissatisfaction, and gives the technician the opportunity to learn how to improve. This is a chance to discuss anything that did or did not go as smoothly as possible so that the client will consider returning another time. One of the most important questions to ask in a follow-up call is, "Is there anything that could have made your experience better?" Even if it was a great experience, there is always room for improvement. Two effective follow-up procedures are care calls and thank-you notes.

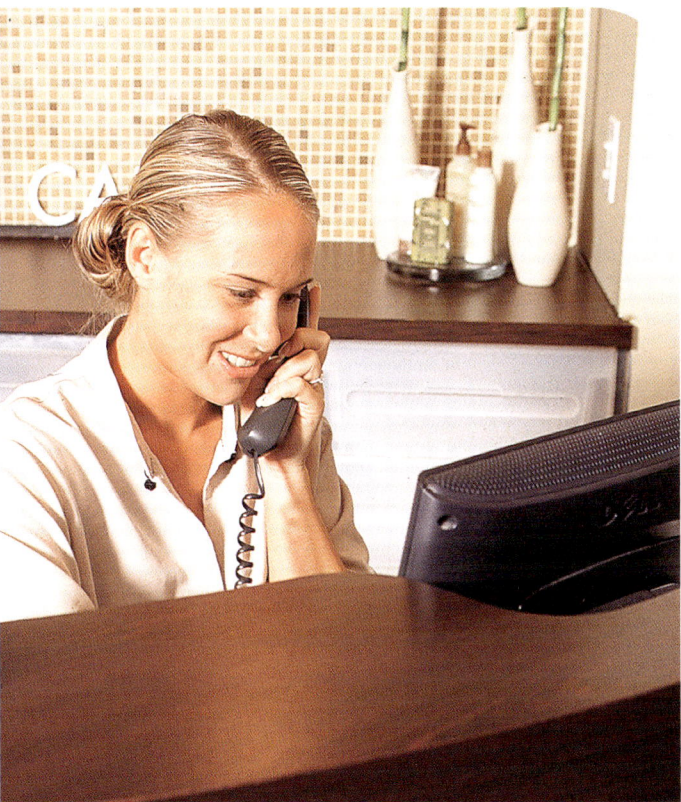

Care Calls

There are many different ways to follow up with a new client after a service. A phone call—often referred to as "follow-up" or a "care call"—is one of the most personal ways. It is best to try to reach a client when you believe he or she will be home, but that is generally evenings

and weekends, when technicians are the busiest. If you need to call during the day and no one is available to take your call, leaving a pleasant message is also impressive. Remember, the purpose of your call is to find out:

- If the client was satisfied with the experience;
- How the client's nails and skin reacted;
- How the products are working;
- If there are any questions that he or she has;
- If there is anything that could have made it a more enjoyable experience.

The following are ideas to help engage the client during a care call.

- "Hello Mrs. Jones, this is Mandy from ABC Nail Spa. I was just calling to see how your nail enhancements are working for you and to see if you have any questions."
- "How are the new cuticle oil and hand cream working for you?"
- "Is there anything I could have done to provide you with a more enjoyable experience?"
- "Please feel free to give me a call at your convenience if you have any questions or if there is anything else I can do for you."
- "I look forward to seeing you in two weeks to rebalance your nail enhancements."

Thank-You Notes

Thank-you notes are another way to follow up after a first-time client has had a service. Many businesses have pre-printed thank-you cards that can be quickly signed and addressed. A thank-you note does not need to be lengthy; a brief note addressing the same topics you would during a care call is all that is needed.

7

Here is an example of a follow-up thank-you note written to a first-time client:

Dear Mrs. Jones,

It was a pleasure having the opportunity to meet you and provide your nail care services. I hope you were pleased with the results as well as the service.

Feel free to contact me if you have any questions or concerns, or if there is anything that I can do to make your next visit more enjoyable. I look forward to seeing you for your next service.

Sincerely,

Mandy

Mandy and the Staff from
ABC Nail Spa
555.123.4567

It is recommended that follow-up calls are made and notes are sent within 72 hours following a visit. This allows three days to determine how the client's nails and skin have reacted and how the new products are working.

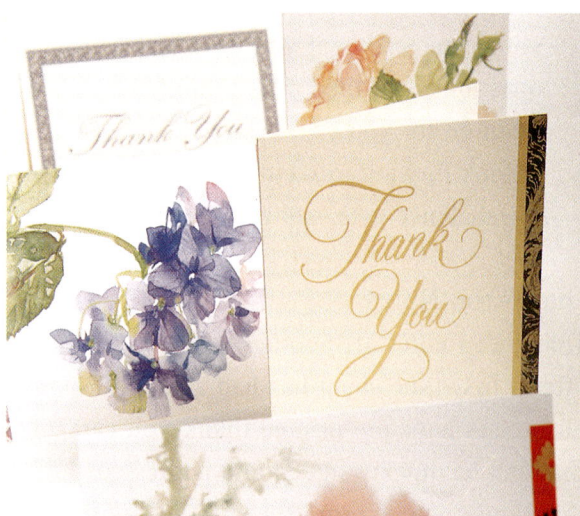

A follow-up call or note should be done for every client who is new to you. Even if you are a new employee in an existing business, it is good to be sure that pre-existing clients are satisfied with the services you deliver. Follow-up is also important with clients who purchase products that they have not used before. This gives you a chance to check and see if the new products are working effectively for this client. A satisfied client will easily express satisfaction, but if a client is dissatisfied with the recommended products, it's an opportunity for you to suggest other options. Clients will view you as a professional who truly cares about achieving results and cares about them. Think of it as a valuable learning tool: You can learn what you do well and what you can improve upon, which helps speed up your learning curve.

As a recap, the five phases of service are as follows:

- Greeting
- Ask, Analyze, Assess
- Agreement
- Delivery
- Completion

The five phases of service described in this chapter can work for all clients and all services. Client care skills, like other techniques and skills, need to be continually practiced to be honed, sharpened and improved.

A rewarding career begins with a commitment to excellence. If you offer your knowledge and your skills to every client, you will be on your way to financial and personal success.

LAST TWO PHASES OF SERVICE

7

Phase Four
Delivery

How
Ensure client's comfort during service; explain steps and actions that are taking place; commit to delivering the highest quality of service.

Why
Satisfy the client's needs.

What
Equipment appropriate for recommended service; recommended products; service skills.

Phase Five
Completion

How
Gain feedback; ask how the client enjoyed the service; discuss home care regimen; suggest purchase of products; schedule next appointment; guide client to front desk, thank him or her and bid goodbye. Document details. Within 72 hours, follow up with a thank-you note and/or a phone call to see if there were any reactions to the service.

Why
Ensure that the client is satisfied and understands how important home care regimen is; increase retail sales; encourage referrals for other clients; ensure that the client had no adverse reactions to the service.

What
Friendly handshake; note cards; business cards; appointment book; service record.

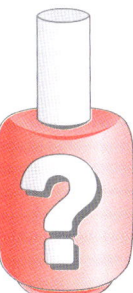

Which phase of service, Delivery or Completion, will be the easiest for you to master? Which phase will be more difficult? Why?

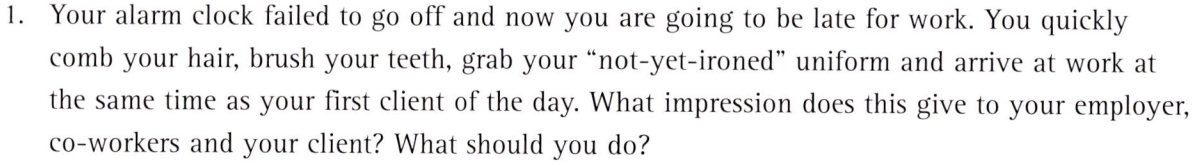

Case Studies

The following situations are designed to help you build your decision-making skills. Using your training to this point, review the following scenarios, then think through and describe how you would handle each challenge.

1. Your alarm clock failed to go off and now you are going to be late for work. You quickly comb your hair, brush your teeth, grab your "not-yet-ironed" uniform and arrive at work at the same time as your first client of the day. What impression does this give to your employer, co-workers and your client? What should you do?

2. During your consultation and analysis, you discover that your client has signs of a bacterial infection under her artificial nails. How do you respond?

3. A new client arrives for a manicure. After the consultation and an initial analysis, you recommend a paraffin treatment with the manicure. Your client asks why you recommend this. How would you reply and why?

In this chapter, you will put your studies into action and learn—step-by-step—how to deliver natural nail manicures and pedicures. In our society, we place a high value on attractive hands and nails. At the same time, a great benefit is that hand and foot services relax and make clients feel pampered. These services produce satisfied clients with positive feelings about the nail salon experience. This translates into repeat business that will keep your appointment book full.

VALUE

The natural nail manicure and pedicure are the core services of the nail technology industry, and the basis from which you can build all of your other services. Mastering these two highly popular services is key to your successful career.

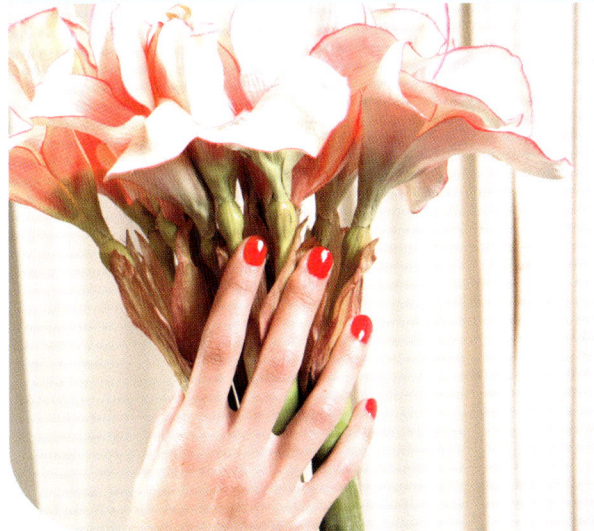

MAIN IDEA

This chapter focuses on two of the most-requested services: the basic natural nail manicure and pedicure procedures. In order to deliver these services at a professional level, nail technicians are expected to master procedures and general massage techniques as well as understand the uses and functions of all products, implements, supplies and equipment. Of all the nail care services you will perform, the ability to perform a relaxing and pleasant manicure or pedicure remains the single-most important entry-level skill for nail technicians.

PLAN		OBJECTIVES
Manicure Essentials	• Massage • Manicure Products • Manicure Implements • Manicure Supplies • Manicure Equipment	Describe the five basic movements of massage for the basic manicure. Name the factors that make performing massage manipulations inadvisable. Identify and describe the functions of manicure products, implements, supplies and equipment.
Basic Manicure	• Basic Manicure Preparation • Basic Manicure Procedure • Basic Manicure Completion	Demonstrate the procedure for the basic natural nail manicure.
Pedicure Essentials	• Massage • Pedicure Products • Pedicure Implements • Pedicure Supplies • Pedicure Equipment	Describe the five basic movements of massage for the basic pedicure. Name the factors that make performing massage manipulations inadvisable. Identify and describe the functions of pedicure products, implements, supplies and equipment.
Basic Pedicure	• Basic Pedicure Preparation • Basic Pedicure Procedure • Basic Pedicure Completion	Demonstrate the procedure for the basic natural nail pedicure.

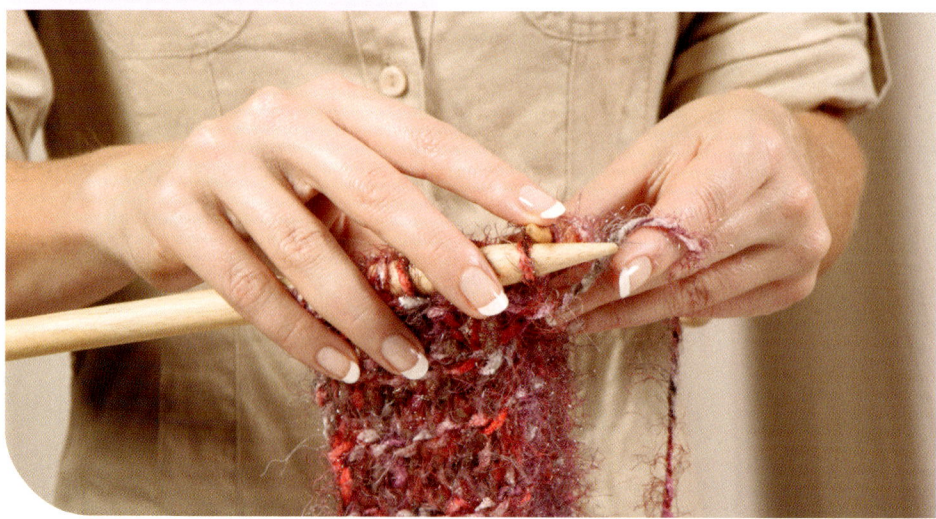

MANICURE ESSENTIALS

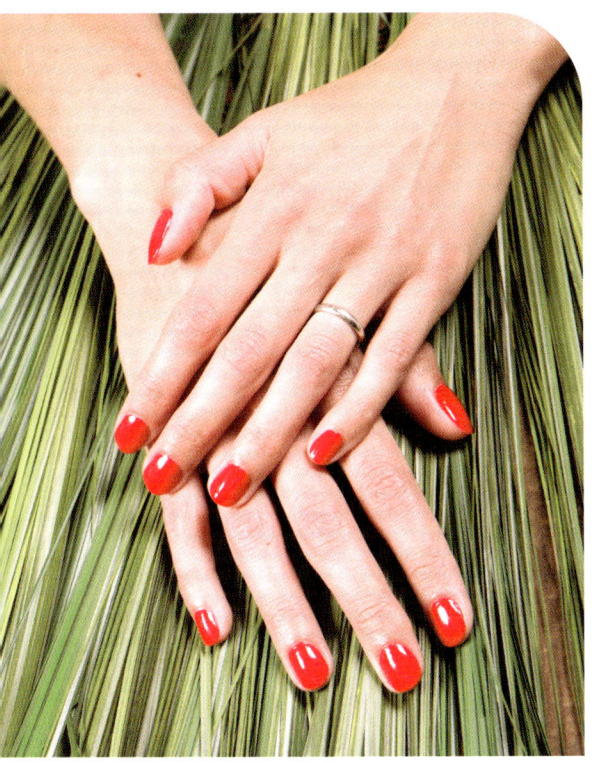

Nail care dates back more than 4,000 years to southern Babylonia. Fingernail polish can be traced even further back to 3,000 B.C. in China, where a person's nail color indicated social status. Today, nail care is an essential for many, and the demand for high-quality care continues to grow, with more than $6 billion spent each year in the United States alone. And women aren't the only ones seeking well-groomed hands and feet. Men are increasingly aware of the positive impact that nicely manicured nails can have both socially and professionally, and account for an ever-growing percentage of nail care clients. In this chapter, you will learn the basic nail services for natural nails in order to provide your clients with safe and beneficial services. Mastering the basics of manicuring and pedicuring will allow you to advance your skills to include artificial nails or enhancements, spa services, mini-services or add-on services.

As a professional nail technician, you will need to be knowledgeable about the essential massage movements, products, implements, supplies and types of equipment used to care for natural nails. It is important to understand the functions and uses of these items in order to provide clients with the best possible services.

Massage

Massage is a systematic, therapeutic method of manipulating the body by rubbing, pinching, tapping, kneading or stroking with hands, fingers or an instrument. In ancient cultures, massage treatments were thought to have magical, therapeutic powers. Men and women had their bodies massaged with animal and vegetable oils to maintain their health and to keep their skin soft, supple and attractive. Today, many people ask: "Is it the mental state derived from the massage that helps a person feel better, or does massage have benefits beyond relaxation?"

Benefits of Massage

As aging occurs, dehydration (loss of fluids) increases. Massage increases circulation to help remove waste from body cells at a more efficient rate. Increased circulation and renewed flexibility are two major benefits of massage. In addition to the physical benefits, massage is also emotionally soothing, since the human body responds well to touch that is safe, caring and confident.

The many benefits of massage include:

- Increased circulation of the blood supply to the skin
- Tighter, firmer muscles
- Stimulation of the glandular activities of the skin
- Stronger muscle tissue
- Relief from pain
- Softer, improved texture of the skin
- Relief of emotional stress and body tension

In most regions, a nail technician is licensed only to massage from the elbow to the fingertips and the knee to the ends of the toes. Be guided by your regulating agency on the areas of the body a nail technician may massage.

The Five Basic Massage Techniques

There are five basic massage movements (manipulations). Each one performs a different function and delivers different results. The use of each movement in combination with others delivers optimal results.

Effleurage

Effleurage is a stroking or circular movement that is light, relaxing, smooth and gentle. This method is carried out with the pads of the fingertips or the palms of the hands. The purpose of effleurage is to soothe muscles and relax the sensory nerve endings at the surface of the skin. Effleurage affects surface muscle tissue and is used on the arms, hands, fingers, legs, feet and toes. Effleurage is often used to begin and end massage.

It is a good practice to lighten your touch and gently remove your hands at the end of a massage. This is referred to as "feathering off."

Petrissage

Petrissage is light or heavy kneading, pinching and rolling of the muscles used on the hands, arms, feet and legs. The purpose of petrissage is to stimulate muscles, nerves and skin glands, which in turn increases the circulation of blood and lymph. Petrissage is performed by kneading the muscles between the thumb and fingers or by pressing the palm of the hand firmly over the muscles, then grasping and squeezing between the heel of the hand and the fingers.

Friction

Friction is a circular or wringing movement with no gliding, usually performed with the fingertips or palms of the hands. Rather than moving across the skin, friction moves the skin either across the muscle or the bone beneath it. The purpose of friction is to stimulate and warm the muscles and this increases circulation.

Tapotement or Percussion

Tapotement is a light tapping or slapping movement applied with the fingertips or partly flexed fingers. The purpose of tapotement is to increase blood circulation, stimulate the nerves and promote muscle contraction. Tapotement assists the skin in releasing carbon dioxide and waste material and is the most stimulating massage movement. This invigorating manipulation should not be used when the primary purpose of the massage is to relax the client.

Vibration

Vibration is a shaking movement achieved when the technician quickly shakes his or her arms while the fingertips or palms are touching the client. Vibration is a very stimulating movement and should be done for only a short period of time.

Massage Cautions

Avoid performing massage manipulations on clients with the following conditions:

- Skin conditions such as redness, swelling, pus, disease, bruises and/or broken or scraped skin
- Heart conditions/High blood pressure
- Stroke
- Pregnancy

Use caution when performing massage manipulations on clients with the following conditions:

- Prominent varicose veins
- Arthritis

When working with clients who are being treated for cancer, it is advisable to find out whether or not their physician has specific recommendations relative to massage. Depending on the doctor or the prescribed course of treatment, it may be necessary to refrain from massage of any kind.

Keep in mind that the massage portion of a nail care service is generally considered to be the most relaxing and enjoyable part. Therefore, perfecting the various massage movements will help ensure that your clients will want to come to you for their future nail care needs.

More and more clients are just as interested in the massage portion of the service as they are in the nail care aspect. To add to your manicure and pedicure services, you may want to study reflexology, Shiatsu and/or Swedish massage. Be guided by your regulating agency as to which services nail technicians can perform.

Avoid removing the hands from the body once the massage manipulation has begun. If you need to remove your hands, use a light, feather-like movement to gently lift the hands off of the body. Replace hands on the skin in the same manner.

Important points to remember when performing massage manipulations:

- Check for conditions mentioned previously.
- Avoid massage that is too deep, aggressive or lengthy.
- Provide an even tempo or rhythm and pressure to ensure a relaxing effect for the client.

Manicure Products

Nail products, also referred to as nail cosmetics, are vital in keeping nails healthy and well-cared for. To best care for your clients' nails, you will need to know how and when to apply each product, as well as how the nails will benefit from each specific one. That's why it is important to know the ingredients—the more you know about the product you are using, the better you will be able to determine what is best for each client. One thing to remember is to always follow the manufacturers' instructions and recommendations; not doing so could cause undesirable results or even adverse reactions. Many of the same products used to perform a manicure are used in providing other nail services as well.

Liquid Soap

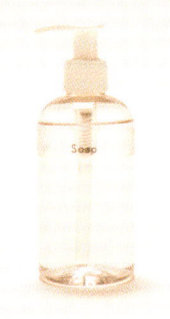

Liquid soap is used to cleanse the technician's and the client's hands before the service. It can also be used in the finger bowl for soaking the client's fingernails. The main purpose of soap is to help fight off harmful surface bacteria. It is recommended to use a liquid soap because bar soap is more likely to become contaminated with bacteria.

Antiseptic Sanitizer

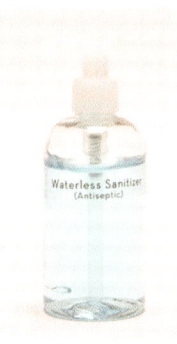

An **antiseptic sanitizer** helps to reduce bacteria on the surface of the skin to aid in the prevention of **cross-contamination**, which is the transfer of bacteria from a contaminated surface or object. This cleanser is also used to cleanse the technician's and client's hands before the service, but should not be used in place of washing hands with soap. The antiseptic sanitizer that is most often used in the salon is a gel-like waterless sanitizer that is applied to the hands like liquid soap, but is not rinsed off. Be guided by your regulatory guidelines regarding the use of antiseptic sanitizers in the salon.

Polish Remover

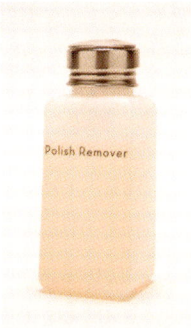

Nail **polish remover** is used to dissolve and remove polish. It is a liquid that sometimes contains acetone, a highly flammable liquid solvent. Pure acetone is used to remove most nail enhancements completely and, therefore, it is recommended that a non-acetone or low-acetone polish remover be used to remove any polish from nail enhancements.

> Did you know that nails can be an indicator of your overall health? Many times doctors can quickly judge a person's health condition by looking at the color of the person's nails. That's why you are asked to remove your nail polish when admitted to the hospital.

REMOVING POLISH

Polish remover is used to remove polish from the nail easily. Here is a quick step-by-step of how to remove polish from the nail plate.

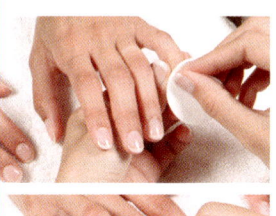

1. Saturate cotton or a lint-free nail wipe with polish remover and place the saturated cotton or wipe on the nail plate.

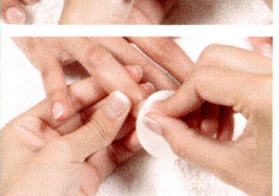

2. Let it stand for a few seconds, and then wipe toward the free edge. Remove all polish from each nail before moving to the next nail.

Cuticle Remover

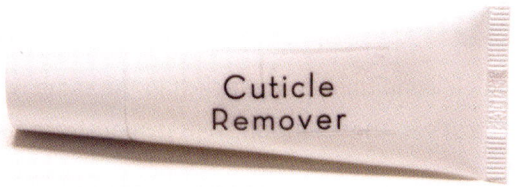

Cuticle remover is used to soften cuticle tissue to allow gentle pushing back and to aid in its removal. It is available in cream or gel form and contains chemical exfoliants, sodium hydroxide or potassium hydroxide at a 2-5% solution. Cuticle remover should not be left on the cuticles longer than 10 minutes because chemical exfoliants do not stop working until they are removed. For this reason, some product lines recommend using cuticle remover before soaking in the finger bowl. Always follow the manufacturer's instructions.

CUTICLE REMOVER APPLICATION

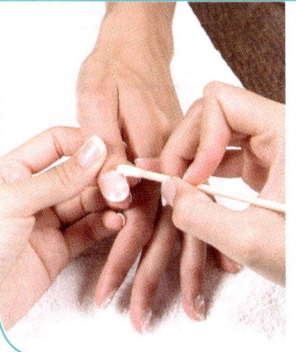

To properly apply cuticle remover, remember these points:

- Apply cuticle remover to the cuticle area using either a cotton-tipped orangewood stick, cotton swab or dropper.

- Avoid having the applicator tip or dropper come into contact with the client's nail or skin if applying the cuticle remover directly from the bottle.

Cuticle Conditioners

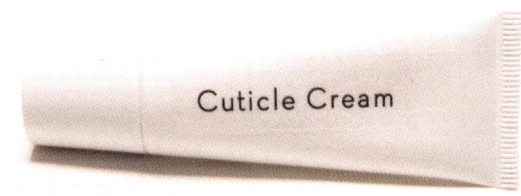

Cuticle conditioners are used to soften cuticles and surrounding skin. They moisturize cuticles and nails to prevent hangnails and dry cuticles, while they add moisture and flexibility to dry, brittle nails. There are two types of conditioners available today: creams and oils. **Cuticle creams**

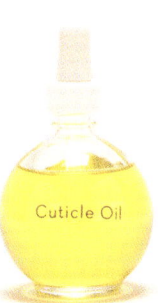

sometimes contain a small amount of alpha hydroxy acids, which help remove dead skin and allow products to penetrate better. Creams also contain ingredients such as lanolin and cocoa butter that help moisturize. **Cuticle oils** also help prevent nails from becoming dry and brittle and contain ingredients such as Vitamin E and jojoba oil. Cuticle conditioners are often used as a finishing touch to a nail service, but can also be used daily as part of a home care regimen.

CUTICLE CONDITIONING

Cuticle conditioners are applied in the same way as cuticle remover—except they are massaged into the cuticle. The following steps demonstrate the application of cuticle conditioner.

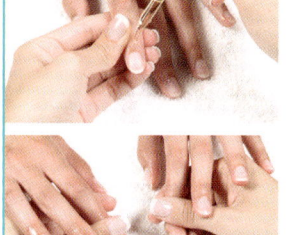

1. Apply cuticle conditioner to the cuticle area using either a cotton-tipped orangewood stick, cotton swab or dropper.

2. Avoid having the applicator tip or dropper come into contact with the client's nail or skin if applying the cuticle conditioner directly from the bottle. Massage the conditioner gently into the cuticle area.

Nail Bleach

Nail bleach is used to remove stains and discoloration on the nail plate. It can be applied under the free edge or on top of the nail plate. The active ingredient is hydrogen peroxide at 6%.

Hairstylists often use 20-volume (6%) developer when coloring hair. The 20-volume developer is hydrogen peroxide at 6% and also works as a nail-bleaching agent.

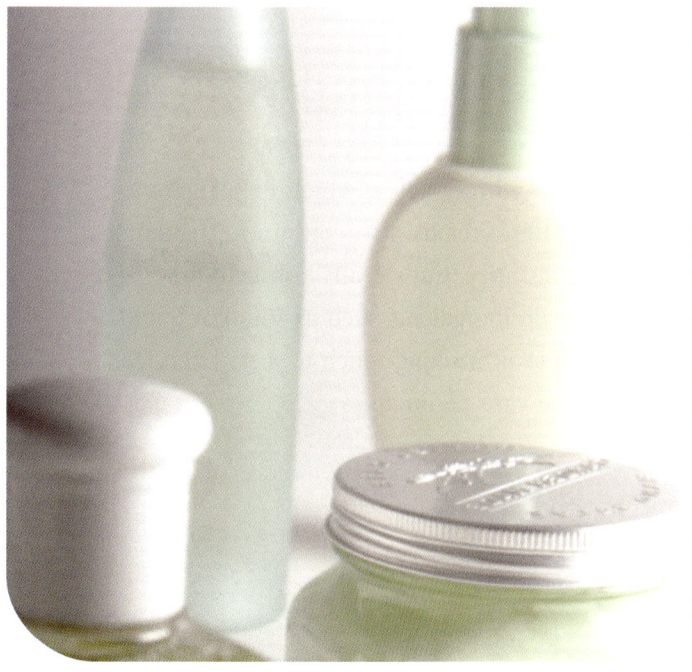

Moisturizing Lotion or Cream

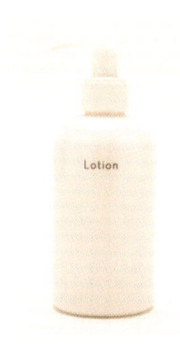

Lotions or **creams** are used to perform hand, arm, foot and leg massage. They help skin retain moisture and prevent or protect it from dryness. The difference between a cream and a lotion is generally that creams are thicker in consistency. Typically, cream is used if the skin is very dry because it contains more moisturizing ingredients. Lotion has a thinner consistency and is typically used if there is excessive arm or leg hair because it is less likely to cling to the hair. Lotion also helps to allow the technician's hands to move more easily over the area.

Nail Preparation Solution

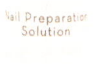

Nail Preparation Solution

Nail preparation solution is a specific product used to remove oil and other products from the nail, prior to applying any polish. This specialized product is designed to help the base coat and polish adhere to the nail plate. Alcohol or nail polish remover may be used in place of a specific nail preparation solution.

Polish

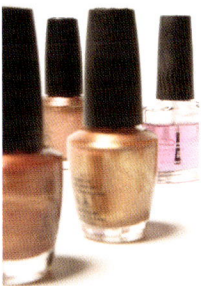

Nail polish is used to strengthen, fill in ridges, and can add shine and/or color to the surface of the nail. Before applying polish, it is important to always roll the bottle of polish between the palms of your hands to make sure that the ingredients are well-mixed. For best results, avoid shaking the bottle, since this can create air bubbles in the polish, which makes the finished polish look bubbly or have a rough texture.

Most polishes contain four major ingredients:

- Polymers—make it hard and shiny
- Plasticizers—increase flexibility and wear
- Solvents—make it spreadable
- Pigments—give it color

Refer to *Chapter 5, Chemistry* for more details on these ingredients.

Nail Strengthener

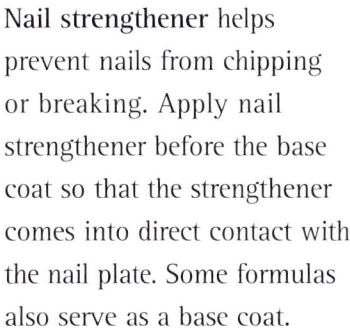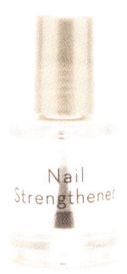

Nail Strengthener

Nail strengthener helps prevent nails from chipping or breaking. Apply nail strengthener before the base coat so that the strengthener comes into direct contact with the nail plate. Some formulas also serve as a base coat.

Often called nail treatment, many strengtheners contain fibers and some contain low levels of formaldehyde, which is a chemical used as a preservative. Though some nail strengtheners may have up to 3% formaldehyde, 1% or lower is a recommended strength to use on nails. Using

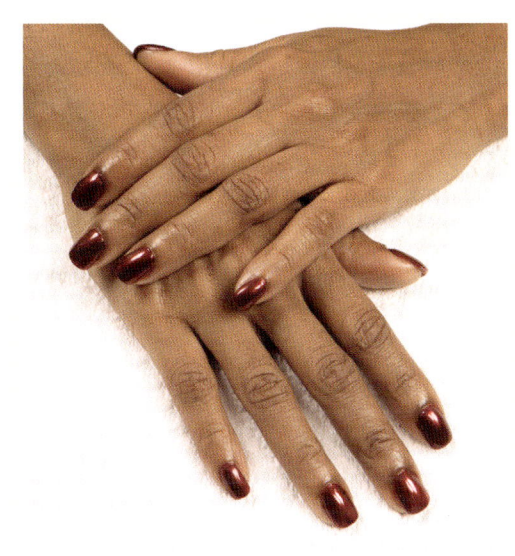

When it comes to nail services, it is the polish that leaves a lasting impression. In fact, polish is the first thing on most clients' minds when they come in to have their nails "done." Often they go right to the polish display to choose a color. Sometimes they bring their favorite polish with them. These days, polishes are available in every imaginable color.

Whether the client wishes to change colors with the seasons or to make a fashion statement, it is this part of the service that gets the client the most involved. What most clients may not know, however, is that nail polishes serve many purposes—they can strengthen and protect the nails, in addition to enhancing the look of the nails.

8

a product that contains more than 1% formaldehyde may cause the nail to become too stiff so that it loses flexibility, making it more likely to chip or break under pressure.

Base Coat

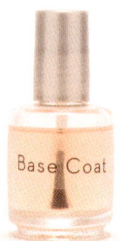

A **base coat** is often used to even out the nail plate and to help polish adhere to the nail while preventing it from staining the nail plate. Base coats contain TSF (toluene sulfonamide formaldehyde) resin, which is a chemical that helps improve adhesion and toughens the polish coating. Though TSF is found in other types of polish, a higher percentage is used in base coats. Some base coats also contain ingredients that help to even out a ridged nail plate. These are called **ridge fillers**.

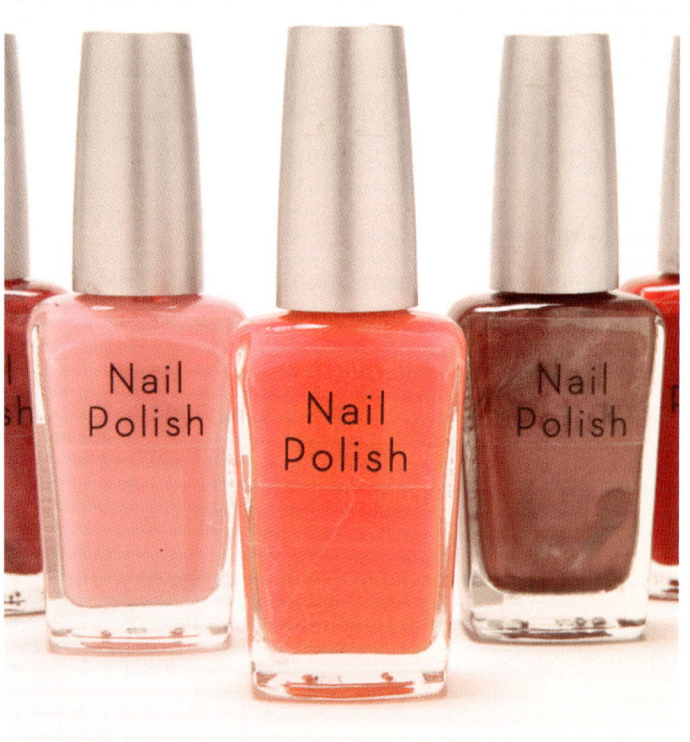

Colored Polish

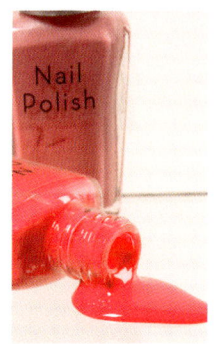

The application of **colored polish** creates a colored effect on the nail plate ranging from subtle and natural to extreme and bold. Colored polish contains pigments that create the different colors and finishes. The **finish** refers to the characteristics such as shimmer, pearl, metallic and matte. Clients usually choose the polish they want based on the color and on the look of the finish.

Top Coat

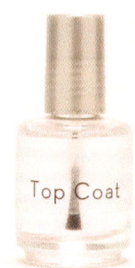

A **top coat** is used to seal the colored polish or base coat (if no color is used), and to help prevent the polish from chipping. Top coats also add shine, which is a result of having a greater amount of nitrocellulose polymer and plasticizer than contained in other types of polish. Unlike colored polishes, top coats contain no pigments, making them colorless. Clients can reapply the top coat at home between visits to maintain their polish and make it last longer. Sharing this advice with your clients may help increase retail sales. If the client is informed that the top coat will extend the results of the service, she will be more likely to purchase a bottle of top coat on her way out.

Polish should be applied in the following order:

1. 1 coat of nail strengthener (optional)
2. 1 coat of base coat or ridge filler
3. 2 coats of colored polish (optional)
4. 1 coat of top coat
5. 1 coat of speed dry (optional)

Speed Dry

Speed Dry

An important part of the service is allowing the polish to dry completely before the client leaves. **Speed dry** is a drying agent used to help polish dry faster. It is available in spray, polish or drop form and is applied over the finished nails. The reason speed dry is helpful is that once the polish is applied, most clients are ready to get on with their day. While this helps the polish dry quicker, it is still a good idea to allow adequate time before the client leaves and to remind the client to be careful not to smudge the polish.

> A "coat" of polish refers to the application of a thin layer of polish that covers the entire nail plate.

POLISH APPLICATION

Applying polish correctly requires practice. It's important to avoid applying too much product to prevent polish from touching the cuticle or sidewalls. Polish is typically applied in three strokes, beginning in the middle of the nail plate, and then on each side. Usually there is enough polish on the brush so that you won't have to add more polish between strokes. Here are some guidelines for a flawless application:

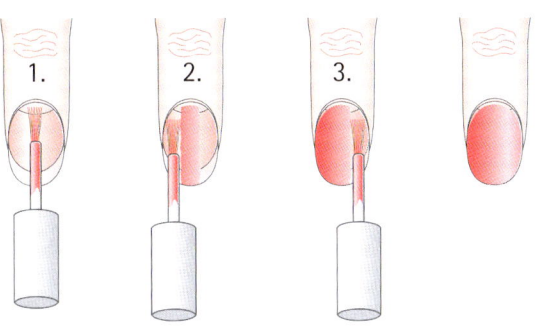

1. Hold the finger between your index finger and thumb and pinch slightly to move the sidewalls away from the nail plate.

2. Remove the brush from the polish bottle. Wipe the side of the brush that faces away from you on the inside of the neck of the bottle. This creates a "bead" of polish on the end of the brush.

3. Place the brush at the middle of the base of the nail at an angle. Brush toward the free edge. The brush handle remains at an angle while the brush itself flattens to the nail.

4. Apply the polish approximately 1/16" (.2 cm) from the cuticle to avoid getting any polish on the cuticle or sidewalls.

5. Repeat on each side of the nail plate with a three-stroke application —1) Middle, 2) Side, 3) Side.

6. If the free edge extends past the tip of the finger, wrap the polish around the free edge to help prevent chipping of the polish.

Typically there are four coats of nail polish applied: base coat, two coats of colored polish and a top coat. Alternating hands during polishing allows time for each coat of polish to dry sufficiently before the next coat is applied.

MANICURE PRODUCTS

The following is a list of all of the products needed for a manicure service.

Product	Function
Liquid Soap	Fights off harmful surface bacteria from the skin; may be used in finger bowl for soaking client's fingernails
Antiseptic Sanitizer	Reduces bacteria on the surface of the skin; aids in the prevention of cross-contamination
Polish Remover	Dissolves polish
Cuticle Remover	Softens dead cuticle tissue to allow gentle pushing back and to aid in its removal
Cuticle Conditioner	Softens and moisturizes cuticles and surrounding skin
Nail Bleach	Removes stains and discoloration on the nail plate
Moisturizing Lotion or Cream	Helps skin retain moisture and prevents or protects it from dryness
Nail Preparation Solution	Removes oil and product to help polish adhere to the nail plate
Polishes	**Base Coat:** Evens out nail plate and prevents polish from staining the nail plate **Nail Strengthener:** Prevent nails from chipping or breaking **Colored Polish:** Creates a colored effect on the nail **Top Coat:** Seals colored polish and helps prevent chipping
Speed Dry	Decreases polish drying time

Manicure Implements

Implements are tools that can be disinfected after each service. Many of the implements have multiple uses and are interchangeable. It is in your best interest to understand the features and benefits of each one so you will be able to determine which is best to use during nail services. Preventing the spread of bacteria and infection in the salon is a priority at all times. Sanitation and disinfection of all implements that are used are critical in the salon environment. If you are busy, it is a good idea to have multiple sets of implements—you can use one set while disinfecting the others.

Many of the same implements used to perform a manicure are used in providing other nail services as well.

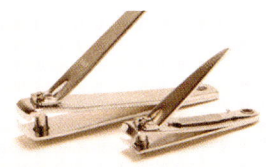

Nail Clippers

Nail clippers are used to shorten nails in order to save time that would be spent filing the nails. There are two types of nail clippers: **fingernail clippers** and **toenail clippers**. The main difference between fingernail clippers and toenail clippers is that toenail clippers are larger. They are available with straight or curved blades. Using straight toenail clippers helps to prevent cutting into the corners of the nail plate. All clippers require disinfection after every service. Always be sure to thoroughly dry the joint of the clippers, as leaving moisture can cause the joint to rust.

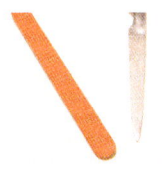

Nail Files

Most people are familiar with **nail files** because they use them at home to file their nails. Nail technicians use nail files to shorten and shape the nails. To properly file the nails, the file is moved from corner to center. Nail technicians should avoid sawing back and forth across the entire free edge because this causes the layers of the nail plate to separate, which can lead to breakage. Files are also used to bevel the nails once they have been shortened and shaped.

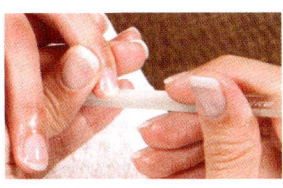

Beveling means holding the file vertically at a 45° angle to the tip of the nail and using upward strokes to remove ragged pieces of nail and to smooth rough edges. Beveling can only be performed on nails that extend past the tip of the finger.

Although there are many different types of nail files, they are primarily differentiated by **grit**, which refers to the number of granules per square inch. The higher the number, the finer the grit is; and the finer the grit is, the less abrasive it is. The lower the number, the more coarse the grit is. It is advisable to file natural nails with a file of 240 grit or above because damage to the natural nail could occur using below 240 grit.

There are several types of files made of different materials that are used for specific purposes. The following are the three most common files used on natural nails:

Emery Boards

An **emery board** is used to smooth and shape natural nails. It is a double-sided

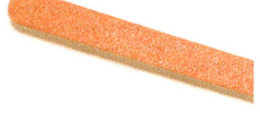

cardboard stick, much like a popsicle stick, usually with a fine side, which is used to file, bevel and smooth the free edge of the nails; and a coarse side, which is used to shorten the nails. Emery boards are disposable and are discarded after every service. Do not save an emery board in a bag for your client's next visit—doing so can create a breeding ground for bacteria.

Glass Files

A **glass file** is used to smooth and shape natural nails just as emery boards are; however, glass files can be disinfected and are not considered disposable. They are gentle on soft, fragile nails and are designed for natural nail care as opposed to artificial nail care. Glass files are long-lasting and easy to disinfect after every service.

8

Metal Files

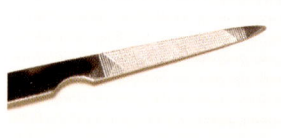

A **metal file**, sometimes referred to as a diamond file, is used to smooth and shape natural nails. However, some metal files can be too abrasive for natural nails and cause the layers to separate, creating rough edges and leading to breakage. Metal files require disinfection after every service.

Buffer

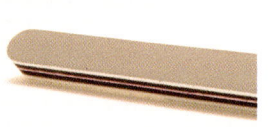

A **buffer** is used to smooth out ridges or corrugations on the nail plate. It is important to buff in the direction of nail growth to help prevent the layers of the nail from separating. There are several different types of buffers including three-way buffers, chamois buffers, buffing blocks, finishing buffers and many more. Both disposable and disinfectable buffers are available. Buffers need to be disinfected, if possible, or discarded after every service. Chamois buffers are not permitted by some regulating agencies because they cannot be disinfected and are not considered disposable, so be guided by your regulatory guidelines.

Cuticle Pusher

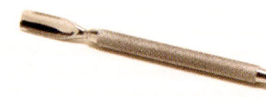

A **cuticle pusher**, also referred to as a **steel pusher**, is used to loosen and push back the cuticles. The metal, spoon-shaped end is designed to follow the natural curve of the nail, making it easier to lift dead cuticle from the nail plate. The cuticle pusher requires disinfection after every service.

Cuticle Nippers

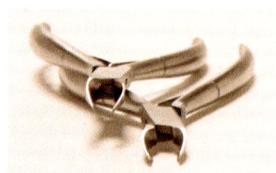

Cuticle nippers are a metal instrument with two blades that pinch together, used to trim excess cuticle and hangnails. There are many different types of nippers available, including: 1/4" (.6 cm) jaw; 1/2" (1.3 cm) jaw; box joint; lap joint; single or double spring; rubber-handled and many more. The smaller the blade, the more precise the instrument will be, especially for a beginner. Cuticle nippers are used with the blades parallel to the cuticle, as indicated in the illustration on the following page. In general, using the tips or points of the nippers to trim is not recommended since it may increase the risk of cutting into living tissue and injuring the

---

A common implement for smoothing nails is called a **three-way buffer**, which is comprised of three different grits. These buffers are usually designed using three colors, to indicate the grits used.

For example:
  Black (Roughest) 2400 grit
  White (Medium) 4000 grit
  Gray (Finest) 12000 grit

To achieve a natural shine, move the buffer from the base of the nail to the free edge. Be sure to lift the buffer from the nail between strokes. Breaking contact will help prevent the friction caused by buffing from overheating the nail and causing the client discomfort.

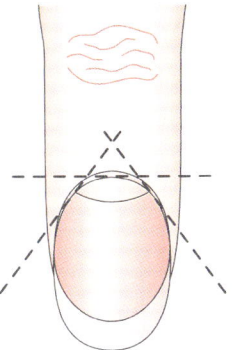

Nail Brush

The **nail brush** is typically used with soap and water to clean the nails and the

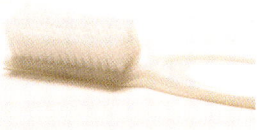

skin surrounding them. A nail brush is made of synthetic bristles and typically has a plastic handle. Brushing the nails can also help remove any remaining bits of non-living cuticle after removing cuticles. Disinfect the nail brush after every service.

client. Pulling at the cuticles with the nippers may also cause tearing and/or injury. The use of nippers to trim cuticles is not permitted by some regulating agencies, so always check regulatory guidelines.

Nippers must be disinfected after every service. Always be sure to thoroughly dry the joint of the nippers, as leaving moisture can cause the joint to rust.

> Some buffers are made from a material called **chamois**, which is a soft leather made from the skin of a sheep or chamois antelope. Always follow regulatory guidelines as this type of buffer may not be allowed or it is disposed of after every client.

MANICURE IMPLEMENTS

The following is a list of all of the implements needed for a manicure service.

Implement	Function
Nail Clippers	Shorten nails
Nail File	Shortens and shapes nails **Emery Board:** Smoothes and shapes natural nails; disposable **Glass File:** Smoothes and shapes natural nails; disinfectable **Metal File (Diamond File):** Smoothes and shapes natural nails; disinfectable
Cuticle Pusher (Steel Pusher)	Loosens and pushes back cuticles
Cuticle Nippers	Trim excess cuticle and hangnails
Nail Brush	Cleans the nails and surrounding skin
Buffer	Smoothes ridges or corrugations on the nail plate

Be sure to pre-clean or sanitize all implements before placing them in an EPA-registered, broad spectrum (hospital-level) disinfectant.

Manicure Supplies

Supplies are materials that are discarded or replaced after each service. It is important to always have extra supplies on hand since they cannot be reused. Many of the same supplies used to perform a manicure are used in providing other nail services as well.

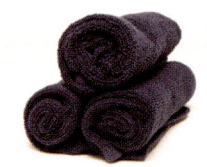

Towels

Clean **towels** are used to dry the client's hands or feet. Towels provide a clean, soft surface when folded and used as a cushion for resting clients' hands or feet. Soiled towels require storage in a covered hamper or container after use. Be guided by your regulatory guidelines on storing and handling towels.

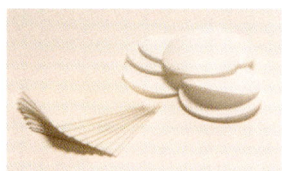

Cotton or Lint-Free Nail Wipes

Cotton is used to remove polish and oils from the nail plate. Cotton can also be wrapped around the end of an orangewood stick to create a softer edge and to absorb product. **Lint-free nail wipes**, also referred to as **pledgets**, serve the same purpose and are often preferred by technicians. Always check regulatory guidelines on proper storage of cotton and lint-free nail wipes.

Cosmetic Spatula

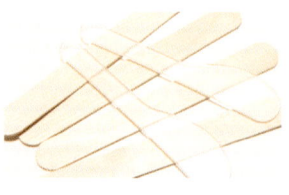

A **cosmetic spatula** is used to remove product from jars to prevent contamination of the product by using fingers. Spatulas are made of plastic, metal or wood; plastic and metal spatulas can be disinfected; wood spatulas cannot be disinfected and are discarded after use.

Orangewood Stick

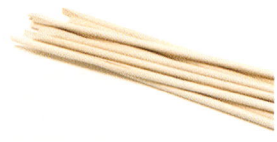

An **orangewood stick,** also known as a birchwood stick, is a thin, round wooden stick with a flat end and sometimes a pointed end. Orangewood sticks are used to loosen and push back the cuticles, apply cosmetics, clean under the free edge and to remove polish from the sidewalls of the nails. Generally, the flat end of an orangewood stick is wrapped in cotton to create a softer edge and to absorb more product. Orangewood sticks are disposable and are discarded after each use.

MANICURE SUPPLIES	
The following is a list of all of the supplies needed for a manicure service.	
Supplies	**Function**
Towels	Dry client's hands and feet; can be folded into a cushion
Cotton or Lint-Free Nail Wipes	Remove polish and oils from the nail plate
Cosmetic Spatula	Removes product from jars
Orangewood Stick	Loosens and pushes back cuticles; applies cosmetics; cleans under the free edge; removes polish from sidewalls

Manicure Equipment

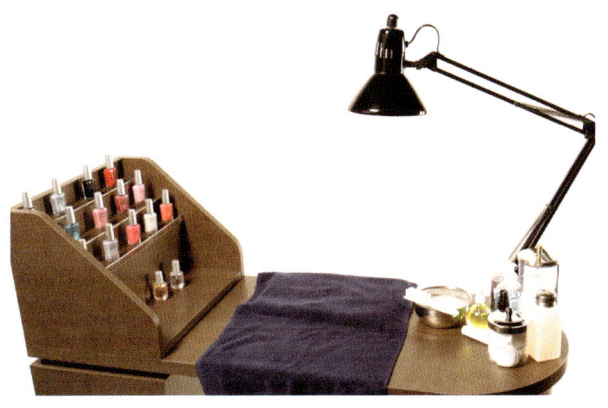

Equipment refers to the furniture and implements that are considered permanent in the salon or spa. Depending on the space available and the services offered, equipment can be very basic or very elaborate. Some salons may have simple manicure tables, while others offer more technically advanced, vented tables. This varies in each salon or spa. However, it is important that all equipment is able to be properly disinfected no matter how basic or elaborate. Several pieces of equipment used to perform a manicure are used in providing other nail services as well.

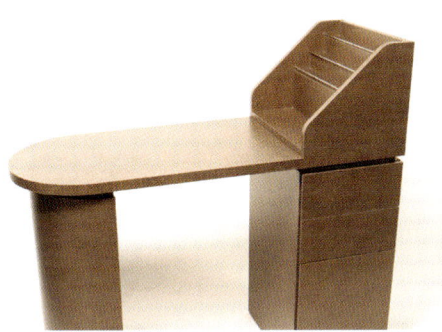

Manicure Table

A **manicure table** provides a flat, nonporous area to perform services on the hands. Most tables will have a drawer for storing cosmetics and disinfected implements. There are many different types of manicure tables, from basic to elaborate, that can be custom-designed to fit the needs of a salon or spa.

For better long-term health, chairs, tables and pedicure stations should be ergonomically correct, meaning specially designed to accommodate the technician's constantly reaching arms and to provide proper back support.

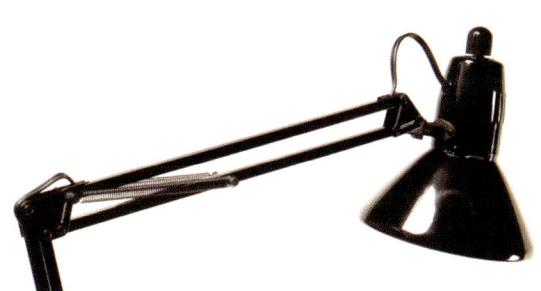

Table Lamp

A **table lamp** is used to provide additional light while performing a service. It usually attaches to the table and utilizes a 40-watt bulb. If a higher wattage bulb is used, there is a chance the heat generated from the bulb could interfere with the performance of the products being used.

Glass Container

A **glass container** is used to hold supplies such as cotton or lint-free wipes and spatulas. It is best to use smaller containers for space-saving purposes. To help prevent cross-contamination, all containers should have lids. Always check regulatory guidelines on proper storage of materials such as cotton.

Lint Free Wipes

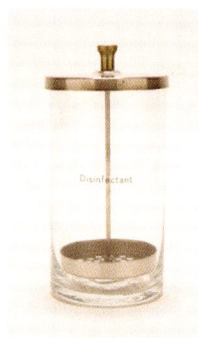

Disinfection Container

A **disinfection container** holds an EPA-registered, broad spectrum (hospital-level) disinfection solution and is used to disinfect implements. The container has to be large enough to allow complete immersion of clean tools in the solution. Some containers have a lift tray, which allows the disinfectant to be drained off before removing the implements from the tray; if not, implements need to be removed with tongs to prevent skin from coming into contact with the disinfection solution. A spray bottle filled with an EPA-registered, broad spectrum (hospital-level) disinfection solution is used to clean the service area and equipment.

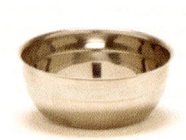

Finger Bowl

The **finger bowl** is used to soak the client's fingernails in order to clean under the free edge and to soften the cuticles. Soap or an antibacterial soaking solution is added to warm water in the bowl. Finger bowls are available in a variety of colors, shapes and materials. The most typical finger bowls are plastic with indentations for the client's fingers to rest. The bowl is disinfected after each use and filled with new soaking solution for every client.

You may place nonporous marbles in the bottom of the finger bowl. The client can move them around while the fingers are soaking. Marbles can also make it more comfortable for clients to rest their fingers in the bowl— and add a unique and colorful touch to your service!

Client Cushion

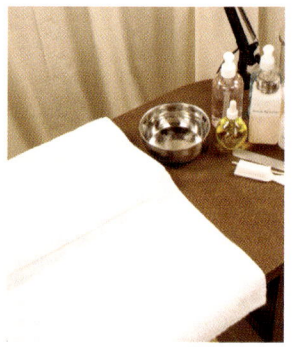

A **client cushion** is used for the client to rest his or her elbows on during a hand care service and is usually positioned on the table in front of the client. Cushions typically measure approximately 8" x 12" (12 x 19 cm). If the table does not have a cushion already attached, one can be made by folding a towel to the approximate cushion size. The cushion needs to be covered by a clean towel or disposable towel for every client.

Technician and Client Chairs

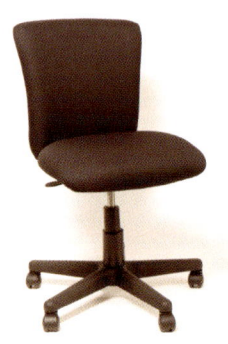

The **technician's chair** should be adjustable and allow easy access to all equipment and tools. Generally, the technician's chair will have wheels, the ability to swivel and offer height adjustment as well as provide proper back support to prevent straining when reaching for implements and supplies. The **client's chair** should be comfortable and

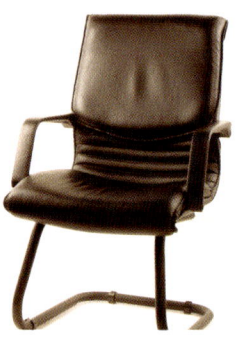

provide proper back support; it may also include arm rests. Both chairs require proper disinfection.

Some salons have drying stations where clients can sit comfortably and wait for their nails to dry. Often these stations include a nail dryer which is a piece of equipment that helps dry the nails faster. For more on nail dryers, see *Chapter 10, Specialty Nails.*

MANICURE EQUIPMENT

The following is a list of all of the equipment needed for a manicure service.

Equipment	Function
Manicure Table	Provides a flat area to perform hand care services
Table Lamp	Provides additional light while performing services
Glass Container	Holds supplies
Disinfection Container	Holds EPA-registered, broad spectrum (hospital-level) disinfection solution; must be large enough for complete immersion of implements
Finger Bowl	Serves as a container to soak client's fingernails in order to clean under the free edge and soften cuticles
Client Cushion	Supports client's elbows during hand care services
Technician Chair	Provides adjustable seat for technician performing service; allows for easy access to all equipment
Client Chair	Comfortable seat for client receiving services; provides proper back support

8

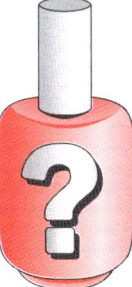

After reviewing the previous information on the different products, implements, supplies and equipment used for a manicure, which ones have you used or had used on you? Do you feel this was the best choice for what you were trying to achieve?

BASIC MANICURE

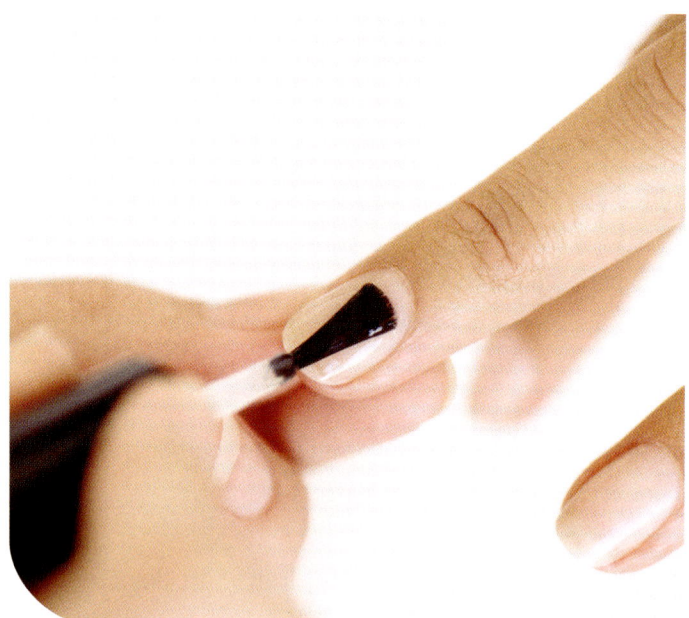

Think about how much we use our hands on a daily basis. From hitting the button on the alarm clock in the morning to turning out the light at night, our hands have a variety of uses. We use our hands to greet one another as well as to gesture and express ourselves. It is for all these reasons that we should practice the proper care and treatment to keep them looking their best at all times.

Every personal care establishment offers what is referred to as a "bread and butter" service. These are basic services that strengthen the entire menu of services. For nail technicians, manicures are one of the most requested services.

A **manicure** is the cosmetic care of the hands and fingernails. The word "manicure" comes from the Latin words *manus*, meaning, "hand," and *cura* meaning "care." A basic manicure typically includes filing and shaping of the nails, cuticle care, massage and polish.

Manicures are also the starting point for all other hand care services. It is highly beneficial to sharpen your skills early in your career by practicing and perfecting the steps of the basic manicure.

Remember, the nail technician does not diagnose or treat nail or skin diseases. If there is a visible sign of a nail or skin disease, the client must be referred to a physician.

FIVE PHASES OF SERVICE

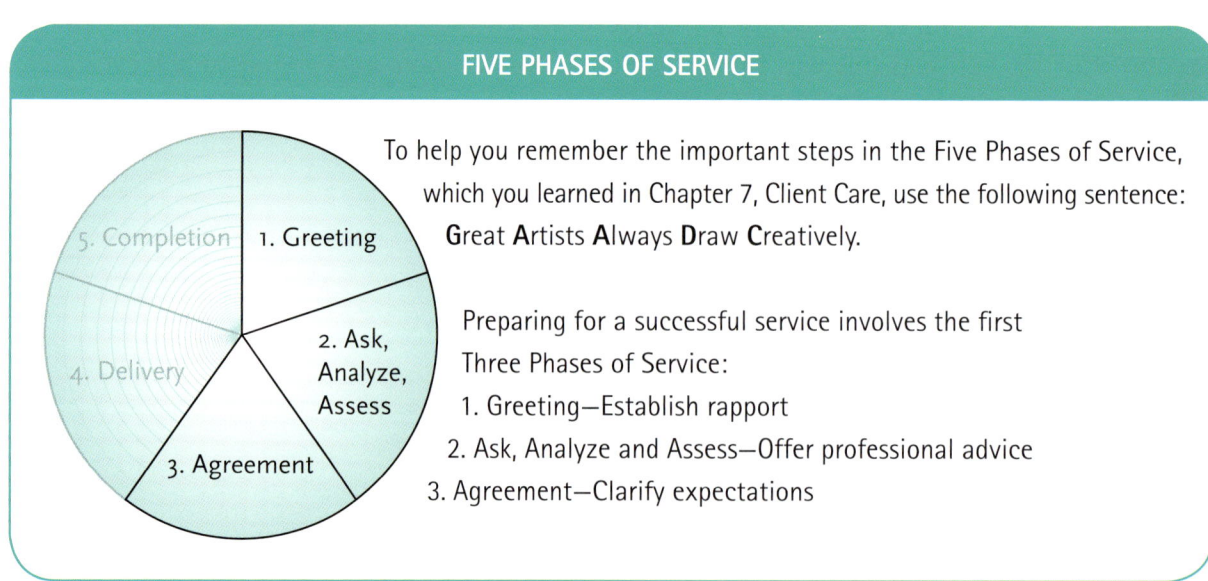

To help you remember the important steps in the Five Phases of Service, which you learned in Chapter 7, Client Care, use the following sentence: **G**reat **A**rtists **A**lways **D**raw **C**reatively.

Preparing for a successful service involves the first Three Phases of Service:
1. Greeting—Establish rapport
2. Ask, Analyze and Assess—Offer professional advice
3. Agreement—Clarify expectations

5. Completion   1. Greeting
2. Ask, Analyze, Assess
4. Delivery
3. Agreement

BASIC MANICURE PREPARATION

As with any professional service, it is important to have the service area, products, implements, supplies and equipment in proper order prior to the client's arrival.

After completing the consultation, it is advisable to ask the client to remove any jewelry from hands and wrists. Remind clients to put it in a safe place such as a pocket or purse, and **require that hands be washed with liquid or foam soap**.

Determine the client's dominant hand by asking which hand he or she writes with. Generally, you will begin on the client's non-dominant hand. This allows the dominant hand, which often requires more cuticle care, to remain in the finger bowl longer.

8

Products
- Liquid soap
- Antiseptic sanitizer
- Polish remover
- Cuticle remover
- Cuticle conditioner
- Hand lotion or cream
- Nail preparation solution
- Nail strengthener
- Base coat
- Colored polish
- Top coat
- Speed dry

Implements
- Fingernail clippers
- Emery board/glass file/metal file
- Cuticle pusher
- Cuticle nippers
- Nail brush
- Buffer

Supplies
- Orangewood sticks
- Towels
- Cotton or lint-free wipes in a disinfected glass container

Equipment
- Finger bowl
- Manicure table
- Table lamp
- Glass container
- Disinfection container filled with EPA-registered, broad spectrum (hospital-level) disinfectant
- Technician and client chair

Basic Manicure Table Set-Up
- Clean and disinfect the surface of the table with an EPA-registered, broad spectrum (hospital-level) disinfectant.
- Place polishes on the left side of the table.
- Place all other products on the right side of the table in the order of use.
- Place the disinfection container filled with an EPA-registered, broad spectrum (hospital-level) disinfectant on the right side of the table.
- Disinfect all implements properly before beginning.
- Place a clean towel on the table, making sure to cover the client cushion, if there is one. Place all implements on a towel.
- Place the finger bowl and nail brush on the left side or in the middle of the table.
- Place a covered trash can on the floor to the right. If a trash can is not available, fasten a plastic bag to the right side of the table and discard the bag after every service.
- The drawer is used to store new materials in the original container or a sealed bag. Never place used or unsanitized items in the drawer. Store additional clean implements in a covered container in the drawer.

This set-up is for a right-handed technician. Reverse the process if you are a left-handed technician. Table set-up can vary according to preference and the area regulating agency.

NAIL SHAPES

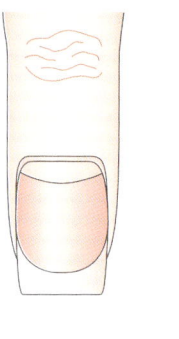
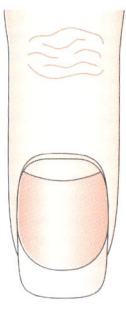
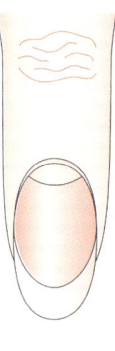
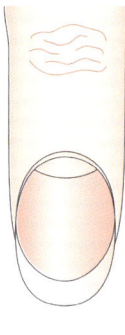
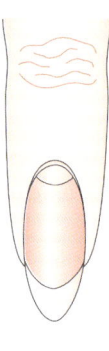

Square   Squoval   Oval   Round   Point

Part of beautifying the hands is the shaping of the nails. To offer clients the best shape for their nails, use the shape of their cuticles as a guide. For example, if they have oval-shaped cuticles, an oval-shaped nail will usually look the best on them. It is also important to take into consideration the client's occupation, daily activities and hobbies. There are five basic fingernail shapes:

1. **Square-shaped** nails are straight across at the free edge and squared at the corners. The square shape has a full width at the tip of the nail, which makes it sturdy, but the corners, though smooth, can break easily because they are more likely to catch on clothing and other surfaces.

2. **Squoval-shaped** nails are a combination of square and oval. They are straight across at the free edge, but have slightly rounded or tapered corners. Squoval, sometimes referred to as "soft-square" or "rounded-square," is a sturdier nail shape because the nails are typically kept shorter and still have a full width at the tip. For people who are more active, squoval-shaped is a good choice.

3. **Oval-shaped** nails are tapered and rounded at the tip. The oval shape is typical for longer nails and is considered more elegant and a good choice for people whose hands are on display, such as salespeople and hand models.

4. **Round-shaped** nails are slightly tapered and generally kept shorter in length. The most common shape for men is round-shaped, because it is the most natural-looking.

5. **Point-shaped** nails are tapered to a slightly rounded point at the tip of the free edge. This shape is well-suited for women with slender nail beds and are generally worn at a longer length, though they tend to break more easily.

BASIC MANICURE PROCEDURE

The basic manicure is one of the most requested nail services. By following and practicing the steps on the following pages, you will be prepared to give a basic manicure. Note that the procedure below corresponds with the step-by-step technical images that follow.

4. Delivery - Meet client's expectations

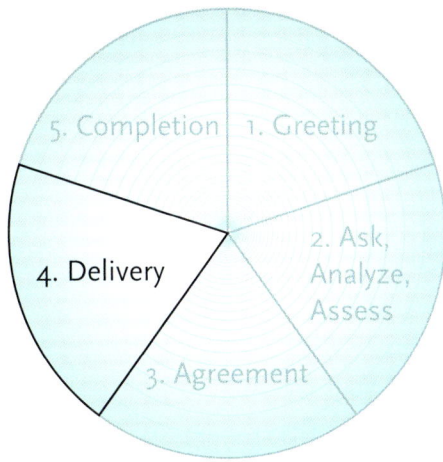

SANITIZE

1. Wash and sanitize your hands
2. Sanitize client's hands

ANALYZE

3. Perform visual analysis of hands
4. Remove polish
5. Perform visual analysis of nails

SHAPE

6. Determine nail shape
7. File and shape
8. Place left hand in finger bowl

REPEAT SHAPE (Step 7) on right hand

9. Remove left hand from finger bowl
10. Place right hand in finger bowl

CUTICLE CARE

11. Apply cuticle remover
12. Push back cuticles
13. Nip cuticles/hangnails if necessary
14. Clean under free edge
15. Remove right hand from finger bowl
16. Brush nails

REPEAT CUTICLE CARE (Steps 11–16) on right hand

17. Buff nails (optional)
18. Apply cuticle oil
19. Bevel nails

MASSAGE

20. Obtain product
21. Apply product
22. Establish control
23. Perform massage movements

REPEAT MASSAGE (Steps 20–23) on right hand

POLISH

24. Remove oils from each nail plate
25. Apply base coat
26. Apply colored polish
27. Apply second coat
28. Apply top coat
29. Clean up excess polish
30. Apply speed dry

8

BASIC MANICURE

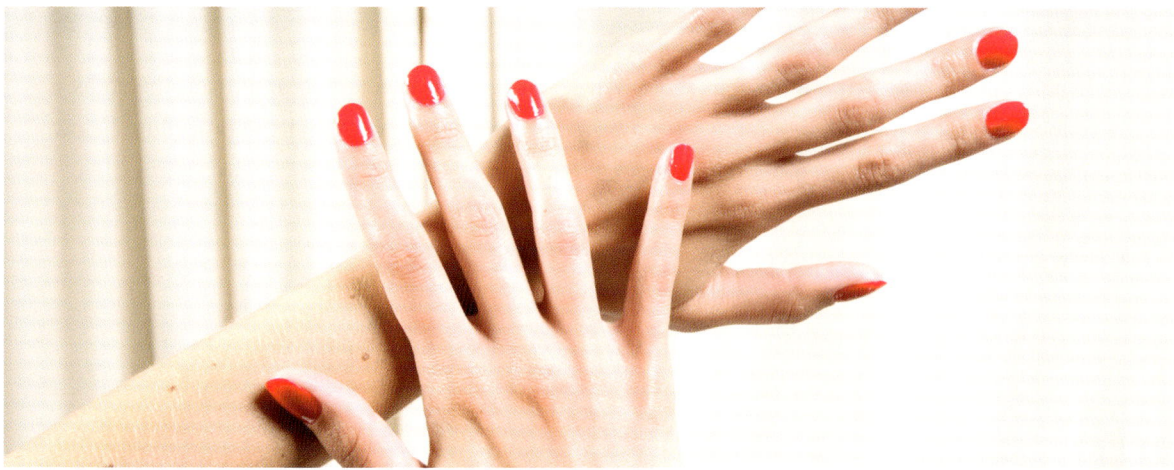

 A checkmark next to a step indicates an ideal time to check on your client's comfort, and to take extra safety precautions.

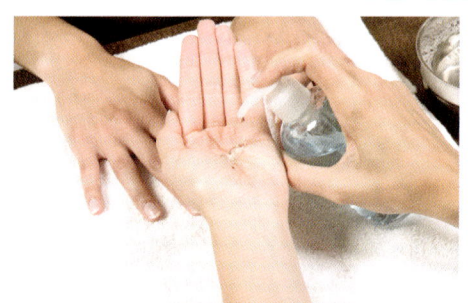

1. **Wash and sanitize your hands.**
   - Use liquid or foam soap.
   - Wear protective gloves if required by regulating agency.
   - Use waterless sanitizer or topical antiseptic if required by regulating agency.

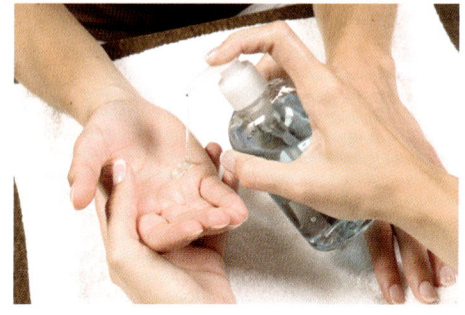

2. **Sanitize client's hands.**
   - Use waterless sanitizer or topical antiseptic if required by regulating agency.

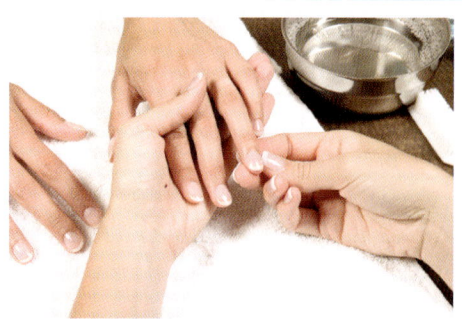

ANALYZE

3. **Perform visual analysis of hands.**
   - Continue with service if hands are free of any visible signs of diseases or disorders.

NOTE: As a nail technician, you cannot diagnose or treat diseases or disorders. You can only refer the client to a physician.

Skin: Signs to look for during analysis on hands include open skin, redness, swelling, discoloration or any other signs of an infection that would prevent the service from being performed.

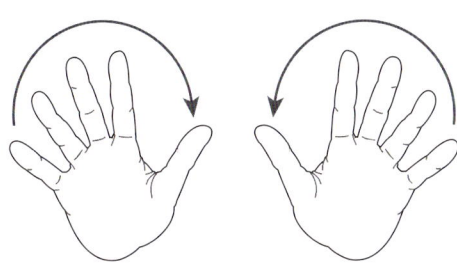

Any procedure that will be performed on all 10 fingers will always be done in the same order: On the non-dominant hand from the little finger to the thumb; then on the dominant hand from the little finger to the thumb.

For this procedure, the client is right-handed. So, we will work the left hand, little finger to the thumb; then the right hand, little finger to the thumb.

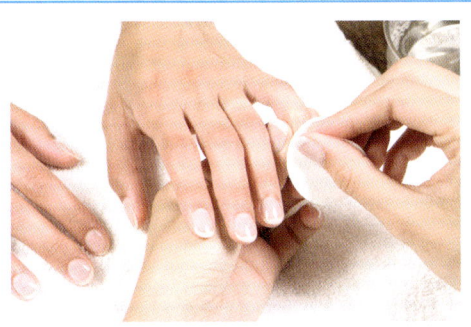

4. **Remove polish.**
    - Use a lint-free wipe or cotton, saturated with polish remover, on the nail plate.
    - Let remover set for a few seconds.
    - Wipe toward the free edge.
    - Remove all polish from each nail before moving to the next nail. Repeat on the right hand.

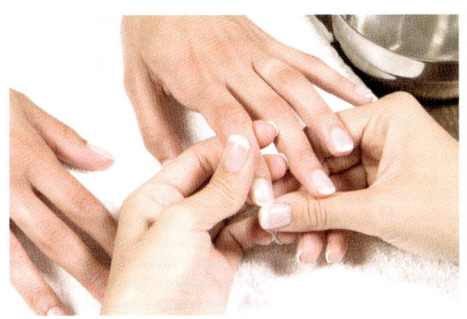

5. **Perform visual analysis of nails.**
    - Continue with service if nail plates are free of any visible signs of diseases or disorders.

Nails: Signs to look for during analysis on fingernails include discoloration, flaking, swelling, pain indicators, pus, detached nail plate, growth under the nail or any other signs of an infection that would prevent the service from being performed.

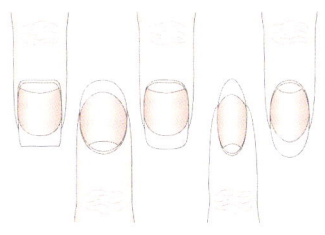

SHAPE

6. **Determine nail shape.**
    - Confirm desired nail shape.
    - Keep in mind factors discussed in consultation.

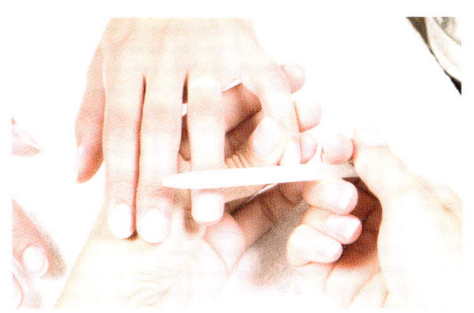

7. **File and shape** free edge of each nail.
    - Always file from each corner of nail to center.
    - Get client's approval (length and shape) after shaping left hand.
    - Use fingernail clippers to remove length if free edge needs to be shortened considerably.
    - Shape nail with file after clipping.

8

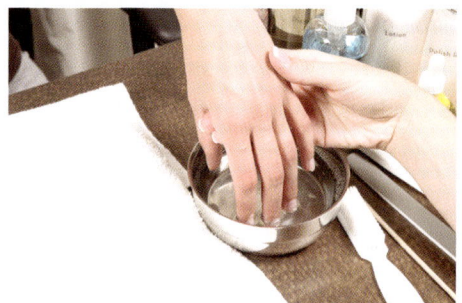

8. Place left hand in finger bowl.

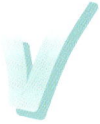

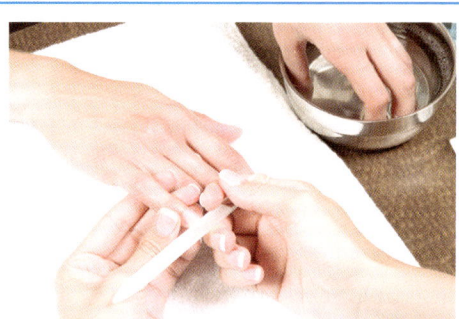

REPEAT SHAPE (Step 7) on right hand.
- File and shape free edge of each nail.

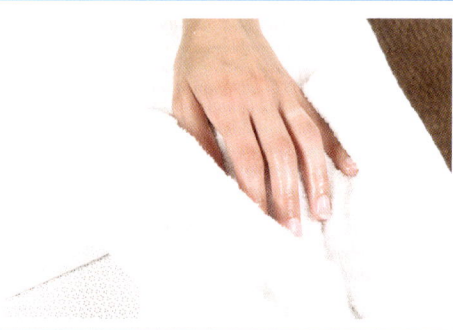

9. Remove left hand from finger bowl.
- Place hand on towel.
- Use towel to dry hand.

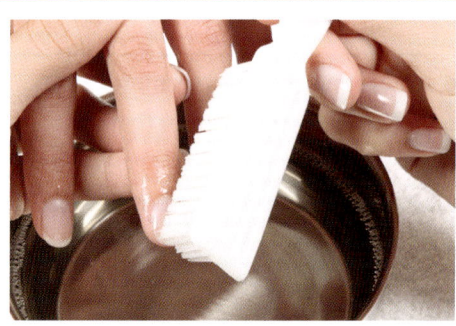

*Optional:
- Brush the nails to help to clean fingers and nail plate.
- Hold hand over finger bowl.
- Use a damp brush.
- Brush down each finger, toward tip.
- Place hand on towel.
- Use towel to dry hand.

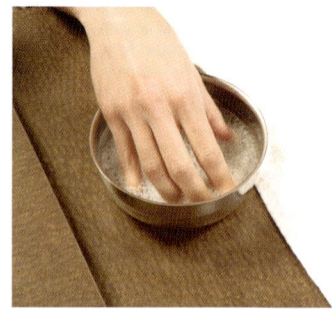

10. Place right hand in finger bowl.
- Perform following steps on left hand (while right hand is soaking).

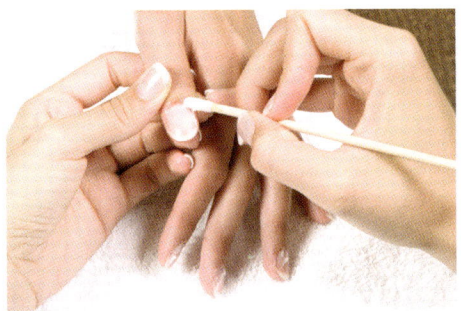

CUTICLE CARE

11. Apply cuticle remover.

- Use cotton-tipped orangewood stick, cotton swab or dropper.
- Begin with little finger.

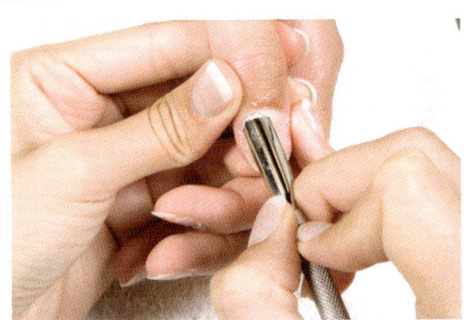

12. Push back cuticles.

- Use cotton-tipped orangewood stick or metal cuticle pusher.
- Use light, quick, circular movements along cuticle.
- Work from one side of nail toward center; then from other side toward the center.
- Use a gentle, non-aggressive touch.
- Move orangewood stick or pusher along nail plate without applying downward pressure to avoid damaging the nail matrix.

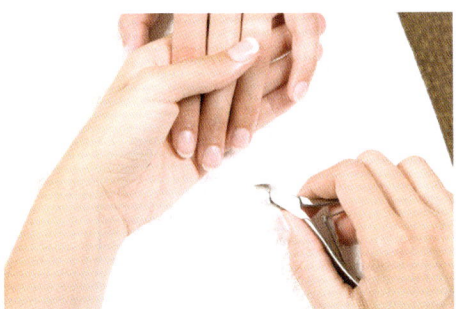

Optional:

13. Nip cuticles/hangnails if necessary.

- After loosening, the excess cuticle will appear translucent.
- Use cuticle nippers to remove lifted or loosened excess cuticle.
- Position blades parallel to cuticle.
- Squeeze handles to cut; release the nippers before moving on.
- Avoid using the point of the nippers and/or pulling at the cuticles.
- Remove cuticle in one piece if at all possible.
- The nippers may also be used to remove hangnails.

NOTE: Be guided by your regulatory guidelines regarding the use of cuticle nippers.

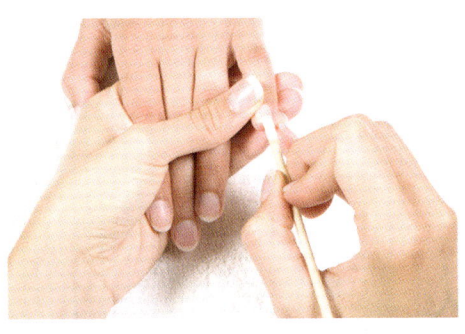

14. Clean under free edge.

- Use cotton-tipped orangewood stick dampened with polish remover or water.

NOTE: At this point, nail bleaching can be an option using a 20-volume (6%) developer or prepared nail bleach. Use a cotton-tipped orangewood stick and apply bleach to the nail plate. Do not allow bleach to touch the skin—it can cause irritation.

8

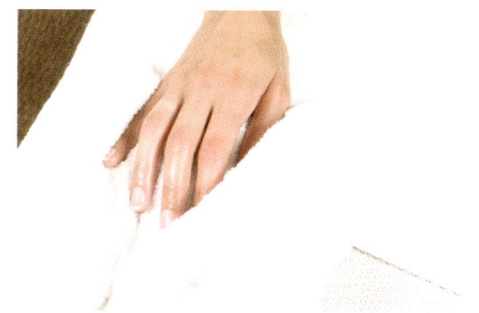

15. Remove right hand from finger bowl.

- Place hand on towel.

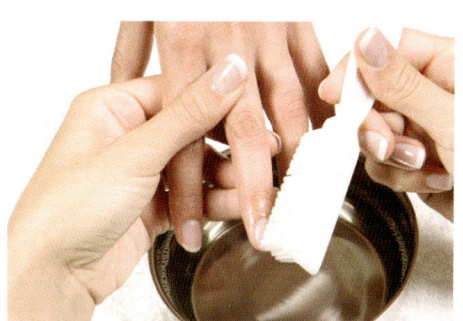

16. Brush nails.

- Hold left hand over finger bowl.
- Remove remaining bits of excess cuticle.
- Option: Spray nails with water and wipe each nail plate with towel.
- This will also help to remove any remaining cuticle solvent.
- Place left hand on towel and dry both hands.

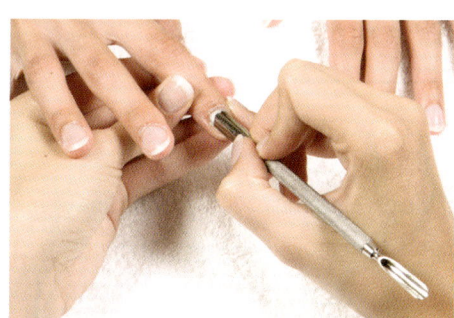

REPEAT CUTICLE CARE (Steps 11–16) on right hand.

- Apply cuticle remover.
- Push back cuticles.
- Nip cuticles if necessary.
- Clean under free edge.
- Brush nails.

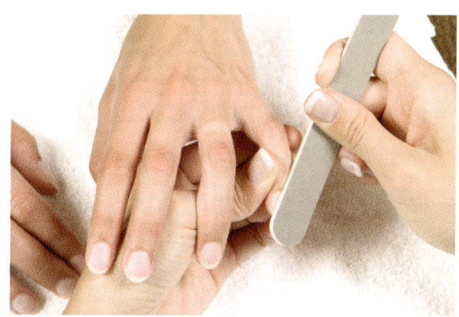

Optional:

17. Buff nails.

- Use buffer.
- Buff in direction of nail growth, toward the free edge.

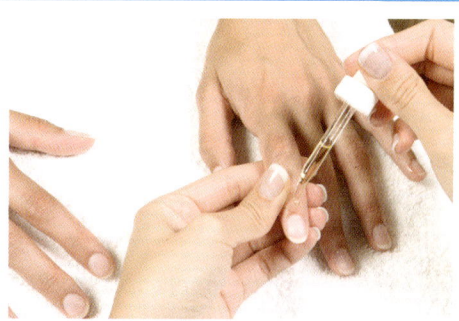

18. Apply cuticle oil.

- Use cotton-tipped orangewood stick, cotton swab or dropper.
- Apply to all 10 fingers.
- Gently massage oil into cuticle area.

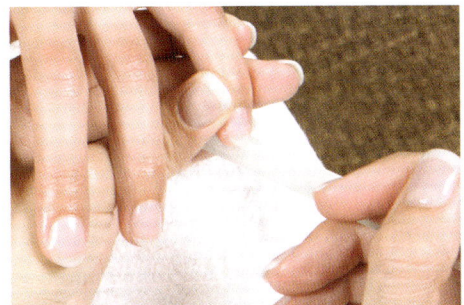

19. **Bevel nails.**

- Hold file vertically (45° angle to underside of free edges).
- File with upward stroke. Do not move the file back and forth—only upward.
- Bevel nails on both hands.

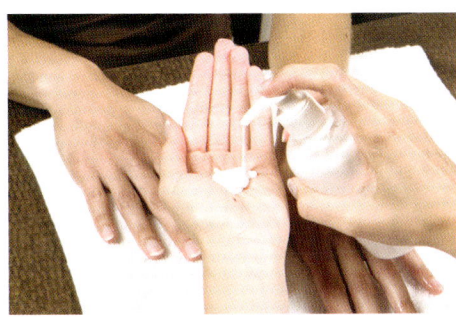

MASSAGE

20. **Obtain product** (massage cream, lotion or oil).

- Use spatula if necessary.
- Distribute product into both of your hands.

8

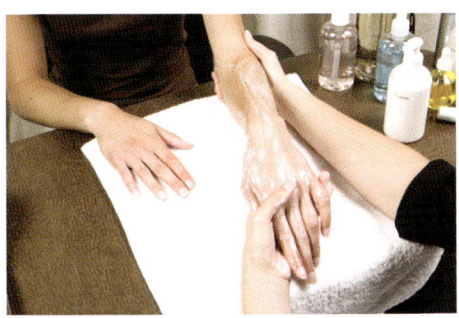

21. **Apply product.**

- Apply over client's entire hand, wrist and lower arm, up to elbow.
- Begin with client's left hand.
- Move your hand in rotating friction motion.
- Massage elbow 3-5 times.

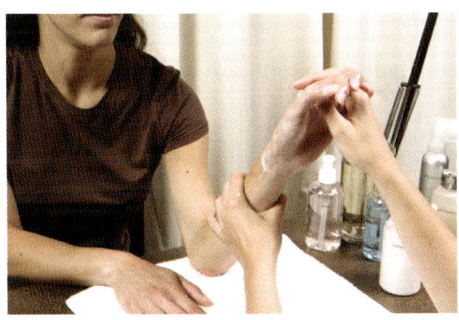

22. **Establish control** of client's hand and arm.

- Place client's elbow on towel.
- Raise arm and hand.
- Intertwine your fingers with client's.
- Move hand in circular movement.
- This may be referred to as a relaxer movement.
- Repeat movement 3-5 times, clockwise and counter-clockwise.
- Gently place hand on table, palm down.

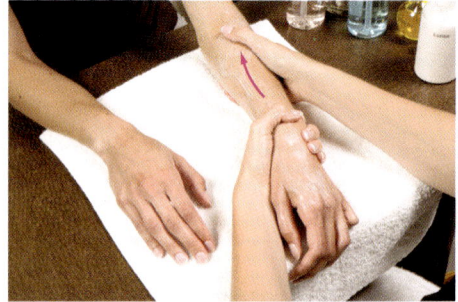

23. **Perform massage movements.**

Perform effleurage, palm down.

- Place one of your hands over client's wrist with your fingers curling over arm and your thumb resting on top.
- Move your hand up toward elbow.
- Keep your thumb on top and move back down arm to wrist in smooth, fluent effleurage movements.
- Perform movement alternating your right and left hand while holding client's wrist with your opposite hand.
- Repeat sequence 3-5 times.

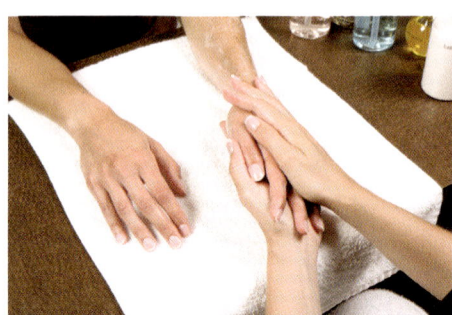

Rotate client's hand, palm up.

- Take client's hand between your hands (one on top, one underneath).
- Rotate arm slowly so palm faces upward.
- Gently place arm back onto towel without losing contact.

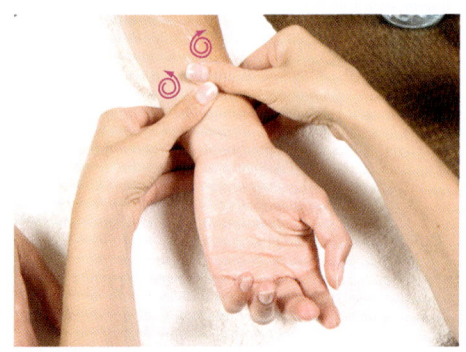

Perform effleurage, palm up.

- Place your thumbs side-by-side on inside of client's wrist (with your fingers underneath wrist).
- Move up arm toward elbow.
- Use your thumbs to make circular effleurage movements in opposite directions.
- Slide your hand back down arm without losing contact.
- Repeat sequence 3-5 times.

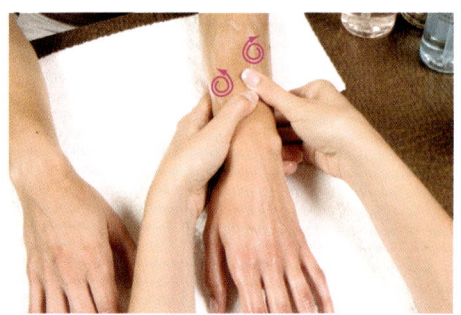

Perform effleurage, palm down.

- Grasp client's hand between your hands and gently turn arm over (palm faces downward). The palm will remain in this position for the remainder of the massage procedure.
- Use your thumbs to make same circular or rotating effleurage movements (without breaking contact).
- Move up toward elbow then back down arm to wrist.
- Repeat sequence 3-5 times.

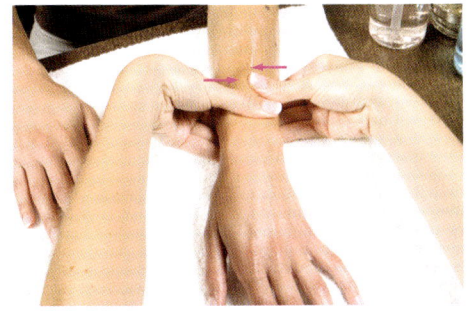

Perform petrissage, palm down.

- Place both thumbs horizontally on top of client's wrist (with your fingers underneath wrist).
- Move up arm toward elbow.
- Slide your thumbs over and under each other in half-circle, kneading movements (petrissage).
- Work back toward wrist using same movement.
- Repeat this sequence 3-5 times.

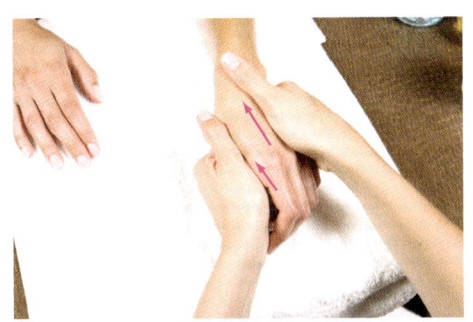

Knead palm.

- Take client's hand in both of your hands (your thumbs on top and your fingers in palm of hand).
- Use your fingers to knead palm.
- Rotate your fingers over sides of hand and wrist.
- Alternate movement between your right and left hands.
- Repeat sequence 3-5 times.

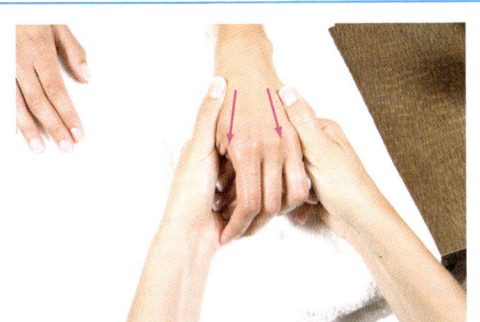

Slide down metacarpals.

- Squeeze hand (your thumbs still on top and fingers in palm).
- Apply pressure between metacarpals.
- Move toward fingers.
- Move down thumb and little finger simultaneously.
- "Pinch off" at tips of fingers.
- Repeat on pointer and ring fingers.
- Repeat on middle finger.
- Repeat sequence 3-5 times.

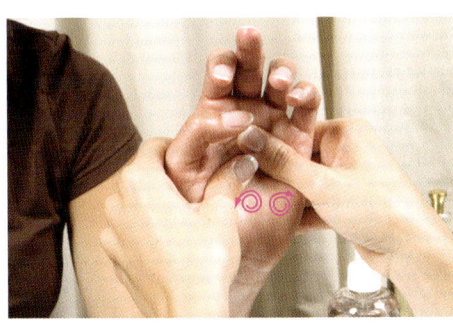

Perform effleurage in palm.

- Raise client's arm upward with palm facing you.
- Place your thumbs on palm and your fingers on top of hand.
- Use your thumbs to make circular effleurage movements in opposite directions (over entire palm).
- Repeat sequence 3-5 times.

8

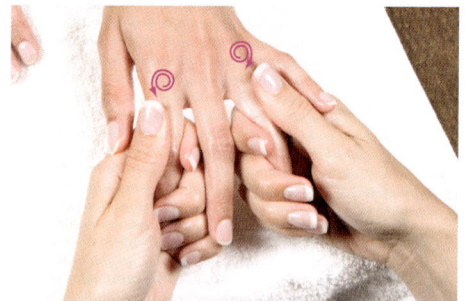

Perform effleurage on fingers.

- Bring arm down.
- Place your thumbs on top of client's fingers.
- Begin with thumb and little finger.
- Use circular effleurage movements on fingers, pinching off at tips.
- Repeat on pointer and ring fingers.
- Repeat on middle finger.
- Repeat sequence 3-5 times.

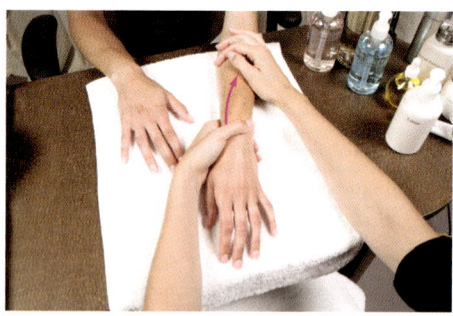

Perform effleurage and feather off.

- Repeat relaxing movement (used earlier) 3-5 times with client's palm facing downward.
- Redistribute hair on client's arm in direction of natural growth (last movement).
- Grasp client's hand.
- Feather off gently (one of your hands on top, one underneath). This completes the massage portion of the manicure on the left hand.

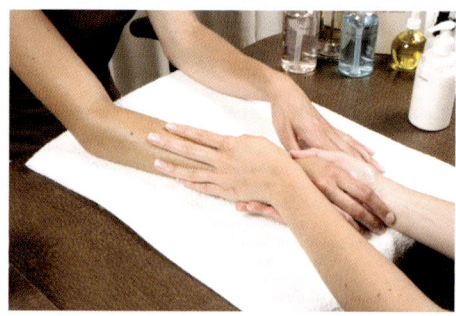

REPEAT MASSAGE (Steps 20–23) on right hand.

- Obtain product.
- Apply product.
- Establish control of client's hand and arm.
- Perform massage movements.

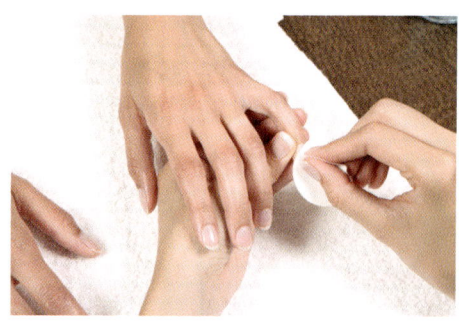

POLISH

24. Remove oils from each nail plate.

- Use lint-free wipe or cotton.
- Saturate with nail preparation solution, alcohol or polish remover.
- Wipe nail plate.

NOTE: Prior to the application of nail polish, you may ask the client to put jewelry back on. If the client has not pre-paid before the service, you may want to do this now to avoid smudging the polish at the end of the service. Just ask, "Would you like to pay before your polish is applied?"

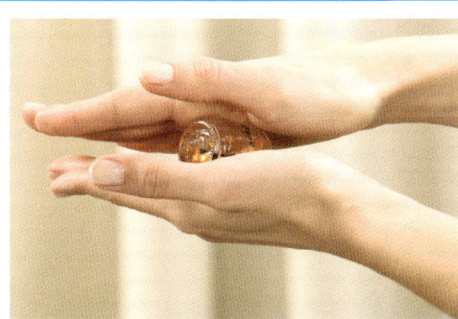

Remember:
- Mix polish by rolling bottle between your palms.

8

Since the polishing procedure will be performed on all 10 fingers, polish in this order: From the little finger of the left hand to the thumb; then the right hand, from the little finger to the thumb.

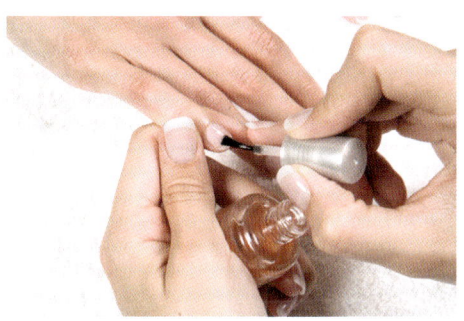

25. **Apply base coat** to each nail.
- Remove brush from polish bottle.
- Wipe side of brush (facing away from you) on inside neck of bottle.
- This creates a "bead" of polish on the end of the brush.
- Hold client's finger between your index finger and thumb.
- Pinch slightly to move sidewalls away from nail plate.

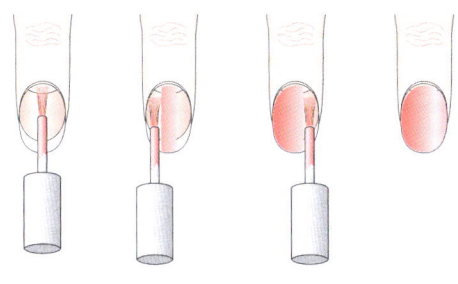

NOTE: Apply the polish 1/16" (.2 cm) from the entire cuticle. With the bead of polish toward the nail plate, place the brush at middle of the base of the nail at approximately a 35° angle. Brush toward the free edge. Repeat on each side of the nail plate with a 3-stroke application: 1). Middle, 2). Side, 3). Side. Note that the brush handle remains at a 35° angle, while the brush itself flattens to the nail.

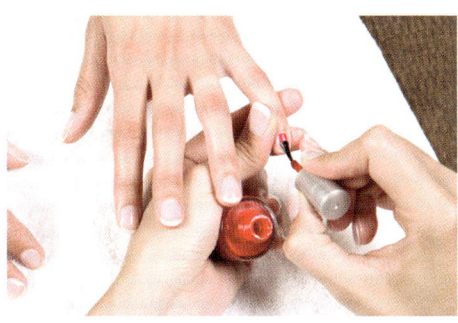

26. **Apply colored polish.**
- Use same technique to apply chosen colored polish.
- Begin with little finger of left hand.
- Work toward thumb.
- Repeat on right hand.

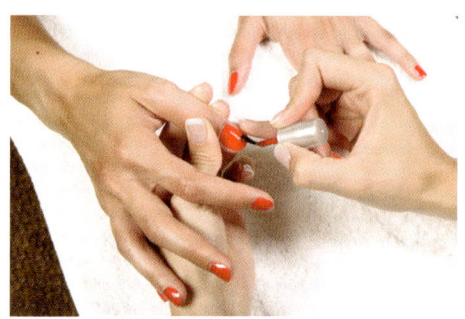

27. **Apply second coat** of colored polish.

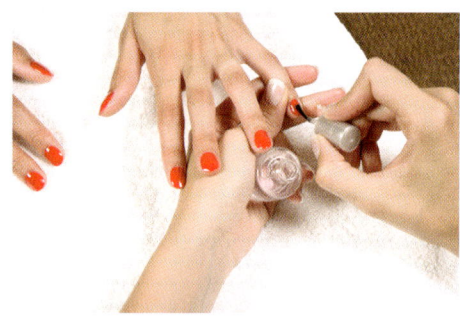

28. **Apply top coat** using same technique.

NOTE: Move directly from base coat to top coat if no colored polish is desired, for a total of two coats.

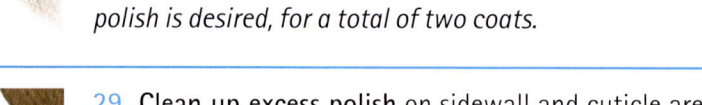

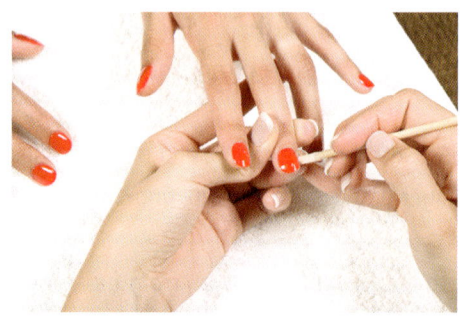

29. **Clean up excess polish** on sidewall and cuticle areas (if necessary).
  - Use cotton-tipped orangewood stick or synthetic fiber brush.
  - Dampen with polish remover.
  - Remove polish from skin carefully.

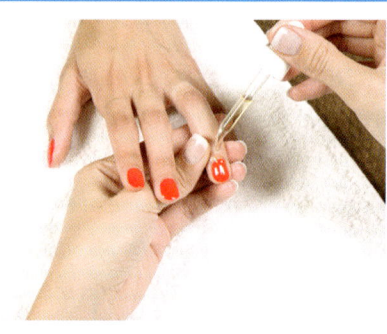

30. **Apply speed dry** to each nail if desired.
  - Optional: Apply small amount of cuticle oil to each cuticle.
  - Rub oil gently into cuticle area without pressure to freshly polished nail plate.

BASIC MANICURE COMPLETION

- Escort client to reception area.
- Discuss retail products.
- Rebook next appointment.

Infection Control and Safety
- Disinfect all implements.
- Discard any disposable items.
- Replenish supplies.
- Disinfect the table and the service area using an EPA registered, broad spectrum (hospital-level) disinfectant.
- Set up for the next client.
- Empty finger bowl and disinfect after every client
- Practice blood spill procedures if a blood spill occurs, refer to page 67.

5. Completion - Gain feedback; infection control and safety

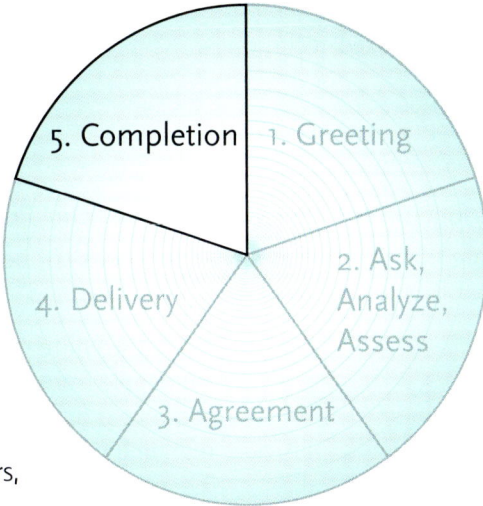

5. Completion
1. Greeting
2. Ask, Analyze, Assess
3. Agreement
4. Delivery

8

REMEMBER:
- Remove all product from jars with a spatula and keep lids tightly closed to avoid contamination.
- Keep labels on all containers and store products in a cool place to lengthen shelf-life.
- Keep tools dry to avoid rust.
- Place soiled towels in a covered container; use clean towels on each client.
- Complete the Service Record on the Client Consultation Form.

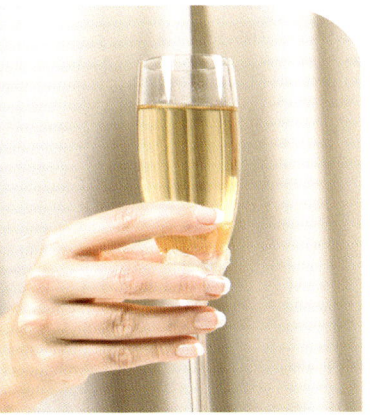

French Manicure

A **French manicure** is a style used to polish the nails creating a stylized natural-looking effect on the nail by covering the free edge, or tip, of the nail with white and then coating the entire nail with a sheer pink or beige color. The natural look of the nail is enhanced by emphasizing the white area of the nail. The white area is the part of the nail plate from the free edge up to the visible crescent-shape created by the hyponychium, or point where the nail plate attaches to the nail bed. This point is often referred to as the nail's natural "smile line" because from the nail technician's point of view, the ends of the line curve up, and the nail appears to be smiling.

White polish is applied to the nail to accentuate the tip of the nail and to create a smooth smile line. The sheer polish enhances the healthy pink or beige color of the nail plate under which the nail bed is attached. There is a wide variety of sheer tinted polishes available for clients to choose from. Some manufacturers offer entire collections of colors appropriate for use on a French manicure.

Although a French application takes a little more time to perform than a one-color application, it is to your benefit to practice and perfect a French manicure because it is usually considered an add-on cost. Many brides choose to wear a French manicure on their wedding day because it helps create subtle, yet elegant-looking hands without the distraction of bold colors. The neutral look of a French manicure can also provide a great base for nail art. There are many different ways to achieve a similar effect, but the following is an effective way to learn and begin developing your own personalized techniques.

FRENCH MANICURE

Perform Steps 1-24 of the Basic Manicure Procedure, then follow these steps for applying the polish. Note that this French application does not begin with a base coat.

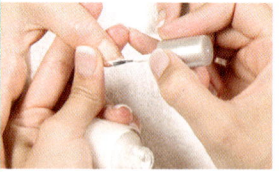

1. Apply the white polish to the free edge, before applying the base coat. First apply from one side of the free edge to the middle of the free edge and repeat on the other side to create a rounded "V-shape." Then finish rounding out the middle or point of the "V" to create a smooth, wide "U-shaped" smile line.

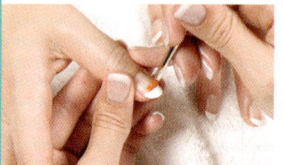

2. Refine the smile line using a synthetic bristle brush or cotton-tipped orangewood stick saturated with polish remover. Clean up the white polish as needed.

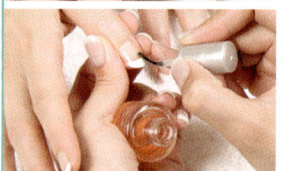

3. Apply the base coat over the entire nail, using the standard nail polish application.

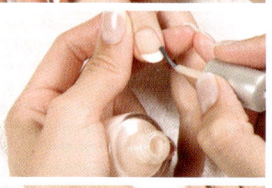

4. Apply a sheer pink, beige or neutral color over the entire nail plate. Be sure the color is sheer enough to only slightly tint, not discolor, the white polish. Most of the time only one coat of color is applied over the entire nail, but it is acceptable if your client prefers two coats.

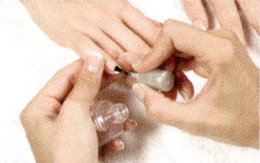

5. Apply the top coat to complete the French manicure.

With this application method, you can experiment using other colors to create interesting and eye-catching variations. Eventually, as you try different ways to perform this service and as you gain more experience, you will want to develop your own method.

In the 1920s, a product was introduced to create this same effect. A chalky white liquid was applied underneath the free edge of the nail and allowed to dry, giving the tips a clean, natural look.

Male Manicure

The number of male clients seeking nail services is steadily growing, especially with more spas and salons catering to male clientele. Male manicures vary only slightly from female manicures, but there are some important considerations that technicians need to be aware of. When performing a male manicure, one of the most important things to consider is the fragrance of products; most men prefer a woodsy or fresh scent versus a floral or fruity scent, so you may need separate lines of product. Men typically have drier, more damaged cuticles, so during the manicure keep a sharp focus

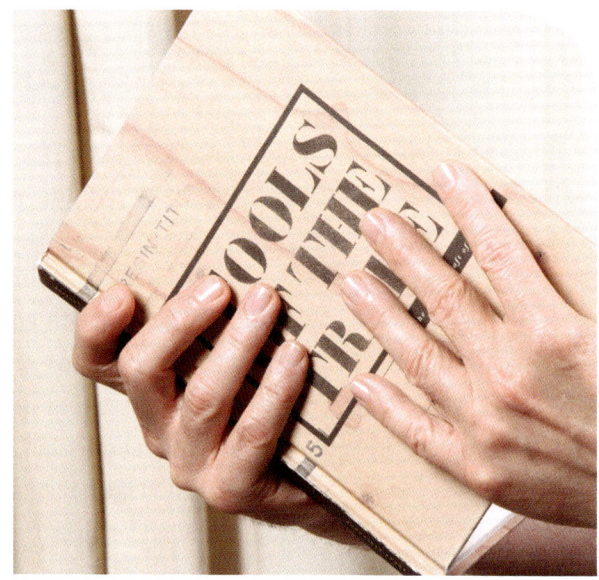

on the cuticle area—you may have to spend a little extra time on them. Men tend to take less care of their hands than women do, so they may have more callused areas on their hands or drier skin. Therefore, it is important to apply a lotion or cream to the hands of male clients. In addition, men don't typically wear a colored polish. They may want their nails buffed to a shine, or they may prefer to have a clear matte-finish polish applied. Many nail product companies are making nail products specifically designed with the male client in mind.

MALE MANICURE

Follow the Basic Manicure Procedure (Steps 1-30 with polish; Steps 1-23 without polish) as demonstrated earlier in the chapter (pages 205-216), while focusing on the following:

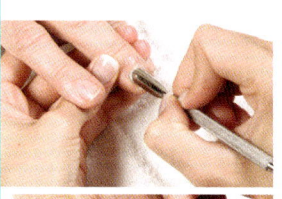

1. **Cuticle Care:** Focus on pushing the cuticles back, being careful not to create an opening or tear in the skin.

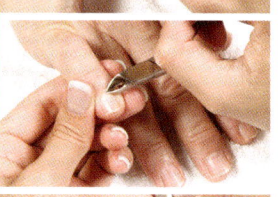

2. **Nip Cuticles/Hangnails:** If permitted by your regulating agency. Again, be careful not to cut into living tissue.

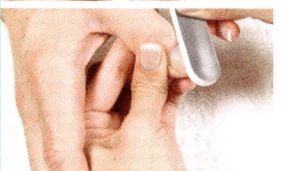

3. **Buff Nails:** At the end of the manicure if the client prefers not to have colored polish applied; buff nails to a shine or apply a clear matte-finish polish.

CHILDREN'S MANICURE

Children also like receiving manicure services. Whether it's a mother-daughter day or a birthday party at the salon, children are now lining up for natural nail services. You will want to consider the following:

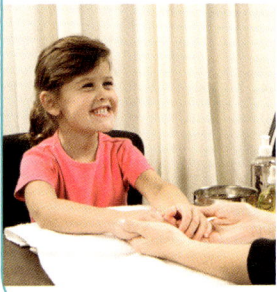

- Use adjustable-height chairs.
- Use a light touch and a cotton-tipped orangewood stick for additional comfort, and shorten the massage steps using less pressure.
- Use products that are age appropriate, and always have parental permission.
- Have a clear policy addressing the youngest age limit for children receiving services.

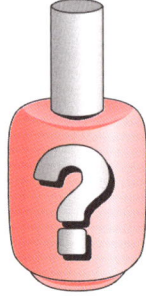

Which part of the Basic Manicure Procedure explained in this section do you feel is most important? Why?

PEDICURE ESSENTIALS

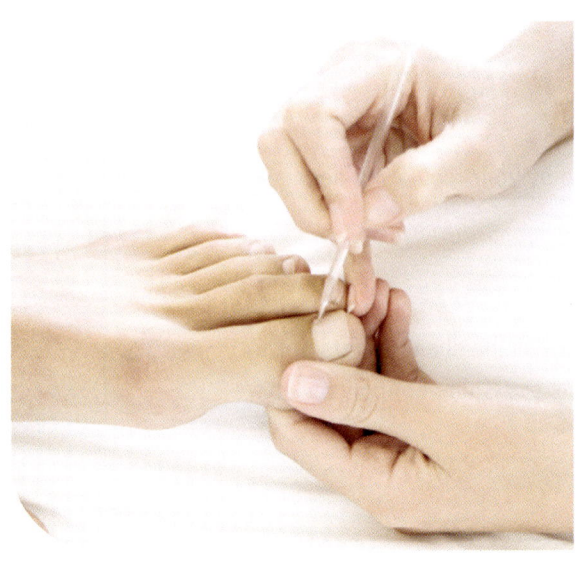

A **pedicure** is the cosmetic care of the feet and toenails. The word "pedicure" comes from the Latin words *ped*, meaning, "foot," and *cura*, meaning "care." In other words, it is a manicure for the feet. Just as our hands need special attention, so do our feet.

Pedicure services make up roughly 25% of nail services performed by nail technicians, so it is valuable to practice and perfect the steps of the basic pedicure early in your career. Mastering the basics of pedicuring will allow you to advance your skills to include spa services and mini-services or add-on services.

As a professional nail technician, you will need to be knowledgeable about the essential massage movements, products, implements, supplies and types of equipment used to care for natural nails. It is important to understand the function and use of each item in order to provide clients with the best possible services.

Massage

In the previous section, Manicure Essentials, you learned that massage is a systematic, therapeutic method of manipulating the body by rubbing, pinching, tapping, kneading or stroking with hands, fingers or an instrument. The following information reviews the types of massage and the benefits received from each. (Turn to page 185 for more information on massage.)

8

THE FIVE BASIC MASSAGE TECHNIQUES

There are five basic massage movements (manipulations). Each one performs a different function and delivers different results. The use of each movement in combination with others delivers optimal results.

Type	Description	Function
Effleurage	Stroking or circular movement that is light, relaxing, smooth and gentle; often used to begin or end massage	Soothes muscles; relaxes sensory nerve endings at the surface of the skin
Petrissage	Light or heavy kneading; pinching and rolling of the muscles	Stimulates muscles, nerves and skin glands, which in turn increases circulation of blood and lymph
Friction	Circular or wringing movement with no gliding, usually performed with the fingertips or palms of the hands	Stimulates and warms the muscles, which in turn increases circulation
Tapotement or Percussion	Light tapping or slapping movement applied with the fingertips or partly flexed fingers	Increases blood circulation, stimulates nerves and promotes muscle contraction
Vibration	Shaking movement achieved when the technician quickly shakes his or her arms while the fingertips or palms are touching the client	Very stimulating movement and should be done for only a short period of time

Massage Cautions

Avoid performing massage manipulations on clients with the following conditions:

- Skin conditions such as redness, swelling, pus, disease, bruises and/or broken or scraped skin
- Heart conditions/High blood pressure
- Stroke
- Pregnancy

Use caution when performing massage manipulations on clients with the following conditions:

- Prominent varicose veins
- Arthritis

Important points to remember when performing massage manipulations:

- Check for conditions mentioned above.
- Avoid massage that is too deep, aggressive or lengthy.
- Provide an even tempo or rhythm and pressure to ensure a relaxing effect for the client.

Keep in mind that the massage portion of a pedicure service is generally considered to be the most relaxing and enjoyable part. Therefore, perfecting the various massage movements will help ensure that your clients will want to come to you for their future nail care needs.

DIABETES CAUTION

People with diabetes may experience a loss in feeling in their feet, have thin skin and an increased risk of infection. Therefore, a diabetic client may not be able to tell you if something is hurting and you could accidentally create an opening in the skin. If the client remains unaware of an opening in the skin, it could become infected and require medical attention. Therefore, it is advisable for clients with diabetes to get a doctor's permission before receiving a pedicure.

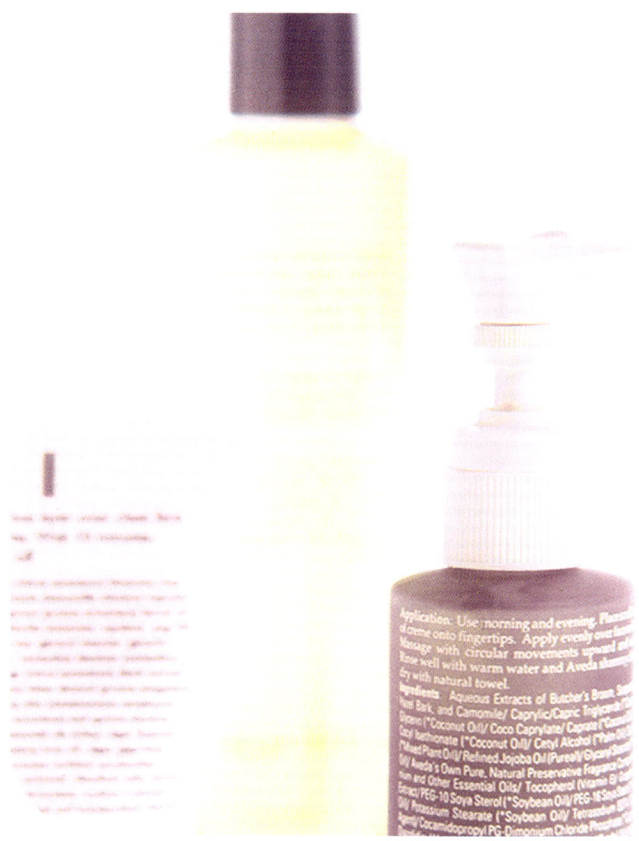

Pedicure Products

Nail products, also referred to as nail cosmetics, are vital in keeping nails healthy and well-cared for. To best care for your clients' toenails and feet, you will need to know how and when to apply each product, as well as how the nails will benefit from each specific one. That's why it is important to know the ingredients in each— the more you know about the product you are using, the better you will be able to determine what is best for each client. One thing to remember is to always follow the manufacturers' instructions and recommendations; not doing so could cause undesirable results or even adverse reactions.

Many of the same products used to perform a manicure are used in providing pedicure services as well. To perform a pedicure service you will need to know about the following additional products.

Foot Spray

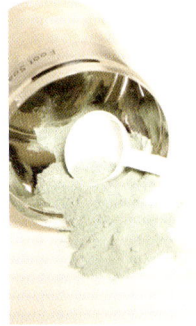

Antiseptic **foot spray** is used to sanitize the feet before examining them and placing them in the pedicure basin. It contains an antifungal agent and a mild antiseptic that is used to aid in the prevention of cross-contamination in the salon or spa. Foot spray should not be used alone in place of soaking the feet.

Foot Soak

A **foot soak** is a gentle soap solution used to cleanse, deodorize, sanitize and soften the feet, allowing for deeper penetration of skin and nail products. It is used in the pedicure basin with water at the beginning of a pedicure to wash and sanitize the feet. Foot soak is available in several forms including crystals, gels, powders and tablets.

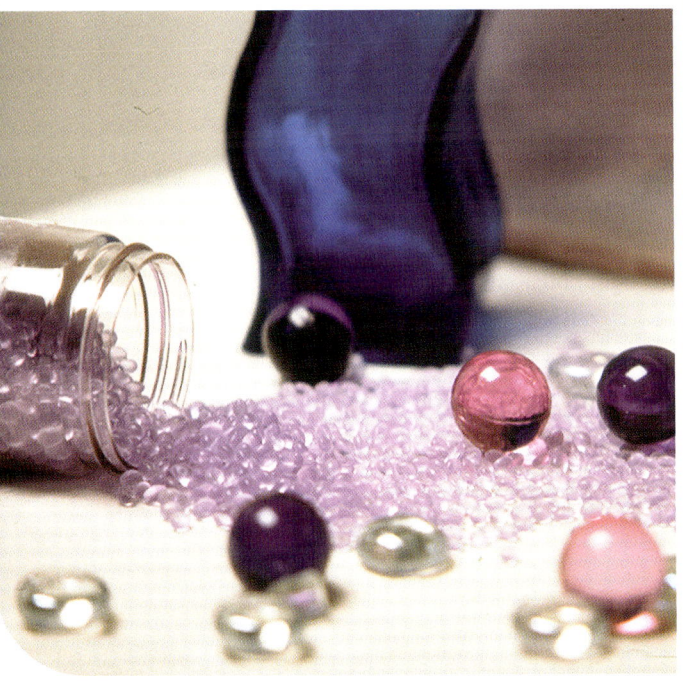

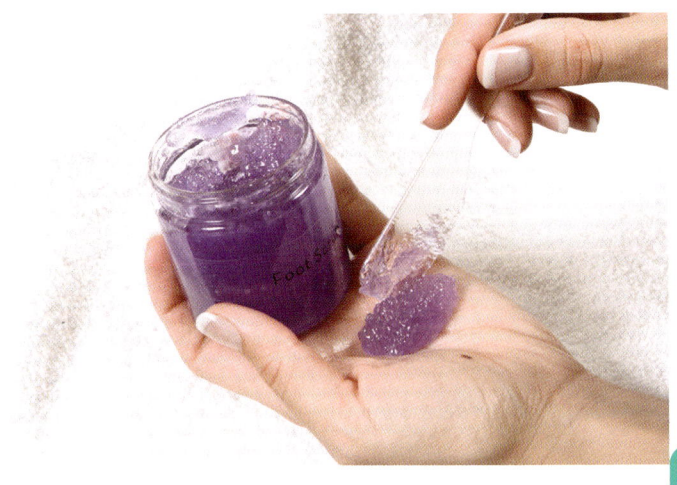

8

Exfoliants

Foot scrub and sloughing (SLUFF-ing) lotion are two examples of manual exfoliants used during a pedicure service. A foot scrub is a granular substance with a slightly grainy or rough texture that helps remove superficial dead skin cells. Sloughing lotion is a substance that is applied to the skin in a thin layer, allowed to dry, and then rubbed off, taking with it dead skin cells from the surface of the skin. Using an exfoliant allows for deeper cleansing, increases moisture retention and smoothes the skin.

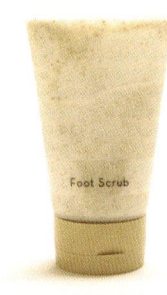

Massage Oil

Massage oil is used to moisturize and hydrate the skin when performing a foot and leg massage during a pedicure service. Most massage oils used by nail technicians contain a blend of aromatherapy oils, which can also be blended by the technician. For more on aromatherapy, see *Chapter 10, Specialty Nail Services.*

PEDICURE PRODUCTS

The following is a list of all of the products needed for a pedicure service.

Product	Function
Liquid Soap	Fights off harmful surface bacteria from the skin
Antiseptic Sanitizer	Reduces bacteria on the surface of the skin; aids in the prevention of cross-contamination
Antiseptic Foot Spray	Sanitizes feet before placing them into pedicure basin
Foot Soak	Softens the feet allowing for deeper penetration of skin and nail products
Polish Remover	Dissolves polish
Cuticle Remover	Softens dead cuticle tissue to allow gentle pushing back and to aid in its removal
Exfoliant	Helps remove dead skin cells from the surface of the skin
Cuticle Conditioner	Softens and moisturizes cuticles and surrounding skin
Nail Bleach	Removes stains and discoloration on the nail plate
Moisturizing Lotion or Cream	Helps skin retain moisture and prevents or protects it from dryness
Massage Oil	Moisturizes and hydrates the skin
Nail Preparation Solution	Removes oil and product to help polish adhere to the nail plate
Polishes	**Base Coat:** Evens out nail plate and prevents polish from staining the nail plate **Nail Strengthener:** Prevents nails from chipping or breaking **Colored Polish:** Creates a colored effect on the nail **Top Coat:** Seals colored polish and helps prevent chipping
Speed Dry	Decreases polish drying time

Pedicure Implements

Pedicure implements are generally considered to be non-disposable since they are nonporous and able to be disinfected and reused. Many of the same implements used to perform a manicure are used in providing pedicure services as well. To perform a pedicure service you will need to know about the following additional implements.

Curette

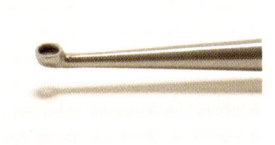

A **curette** is a spoon-shaped metal instrument used for the removal of debris from the nail margins. It's typically used for pedicures. A curette requires disinfection after every service.

Nail Rasp

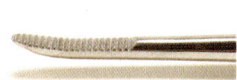

A **nail rasp** is a metal instrument used to smooth the edges of the toenail in the nail groove, especially for slightly rounding the corners on toenails. The nail rasp is designed to file only in one direction, like a cheese grater, and is used by filing from corner to center. A nail rasp is disinfected after every service.

Foot File

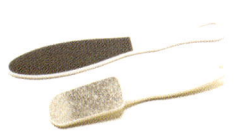

A **foot file** is used to remove dry, flaky skin and to smooth calluses. Also referred to as a **foot paddle**, there are a variety of foot files made from different materials that are either disinfected or discarded. Some types of foot files have abrasives on a sticker-like backing that can be peeled off and discarded after each client. Always follow regulatory guidelines and manufacturer's recommendations for using foot files.

Toenail Nippers

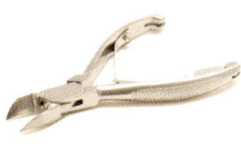

Toenail nippers resemble cuticle nippers, but are used to trim toenails rather than cuticles.

Toenail nippers are different than toenail clippers because they open wider and give more leverage to the technician, which make them especially good for trimming thick toenails. The blades can be curved or straight and the ends can be blunt or pointed. Toenail nippers require disinfection after every service. Always be sure to thoroughly dry the joint of the toenail nippers, as leaving moisture can cause the joint to rust.

CREDO BLADE

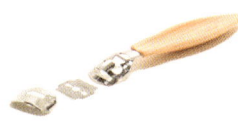

A **credo blade** is a metal instrument that holds a blade and is used for "cutting" calluses similar to how a potato peeler is used. The credo blade is prohibited by most regulatory agencies because it removes calluses by cutting the skin, which is typically only legally performed by a physician. Also, by removing the callus, the skin reacts by regenerating the skin cells rapidly to compensate for the loss—so most often, the callus comes back thicker. Calluses develop for a reason—protection—and so it is not recommended to remove them, only to smooth and reduce them.

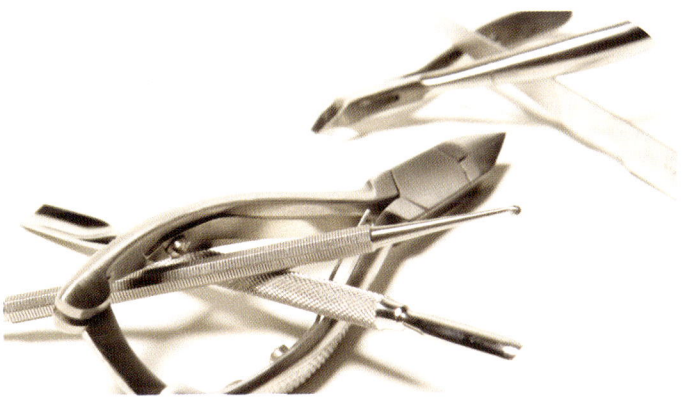

PEDICURE IMPLEMENTS

The following is a list of all of the implements needed for a pedicure service.

Implements	Function
Nail Clippers	Shorten nails
Nail File	Shortens and shapes nails
	Emery Board: Smoothes and shapes natural nails; disposable
	Glass File: Smoothes and shapes natural nails; disinfectable
	Metal File (Diamond File): Smoothes and shapes natural nails; disinfectable
Cuticle Pusher (Steel Pusher)	Loosens and pushes back cuticles
Cuticle Nippers	Trim excess cuticle and hangnails
Nail Brush	Cleans the nails and surrounding skin
Buffer	Smoothes ridges or corrugations on the nail plate
Curette	Removes debris from the nail margins
Nail Rasp	Smoothes the edges of the nails in the nail grooves
Foot File (Foot Paddle)	Removes dry, flaky skin and smoothes calluses
Toenail Nippers	Trim thick toenails

Be sure to pre-clean or sanitize all implements before placing them in an EPA-registered, broad spectrum (hospital-level) disinfectant.

Pedicure Supplies

While pedicure implements are able to be disinfected and reused, pedicure supplies are items that are discarded after each use. The following supplies are specifically used to perform pedicure services.

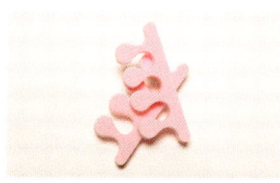

Toe Separators

Toe separators are used to separate the toes during the polishing steps of a pedicure service. There are many different types of toe separators available, but typically a foam rubber material is the most common. Cotton or tissue can also be used to separate the toes by placing it (sometimes by twisting it) between the toes that need to be spread apart. Toe separators are not able to be disinfected and are discarded after each service.

Pedicure Slippers

Pedicure slippers are open-toed sandals worn instead of shoes to help protect the

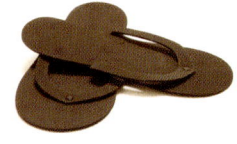

polish while it dries. They are placed on the client's feet before polishing the toenails. The most common pedicure slippers are made of paper or porous foam rubber. Some slippers are made of non-porous rubber or plastic and can be disinfected after each service and reused; however, paper or porous foam rubber slippers are discarded after each use. Some clients will bring their own open-toed shoes or sandals.

Placing pedicure slippers on your client's feet before inserting toe separators helps ensure that the slippers won't fall off!

PEDICURE SUPPLIES

The following is a list of all of the supplies needed for a pedicure service.

Supplies	Function
Towels	Dry client's feet; can be folded to make a cushion
Cotton or Lint-Free Nail Wipes	Remove polish and oils from the nail plate
Cosmetic Spatula	Removes product from jars
Orangewood Stick	Loosens and pushes back cuticles; applies cosmetics; cleans under the free edge; removes polish from sidewalls
Toe Separators	Separate toes for polishing
Pedicure Slippers	Help protect the polish while it dries

8

Towels are especially important for use during pedicures. Bare feet should never come into direct contact with either the floor or the foot rest—there should always be a towel in between, protecting the foot.

Pedicure Equipment

Pedicure equipment includes the furnishings and provisions necessary to provide a professional pedicure service. The equipment needed to perform a pedicure follows.

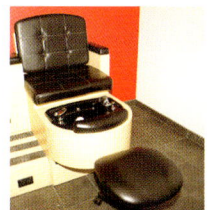

Pedicure Station

Pedicure stations consist of a comfortable client chair with arm rests, a foot rest and a chair or stool for the technician. Client chairs sometimes have massaging and heating elements for added comfort. A **pedicure stool** is made for the technician, and is basically a low stool that sometimes has a foot rest attached for the client. Having a low stool makes it easier for the technician to work on the client's feet without straining. If there is not a foot rest attached, a separate one can be used.

Pedicure Basin or Bath

A **pedicure basin** or **bath** is used to soak the client's feet during a pedicure service. A pedicure basin needs to be large enough to completely immerse the client's feet in warm water and a foot-soaking solution. Some regulating agencies require a separate basin filled with clean water to rinse the feet after soaking, so check regulatory guidelines.

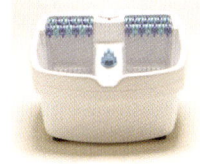

There are many different types of basins or baths available for use in the salon, with some being portable and others attached to the pedicure station with running water in them. Many salons and spas have what is known as a **"pedicure throne."** This means it is an all-inclusive unit that includes a client chair, a basin or bath and a foot rest all in one. The pedicure throne is stationary, making it a fixed station connected to running water. Some pedicure thrones include jets or propellers in the basin to create a whirlpool effect, which creates a relaxing, enjoyable time for the client.

Proper disinfection procedures are critical to prevent the growth of bacteria and fungus in the screens and filters or other areas of the pedicure basins or baths. Always be sure to follow manufacturer's instructions and follow regulatory guidelines.

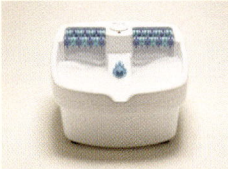 Before preparing the foot bath, always be sure it is properly disinfected. Check the temperature of the water, as it may take a few seconds for warm water to reach a comfortable level. After checking the temperature of the water, close the drain if necessary and place the recommended amount of foot soak in the basin. If it is a foaming soak and the basin has jets or a vibrating movement, you might want to add less product to prevent the bubbles from overflowing. Fill the water to the manufacturer's recommended level and check the water temperature again in preparation for the client.

PEDICURE EQUIPMENT

The following is a list of all of the equipment needed for a pedicure service.

Equipment	Function
Glass Container	Holds supplies
Disinfection Container	Holds EPA-registered, broad spectrum (hospital-level) disinfection solution; must be large enough for complete immersion of implements
Pedicure Station	Provides comfortable seat with arm rests, pedicure basin, foot rest and technician stool for pedicure services
Pedicure Basin or Bath	Serves as a water container used to soak client's feet during a pedicure service

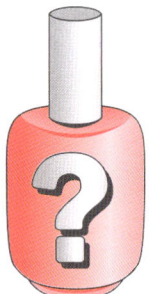 Why is it important to be familiar with different pedicure products, implements, supplies and equipment that are available to nail technicians?

BASIC PEDICURE

Though they aren't on display as often as our fingernails, colorful toenails can be a perfect way to accessorize when wearing sandals or open-toed shoes. While pedicures are often seen as a way to pamper oneself or relieve stress, it's the overall health and care of the foot that people often associate with pedicures.

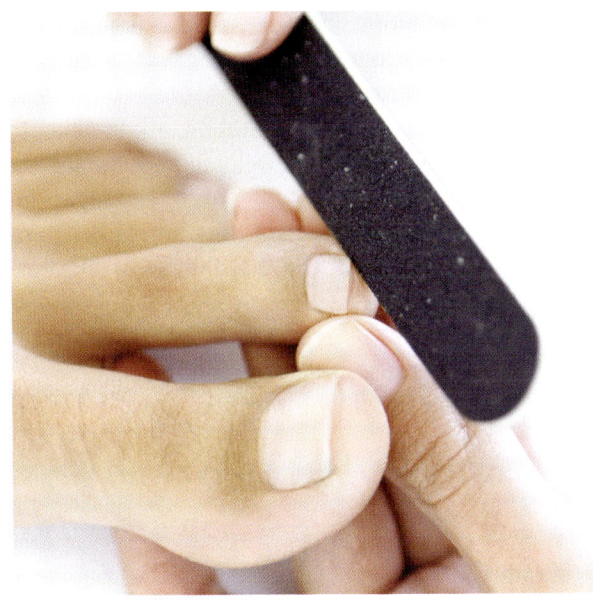

As a nail technician, you can help your clients care for their feet by noticing any changes and also by properly trimming and shaping their toenails. Toenails should be trimmed to the tip of the toe, generally straight across with the corners slightly rounded, which helps avoid ingrown toenails.

A basic pedicure includes trimming and shaping the nails, cuticle care, massage and polish. There are many different types of pedicures offered using extra products to pamper the feet, such as exfoliants, foot masks, fresh fruit and much more! Learning the basic pedicure will allow you to build your skills to incorporate more advanced pedicure services that will enhance your career.

FIVE PHASES OF SERVICE

To help you remember the important steps in the Five Phases of Service, which you learned in *Chapter 7, Client Care*, use the following sentence: **G**reat **A**rtists **A**lways **D**raw **C**reatively.

Preparing for a successful service involves the first Three Phases of Service:
1. Greeting—Establish rapport
2. Ask, Analyze and Assess—Offer professional advice
3. Agreement—Clarify expectations

(Pie chart:)
- 1. Greeting
- 2. Ask, Analyze, Assess
- 3. Agreement
- 4. Delivery
- 5. Completion

Remember, the nail technician does not diagnose or treat nail or skin diseases. If there is a visible sign of a nail or skin disease, the client must be referred to a physician.

BASIC PEDICURE PREPARATION

As with any professional service, it is important to have the service area, products, implements, supplies and equipment in proper order prior to the client's arrival.

After completing the consultation, ask the client to remove shoes, socks and jewelry, if applicable. Remind clients to store jewelry in a safe place, such as a pocket or purse.

If the client is wearing pants, ask him or her to roll them up to the knee. For repeat clients, you may want to recommend that they wear short or loose-fitting pants for their next appointment.

- Suggest to your repeat pedicure clients that they not shave their legs the day of the pedicure. Shaving causes small tears in the skin, which could allow some products to irritate the skin and increase the risk of infection.

- NOTE: You may need to get a doctor's permission to perform a pedicure service on a diabetic client.

Products
- Liquid soap
- Antiseptic sanitizer
- Foot soak
- Foot spray
- Polish remover
- Cuticle remover
- Cuticle conditioner
- Exfoliant (optional)
- Foot lotion or cream
- Nail preparation solution
- Base coat
- Colored polish
- Top coat
- Speed dry

Implements
- Toenail clippers
- Emery board/metal file/glass file
- Cuticle pusher
- Cuticle nippers
- Nail brush
- Foot file or paddle
- Buffer

Supplies
- Orangewood sticks
- Towels
- Cotton or lint-free wipes in a disinfected glass container

Equipment
- Glass container
- Disinfection container filled with EPA-registered, broad spectrum (hospital-level) disinfectant
- Pedicure station
- Pedicure basin or bath
- Technician chair or stool

Basic Pedicure Set-Up
- Disinfect the pedicure basin properly before beginning.
- Clean and disinfect the surface of the table and foot rest with an EPA-registered, broad spectrum (hospital-level) disinfectant.
- Organize all products in the order of use.
- Place the disinfection container filled with an EPA-registered, broad spectrum (hospital-level) disinfectant on the table.
- Disinfect all implements properly before beginning.
- Place a clean towel on the table and place all implements on the towel.
- Place a clean towel on the foot rest.
- Place a covered trash can on the floor to the right of you. If a trash can is not available, fasten a plastic bag to the table and discard the bag after every service.

Pedicure set-up can vary for each person's preference and regulating agency.

BASIC PEDICURE PROCEDURE

The basic pedicure is one of the most-requested nail services. By following and practicing the steps on the following pages, you will be prepared to give a basic pedicure. Note that the procedure below corresponds with the step-by-step technical images that follow.

4. Delivery - Meet client's expectations

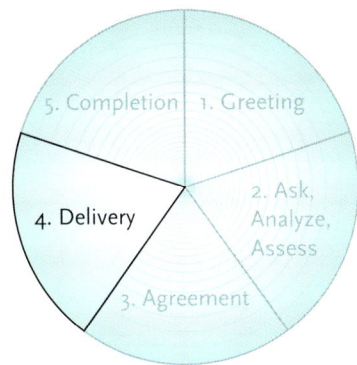

SANITIZE
1. Wash and sanitize your hands
2. Sanitize client's feet

ANALYZE
3. Perform visual analysis of client's feet
4. Soak feet
5. Remove both feet and dry
6. Remove polish
7. Perform visual analysis of nails

SHAPE
8. Trim free edge of each nail
9. File and shape, return left foot to foot bath

REPEAT SHAPE (Steps 8–9) on right foot, and return to foot bath

CUTICLE CARE
10. Remove left foot from foot bath
11. Apply cuticle remover
12. Push back cuticles
13. Nip cuticles if necessary
14. Clean under free edge
15. Buff nails (optional)

16. Brush nails, return left foot to foot bath
17. Remove right foot from foot bath

REPEAT CUTICLE CARE (Steps 11–16) on right foot, and return to foot bath

EXFOLIATION
18. Remove left foot from foot bath
19. Exfoliate the foot (optional)
20. File foot using foot file or paddle
21. Rinse foot, return left foot to foot bath
22. Remove right foot from foot bath

REPEAT EXFOLIATION (Steps 19–21) on right foot

CUTICLE OIL APPLICATION
23. Apply cuticle oil

MASSAGE
24. Obtain product
25. Apply product
26. Establish control
27. Perform massage movements

REPEAT CUTICLE OIL APPLICATION AND MASSAGE (Steps 23–27) on right foot

POLISH
28. Remove oils from each nail plate
29. Position slippers and toe separators
30. Apply base coat
31. Apply colored polish
32. Apply second coat
33. Apply top coat
34. Clean up excess polish
35. Apply speed dry

BASIC PEDICURE

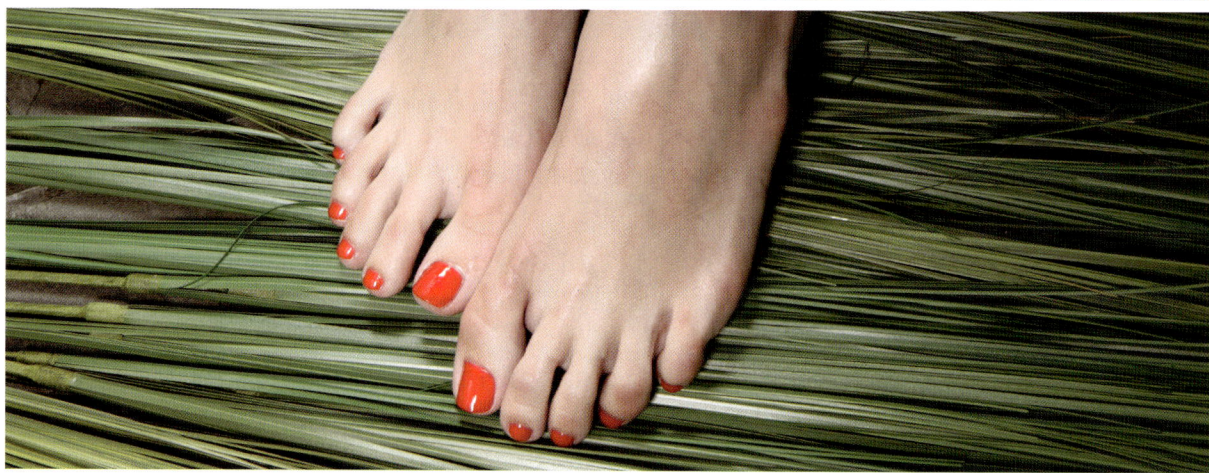

> A checkmark next to a step indicates an ideal time to check on your client's comfort, and to take extra safety precautions.

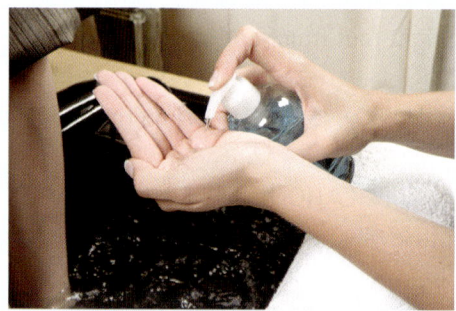

1. **Wash and sanitize your hands.**
   - Use liquid or foam soap.
   - Wear protective gloves if required by regulating agency.
   - Use waterless sanitizer or topical antiseptic if required by regulating agency.

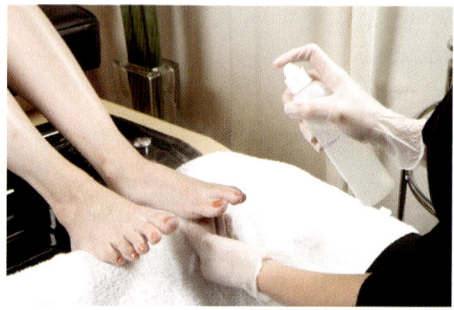

2. **Sanitize client's feet.**
   - Use waterless sanitizer or topical antiseptic if required by regulating agency.

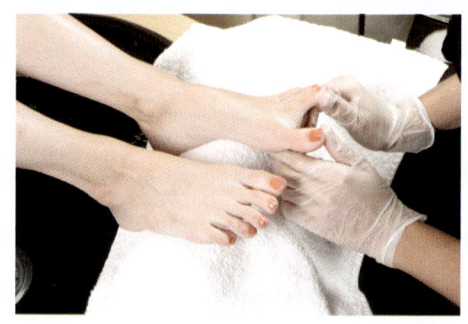

ANALYZE

3. **Perform visual analysis of client's feet.**
   - Continue with service if feet are free of any visible signs of diseases or disorders.

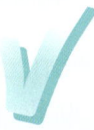

NOTE: As a nail technician, you cannot diagnose or treat diseases or disorders. You can only refer the client to a physician.

Skin: Signs to look for during analysis on feet include open skin, redness, swelling, discoloration or any other signs of an infection that would prevent the service from being performed.

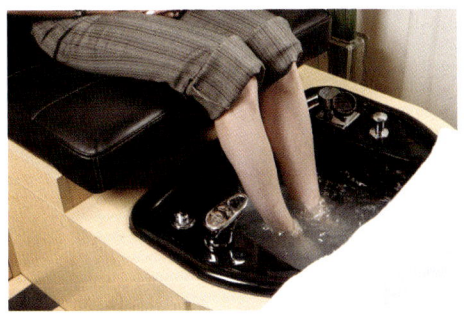

4. **Soak feet.**
   - Place both of client's feet in prepared foot bath.
   - Check if water temperature is comfortable for client.
   - Soak approximately 5-10 minutes.

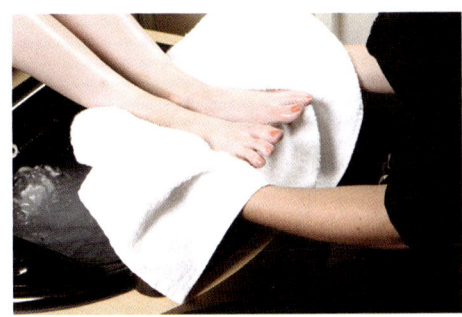

5. **Remove both feet and dry.**
   - Help client remove both feet from foot bath.
   - Place feet on foot rest (covered by towel).
   - Dry feet thoroughly.
   - Take extra care to dry between toes.

8

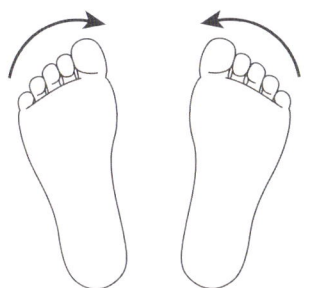

NOTE: Any procedure that will be performed on all 10 toes will always be done in the same order: From the little toe of the left foot to the big toe. Then the right foot, from the little toe to the big toe.

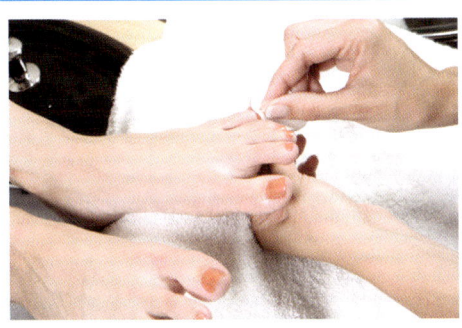

6. **Remove polish.**
   - Begin with left foot.
   - Use a lint-free saturated wipe or cotton on the nail plate.
   - Let remover stand for a few seconds.
   - Wipe toward the free edge.
   - Remove all polish from each nail before moving to the next nail. Repeat on the right foot.

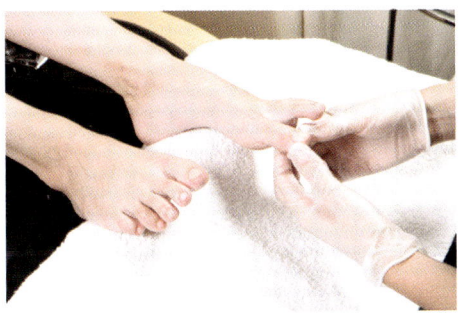

7. **Perform visual analysis of nails.**
   - Continue with the service if nail plates are free of any visible signs of diseases or disorders.

Nails: Signs to look for during analysis include discoloration, flaking, swelling, pain indicators, pus, detached nail plate, growth under the nail or any other signs of an infection that would prevent the service from being performed.

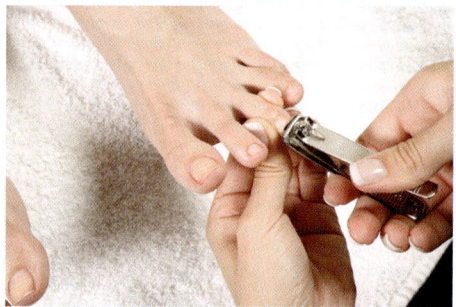

SHAPE

8. Trim free edge of each nail.

- Begin with little toe of left foot.
- Use toenail clippers to trim toenails.
- Work toward big toe.
- Begin with emery board or glass file (instead of clippers) if minimal length to be removed.

NOTE: Toenails are trimmed to the tip of the toe and are shaped straight across with the corners slightly rounded to avoid ingrown nails.

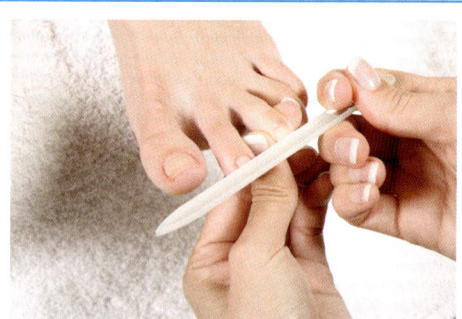

9. File and shape free edge.

- Use emery board or glass file.
- Get client's approval after shaping.
- Place left foot back in foot bath.

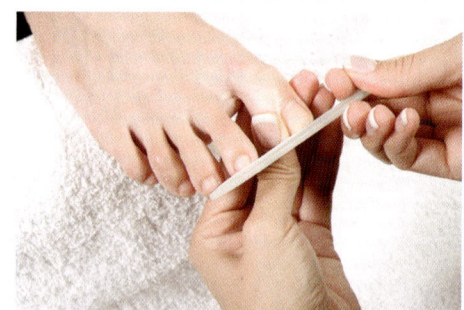

REPEAT SHAPE (Steps 8–9) on right foot.

- Trim free edge of each nail.
- File and shape free edge.
- Place right foot back in foot bath.

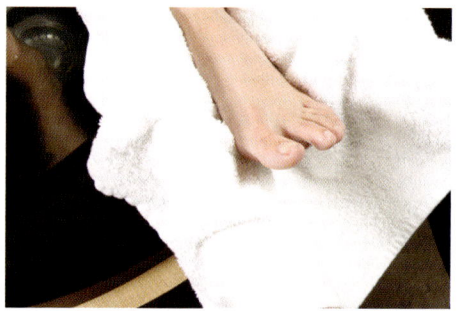

CUTICLE CARE

10. Remove left foot from foot bath and dry thoroughly.

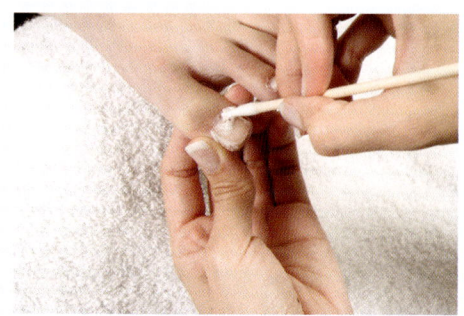

11. Apply cuticle remover to cuticle area.

- Use cotton-tipped orangewood stick, cotton swab or dropper.
- Begin with little toe.

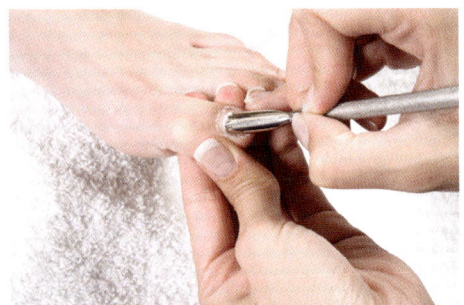

12. Push back cuticles.

- Use cotton-tipped orangewood stick or metal cuticle pusher.
- Use light, quick, circular movements along cuticle.
- Work from one side of nail toward center; then from other side toward center.
- Use a gentle, non-aggressive touch.
- Move orangewood stick or pusher along nail plate without applying downward pressure to avoid damaging the nail matrix.

If there is excessive skin under the free edge you can use cuticle remover to soften it, but never try to remove or push this skin back. This increases the risk of tearing the skin and can be painful for the client.

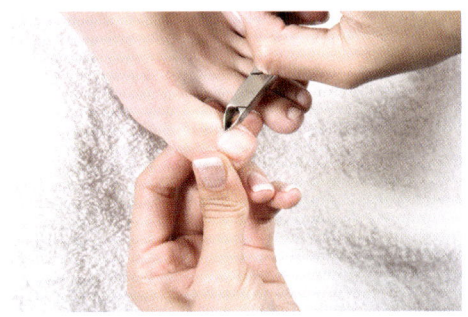

13. Nip cuticles/hangnails if necessary.

- After loosening, the excess cuticle will appear translucent.
- Use cuticle nippers.
- Remove any lifted or loosened excess cuticle.
- Position blades parallel to cuticle.
- Squeeze handles to cut; release the nippers before moving on.
- Remove cuticle in one piece if at all possible.
- The nippers may also be used to remove hangnails.
- Avoid using the point of the nippers and/or pulling at the cuticles.

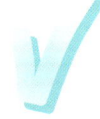

NOTE: Be guided by your regulatory guidelines regarding the use of cuticle nippers.

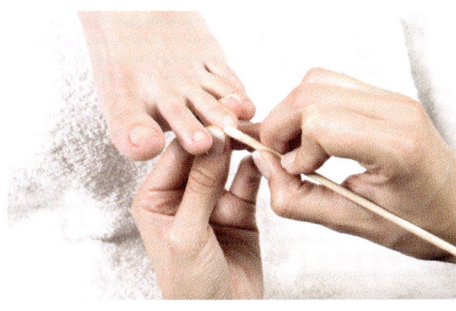

14. Clean under free edge.

- Use cotton-tipped orangewood stick or curette.
- Dampen cotton with polish remover or water (if using orangewood stick).
- Clean nail folds as well.

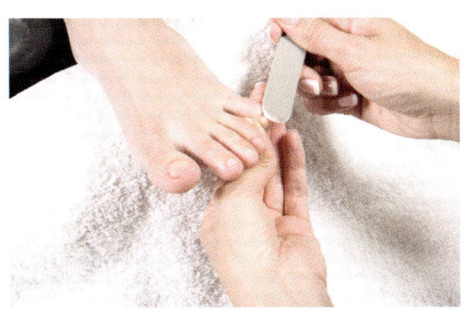

Optional:
15. Buff nails.

- Use buffer.
- Buff in direction of nail growth, toward free edge.

8

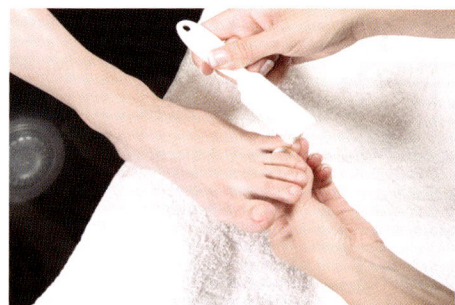

16. Brush nails.

- Use damp nail brush.
- Remove remaining bits of excess cuticle.
- Return left foot to foot bath.

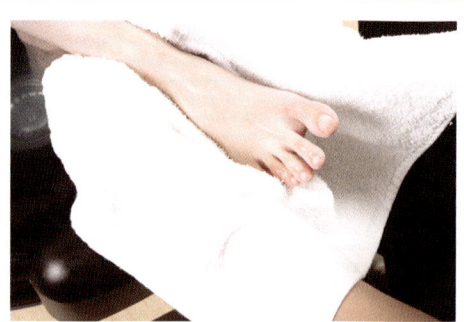

17. Remove right foot from foot bath and dry thoroughly.

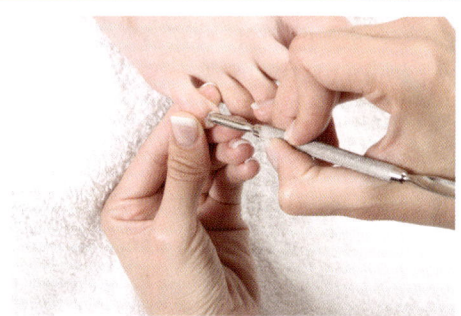

REPEAT CUTICLE CARE (Steps 11–16) on right foot.

- Apply cuticle remover.
- Push back cuticles.
- Nip cuticles if necessary.
- Clean under free edge.
- Buff nails.

- Brush nails.
- Place right foot back in foot bath.

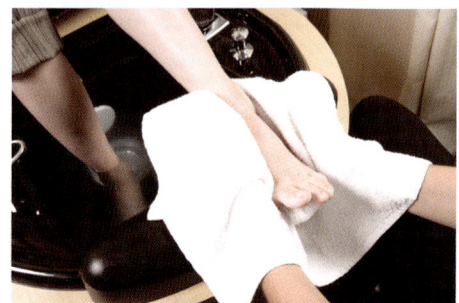

EXFOLIATION

18. Remove left foot from foot bath and dry thoroughly.

Some regulating agencies require that the feet are rinsed in a separate basin filled with clean water. Check regulatory guidelines.

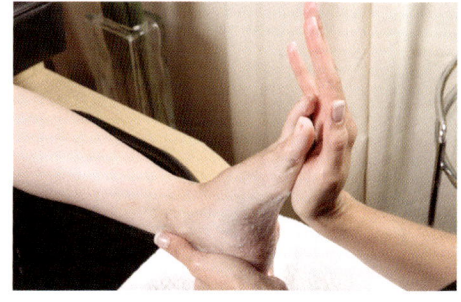

19. Exfoliate foot (optional).

- Use foot scrub or sloughing lotion.
- Apply product with your hands.
- Use with caution on top of foot (if product is granular).
- Focus on dry, callused areas.

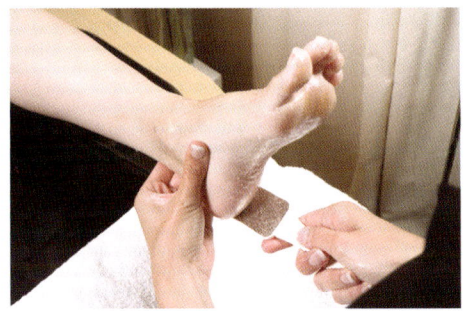

20. File foot using foot file or paddle.

- Move file back and forth across callused areas.
- Focus on the dry, callused areas.
- Soften and smooth calluses without removing.

NOTE: Some products or foot files may require the removal of the foot scrub before using the foot file. Always follow manufacturer's instructions.

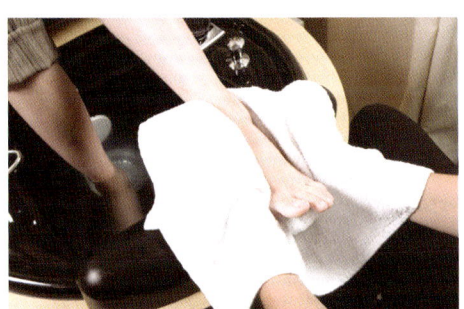

21. Rinse foot and return left foot to foot bath.

- Remove debris and product completely.
- Dry foot with clean towel.
- Wrap foot in same towel.
- Place foot off to side on a towel on foot rest or floor.

8

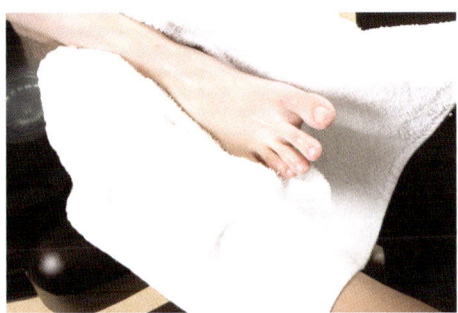

22. Remove right foot from foot bath and dry thoroughly.

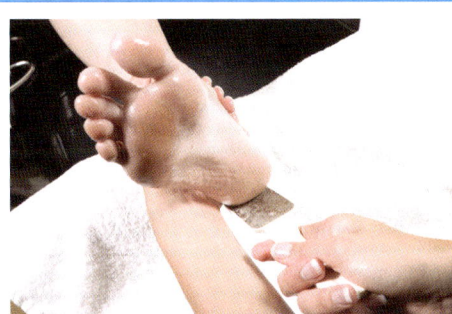

REPEAT EXFOLIATION (Steps 19–21) on right foot.

- Exfoliate foot (optional).
- File foot using foot file or paddle.
- Rinse foot.

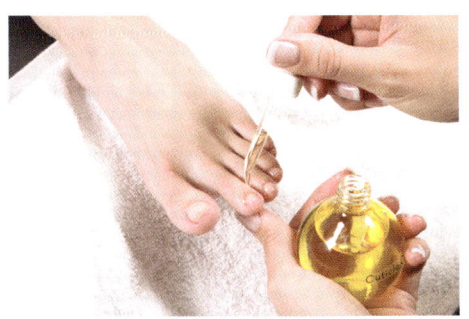

CUTICLE OIL APPLICATION

23. Apply cuticle oil.

- Unwrap left foot.
- Use cotton-tipped orangewood stick, cotton swab or dropper.
- Begin with little toe.
- Gently massage oil into cuticle area.
- Avoid having the bottle tip come into contact with the client's nail or skin if applying the cuticle oil directly from the bottle.

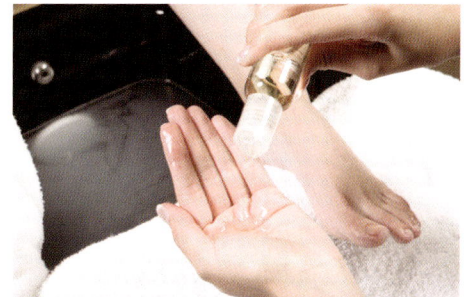

MASSAGE

24. Obtain product (massage cream, lotion or oil).
- Use spatula if necessary.
- Distribute product into both of your hands.

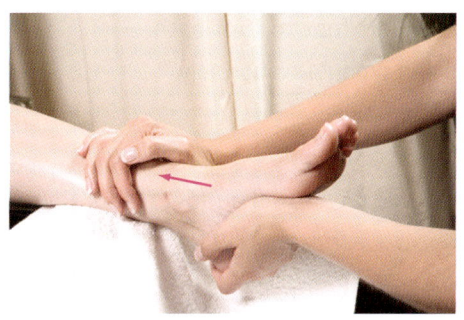

25. Apply product.
- Apply over client's entire foot, ankle and lower leg.
- Begin at bottom of foot.
- Work over top then toward ankle.
- Continue up the lower leg to below knee.
- Move your fingers around back of calf muscle, then back down toward ankle.
- Alternate your right and left hands while holding client's foot or ankle with your opposite hand.
- Repeat movement on lower leg 3-5 times.

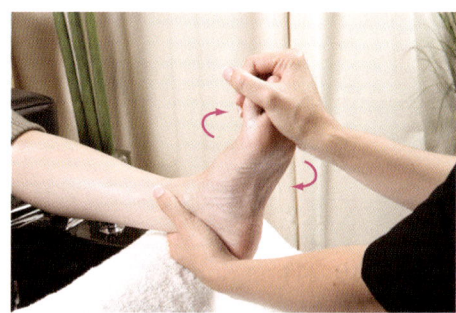

26. Establish control of client's foot.
- Cup heel in one hand.
- Use other hand to rotate foot in circular movement. This may be referred to as a relaxer movement.
- Repeat movement 3-5 times, clockwise and counter-clockwise.
- Place foot back on foot rest.

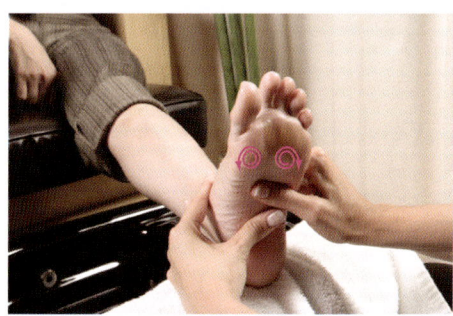

27. Perform massage movements.
Perform effleurage, thumbs on bottom, fingers on top.
- Place your thumbs on bottom of foot and your fingers on top (heel resting on foot rest).
- Use thumbs to perform circular effleurage movements (opposite directions).
- Work from heel to ball of foot and back down to heel.
- Repeat sequence 3-5 times.

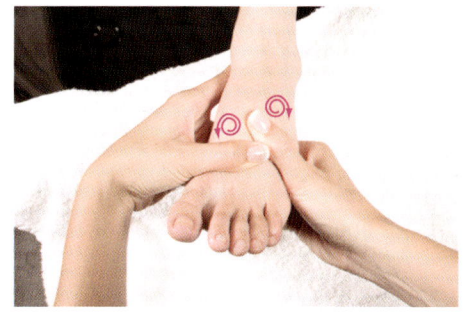

Perform effleurage, thumbs on top, fingers on bottom of foot.
- Place your thumbs on top of foot and your fingers on bottom, with heel resting on foot rest.
- Begin at base of toes.
- Use your thumbs to make circular effleurage movements on top of foot.
- Work up toward ankle and back down.
- Repeat sequence 3-5 times.

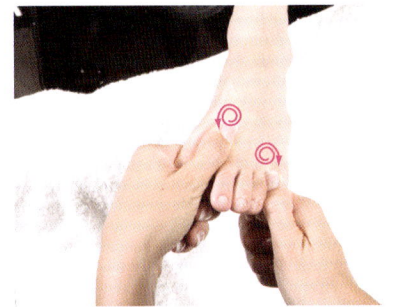

Perform effleurage, thumbs on top, fingers beneath toes.

- Position your thumbs on top of and between toes (heel resting on foot rest).
- Start at outside of foot (big and little toes).
- Use effleurage movements.
- Work from first joint to tips of toes.
- Work toward center and back toward outside of the foot.
- Alternate hands to avoid breaking contact with client's foot.
- Repeat sequence 3-5 times.

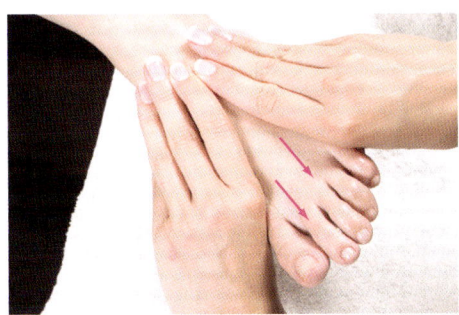

Perform petrissage, thumbs on bottom, fingers on top-in a diamond-shape-with heel resting on foot rest.

- Use kneading petrissage movement.
- Work from heel, over instep, to base of the toes moving both hands at same time.
- Move back to heel using less pressure.
- Repeat sequence 3-5 times.

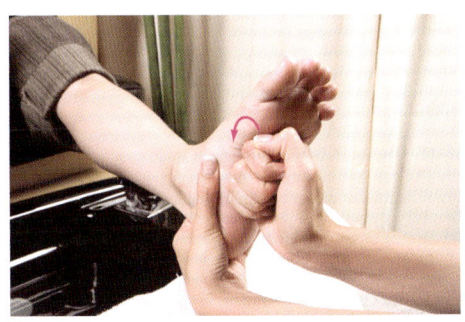

Perform friction.

- Hold back of heel with one hand.
- Position knuckles of other hand on bottom of foot.
- Rotate your wrist.
- Work from heel to ball of foot and back to the heel.
- Repeat this sequence 3-5 times.

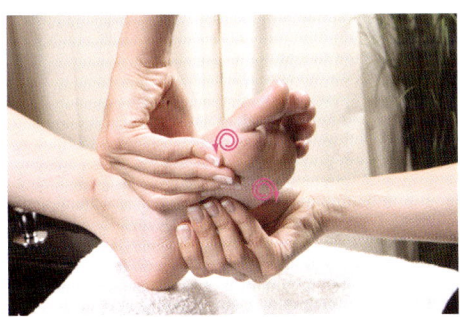

Perform effleurage, thumbs on top, fingers on bottom of foot.

- Use circular effleurage movements throughout instep area, with heel resting on foot rest.
- Alternate movement between right and left hands.
- Repeat sequence 3-5 times.

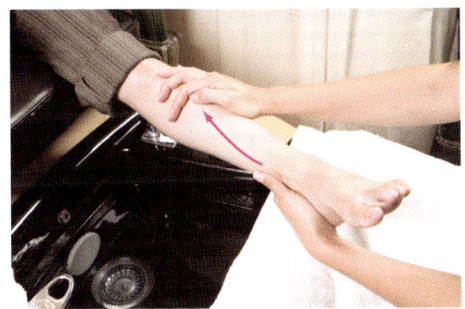

Perform effleurage, with heel remaining on foot rest.

- Use long, fluent effleurage strokes up front of the leg, around calf muscle and back down to ankle.
- Alternate right and left hands while holding client's foot or ankle with opposite hand.
- Repeat movement 3-5 times.

8

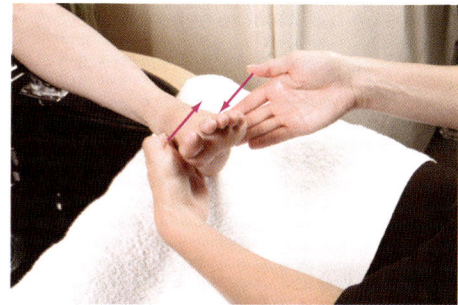

Perform tapotement.

- Use tapotement on sides of foot with heel resting on foot rest.
- Use soft, slapping movement.
- Push foot back and forth between hands.

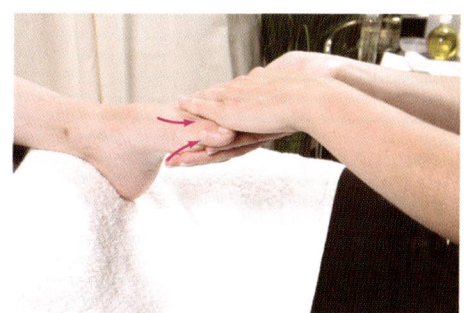

Feather off.

- Place one hand on top of foot, other hand on bottom.
- Feather off to complete massage portion of pedicure.
- Place foot off to the side on a towel, either on the foot rest or floor.

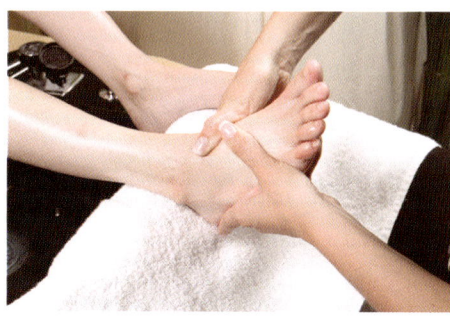

REPEAT CUTICLE OIL APPLICATION and MASSAGE (STEPS 23–27) on right foot.

- Unwrap right foot.
- Obtain product.
- Apply product.
- Establish control.
- Perform massage movements.

*Optional: You can apply powder to your client's feet at this time, if preferred.

At this point, the foot bath is no longer needed. Both feet can rest on the foot rest covered with one of the towels used to wrap the feet. You may also begin the sanitation process. If you are working on a pedicure 'throne,' move the client's feet to the side, then empty, rinse and disinfect the pedicure basin. You can allow the pedicure basin to run while you polish the toenails. If using a portable pedicure basin, move it to the side if necessary.

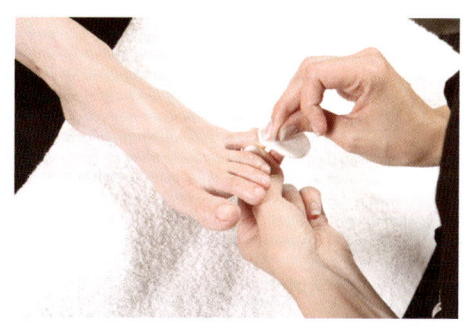

POLISH

28. Remove oils from nail plate.

- Saturate lint-free wipe or cotton with nail preparation solution, alcohol or polish remover.
- Wipe nail plate.
- Repeat on opposite foot.

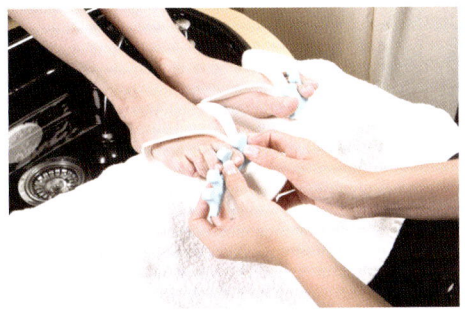

29. **Position slippers and toe separators** on feet.
- Place slippers on client's feet.
- Insert toe separators.
- Option: Put client's shoes on if open-toed.
- Place towel or paper towel between bottom of toes and shoes to protect shoes from product.
- Check with the client before doing this.

Since the polishing procedure will be performed on all 10 toes, polish in this order: From the little toe of the left foot to the big toe; then the right foot, from the little toe to the big toe.

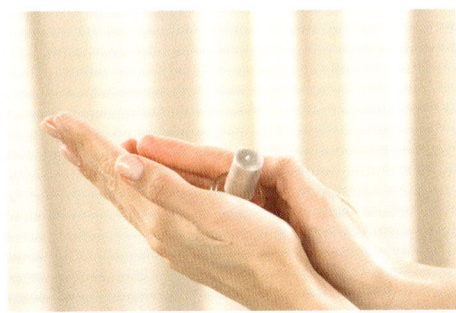

Remember:
- Mix polish by rolling bottle between your palms.

8

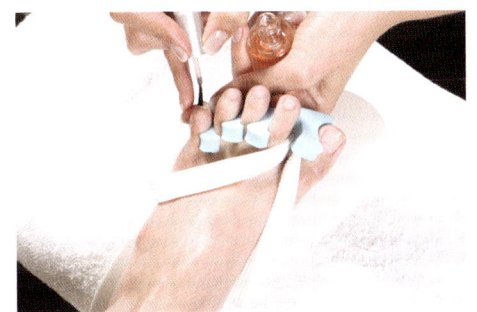

30. **Apply base coat** to each nail.
- Remove brush from polish bottle.
- Wipe side of brush (facing away from you) on inside bottle neck to create a "bead" of polish on the end of the brush.
- Hold client's little toe between your index finger and thumb.
- Pinch slightly to move sidewalls away from nail plate

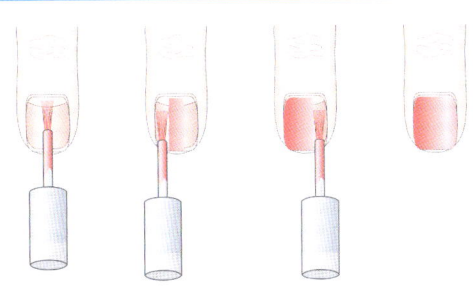

NOTE: Apply the polish 1/16" (.2 cm) from the entire cuticle. With the bead of polish toward the nail plate, place the brush at middle of the base of the nail at approximately a 35° angle. Brush toward the free edge. Repeat on each side of the nail plate with a 3-stroke application: 1). Middle, 2). Side, 3). Side. Note that the brush handle remains at a 35° angle, while the brush itself flattens to the nail.

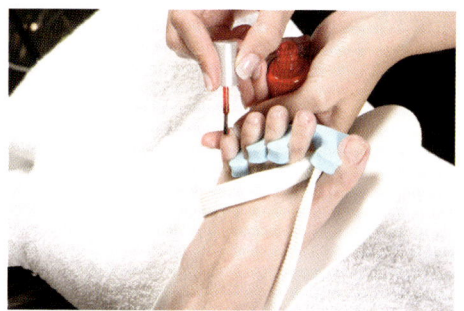

31. Apply colored polish.

- Use same technique to apply chosen colored polish.
- Begin with the little toe of the left foot.
- Work toward the big toe.
- Repeat on the right foot.

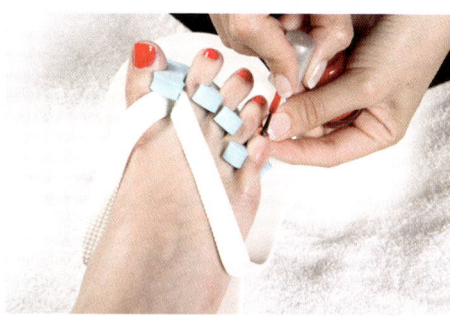

32. Apply second coat of colored polish.

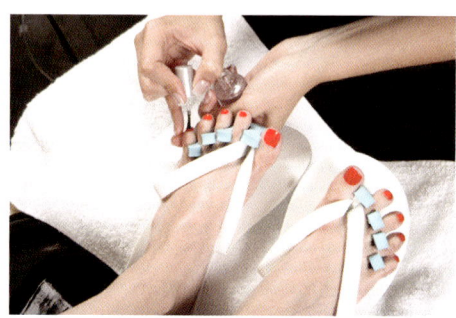

33. Apply top coat, using the same technique.

NOTE: Move directly from base coat to top coat if no colored polish is desired, for a total of two coats.

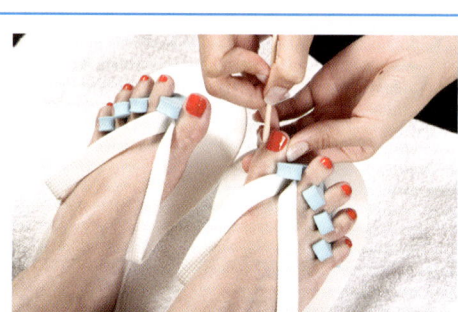

34. Clean up excess polish on sidewall and cuticle areas (if necessary).

- Use cotton-tipped orangewood stick or synthetic fiber brush.
- Dampen with polish remover.
- Remove polish from the skin carefully.

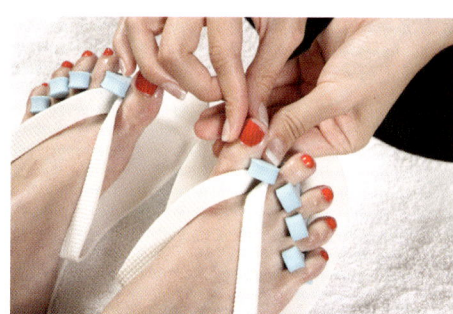

35. Apply speed dry to each nail if desired.

- Optional: Apply small amount of cuticle oil to each cuticle.
- Rub oil gently into cuticle area without pressure to freshly polished nail plate.

BASIC PEDICURE COMPLETION

- Escort client to reception area.
- Discuss retail products.
- Rebook next appointment.

Infection Control and Safety
- Disinfect all implements.
- Discard any disposable items.
- Replenish supplies.
- Disinfect the service area using an EPA-registered, broad spectrum (hospital-level) disinfectant.
- Empty and disinfect the pedicure basin after every client.*
- Set up for the next client.
- Practice blood spill procedures if a blood spill occurs, refer to page 67.

5. Completion - Gain feedback; infection control and safety

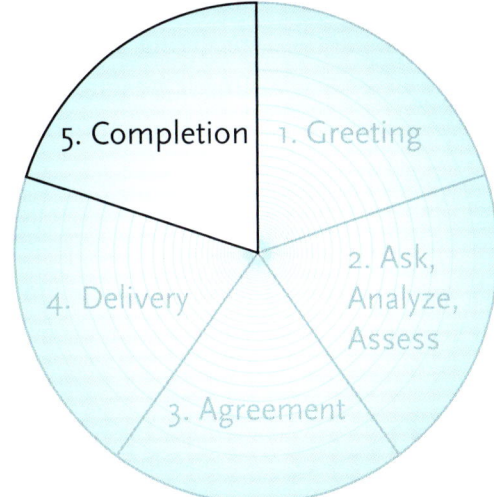

REMEMBER:
- Remove all product from jars with a spatula and keep lids tightly closed on product jars to avoid spillage and contamination.
- Keep labels on all containers and store products in a cool place to lengthen shelf-life.
- Keep tools dry to avoid rust.
- Place soiled towels in a covered container; use clean towels on each client.
- Complete the Service Record on the Client Consultation Form.

* Since there are so many different types of pedicure basins, it is important to follow the manufacturer's instructions as well as regulatory guidelines for disinfection after each use.

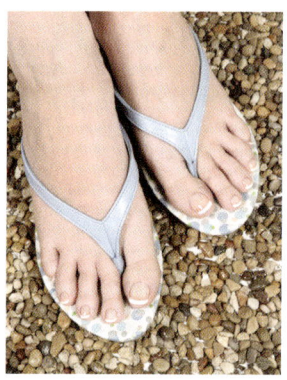

French Pedicure

As with a French manicure, a **French pedicure** is also a very popular service. The unique application remains the same as the French manicure and also creates an enhanced, natural effect. To prevent the toenail from appearing "stubby," it is better if clients do not have their toenails clipped too short. Some clients might choose to grow their nails out before receiving a French pedicure. The main difference is that the smile line is generally less arched than on the fingers, and the white polish is applied to a proportionately smaller area of the nail.

FRENCH PEDICURE

Perform Steps 1-29 of the Basic Pedicure Procedure, then follow these steps for applying the polish. Note that French application does not begin with a base coat.

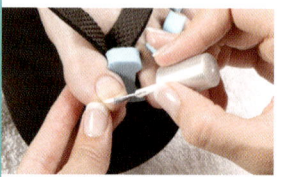

1. Apply the white polish to the free edge before applying the base coat. First apply from one side of the free edge to the middle of the free edge and repeat on the other side to create a rounded shape. Then finish rounding out the smile line. If the free edge is limited in length, use the natural smile line as a guide.

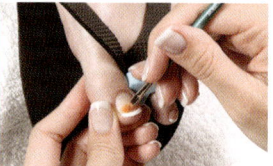

2. Clean up the white polish using a synthetic bristle brush or cotton-tipped orangewood stick saturated with polish remover to refine the smile line.

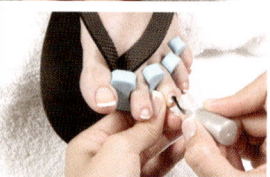

3. Apply the base coat over the entire nail.

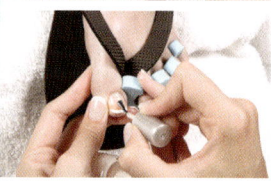

4. Apply a sheer pink, beige or neutral color over the entire nail plate. Be sure the color is sheer enough not to discolor the white polish. Most of the time only one coat of color is applied over the entire nail, but if your client prefers two coats this is acceptable.

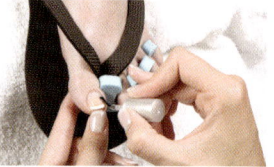

5. Apply the top coat to complete the French pedicure.

As mentioned before, there are many different ways of perfecting this very popular service and as you gain experience, you may develop your own personal method.

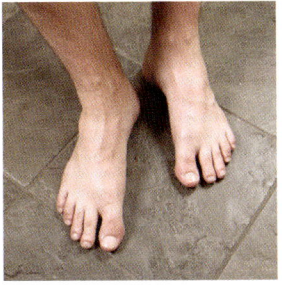

Male Pedicure

With more male clients in salons and spas than ever before, they are not only getting manicures but pedicures as well. Male pedicures follow the same procedures as female pedicures, but as mentioned previously, focus on cuticle care and callused areas. Again, avoid using fruity or floral-scented products. Typically, male pedicure clients do not want to wear colored polish. Instead the toenails may be buffed to a shine or a clear matte polish may be applied.

MALE PEDICURE

Follow the Basic Pedicure Procedure (Steps 1-35 with polish; Steps 1-27 without polish) as demonstrated earlier in the chapter, while focusing on the following:

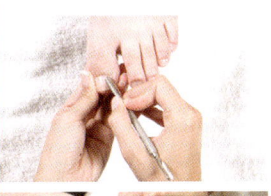

1. **Cuticle Care:** Focus on pushing the cuticles back, being careful not to create an opening or tear in the skin.

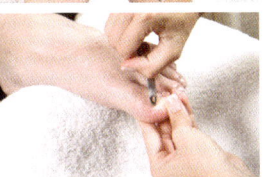

2. **Nip Cuticles:** If permitted by your regulating agency. Again, be careful not to cut into living tissue.

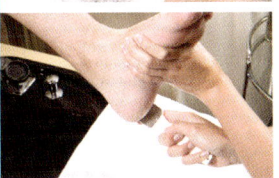

3. **Smooth Calluses:** Concentrate on the callused areas of the feet using either a foot file or foot scrub.

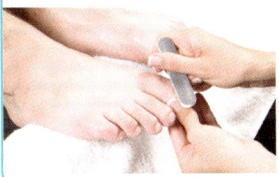

4. **Buff Nails:** At the end of the pedicure if the client prefers not to have colored polish applied; buff nails to a shine or apply a clear matte polish.

CHILDREN'S PEDICURE

Children also like receiving pedicure services. As mentioned previously in the Children's Manicure, you will want to consider the following:

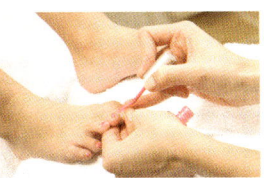

- Use adjustable-height chairs so their feet can reach the foot bath.
- Use a light touch and a cotton-tipped orangewood stick for additional comfort, and shorten the massage steps using less pressure.
- Use products that are age appropriate and always have parental permission.
- Have a clear policy addressing the youngest age limit for children receiving services.

8

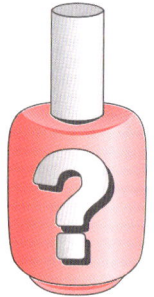

Which of the nail services explained in this chapter have you received? Which ones would you like to receive? Why?

DECISION-MAKING SKILLS

Case Studies

The following situations are designed to help you build decision-making skills. Using your training to this point, review the following scenarios, then think through and describe how you would handle each challenge.

1. A new client comes in for a manicure. During the consultation you discover that her nails are dry and brittle. What are some additional questions you can ask this client? What would you recommend?

2. While performing a pedicure on a new client, she questions your use of a foot file rather than a credo blade. How would you explain the difference and the reason for your choice?

Beautiful nails are what your clients want, and that's why they come to you. From a wedding event to a broken nail repair, artificial nails can beautify, strengthen, lengthen, conceal and protect. Whatever their purpose, artificial nails offer your clients a variety of benefits for beautifying or enhancing the appearance of their hands and nails. The nail industry is ever-evolving when it comes to producing new products for the nails, and artificial nail services continue to expand in fresh and exciting ways. Keeping yourself ahead of the curve when it comes to these services is a smart career move.

VALUE

Artificial nail services are a billion-dollar industry that continues to draw huge revenue. As a professional nail technician, knowing how to perform these higher-priced services efficiently will dramatically increase your income in the salon.

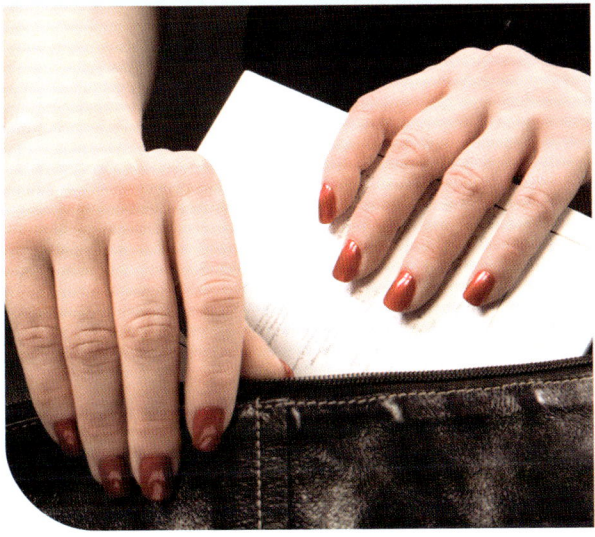

MAIN IDEA

This chapter will lead you through the most common artificial nail systems—nail wraps, acrylic nails and gel nails—and teach you how to apply them. You will also learn about the uses and functions of all products, implements, supplies and equipment needed for these services. Knowing the differences among the varieties available and how each is applied will help you recommend the type that best suits each individual client's needs.

PLAN	OBJECTIVES
Fundamentals of Artificial Nails • Basic Artificial Nail Preparation • Nail Tips • Basic Artificial Nail Balancing • Basic Artificial Nail Finishing	Identify the main purpose of a proper artificial nail preparation. Describe the structure of a nail tip and how to properly fit it. Explain the importance of a well-balanced nail. State the two ways an artificial nail can be finished.
Artificial Nail Systems • Nail Wraps • Acrylic Nails • Gel Nails	Explain how resin helps create a nail wrap overlay. Describe how to form an acrylic bead. Identify the major difference between how acrylic nails and gel nails harden.
Artificial Nail Procedures • Fundamental Procedures • Nail Systems Procedures	Demonstrate the procedures for artificial nail preparation, nail tip application, balancing, and finishing. Demonstrate the application and maintenance procedures for nail wrap, acrylic nail and gel nail systems.

FUNDAMENTALS OF ARTIFICIAL NAILS

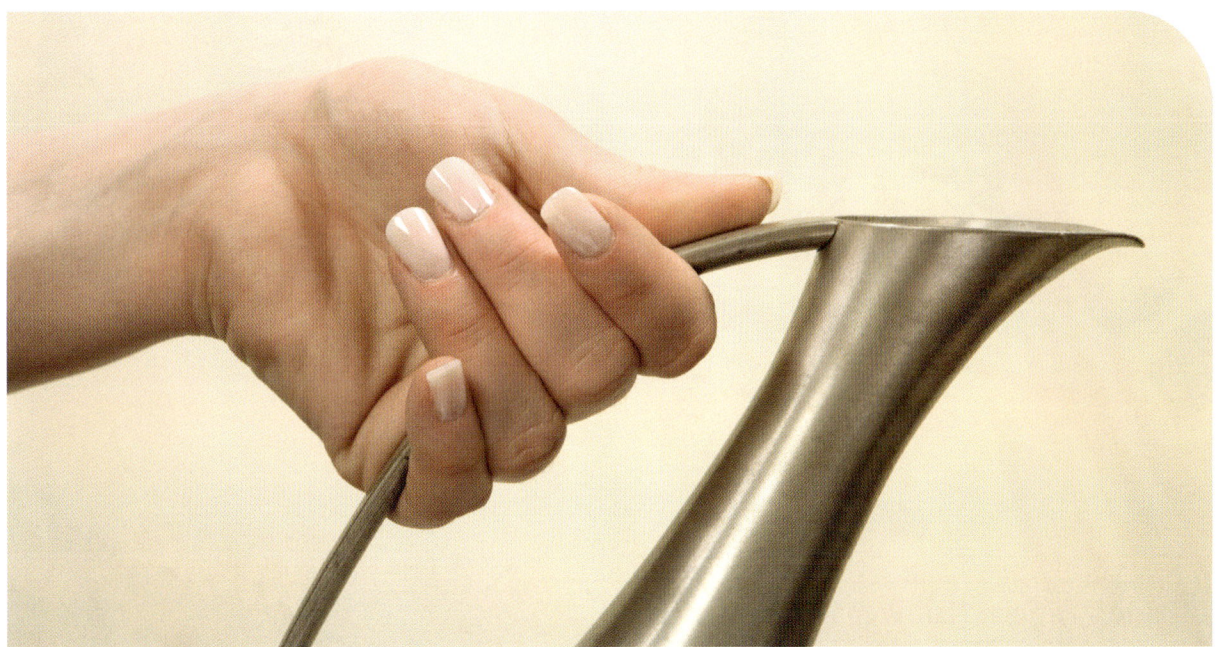

9

There are many reasons for wearing artificial nails, which are also referred to as nail enhancements. Nail enhancements offer clients a variety of benefits and options for changing the appearance of their hands and nails. Some clients also use artificial nails to add strength to their thin or weak natural nails while others apply them to add length, conceal or repair broken nails. Since these highly popular services require regular maintenance, they can help you build your clientele and your profitability in the salon.

As you will learn in this chapter, there are three major systems of artificial nail products: nail wraps, acrylics and gels. These products can use two types of applications: overlays or sculptured nails. Overlays are created by applying any of these products over the natural nail or a nail tip, which are fingernail extensions applied to extend the natural nail. Conversely, sculptured nails are built on top of a nail form, which is a temporary attachment placed under the free edge of the natural nail to help create and sculpt an artificial nail and free edge.

The main difference between an overlay and a sculptured nail is that the product is applied past the tip of the nail when creating a sculptured nail. When performing an overlay service, the product is applied over existing nail structure, whether it is the natural nail or the natural nail with a tip. To remember easily, think of sculpting as "creating" and overlays as "laying over."

The secret to providing a safe and successful artificial nail service is found in two important steps: (1) The preparation of the client's nails before the service; and (2) the completion when the nails are balanced and finished. These two key steps, in addition to nail tip application if your client chooses to use them, will remain the same for any artificial nail service.

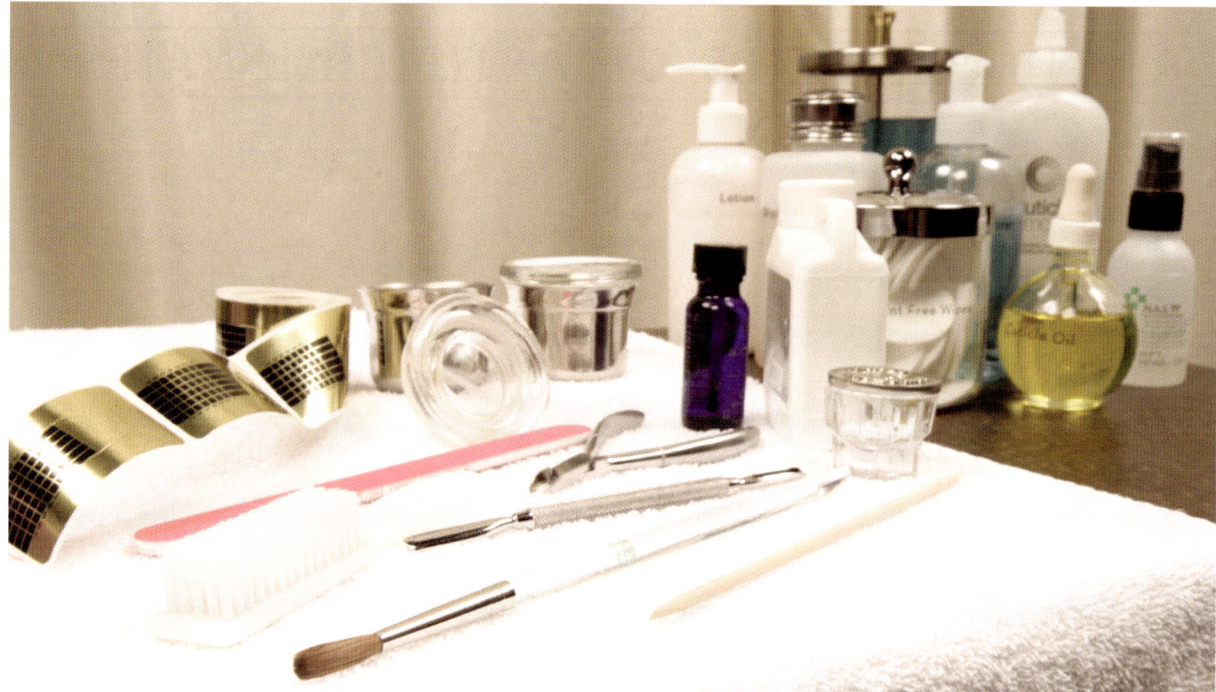

Basic Artificial Nail Preparation

The first and most important step of any artificial nail application is the proper preparation of the natural nail plate. Performed correctly, this can be done without causing any harm to the nail. In fact, the main purpose of artificial nail preparation is to protect the natural nail from potential damage or infection and to ensure proper adhesion.

To prepare natural nails for any artificial nail application, a basic "waterless" manicure is performed, which means that it is performed without soaking the nails. The process is then followed by the removal of "shine" (oil and residue) from the surface of the nail plate. It is important not to touch the nail once the nail preparation solution has been applied in order to avoid transferring oil back onto the nail plate. Finally, unlike the Basic Manicure Procedure as demonstrated in *Chapter 8, Natural Nail Services*, cuticle conditioner, moisturizers and polish are not applied until after the artificial nails have been applied.

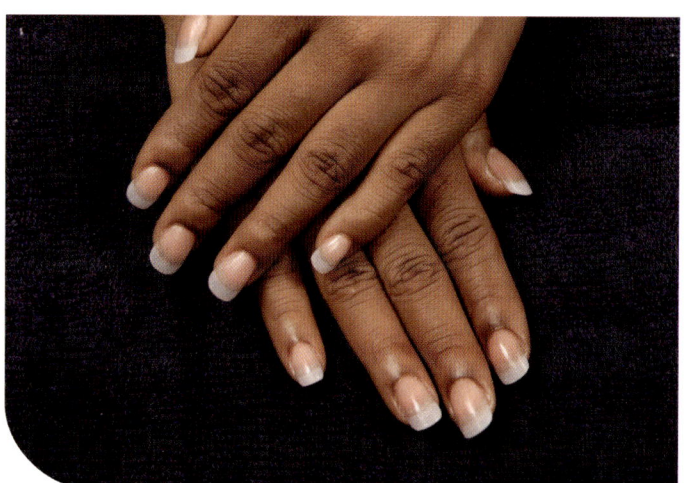

Basic Artificial Nail Preparation Essentials

Many of the same products, implements, supplies and equipment used for a basic manicure are also used to prepare the natural nail for the application of artificial nails. The following charts include the preparation essentials for artificial nail services.

BASIC ARTIFICIAL NAIL PREPARATION PRODUCTS

The following is a list of the products needed to prepare the nails before an artificial nail service.

Product	Function
Liquid Soap	Fights off harmful surface bacteria on skin
Antiseptic Sanitizer	Reduces bacteria on surface of skin; aids in prevention of cross-contamination
Polish Remover	Dissolves polish
Cuticle Remover	Softens dead cuticle tissue to allow gentle pushing back and to aid in its removal
Nail Preparation Solution	Removes oil and polish remnants to help product adhere to nail plate; dehydrates the nail plate

9

BASIC ARTIFICIAL NAIL PREPARATION IMPLEMENTS

The following is a list of the implements needed to prepare the nails before an artificial nail service.

Implement	Function
Nail Brush	Cleans nails and surrounding skin
Cuticle Pusher	Loosens and pushes back cuticles
Cuticle Nippers	Trim excess cuticle and hangnails
Nail Clippers	Shorten nails
180–240 Grit File	Removes shine, shapes nails and blends nail tips

BASIC ARTIFICIAL NAIL PREPARATION SUPPLIES

The following is a list of the supplies needed to prepare the nails before an artificial nail service.

Supplies	Function
Cotton or Lint-Free Nail Wipes	Remove polish and oils from nail plate
Towels	Dry client's hands; can be folded into a cushion
Orangewood Stick	Loosens and pushes back cuticles; applies cosmetics; cleans under free edge

BASIC ARTIFICIAL NAIL PREPARATION EQUIPMENT

The following is a list of the equipment needed to prepare the nails before an artificial nail service.

Equipment	Function
Manicure Table	Provides flat area to perform hand care services
Table Lamp	Provides additional light while performing services
Glass Container	Holds supplies
Disinfection Container	Holds EPA-registered, broad spectrum (hospital-level) disinfection solution; must be large enough for complete immersion of implements
Client Cushion	Supports client's elbows during hand care services
Technician Chair	Provides adjustable seat for technician performing service; allows for easy access to all equipment
Client Chair	Comfortable seat for client receiving services; provides proper back support

ARTIFICIAL NAIL MYTHS

There are many myths about the negative effects of wearing artificial nails. The truth is, many are due to the improper preparation and filing steps done by a nail technician. You can help educate clients and dispel these myths by knowing how to address clients' questions about artificial nails.

Myth #1: *Artificial nails cause mold, bacterial growth or infection.*

When properly applied, artificial nails don't cause these problems. A technician who improperly prepares the nails, fails to follow the manufacturer's instructions for application, or who uses contaminated implements may create an opportunity in which these problems can develop.

Make sure that clients clean their nails with a liquid soap using a nail brush. This will ensure the removal of surface oils and bacteria, which, when trapped under artificial nails, are a major cause of infection.

Another critical step in the preparation process is to use a temporary dehydrator or a nail preparation product, as recommended by the manufacturer of the product. The dehydrator or preparation product generally removes any remaining moisture from the surface of the nail. This helps the artificial nail adhere to the natural nail. It also reduces the risk of moisture becoming trapped between the enhancement and the natural nail plate, which can also create a breeding ground for bacteria.

Myth #2: *Artificial nails cause natural nails to become thin.*

This common misconception stems from the belief that the nail must be "roughed up" to ensure product adherence. Over-filing, filing with too much pressure or using an abrasive that is too coarse will thin the nail plate.

To ensure product adherence, only the "shine" must be removed from the surface of the nail using a 240-grit file. This removes the uppermost layer of the natural nail, which contains oils, bacteria, moisture and daily residue, such as nicotine from smoking.

Over-filing the natural nail can actually create several different problems with artificial nails. A thin nail plate creates a weak structure for the enhancement to be built upon. If the structure of the nail is weakened, it may become too flexible. This may cause the applied product to crack since it is less flexible than the weakened nail it is attached to.

Over-thinning the nail plate also increases the risk of an allergic reaction by allowing product to penetrate the nail plate and come into contact with the nail bed. Depending on the products being used, it is also possible for them to cause a chemical burn on the nail bed. Any damage to the nail bed increases the risk for infection. For example, onycholysis (loosening of the nail plate) can occur if the nail is over-filed, which may expose the nail bed, leaving it at a greater risk of becoming infected.

9

Nail Tips

Nail tips are plastic, nylon or acetate fingernail-shaped extensions that are applied to the natural nail using a nail adhesive. Nail tips can provide a temporary length enhancement, but they are more often used as a base for nail wrap, acrylic or gel products. The application of these products over tips or natural nails is known as an overlay. Nail tips without an overlay are considered temporary because the stress area is weak without an overlay to strengthen it.

Structure of a Nail Tip

There are many different types of nail tips available today. They come in a variety of shapes, sizes and colors. Nail tips have two important structural features:

1. **Tip well:** The area that adheres to the natural nail plate.
2. **Position stop:** A ridge underneath the nail tip where the free edge of the natural nail fits into place.

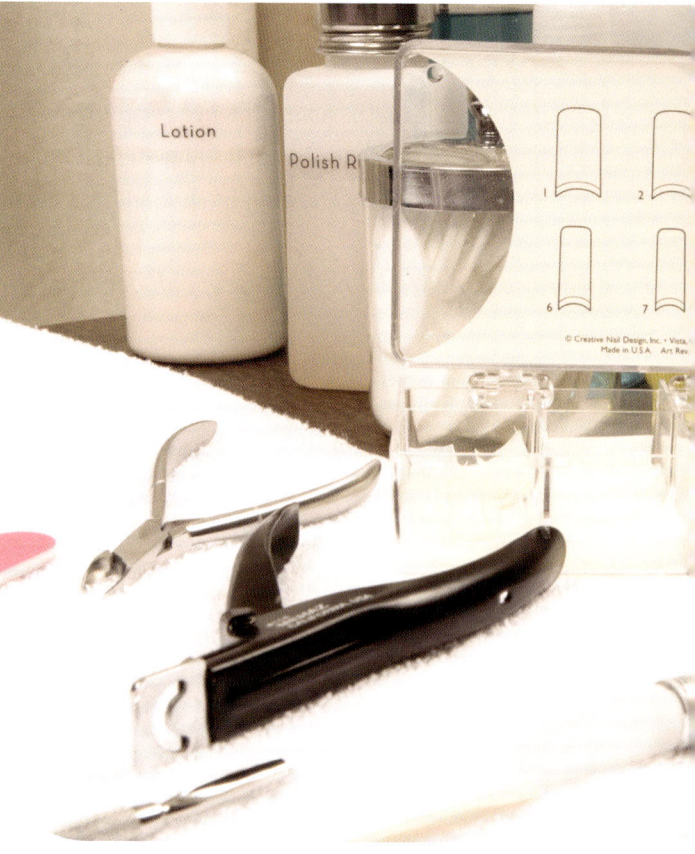

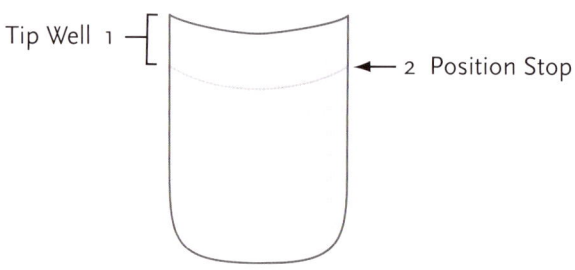

Tip Well 1 ⟶ ⟵ 2 Position Stop

When working with artificial nails, keep in mind that the end of the nail tip or sculpture is often referred to as the free edge, which should not be confused with the free edge of the natural nail.

There are two types of tip wells: full-wells and half-wells. The tip well should only cover half of the nail plate since the length of the natural nail determines which type to use. For example, a long natural nail bed may require the use of a full-well tip, while a short natural nail bed may only need a half-well tip.

To achieve the best fit, it is recommended to give the natural nails a more rounded shape prior to nail tip application. A round-shaped nail tends to fit better against the position stop.

"Ring of fire" is a phrase that refers to a burn caused by filing too aggressively. This occurs when the natural nail is over-filed and a visible redness appears and the client may feel heat on the nail. This typically happens either when blending tips, or when blending product preparing for a fill, if the file is not held flat against the nail.

Sizing a Nail Tip

Correctly sizing nail tips is crucial to creating an attractive and strong nail enhancement. There are three areas that guide you in finding the appropriate size and type of nail tip to use for best results on each client.

1. **C-Curve**

   The horizontal curve of the nail from sidewall to sidewall is called the **c-curve**. The best fit is achieved by matching the c-curve of the nail tip with the curve of the natural nail. If the c-curve of the tip is greater than the client's natural c-curve, the tip will fit too tightly on the nail and may be uncomfortable for the client. It may also create gaps between the natural nail and the tip.

2. **Contact Area**

   The **contact area** is the portion of the nail where the tip well is adhered to the nail plate. The well of the nail tip should never cover more than half of the length of the nail plate; therefore, the contact area should not be more than half the length of the nail. In some instances, such as with clients who have small nail beds, a half-well tip may still cover more than half of the natural nail. In this situation, the tip can be customized by trimming the well of the tip using a pair of small scissors. If just a slight adjustment is desired, a file can be used by holding the file at a 45° angle against the well and filing to reduce the length of the well area.

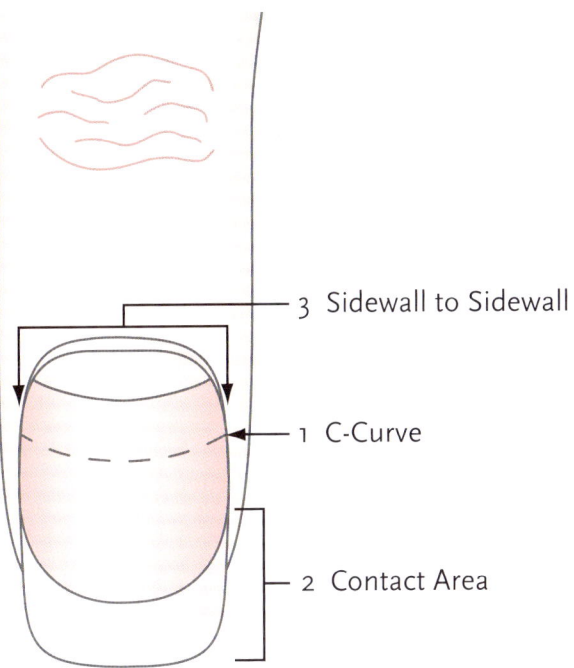

3 Sidewall to Sidewall

1 C-Curve

2 Contact Area

3. **Sidewall to Sidewall**

   The nail tip needs to fit the width of the nail, sidewall to sidewall. If the tip is too big for the nail, gaps will occur. If it is too small, the tip may crack. If the client is between sizes, use the larger size and file the sides down to fit the natural nail as closely as possible.

Nail tips are blended to the surface of the natural nail to eliminate the seam where they are attached, creating a completely smooth surface. Once the tip is applied to the nail, it is blended with a file held flat against the nail tip on top of the natural nail plate. The most important thing to remember while blending the tip is to avoid filing the natural nail plate, which can unnecessarily thin the nail plate, or cause a "ring of fire."

9

Nail Tip Application Essentials

Many of the same products, implements, supplies and equipment used to prepare the natural nail for the application of artificial nails are also used to apply nail tips. To apply tips to natural nails, you will need to know about the following additional products, implements, supplies and equipment.

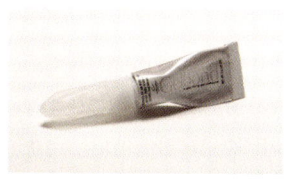

Nail Adhesive

A **nail adhesive** is a type of glue or bonding agent used to adhere nail tips to the natural nail. It is available in a squeezable tube or in a bottle with a brush. Different brands of adhesive vary slightly in drying time, but they usually only differ by a few seconds. Nail adhesive tends to dry out fast, so it is important to replace the cap immediately after use. Nail adhesive can be removed with acetone.

When handling nail adhesive, be very careful not to allow the product to come into contact with the skin. It is especially important to take great care in preventing the product from coming into contact with the eyes. It is recommended to always use safety glasses and even to offer a pair to your client.

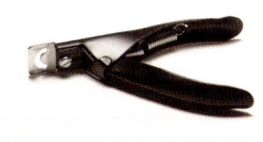

Tip Cutter

A **tip cutter** is a specially designed tool used to trim the length of nail tips. Tip cutters are designed to match the c-curve of the tip when cutting. This keeps the tip from flattening out, reduces the chance of separation at the contact area and also prevents stress cracks. Some tip cutters have a guide to help the technician cut the tips to all the same length. Always use a tip cutter with the blade facing away from the client's finger to prevent injury. Tip cutters require disinfection after every service. Always be sure to thoroughly dry the joint of the cutter, as leaving moisture can cause the joint to rust.

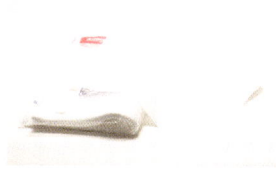

Disposable Towel

A **disposable towel** has many uses when performing any artificial nail procedure. The main purpose is to protect the manicure table from products, such as nail adhesive. They are also used for cleaning and removing excess product from brushes. Disposable towels are often chosen over cloth towels because many artificial nail products cannot be washed out. Some manufacturers make lint-free disposable towels, which are recommended when performing acrylic services. Disposable towels are discarded after every service.

Nail Tips

Nail tips are used to add length to natural nails. After tips are applied to the natural nail, a wrap, acrylic or gel overlay is applied to add strength to the natural nail. Nail tips are considered temporary nails unless an overlay is used. They come in a variety of shapes and sizes to get the perfect fit for every client. Nail tips are offered in natural, clear, white or a variety of other colors to create different effects.

NAIL TIP APPLICATION ESSENTIALS

You are already familiar with the products, implements, supplies and equipment mentioned previously in this chapter. Here is a list of additional items you will need for a nail tip application.

NAIL TIP APPLICATION PRODUCTS

Essential	Function
Nail Adhesive	Adheres nail tips to natural nails

NAIL TIP APPLICATION IMPLEMENTS

Tip Cutter	Shortens nail tips

NAIL TIP APPLICATION SUPPLIES

Nail Tips	Provide length and structure for artificial nails
Disposable Towels	Protect surfaces from products that cannot be washed out of cloth towels

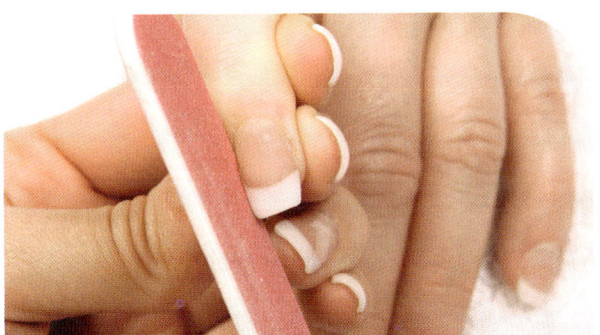

Basic Artificial Nail Balancing

Balancing the nail consists of filing and shaping the nail. The first step in achieving a well-balanced nail is correctly applying the artificial nail product. The second step is filing to remove any imperfections or bumps and to smooth uneven areas once the product has hardened or cured. Finally, the free edge and the surface of the nail are filed into the desired shape. Even the most skilled application of product requires these steps to create a perfectly smooth and evenly balanced nail.

Filing

Once the artificial nail has been applied, it is time to balance it by filing. Filing helps rid the nail of any hard edges and smoothes out any uneven areas between the zones, which is referred to as blending. Properly filing all areas of the nail will help blend Zones 1, 2 and 3 (discussed on page 259) to create beautiful, strong, natural-looking artificial nails. This involves looking at the nail from several angles. When filing, use long strokes that follow the curve of the nail. Use approximately two-thirds of the file. If short, quick strokes are used, too much friction may occur on the nail and your client will feel heat on the nail bed. This may cause a heat burn. Heat burn will also occur if too much pressure is applied when filing. It is always important to check client comfort while filing the nails.

NAIL FILES

The key to expert balancing lies in choosing the best file with the appropriate grit number, and in knowing how to use the chosen file for each step of the balancing process. The grit refers to the number of granules found per square inch—the smaller the number, the coarser the file. In balancing artificial nails, remember to begin with the smaller number grit file and work toward the larger number grit file. Working with the coarse file first helps quickly remove the product that may have been applied unevenly or too thickly. As you work with finer files, the scratches made by the coarse files will smooth out and eventually disappear.

To begin balancing a newly applied set of artificial nails, it is recommended to use a 150-grit file or higher. A list of the files and the typical use for different grits is shown below.

File	Use
Coarse 80–120	Removing length on enhancements; removing excess product for artificial nail maintenance
Medium 130–240	Shaping any nail and refining surface of enhancements
Fine 250–900	Shaping and refining surface of any nail
Extra-Fine 1000–4000	Smoothing surface imperfections on any nail; shining nails

It is important to file all areas of the nail to create a well-balanced nail while making sure to keep Zone 2 the thickest and Zones 1 and 3, thin. Start by filing the parameter areas 1, 2 and 3, making sure the sidewalls (areas 1 and 2) are thin, and blend into the natural nail. Next, move to the cuticle areas 4, 5 and 6 blending to the natural nail so there is no "ledge" felt. Finally, blend areas 7, 8 and 9 to the parameters of the nail.

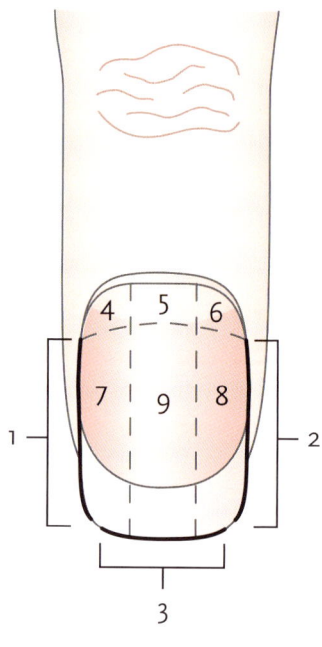

Areas of the Nail

As your client's artificial nails grow out, it will be necessary to balance them during artificial nail maintenance, often referred to as re-balancing. Re-balancing is the act of 1. blending the new product in with the old; 2. making sure that the stress area (Zone 2) remains the thickest; and 3. ensuring the cuticle areas (Zone 3), sidewalls and free edge (Zone 1) are the thinnest. The same techniques used to balance the nails during the first service are used when clients return for maintenance, or re-balancing, services.

NAIL ZONES

For the application of artificial nails, the nail has been divided and labeled into three different sections, or **zones**. These zones of the nail will help you to identify where to work more easily. Throughout the nail industry, these sections are referred to as Zones 1, 2 and 3, as demonstrated in the following illustration.

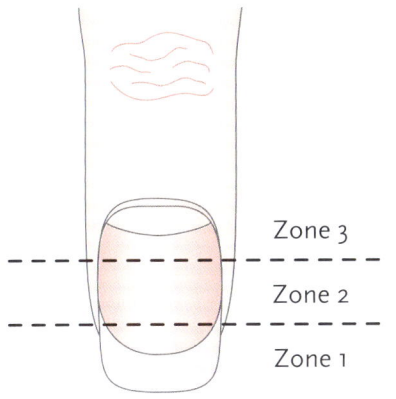

Zone 3
Zone 2
Zone 1

Zone 1: Free edge
Zone 2: Stress area or apex
Zone 3: Cuticle area

These numbered zones will help guide you in balancing the nail. Proper balancing involves making sure that Zones 1 and 3 are the thinnest and Zone 2 is the thickest. When balancing an artificial nail, you are also keeping the areas at the sidewalls thinner than the center area of the nail. This helps the artificial nail match the shape of the natural nail.

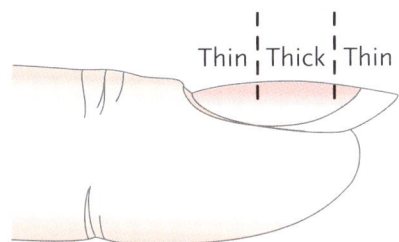

Thin | Thick | Thin

Zone 1: Thin
Zone 2: Thickest application
Zone 3: Thin

The **stress area** flexes when pressure is applied to the free edge. Artificial nail products are applied to be thickest in Zone 2, which covers this stress area. By making this area the thickest, it helps prevent too much flexing. This can cause the artificial product to break, crack or separate from the nail plate, leaving the nail at risk for infection.

Basic Artificial Nail Finishing

Finishing the nail means buffing or polishing to achieve the final look before a client walks out the door. There are two main options available to achieve the desired finished look: buffing and polishing. By buffing the nails to a high shine, your client won't wear polish but will keep the shine until returning for a re-balance. Polishing the nails allows the client to choose a color or look for a special occasion or season.

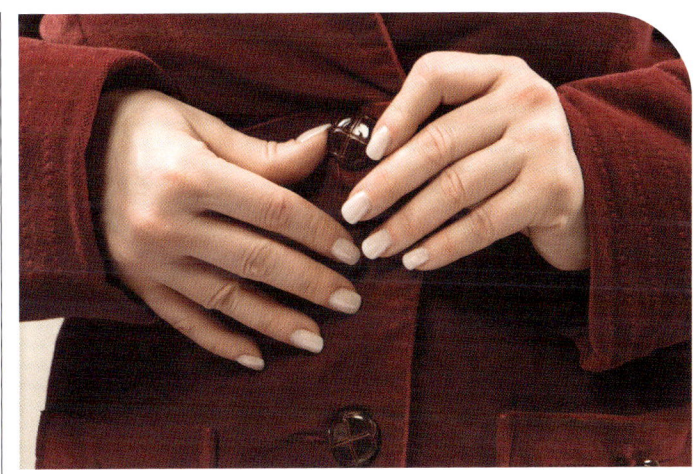

9

Finishing is performed after the nails have been balanced. It is important to have clients wash their hands to remove the residue and dust from the skin. If a hand and arm massage is performed, this would be done before the final finishing of the nails. It's also important to remove all oils and residue from the nail plate before buffing or polishing the nails to secure adhesion of the polish and to prevent the oils from affecting the buffing process.

The lasting impression that clients take away from the salon is the appearance, or final look, of their nails. Artificial nails require maintenance, most often every two to three weeks. Any client's initial experience and satisfaction will be a determining factor in whether he or she chooses to return to you for maintenance. So, your balancing and finishing skills present one of the best opportunities to build a loyal and long-lasting clientele.

BASIC ARTIFICIAL NAIL FINISHING ESSENTIALS

The following is a list of essentials you will need to finish an artificial nail service by either buffing the nails to a shine or polishing the nails, whichever the client desires for the finished look.

BASIC ARTIFICIAL NAIL FINISHING PRODUCTS

Essential	Function
Polishes	Base Coat: Evens out nail and prevents polish from staining the nail plate Colored Polish: Creates a colored effect on the nail Top Coat: Seals colored polish and helps prevent chipping
Cuticle Oil	Softens and moisturizes cuticles and surrounding skin

BASIC ARTIFICIAL NAIL FINISHING IMPLEMENTS

Three-Way Buffer	Smoothes the nail and produces a shine

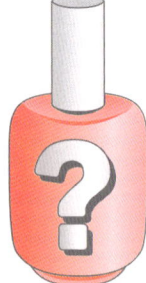

After reviewing the information on balancing an artificial nail, what did you learn that you did not know about how an artificial nail is balanced?

ARTIFICIAL NAIL SYSTEMS

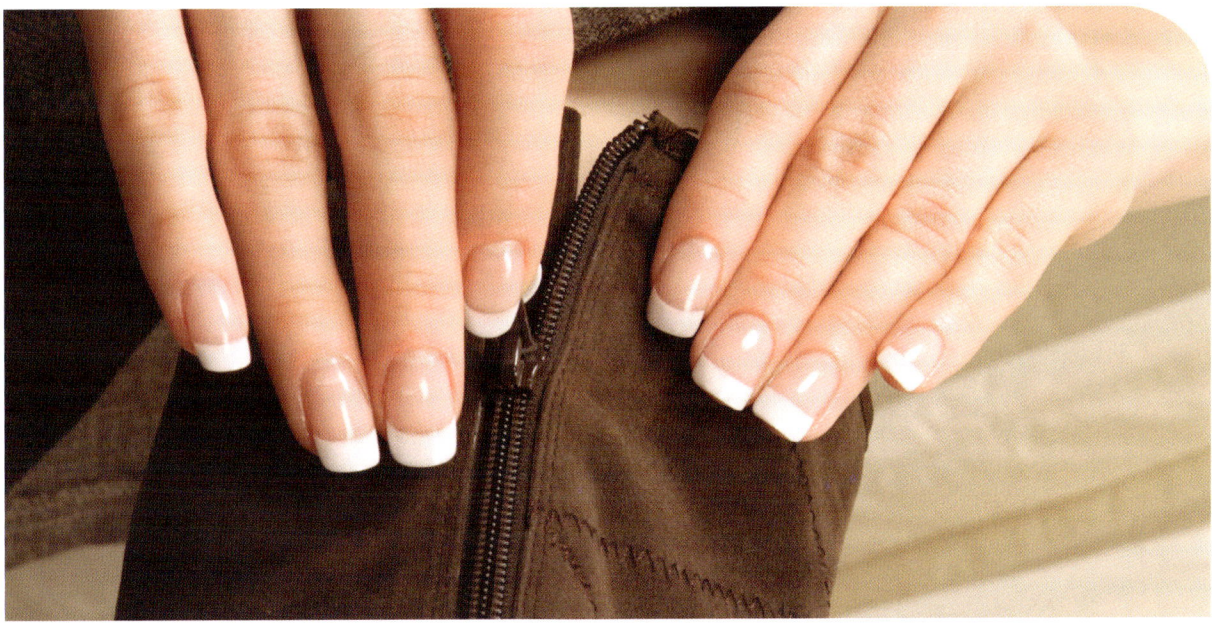

9

Salon clients request artificial nails for a number of reasons. Many use nail enhancements to strengthen and lengthen weak nails. They also are handy for concealing or repairing chipped or broken nails. In this section, you will learn about the three main types of artificial nail systems: nail wraps, acrylic nails and gel nails. All three possess different features and benefits that will help you and your clients determine which finished look will work best for their hands and nails. Along with the application of artificial nails, regular maintenance and repair will serve as excellent ways to build your clientele and increase your profitability and skills as a nail technician.

Nail Wraps

Nail wraps are woven materials that are applied to the natural nails or nails with tips to add strength. The material is held in place and an overlay is created by applying several layers of a thick adhesive called **resin**. The resin is chemically hardened by the application of an **accelerator**.

Many different types of fabric are used for wraps today, including fiberglass, silk, linen and nylon. **Fiberglass** is a synthetic fiber that is loosely woven and is almost invisible once applied. Fiberglass is a very strong and sturdy fabric to use. **Silk** is a natural fiber that is tightly woven. Silk is often recommended for shorter nails with ridges because when applied, it creates a very smooth overlay. **Linen** is a thicker fabric that remains visible on the nail after application. Clients typically wear a polish to hide the fact that they have a linen wrap overlay.

A product that is sometimes referred to as "liquid nail wrap" acts as a nail strengthener. It is basically a polish that contains fibers and is generally applied in the same way as polish.

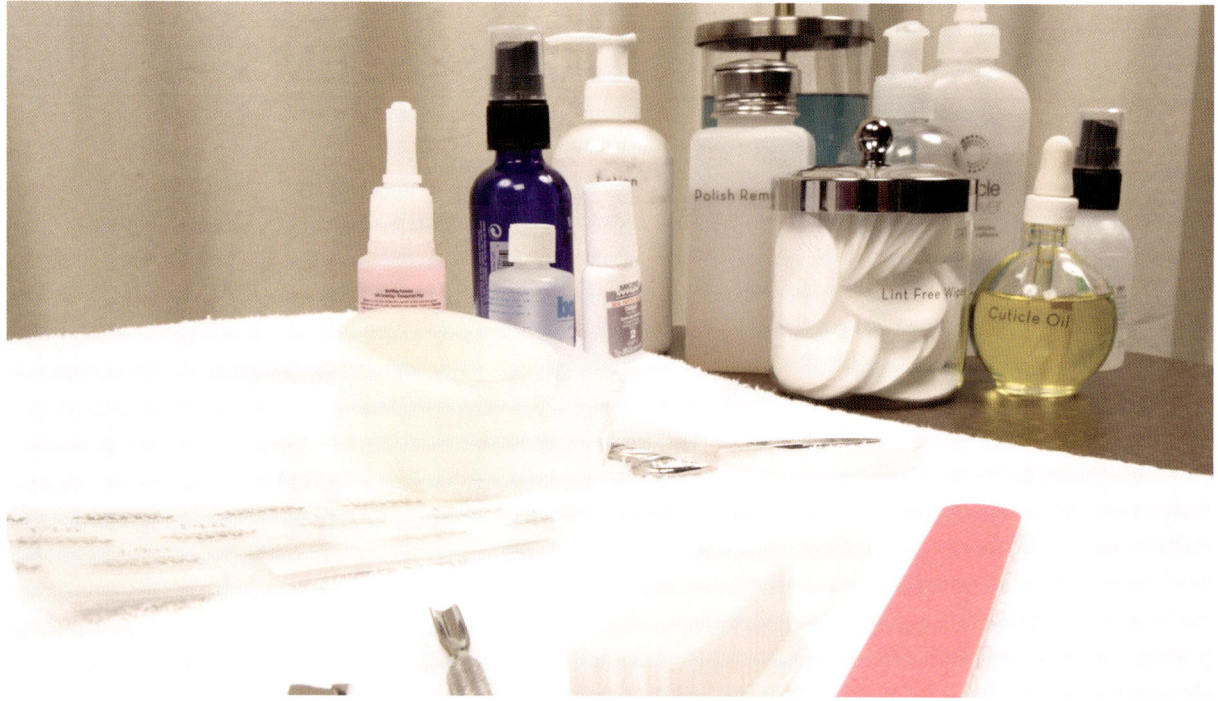

Nail Wrap Overlay Essentials

You wil need the artificial nail preperation essentials, nail tip application essentials (if applicable) and the following additional items to perform a nail wrap overlay.

Resin

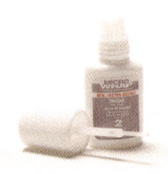

Resin is a thick adhesive product that adheres the fabric wrap to the nail and is layered over the fabric to create a strong overlay. Resin can be used without fabric to do a quick, temporary natural nail repair. Resin is typically available in a squeezable tube or in a bottle with a brush.

Accelerator

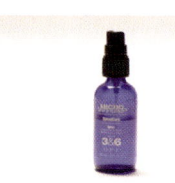

Accelerator is a product that is applied after the resin to help speed up the time it takes to harden the product. An accelerator is known as a catalyst, which is discussed in *Chapter 5, Chemistry*. Accelerator is typically available as a spray or in a bottle with a brush.

Small Scissors

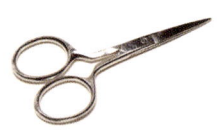

Small scissors are used to trim wrap fabric to the size of the nail. These scissors need to be sharp to evenly cut the fabric. It is also important that the scissors are small enough to trim the fabric around the cuticle and sidewall areas, eliminating the risk of cutting your client. These scissors must be disinfected after every service. Always be sure to thoroughly dry the joint of the scissors, as leaving moisture may cause the joint to rust.

Tweezers

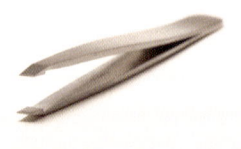

Tweezers are a metal instrument used to help place fabric onto the surface of the nail plate. They are available with a slanted tip, straight tip or pointed tip. Tweezers are disinfected after every service.

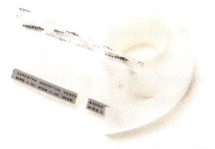

Wrap Fabric

Wrap fabric is typically a woven mesh material that adds strength to the nail. There are several types of fabric used for nail wraps including fiberglass, silk, linen and occasionally certain types of paper. These fabrics are available in long strips or rolls that are then measured and trimmed to match the size and shape of the nail. Some manufacturers supply pre-cut strips that are already sized and shaped to fit the nails. While some fabrics already have an adhesive on one side causing them to stick to the nail, others have to be applied with an adhesive or resin. As you become more experienced with performing nail wraps, you will determine which type of fabric or mesh you prefer.

You can use a small piece of thin plastic to smooth the fabric onto the nail to prevent contaminating the fabric with oils from your fingers. Many manufacturers provide a piece of plastic with the product. If it is not included, a piece of plastic backing from the roll of fabric can be used.

9

NAIL WRAP OVERLAY ESSENTIALS

You are already familiar with some of the the products, implements, supplies and equipment mentioned previously in this chapter. Here is a list of additional items you will need for a nail wrap overlay.

NAIL WRAP OVERLAY PRODUCTS

Essential	Function
Resin	Covers fabric to add strength to nail wrap
Accelerator	Speeds curing of resin

NAIL WRAP OVERLAY IMPLEMENTS

Small Scissors	Trim fabric
Tweezers	Place fabric onto surface of nail plate

NAIL WRAP OVERLAY SUPPLIES

Fabric	Adds strength to nail

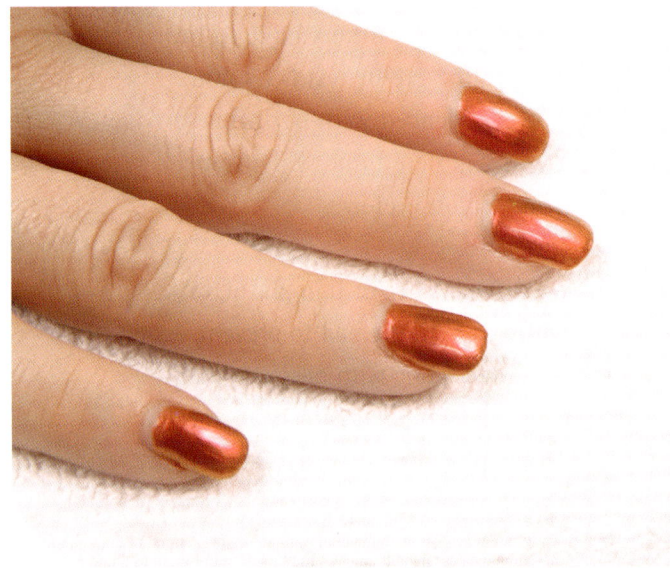

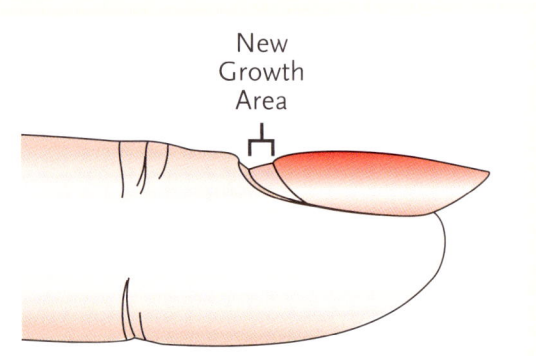

New
Growth
Area

The new growth area refers to the natural nail plate in Zone 3 that becomes exposed as the nail grows. To properly maintain the artificial nail, product needs to be applied to this area and blended into the product that has been previously applied.

Nail Wrap Maintenance

To maintain the strength that nail wraps provide, clients must return regularly to a technician to keep their artificial nails healthy and balanced. Nail wraps are also useful when a client's natural nail becomes cracked or needs repairing. As the nail grows out, it will need to be re-balanced, usually every two weeks. This is also referred to as a **fill-in** or **refill** service. Fill-in means that you will be applying product to the new growth area of the nail. As mentioned earlier, re-balancing is the act of blending the new product in with the old and making sure that the stress area (Zone 2) remains the thickest, and cuticle areas, sidewalls and free edge are the thinnest. This maintenance on wrap overlays is very important to keep up the service to help nails to look their very best. The procedure is similar to the overlay, only the primary focus is on the new growth area.

Before performing maintenance on nail wraps, it is important to analyze the nails carefully to determine if there are any repairs needed. Look for cracks in the nail or lifting, which is the separation of the product from the nail. If there is a crack in the nail, it may require the product to be removed, which is described on page 307,

and reapplied. If the product is lifting or any separation has occurred, carefully file away the product from that area. Avoid using nippers to remove the product. This may damage the natural nail by pulling product off that is still adhered to the nail.

Two-Week Nail Wrap Maintenance

As nail wraps grow out, the natural nail is exposed at the cuticle area. It is necessary to perform maintenance in order to keep the nails balanced. Two-week wrap maintenance is sometimes referred to as a glue-fill because only the resin is being replaced. At this time it is important to be sure that Zone 2 is the thickest. Two-week wrap maintenance is different from a four-week wrap maintenance because no fabric is being replaced, only the resin.

Four-Week Nail Wrap Maintenance

The difference between a two-week wrap maintenance and a four-week wrap maintenance is that after four weeks, the nail has grown out and the fabric must be replaced. Like a two-week fill, the product must be balanced and repaired if necessary, but new fabric must be measured and trimmed to fill the new growth in Zone 3.

Every other fill, or every four weeks, the fabric needs to be placed over the new growth area. The procedure is the same as the overlay procedure, only the primary focus is on the new growth area.

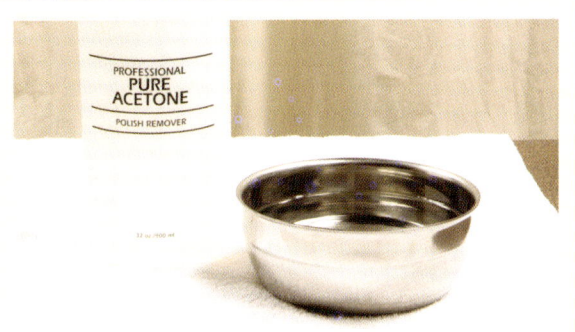

Artificial Nail Product Remover

Artificial nail product remover softens and dissolves most of the products used to create artificial nails. Once the nails are soaked in the chemical, the product softens and is then able to be pushed off of the surface of the nail using an orangewood stick. Pure acetone is a chemical that is commonly used to break down artificial nail products. Many manufacturers offer their own artificial nail product removers which typically include conditioning agents mixed in with the acetone. Since acetone is also sometimes an ingredient in nail polish remover, it is recommended that non-acetone polish remover is used to remove polish from artificial nails.

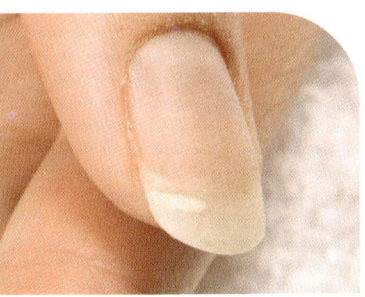

Natural Nail Repair

If a client comes to you with a cracked or torn nail, it is possible to preserve the nail until it grows out. This is most commonly done with a fabric wrap. The nail is prepared as it would be for any other artificial nail service and then a fabric wrap is applied to the area. The piece of fabric or mesh is cut to cover the crack or break in the nail to provide the extra support needed. The wrap is blended with the natural nail and is virtually invisible. If a natural nail repair is necessary, it is applied before soaking the nails in water for a basic manicure or performing any other service such as a hot oil manicure or a paraffin dip. This is necessary because any extra moisture in the nail plate may cause the repair to lift off the natural nail.

Nail Wrap Removal

During the removal of nail wraps it is very important to keep the natural nails in a healthy condition. Fabric wraps can be removed by using acetone or the manufacturer's recommended removal product, which will soften and dissolve the nail wrap. Nail wraps will dissolve easily in the product removers because they are simple polymers as discussed in *Chapter 5, Chemistry.*

Acetone is the main ingredient in most product removers. Artificial nail product removers can have other ingredients to help prevent over–drying the skin and nails. Because removal products can be drying to the skin and nails, it is important to hydrate the skin and nails with lotion and cuticle conditioner after removing artificial nails.

It is recommended to perform a basic manicure and to apply a nail strengthener or treatment to the nails after removing artificial nails. This will help to add moisture and strength back into the nail plates.

Acrylic Nails

When people think of artificial nails, they most likely think of acrylic overlays or sculptured nails. Acrylic nail enhancements have been a staple in the nail industry for decades. An acrylic nail is created by using a combination of an acrylic powder called polymer and an acrylic liquid called monomer. A sable brush is first dipped into the liquid and then the powder to create a bead, or ball, of acrylic on the end or side of the brush. The bead is then pressed into place on the nail to create the overlay or sculpture.

Two common acrylic nail services you will perform in the salon are the single-color acrylic overlay and the pink and white sculptured acrylic nails. A single-color acrylic overlay typically uses either a natural or clear acrylic powder. No matter what color is chosen, only one color is applied over the entire nail when finishing the final look. This can be done over nail tips or natural nails.

Unlike fabric wraps, acrylic can be used to build an acrylic tip without a pre-applied tip to lengthen the nail. This technique, called sculptured nails, is created using a nail form rather than a tip and can be used as an alternative to nail tips.

Unlike the single-color acrylic overlay, you can choose to apply any colored acrylic over the nail forms to create sculptured nails. "Pink and whites," or "permanent French manicure" are phrases often used to describe pink and white sculptured nails. As indicated by the name, pink acrylic powder and white acrylic powder are used. White acrylic powder is used to form Zone 1 and the smile line, just as in a French manicure, while the pink acrylic powder is used to create the rest of the nail. Although this service is demonstrated as a sculptured nail application on page 316, the pink and white acrylic application can also be done over nail tips.

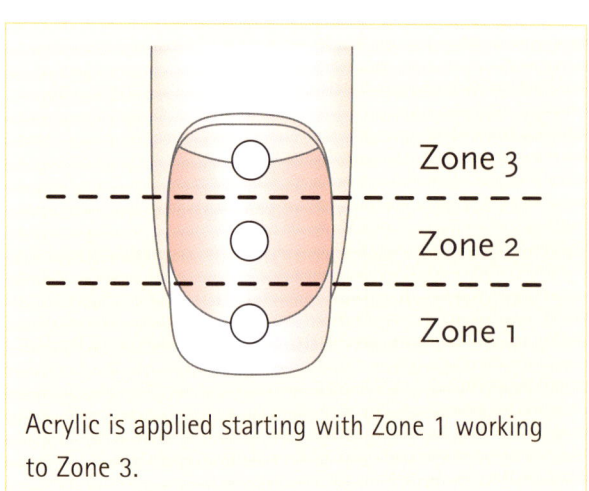

Acrylic is applied starting with Zone 1 working to Zone 3.

Acrylic Nail Essentials

Whether you are using acrylic as an overlay or using acrylic to sculpt the nails over nail forms, the fundamentals of acrylic application remain the same.

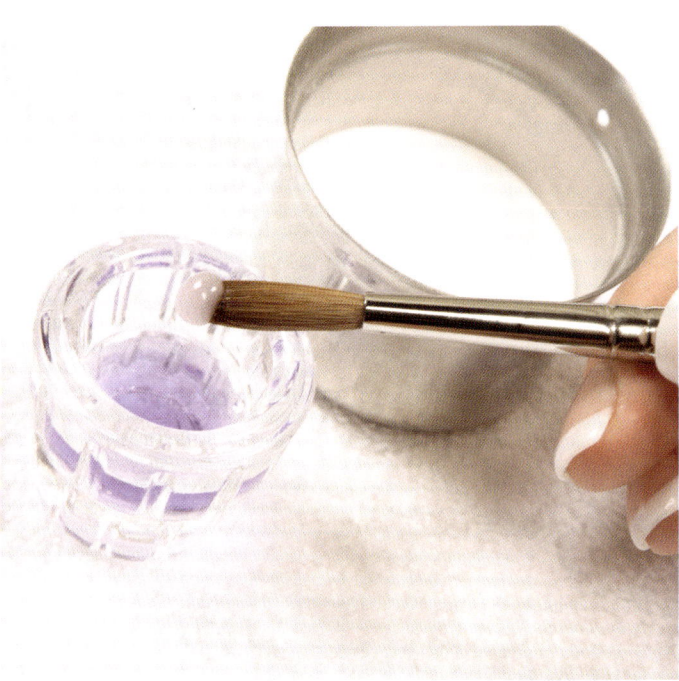

You will need the artificial nail preparation essentials, nail tip application essentials (if applicable) and the following additional items to perform an acrylic nail service.

Polymer or Acrylic Powder

Polymer, or **acrylic powder**, is powdered acrylic that is available in a variety of colors. For a

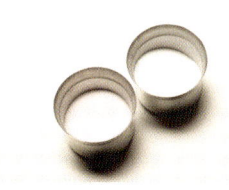

basic acrylic nail application, pink, white, clear or neutral color is typically used. In preparation for an acrylic nail application, polymer is placed into a clean, small glass or metal dish called a **dappen dish**.

One way to remember that the polymer is powdered acrylic is that they both begin with the letter "p."

Keeping the product clean and sanitary is a priority in providing this service to your clients. Make sure that the monomer doesn't appear cloudy at any point during the service. If it does, thoroughly clean the brush and refill the dappen dish with fresh monomer. One way to avoid this contamination is by keeping the brush free of product before placing it into the monomer. Another way to avoid contamination is to dispose of unused monomer. Do not pour it back into the original bottle.

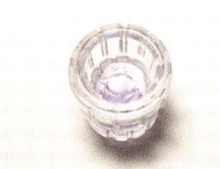

Monomer or Acrylic Liquid

Monomer, or **acrylic liquid**, is a liquid form of acrylic that is combined with the polymer to create an acrylic nail. Monomer is also poured into a clean, small glass or metal dappen dish prior to performing an acrylic service.

Avoid having the monomer come into contact with the nail once the primer has been applied. Brushing monomer on the nail before applying product may cause the product to lift after application.

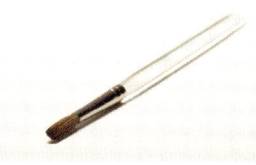

Acrylic Brush

An **acrylic brush**, often called a sable hair brush, typically tapers toward the end of the brush and flattens out when placed against a smooth surface, such as the edge of a dappen dish or a nail. It is important to treat this implement with special care. Avoid touching the hairs of the brush with your fingers. To properly clean the brush and to remove any residue from the brush hairs, submerge it in fresh, clean monomer and wipe product off onto a lint-free paper towel.

9

Be careful not to allow the product to harden and become stuck to the brush hairs. Most manufacturers make brushes to complement their product, which may help you in obtaining the correct liquid to powder ratio. This helps because your brush will have enough liquid to help pick up the correct amount of powder.

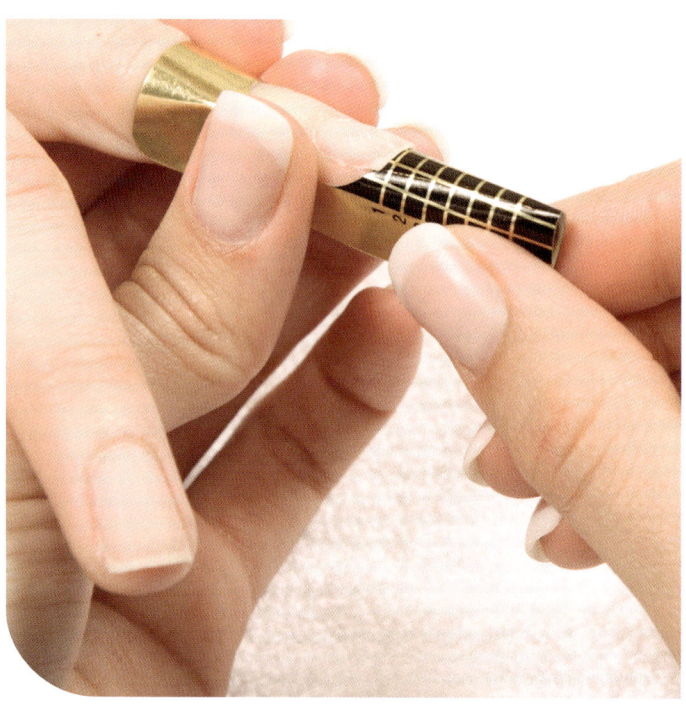

Nail Forms

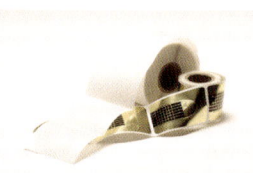

Nail forms are flexible, reusable or disposable items that are placed under the free edge of the natural nail. Artificial nails are sculpted onto the forms, which create a longer free edge without the application of nail tips. Once the nails have been sculpted onto the forms and allowed to dry, the nail forms are carefully removed and either disinfected or discarded.

Dehydrator

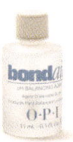

A **dehydrator** is used to eliminate extra moisture from the nail plate so that the product adheres better. The dehydrator should be applied immediately before applying the acrylic because it only functions temporarily. Some manufacturers offer a product that doubles as both a nail preparation solution and dehydrator, while others have separate products. Remember to always follow manufacturer's instructions.

Acrylic Primer

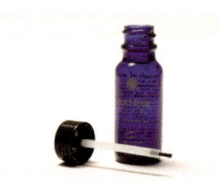

The application of an **acrylic primer** helps the product better adhere to the nail. When using an acid primer, remember to wear goggles and gloves for safety and take great care not to let it come into contact with the client's skin. Only a small amount of product, applied in a very thin layer, is needed to prime the nail. Immediately replace the cap after use. Refer to *Chapter 5, Chemistry* for further information on primers.

For easy application of disposable nail forms with adhesive backing, it helps to slightly bend them so that they take on the shape of the c-curve prior to application. This also makes them more flexible and easier to fit snugly under the free edge. Some forms also have markings that can act as a guide for making the lengths of the nails even.

FORMING AN ACRYLIC BEAD

To place the acrylic onto the nail, the monomer and polymer are combined to form an acrylic bead. This bead is then placed onto the nail, allowed to harden and form the artificial nail. By following the simple steps below, you will see that the acrylic bead is formed by first dipping the brush into the monomer and then into the polymer.

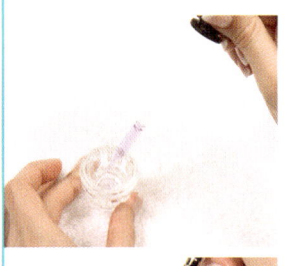

1. **Prepare liquid monomer and powder polymer.**
   - Place small amount of monomer into dappen dish.
   - If necessary or desired, place small amount of powder into separate dappen dish.

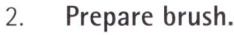

2. **Prepare brush.**
   - Completely submerge hairs of brush into monomer.
   - Press hairs against bottom of dappen dish. Move brush around to release any air trapped between hairs.
   - Wipe both sides of brush on side of dappen dish to flatten brush on both sides.

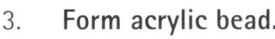

3. **Form acrylic bead.**
   - Dip brush into monomer—for a smaller bead, dip tip of brush; for a larger bead dip brush farther into monomer.
   - Remove brush from dappen dish while wiping against side of dappen dish.
   - Draw a line in acrylic powder with tip of brush or place brush at approximately a 45° angle to pick up powder.

NOTE: *The bead should be on one side of the brush.*

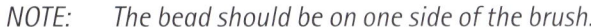

NOTE: *More monomer = larger acrylic bead*
Less monomer = smaller acrylic bead

Monomer surrounds the powder particles creating a shiny yet rough-textured appearance similar to an orange. The acrylic bead should stay solid and not appear to "melt" into the hairs of the brush.

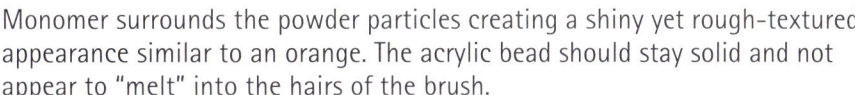

4. **Place bead.**
   - Place bead onto nail.
   - Wiggle brush to release bead.

NOTE: Avoid "wiping" acrylic bead onto nail.

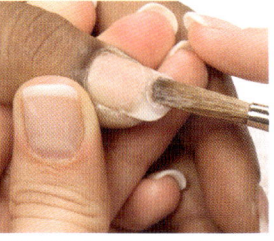

5. **Press bead into place.**
   - Press down middle of bead using side of brush.
   - Press each side of bead following same procedure.
   - Follow c-curve of nail with brush to distribute product.
   - After pressing, blend by lightly stroking brush toward free edge.

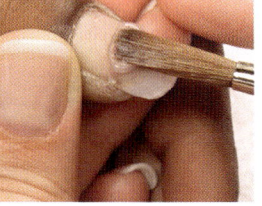

6. **Clean brush.**
   - Wipe brush on a lint-free disposable towel before placing it back into monomer to prevent contaminating monomer.

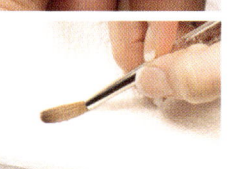

9

ACRYLIC NAIL ESSENTIALS

You are already familiar with the products, implements, supplies and equipment mentioned previously in this chapter. Here is a list of additional items you will need for an acrylic nail service.

ACRYLIC NAIL PRODUCTS

Essential	Function
Monomer	Acrylic liquid
Polymer	Acrylic powder
Primer	Improves adhesion
Dehydrator	Temporarily dehydrates nail

ACRYLIC NAIL IMPLEMENTS

Nail Brush	Cleans nails and surrounding skin
Acrylic Brush	Applies product to nail

ACRYLIC NAIL SUPPLIES

Nail Forms	Provide a temporary base onto which acrylic or gel is applied to create a longer free edge without the application of tips

Acrylic Nail Maintenance

As the natural nails grow, the product moves forward with the growth of the nail. Acrylic nail maintenance is very similar to nail wrap maintenance, because as the nail grows out, a fill-in or re-balancing service is needed. This maintenance on acrylic overlays is very important in keeping the nails looking new. Although the procedure is similar to the overlay, the primary focus is on the new growth area and in making sure that Zone 2 remains the thickest.

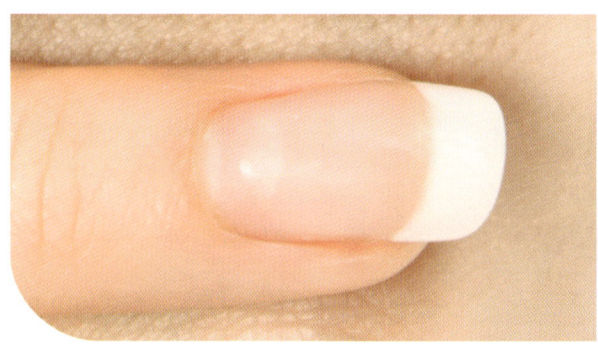

Before performing maintenance on acrylic nails, it is important to analyze the nails carefully to determine if there are any repairs needed. Look for any cracks in the nail or any lifting or separation of the product from the nail. If there is a crack in the nail, it may require that the product be removed, which is described on page 327, and reapplied. If the product is lifting or any separation has occurred, carefully file away the product from that area. Broken or cracked nails can be repaired in the same way between services.

The two-week maintenance is performed in the same way for pink and whites as it is for single-color acrylics. The same color of acrylic used in Zone 3 is used to fill in the new growth area.

Two-Week Acrylic Nail Maintenance

As with nail wrap maintenance, acrylic nails need maintenance also. As the natural nail is exposed at the cuticle area, it is important to re-balance the nail making sure the thickest area is in Zone 2. This is done by using the same color of acrylic that was applied to Zone 3 when the nails were first done. The old product is blended to the natural nail and any lifting is filed off the nail. The new product is then placed into Zone 3 and blended into Zone 2. It is recommended to repair any cracks or lifting at this time to prevent any other problems such as bacteria growth between the natural nail and the acrylic nail. Two-week acrylic nail maintenance is different from four-week only with pink and white acrylic nails. If pink and white acrylic is used, then the white smile lines are replaced or moved back every four weeks.

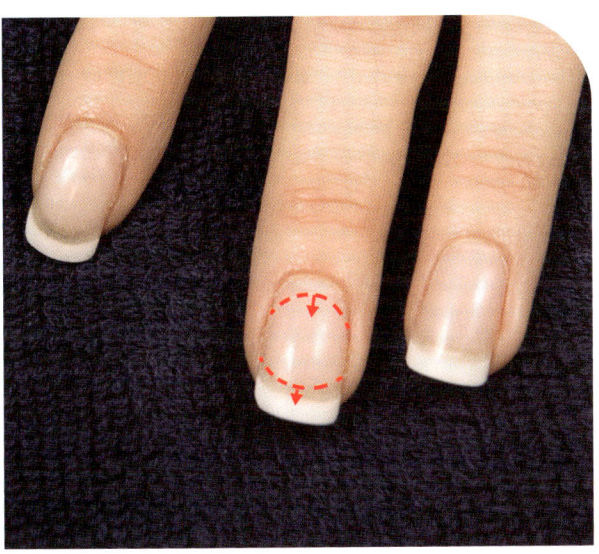

Four-Week Pink and White Acrylic Nail Maintenance

Four-week acrylic nail maintenance only applies to pink and white acrylics. As mentioned previously, the acrylic moves forward with the nail growth. This makes the white smile line move forward on the nail so that it no longer covers the natural smile line. This allows the natural nail's smile line to show through the acrylic product. The four-week maintenance is performed to re-balance the nail, filling in the new growth as well as repositioning the white acrylic smile line. For this procedure, both pink and white acrylic is used. To keep nails looking new and balanced, it is important to reposition the smile line and make sure that the thickest application is in Zone 2.

Four-week maintenance is very similar to the initial pink and white application. The difference is that the acrylic nail is filed down and blended into the new growth. The free edge, where the smile line is located, is thinned out. Thinning out the white acrylic part of the nail makes it possible to add product on top of it without creating a very thick nail. This can be done manually as demonstrated in this chapter, or with an electric file, which is discussed in *Chapter 10, Specialty Nails.*

Acrylic Nail Removal

Like nail wraps, acrylic nails can be removed by using acetone or the manufacturer's recommended artificial nail remover product. This softens and dissolves the artificial nail. Acrylic nail removal is similar to nail wrap removal except it may take longer for the product to dissolve due to the fact that it is comprised of cross-linked polymers as discussed in *Chapter 5, Chemistry.*

It is beneficial for the client to follow up acrylic nail removal with a manicure and a nail strengthener or treatment. This also will help to add moisture and strength back into the nail plate.

9

Gel Nails

When observing the finished looks between gel nails and acrylic nails, it would be difficult to determine which product was initially applied. The two look and feel very similar once finished. However, one major distinction between gel nails and acrylic nails is the way they harden or cure. With acrylics, the chemical reaction between the powder and liquid acrylics causes the product to dry and harden on its own. Gel products, on the other hand, do not fully harden or cure until they are exposed to either an ultraviolet (UV) or halogen light. Another difference is that gel products are in a gel-like form rather than a powder and liquid mixture.

Since gel does not cure until it is exposed to light, it is important to keep the nails level to keep the product from moving. To make it easier for the client to keep the nails level, gel is first applied to the pinky finger through the index finger and cured. The thumbs are done separately and placed under the light together. Similar to acrylics, gels are available in many different colors and can be used as an overlay for natural nails or tips and can also be used to sculpt a nail.

Two common gel nail services are the single–color gel overlay and the pink and white sculptured gel nails. For a single-color gel overlay, either a pink or clear gel is typically used. No matter what color is chosen, only one color is applied over the entire nail. This can be done over nail tips or the natural nails.

Pink gel, white gel and clear gel are used for pink and white sculptured gel nails. A pink and white gel nail application can be done with nail forms and over nail tips. White gel is used to form the smile line in Zone 1, just as in a French manicure. The pink gel is used to create the rest of the nail, Zones 2 and 3, while the clear gel blends the zones together.

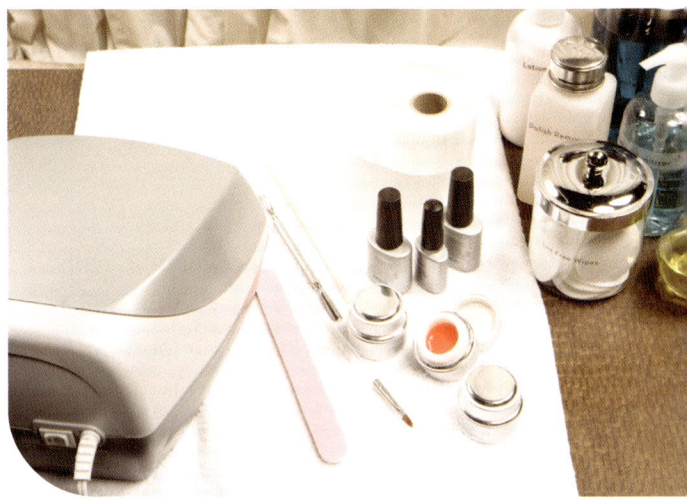

Gel Nail Essentials

You will need the artificial nail preparation essentials, nail tip application essentials (if applicable) and the following additional items to perform a gel nail service.

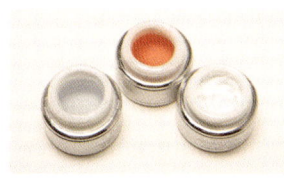

Gel

Gel is an acrylic-based product that is applied to the nail plate, after which the hand is placed under a light (ultraviolet or halogen). This creates a chemical reaction that causes the product to harden or cure. Gel typically comes in a jar or a squeezable tube. It is spread onto the nail with a brush using a very light touch.

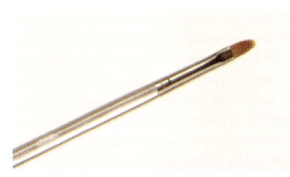

Gel Brush

A brush made from synthetic fibers is the most commonly used **gel brush**. It is important to treat this implement with special care. Avoid touching it with your fingers. Clean the brush following the manufacturer's instructions.

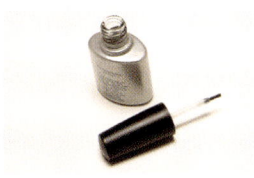

Bonder or Primer

Most gel products also come with a **bonder gel**, which is a bonding agent that helps the product adhere to the nail plate.

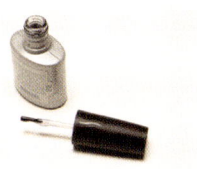

Sealer

Sealer is a thinner gel product, which is applied to the nail after shaping and balancing to finish the nails with a high shine. A sealer is often used to create a tough shield over the final acrylic layer. It is brushed over the entire nail, across the tip of the free edge and then cured under the light. Be sure to follow the manufacturer's instructions.

Curing Light

A **curing light** is an ultraviolet or halogen light used to create a chemical reaction,

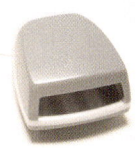

which hardens or cures the product after it is applied to the nails. The unit allows the client to slide her hand or finger into the machine under the light. The correct light must be used for the product to properly cure, so be sure to follow the manufacturer's instructions on which type of light to use and how to use it. Most lights have timers on them that cure the product for the exact amount of time needed. Different gel products may require a different strength and/or amount of light.

> Clients with thin nail plates may feel heat created by the chemical reaction between the gel and the light as the product cures. Be sure to always check for client comfort.

9

GEL NAIL ESSENTIALS

You are already familiar with the products, implements, supplies and equipment mentioned previously in this chapter. Here is a list of additional items you will need for a gel nail service.

GEL NAIL PRODUCTS

Essential	Function
Gel	Forms the artificial nail
Bonder or Primer	Improves adhesion
Sealer	Provides a high-shine finish to gel nails

GEL NAIL IMPLEMENTS

Gel Brush	Applies product to nail

GEL NAIL EQUIPMENT

Curing Light	Cures gel product

Gel Nail Maintenance

As with all artificial nail services, gel nails need to be maintained every two to three weeks depending upon how fast your client's nails grow. Remember to avoid over-filing the natural nails during maintenance in order to keep them healthy. Two-week gel nail maintenance is very similar to two-week acrylic nail maintenance, because as the nail grows out, a fill-in or re-balancing service is needed. It is important to keep up this maintenance on gel nails to keep them looking new. The gel maintenance service is similar to the overlay, except the primary focus is on the new growth area.

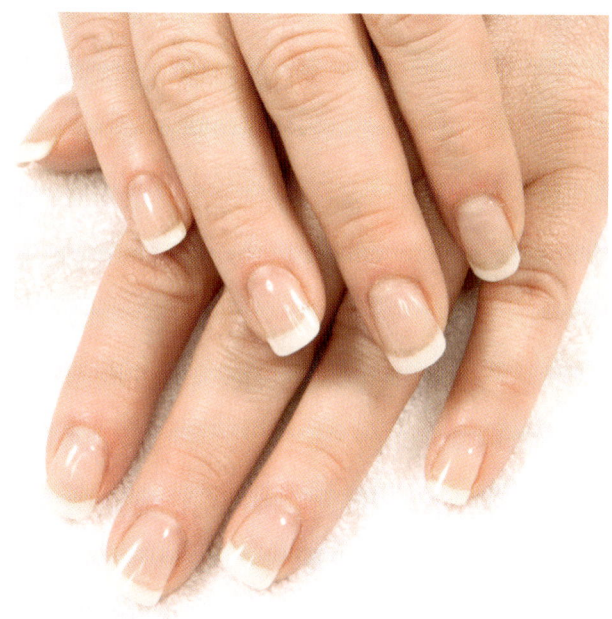

Before performing maintenance on gel nails, analyze the nails carefully to determine if there are any repairs needed. Look for any cracks in the nail or any lifting, which is separation of the product from the nail. If there is a crack in the nail, it may require that the product be removed, which is described on page 352, and reapplied. If the product is lifting or any separation has occurred, carefully file away the product from that area.

The two-week maintenance is performed in the same way for pink and whites as it is for single-color gels. The same color of gel used in Zone 3 is used to fill in the new growth area; then the entire nail is sealed again with clear gel.

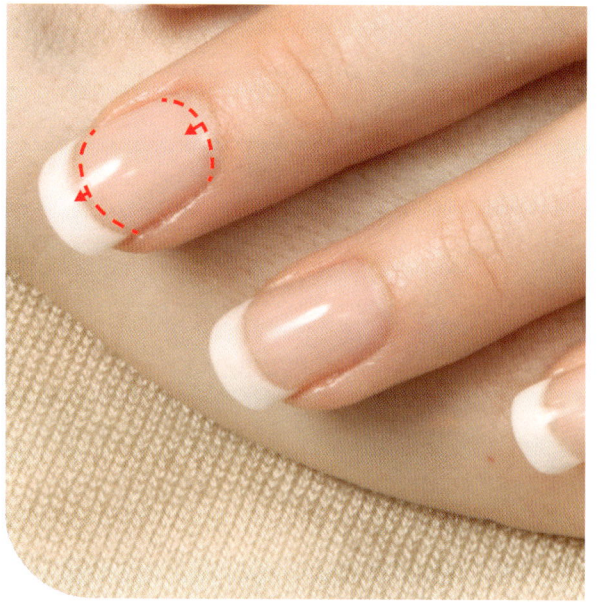

Two-Week Gel Nail Maintenance

Two-week gel maintenance is the same as the two-week acrylic maintenance, except gel is used versus acrylic. The same color of gel that was applied to Zone 3 during the first application is used for two-week gel maintenance. As with acrylics, a two-week and a four-week gel maintenance differs if pink and white gel was used and the smile line needs to be replaced or moved back. It is recommended to prepare the nails properly and check for any lifting or cracks that need to be repaired.

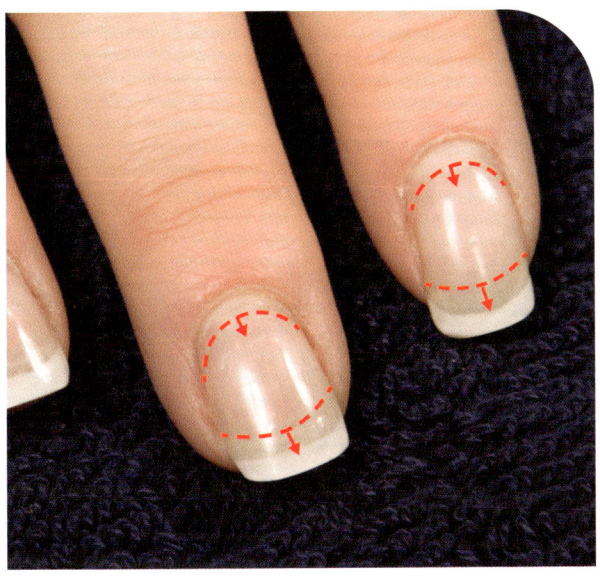

Four-Week Pink and White Gel Nail Maintenance

Four-week gel nail maintenance only applies to pink and white gels. The four-week gel nail maintenance is performed to re-balance the nail and to fill in the new growth as well as to re-position the white gel smile line as with the four-week acrylic maintenance. For this procedure pink, white and clear gel are used.

Four-week maintenance is very similar to the initial pink and white application. The difference is that the gel nail is filed down and blended into the new growth. The free edge, where the smile line is located, is thinned out. Thinning out the white gel part of the nail makes it possible to add product on top of it without creating a very thick nail. This can be done manually as demonstrated in this chapter, or with an electric file, which is discussed in *Chapter 10, Specialty Nails.*

Gel Nail Removal

Unlike nail wrap and acrylic nail removal, gel nails cannot currently be dissolved by acetone or any other solvent. This is due to gel nails being highly cross-linked polymers as discussed in *Chapter 5, Chemistry.* In order to remove gel nails the product has to be gently filed away. Extra caution is necessary when filing the product off to preserve the health of the natural nail and to not over–file the nail plate. Avoid using a heavy hand or an abrasive that is too coarse.

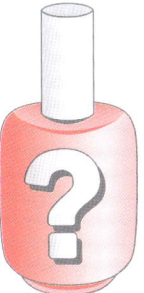

After learning about overlays and sculptured nails, when and why would you recommend one over the other to your client?

ARTIFICIAL NAIL PROCEDURES

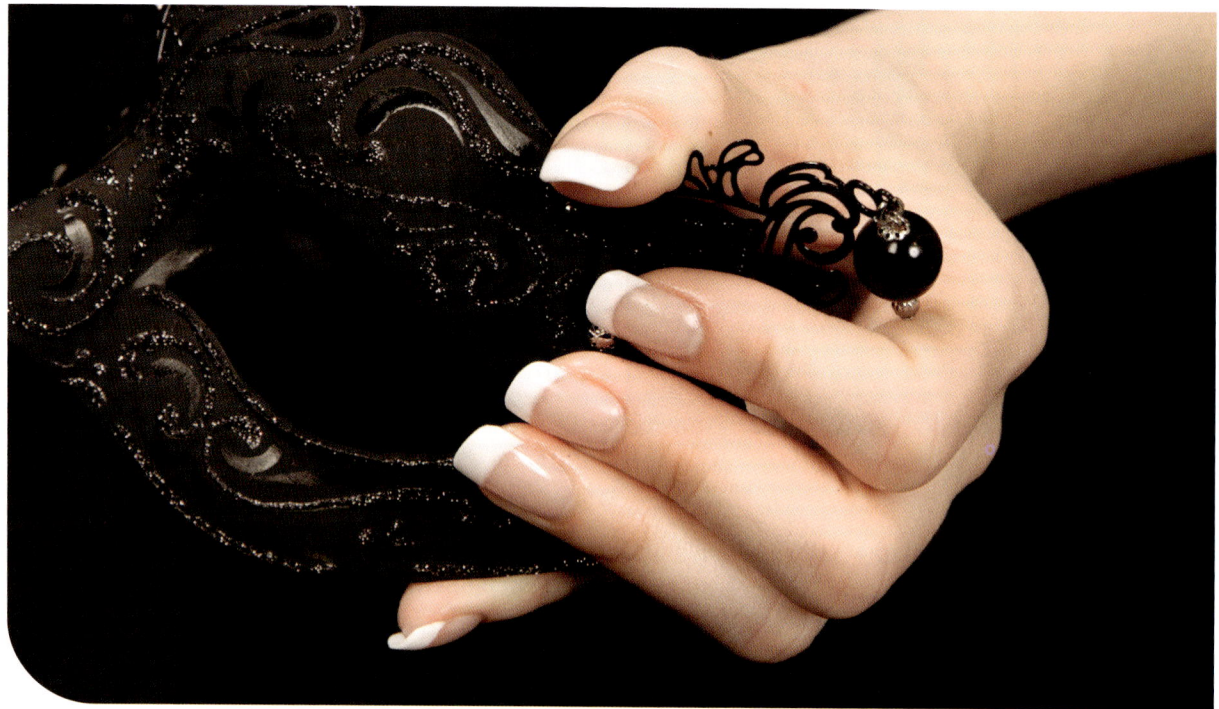

Artificial nail enhancements are a big part of the nail industry and changes are taking place every day. There are several different types of services that can be performed by incorporating different enhancement products. Anything from a permanent French manicure to a colored gel overlay on toenails, which is considered a chip–proof polish, can be done with enhancement products. Gel sealers can be applied over acrylics or wraps to provide a shiny finish until the client returns for maintenance. A multitude of services can be performed after you learn the basic application procedures for artificial nail enhancements.

Today, acrylic powders are available in a variety of colors. Beautiful 3-D nail designs can be created by using various colored acrylics. However, it is important to master the basic skills of using acrylic before venturing into the designs that can be created using colored acrylics.

Fundamental Procedures

Artificial nail preparation, balancing and finishing are fundamental procedures that are performed with artificial nail services. In this section, you will first learn how to perform these three procedures since they will be performed no matter which nail system your client chooses. A nail tip application will only be performed if your client chooses to receive an overlay, but it is an important step in providing the foundation to the nail before applying a wrap, acrylic or gel.

FUNDAMENTAL PROCEDURES
• TABLE OF CONTENTS •

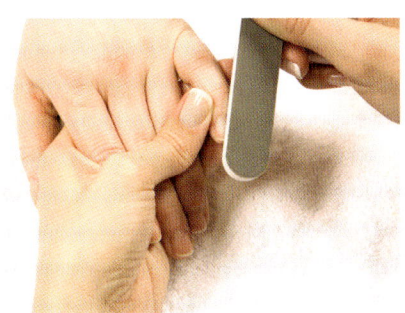

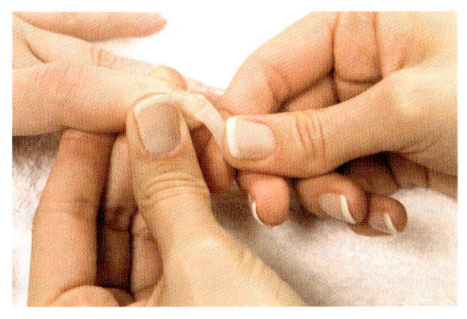

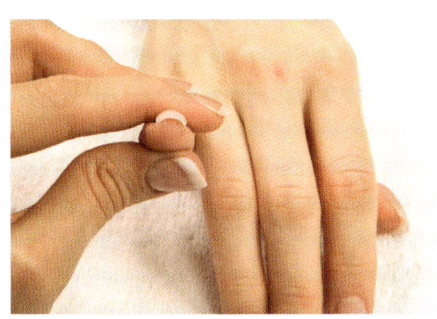

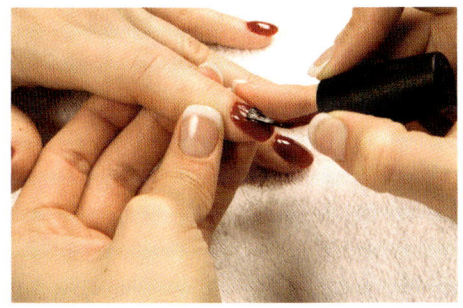

NOTES

BASIC ARTIFICIAL NAIL PREPARATION

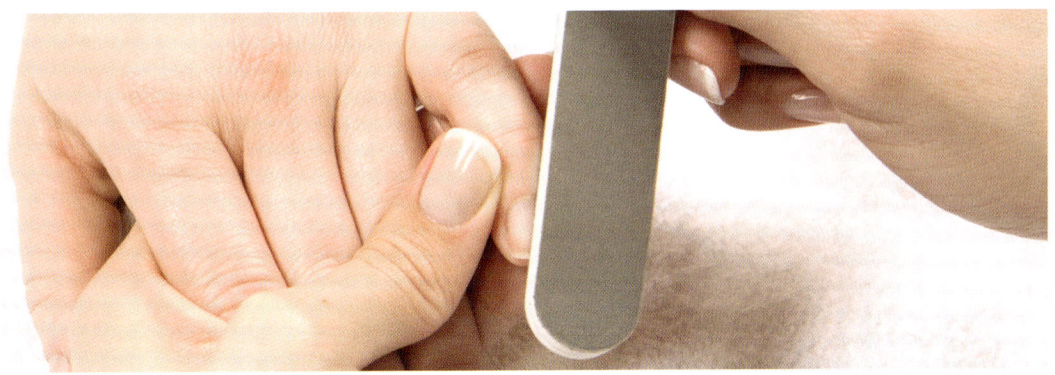

BASIC ARTIFICIAL NAIL PREPARATION PROCEDURE

Proper preparation of the natural nail plate is the most important step of any artificial nail service. The main purpose of this procedure is to protect the natural nail from potential damage or infection. Note that the procedure below corresponds with the step-by-step technical images that follow.

4. Delivery – Meet client's expectations

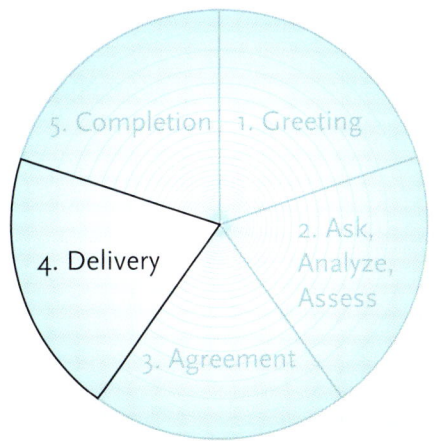

SANITIZE
1. Wash and sanitize your hands
2. Sanitize client's hands

ANALYZE
3. Perform visual analysis of hands
4. Remove polish
5. Perform visual analysis of nails

CUTICLE CARE
6. Apply cuticle remover
7. Push back cuticles
8. Nip cuticles/hangnails if necessary
9. Clean under free edge
10. Remove cuticle remover

FILE
11. Shape nails
12. Remove shine
13. Remove oils and debris from nail plate

BASIC ARTIFICIAL NAIL PREPARATION

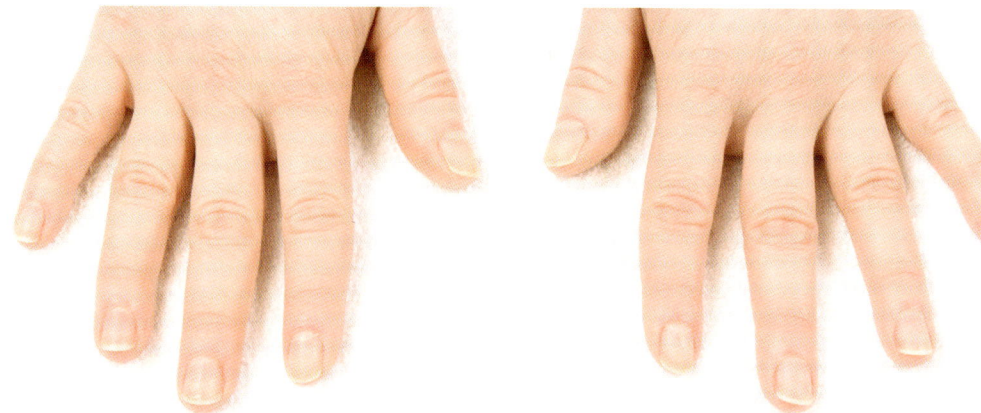

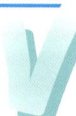 A checkmark next to a step indicates an ideal time to check on your client's comfort, and to take extra safety precautions.

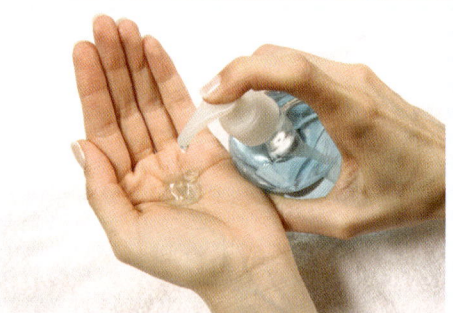

1. **Wash and sanitize your hands.**
   - Use liquid or foam soap.
   - Use waterless sanitizer or topical antiseptic if required by regulating agency.
   - Wear protective gloves if required by regulating agency.

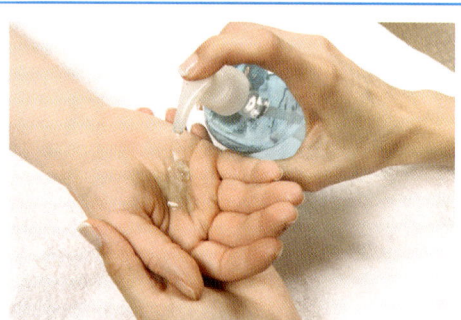

2. **Sanitize client's hands.**
   - Use waterless sanitizer or topical antiseptic if required by regulating agency.

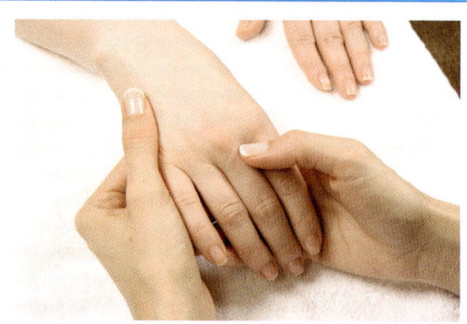

ANALYZE

3. **Perform visual analysis of hands.**
   - Continue with service if hands are free of any visible signs of diseases or disorders.

NOTE: As a nail technician, you cannot diagnose or treat diseases or disorders. You can only refer the client to a physician.

Skin: Signs to look for during analysis on hands include open skin, redness, swelling, discoloration or any other signs of an infection that may prevent the service from being performed.

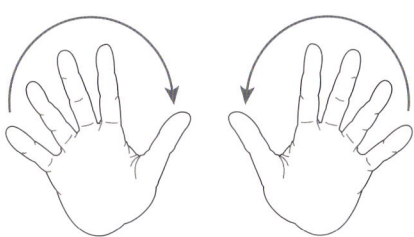

Any procedure that will be performed on all 10 fingers will always be done in the same order: On the non-dominant hand from the little finger to the thumb; then on the dominant hand from the little finger to thumb.

For this procedure, the client is right-handed. So we will work from the left hand, little finger to thumb; then the right hand, little finger to thumb.

9

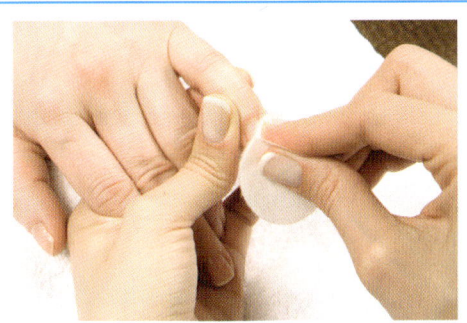

4. **Remove polish.**
   - Use a lint-free wipe or cotton saturated with polish remover on the nail plate.
   - Let remover set for a few seconds.
   - Wipe toward the free edge.
   - Remove all polish from each nail before moving to the next nail. Repeat on the right hand.

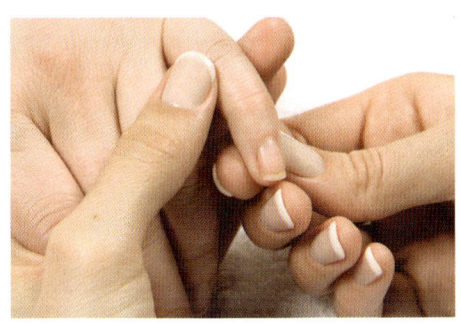

5. **Perform visual analysis of nails.**
   - Continue with service if nail plates are free of any visible signs of diseases or disorders.

Nails: Signs to look for during analysis on fingernails include discoloration, flaking, swelling, pain indicators, pus, detached nail plate, growth under the nail or any other signs of an infection that may prevent the service from being performed.

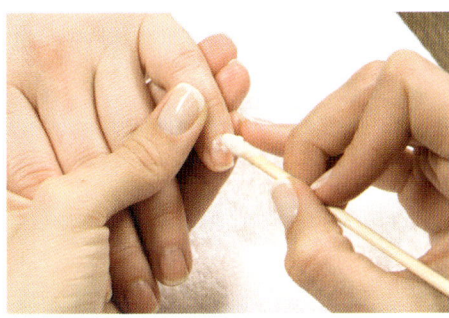

CUTICLE CARE

6. **Apply cuticle remover.**
   - Use cotton-tipped orangewood stick, cotton swab or dropper.
   - Apply to all 10 fingers, beginning with the little finger of the non-dominant hand.

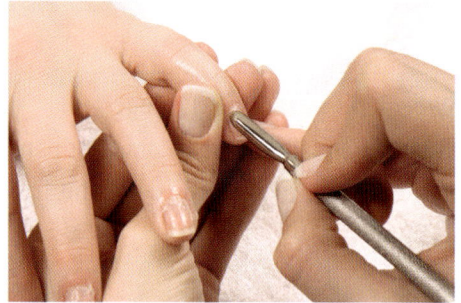

7. Push back cuticles.

- Use cotton-tipped orangewood stick or metal cuticle pusher.
- Use light, quick, circular movements along cuticle.
- Work from one side of nail toward center; then from other side toward the center.
- Use a gentle, non-aggressive touch.
- Move orangewood stick or pusher along nail plate without applying downward pressure to avoid damaging the nail matrix.

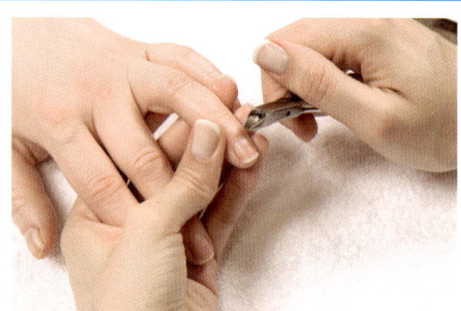

8. Nip cuticles/hangnails if necessary.

- After loosening, excess cuticle will appear translucent.
- Use cuticle nippers to remove any lifted or loosened excess cuticle.
- Position blades parallel to cuticle.
- Squeeze handles to cut; release nippers before moving on.
- Avoid using the point of the nippers and/or pulling at cuticles.
- Remove cuticle in one piece if at all possible.
- Nippers may also be used to remove hangnails.

NOTE: Be guided by your regulatory guidelines regarding the use of cuticle nippers.

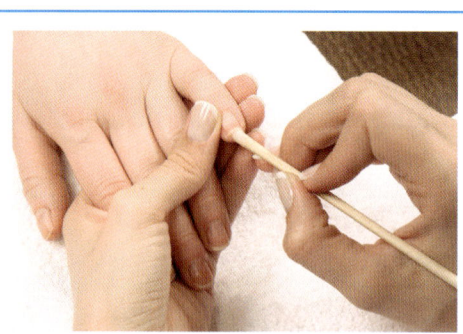

9. Clean under free edge.

- Use cotton-tipped orangewood stick dampened with polish remover or water.

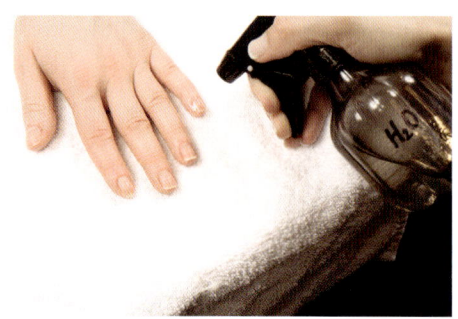

10. Remove cuticle remover.

- Have client wash hands using a nail brush.
- Or, spray nails with water and wipe each nail plate with towel.

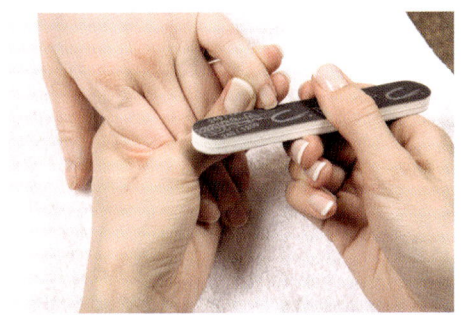

FILE

11. Shape nails.

- Use file to shape nails.
- For nail tip application, create a more rounded shape to fit into the well of the tips.
- For sculptured nail application with forms, create square-shaped nails so forms will fit under the corners of the nails.

NOTE: Remove length using nail clippers if necessary.

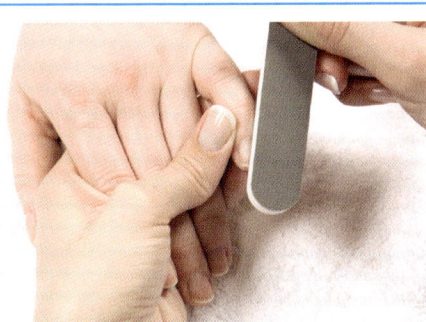

12. Remove shine.

- Use a 240-grit file to lightly buff surface of nail to remove shine.
- Move the file in direction of nail growth.
- Avoid over-filing.

NOTE: Lift file from surface of nail between strokes to avoid overheating nail.

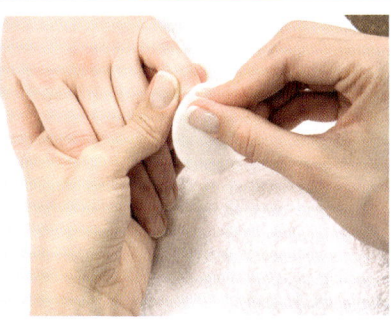

13. Remove oils and debris from nail plate.

- Use a lint-free wipe saturated with nail preparation solution or appropriate product according to the manufacturer's instructions.
- Wipe nail plate making sure to cleanse entire surface.

Proceed with artificial nail service.

9

NAIL TIP APPLICATION

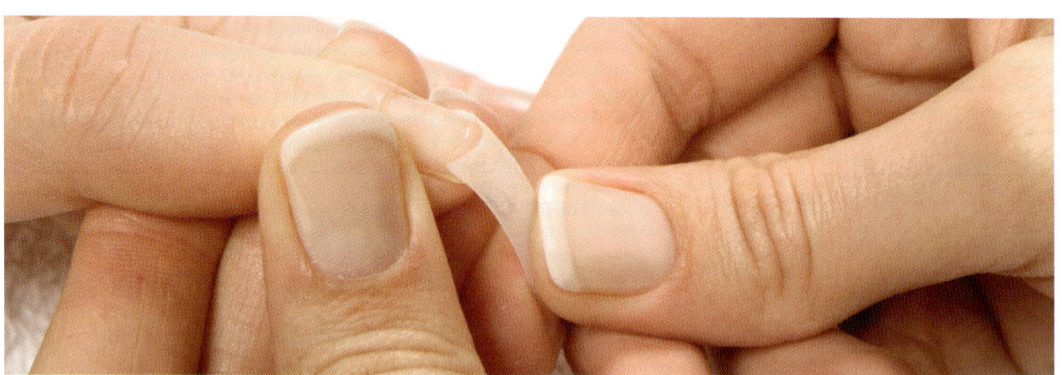

NAIL TIP APPLICATION PROCEDURE

Nail tips, usually made of plastic, nylon or acetate are applied using an adhesive. Nail tips can be a temporary length enhancement or a base for nail wrap, acrylic or gel products. Note that the procedure below corresponds with the step-by-step technical images that follow.

4. Delivery – Meet client's expectations

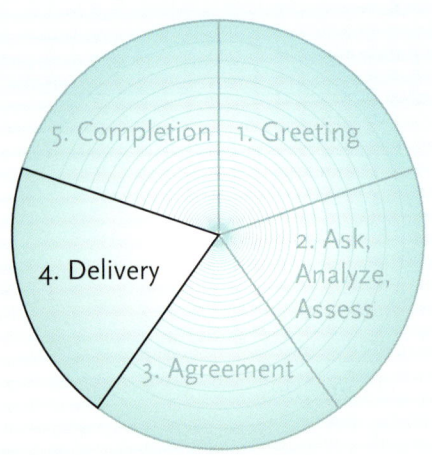

PREPARE NAILS

1. Prepare nails following **Basic Artificial Nail Preparation Procedure** on page 279

PREPARE TIPS

2. Size tips
3. Customize tips
4. Remove oils and debris from nail plate

APPLY TIPS

5. Apply adhesive
6. Apply tip to natural nail
7. Trim tips

FILE TIPS

8. Shape and blend tips
9. Remove oils and debris from nail plate

NAIL TIP APPLICATION

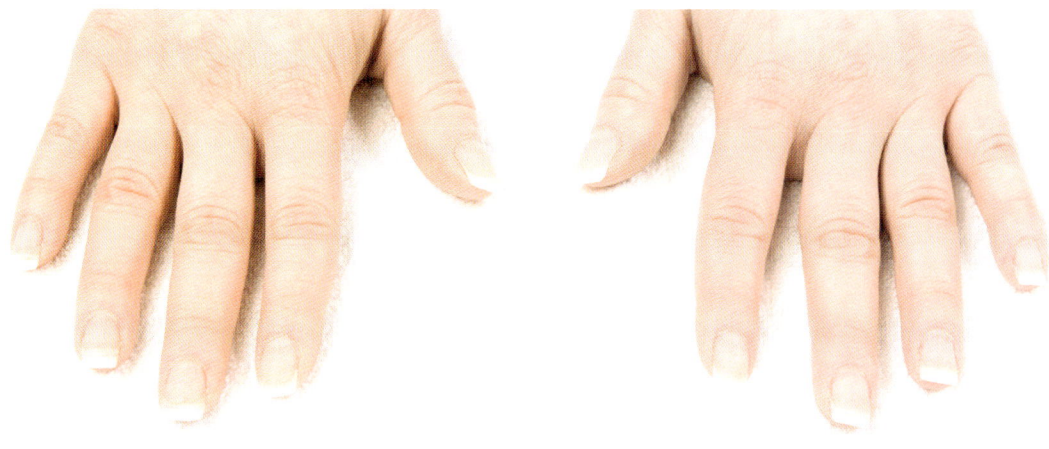

9

 A checkmark next to a step indicates an ideal time to check on your client's comfort, and to take extra safety precautions.

PREPARE NAILS

1. Prepare nails following Basic Artificial Nail Preparation Procedure on page 279.
   - ANALYZE
   - CUTICLE CARE
   - FILE

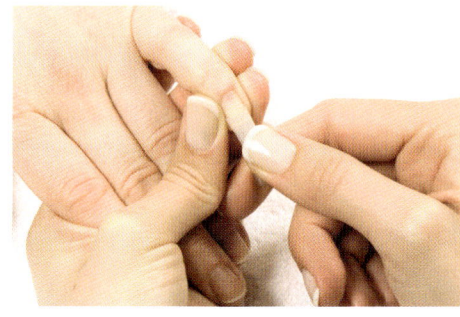

PREPARE TIPS

2. Size tips.
   - Cover natural nail from sidewall to sidewall.
   - Match the c-curve.
   - Size all 10 nails.

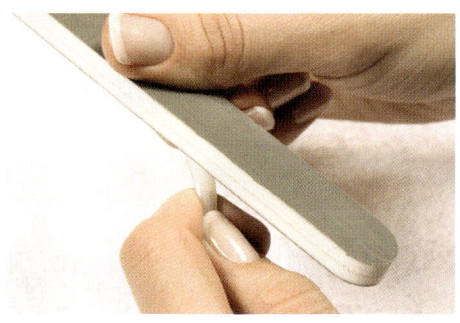

3. Customize tips.
   - Trim the well of the tip (if it covers more than half of the nail plate) using a file or small scissors.
   - Use a file to thin or bevel the entire well of the tip, making sure that the edge closest to the matrix is the thinnest part of the well. This will reduce the amount of filing needed to blend the tip to the natural nail after application.

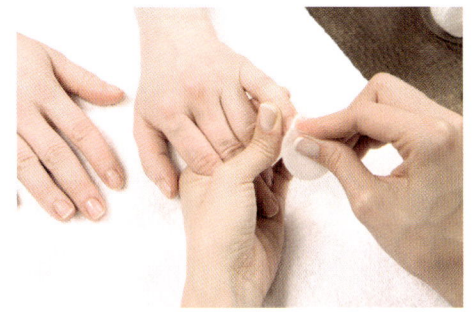

4. **Remove oils and debris from nail plate.**
   - Use a lint-free wipe saturated with nail preparation solution or appropriate product according to the manufacturer's instructions.

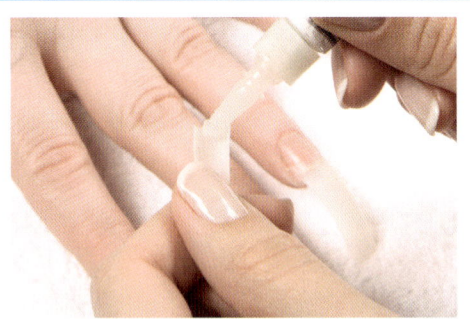

APPLY TIPS

5. **Apply adhesive.**
   - Apply a thin line of adhesive close to free edge of natural nail and to well of tip.
   - Lightly press and drag the well of the tip against the nail toward the free edge using a quick movement to spread adhesive evenly and to help prevent air bubbles.

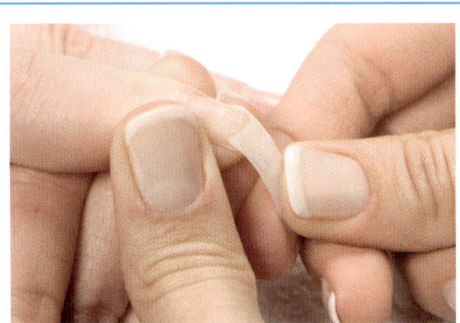

6. **Apply tip to natural nail.**
   - Hold tip at a slight angle, make contact with free edge of nail and slide tip toward cuticle until the free edge is against "position stop."
   - Rock tip down toward nail until it is flat against nail plate.
   - Hold tip in place for a few seconds until adhesive dries.
   - Repeat Steps 5 and 6 on all 10 fingernails.

NOTE: Apply a bead of adhesive to the seam if necessary.

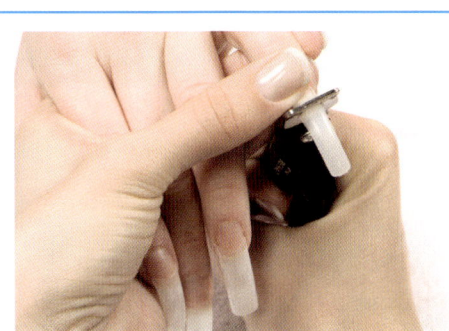

7. **Trim tips.**
   - Use tip cutters, positioning blade toward you.
   - Repeat on all 10 nails.

NOTE: Use fingernail clippers if tip cutters are not available. Trim one side of the tip and then the other to avoid cracking the tip.

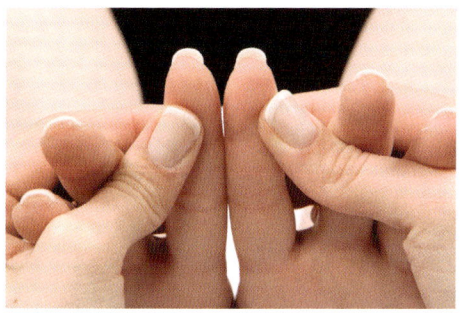

NOTE: You can check the length by holding nails up to compare the length from underneath.

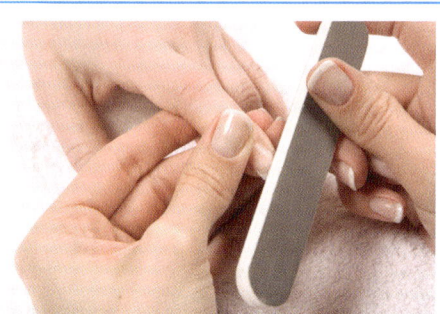

FILE TIPS

8. **Shape and blend tips.**
   - Use 180-grit file or higher to thin edge of the tip that is in contact with natural nail.
   - Hold file flat against nail and use long back-and-forth movements.
   - Refine surface with 180-grit file, then 240-grit file to make sure there is no line of demarcation between natural nail and tip.
   - File free edge of tip to desired shape.

NOTE: To see what the blended area will look like with an overlay product applied, apply antiseptic sanitizer to the surface of the nail.

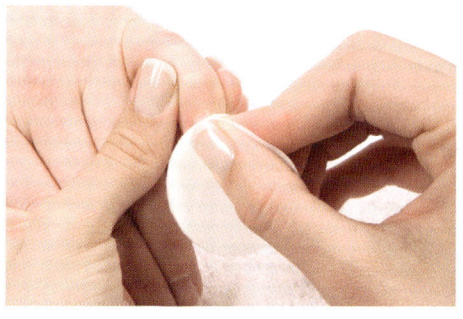

9. **Remove oils and debris from nail plate.**
   - Use a lint-free wipe saturated with nail preparation solution or appropriate product according to manufacturer's instructions.
   - Wipe nail plate making sure to cleanse entire surface.

Proceed with artificial nail service.

BASIC ARTIFICIAL NAIL BALANCING

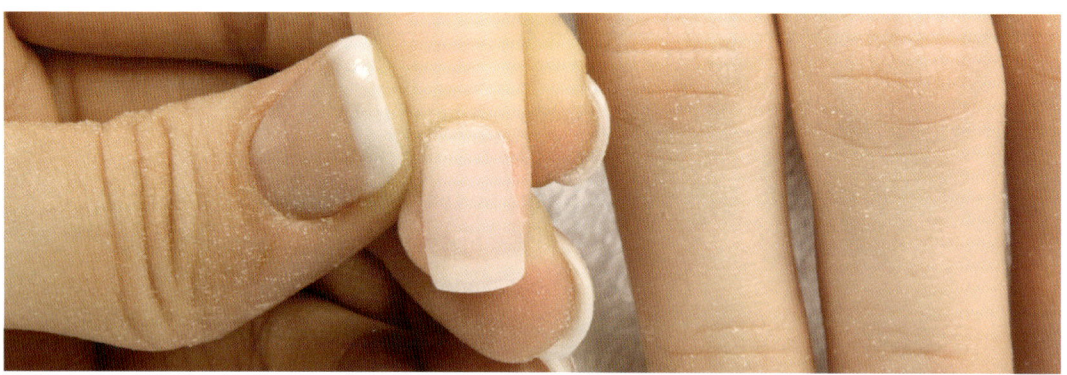

BASIC ARTIFICIAL NAIL BALANCING PROCEDURE

Proper filing and shaping of the nail will contribute to the desired final look expected by your client. Note that the procedure below corresponds with the step-by-step technical images that follow.

4. Delivery - Meet client's expectations

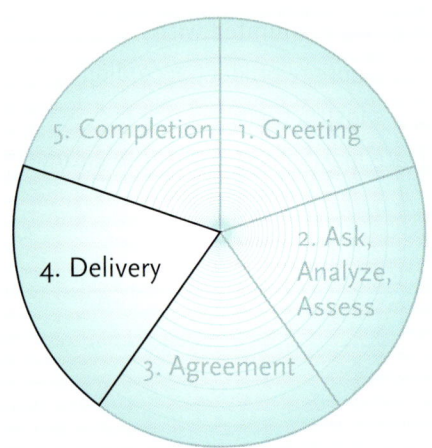

5. Completion   1. Greeting

4. Delivery

2. Ask, Analyze, Assess

3. Agreement

FILE

1. File areas 1 and 2
2. File area 3
3. File areas 4, 5 and 6
4. File areas 7, 8 and 9

BASIC ARTIFICIAL NAIL BALANCING

A checkmark next to a step indicates an ideal time to check on your client's comfort, and to take extra safety precautions.

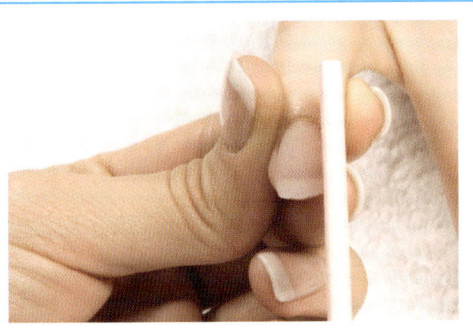

1. **File areas 1 and 2,** which are along each sidewall of the nail.
   - Make sure the sides of the artificial product follow the length of the sidewalls without tapering or fanning out toward the free edge.
   - Pull down on the sidewalls to move them away from the nail and reduce the chance of the file coming into contact with the skin surrounding the nail.

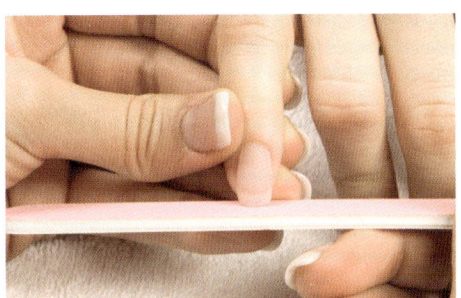

2. **File area 3,** which is the free edge.
   - Shape the free edge to the desired shape and length.

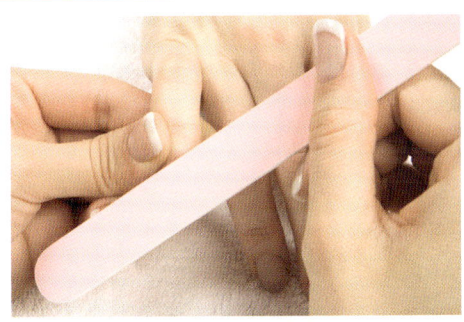

3. **File areas 4, 5** and **6,** which are closest to the cuticle.
   - File these areas to be thinner closest to the cuticle and to gradually become thicker as the areas blend into Zone 2.
   - Use long strokes and keep the file flat against the nail.

NOTE: In these areas it can be difficult to prevent the file from coming into contact with the skin surrounding the nail. Be sure to always check on your client's comfort.

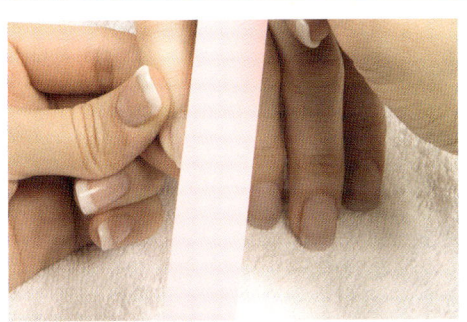

4. **File areas 7, 8** and **9,** which are the center and apex (top) of the nail (extending down to the free edge) where the product should be the thickest.
   - File these areas to create a smooth arc from the cuticle area to the free edge being sure to maintain the thicker part in Zone 2. Remember to keep the highest point of the nail in Zone 2.

Perform these filing techniques on all nails beginning with a lower grit file. Then repeat the steps, using progressively higher grit files to smooth the surface of the nail.

9

BASIC ARTIFICIAL NAIL FINISHING

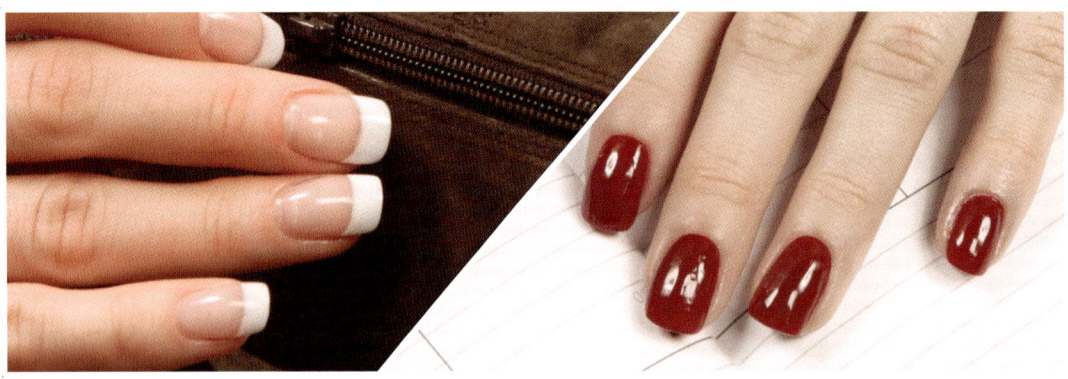

BASIC ARTIFICIAL NAIL FINISHING PROCEDURE

Finishing the artificial nail involves either buffing the nail to a shine or polishing the nail with the client's desired colored polish. The two finishing options will contribute to achieving the final look your client wants. Note that the procedure below corresponds with the step-by-step technical images that follow.

4. Delivery - Meet Client's Expectations

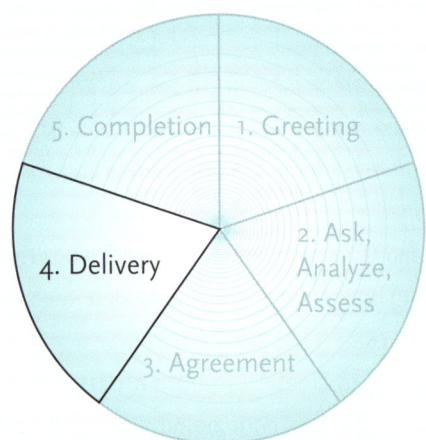

OPTION 1: BUFF NAILS to a shine

1. Use black side of three-way buffer
2. Use white side
3. Use gray side

CUTICLE CARE

4. Apply cuticle oil

OPTION 2: POLISH NAILS

1. Apply base coat
2. Apply two coats of colored polish
3. Apply top coat
4. Clean up excess polish
5. Apply speed dry (if desired)

BASIC ARTIFICIAL NAIL FINISHING

Before finishing nails, perform the following steps:

- Have client wash hands with a nail brush and dry thoroughly.
- Apply cream or hand lotion.
- Remove oils from each nail plate.

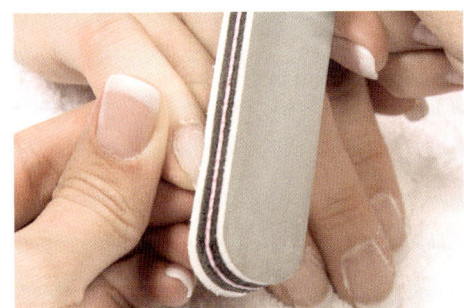

Option 1: BUFF NAILS to a shine

1. **Use black side of three-way buffer.**
   - Buff all nails.

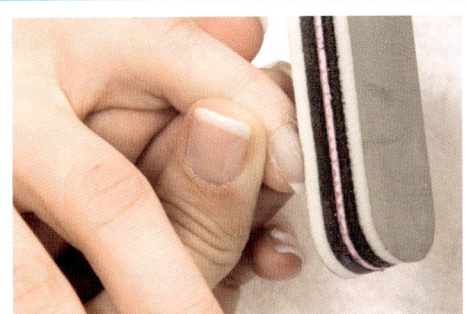

2. **Use white side** of three-way buffer.
   - Buff all nails.

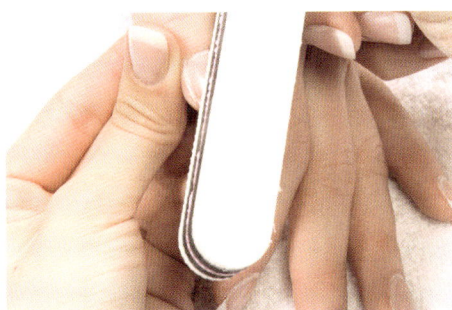

3. **Use gray side** of three-way buffer to finish nails with a shine.
   - Buff all nails.

NOTE: An electric file can also be used to create shine using the appropriate bits. Refer to Chapter 10, Specialty Nail Services, for more information.

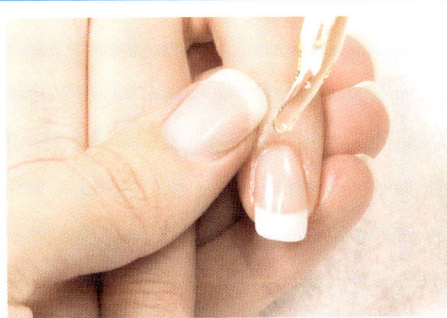

CUTICLE CARE

4. **Apply cuticle oil.**
   - Massage cuticle oil into cuticle area.

9

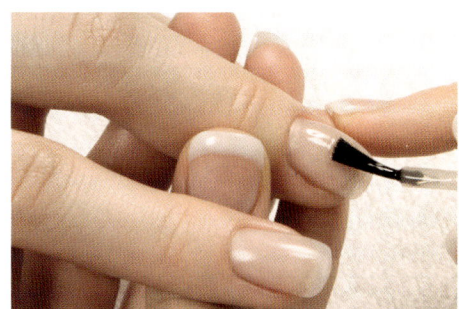

Option 2: POLISH NAILS

1. **Apply base coat** to all nails.
   - Use a base coat made for artificial nails.

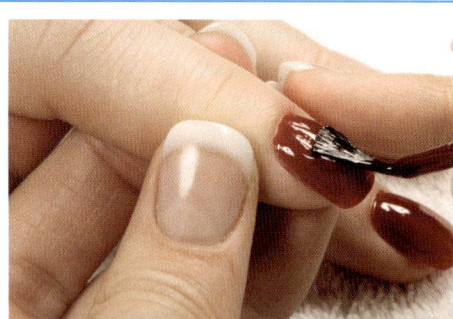

2. **Apply two coats of colored polish** to all nails.

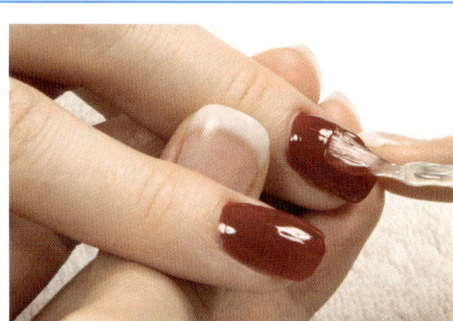

3. **Apply top coat** to all nails.

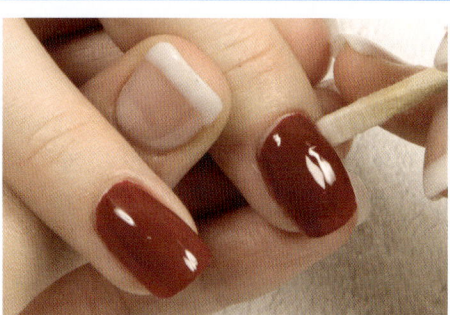

4. **Clean up excess polish** on sidewall and cuticle areas (if necessary).

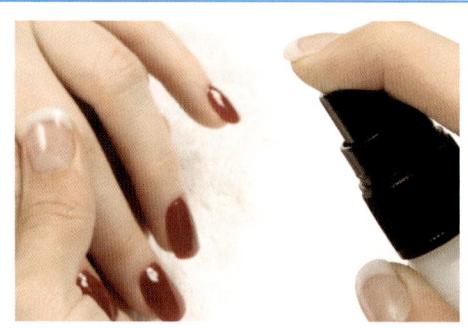

5. **Apply speed dry** to each nail if desired.
   - Optional: Apply small amount of cuticle oil to each cuticle.
   - Rub oil gently into cuticle area without pressure to freshly polished nails.

ARTIFICIAL NAIL COMPLETION

- Escort client to reception area.
- Discuss retail products.
- Rebook next appointment.

Infection Control and Safety
- Disinfect all implements.
- Discard all disposable implements.
- Replenish supplies.
- Disinfect the table and the service area using an EPA-registered, broad spectrum (hospital level) disinfectant
- Set up for the next client.
- Practice blood spill procedures; if a blood spill occurs, refer to page 67.

5. Completion – Gain feedback; infection control and safety

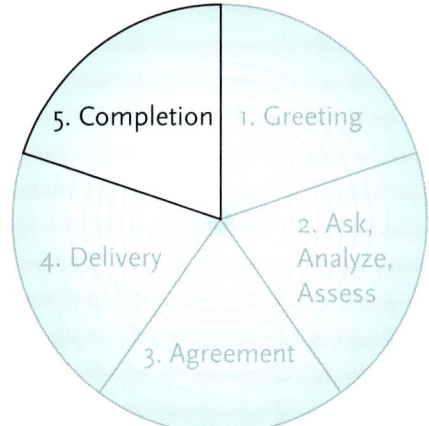

REMEMBER:
- Remove all product from jars with a spatula and keep lids tightly closed to avoid contamination.
- Keep labels on all containers and store products in a cool place to lengthen shelf life.
- Keep tools dry to avoid rust.
- Place soiled towels in a covered container; use clean towels on each client.
- Complete the Service Record on the Client Consultation Form.

Nail Systems Procedures

After learning and practicing the fundamental procedures for artificial nails, you will now look at the procedures for the artificial nail systems. These include wraps, acrylics and gels as well as maintenance and removal procedures for the three systems. The more you practice and perfect the following core services in the nail salon, the more sucessful you will be.

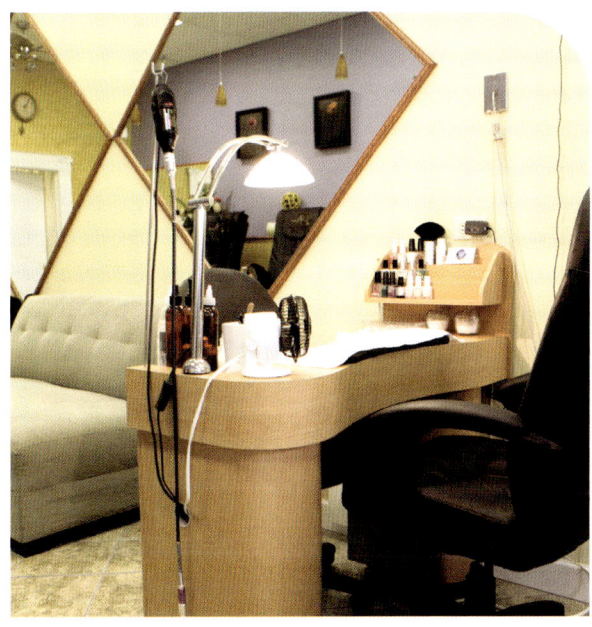

NOTES

NAIL SYSTEMS PROCEDURES
• TABLE OF CONTENTS •

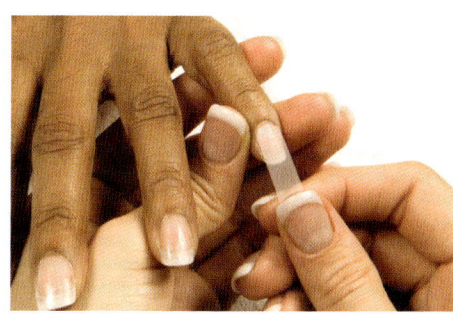

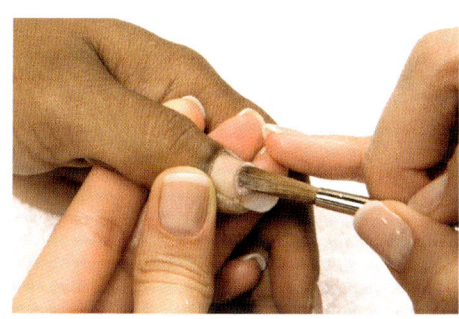

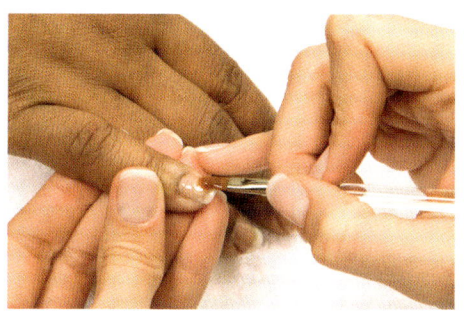

NAIL WRAP OVERLAY

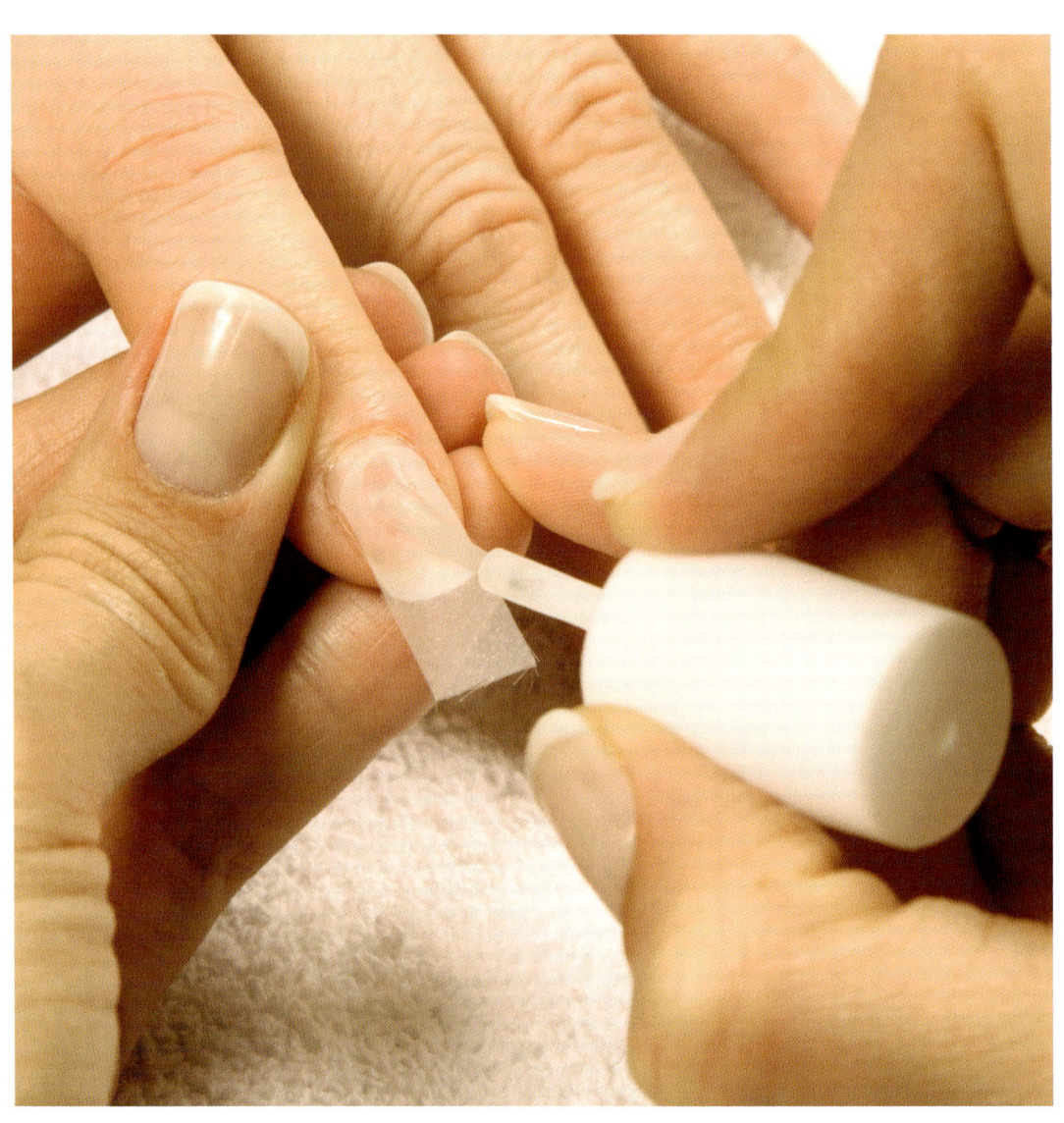

FIVE PHASES OF SERVICE

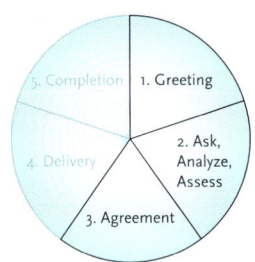

Preparing for a successful service involves the first Three Phases of Service:

1. Greeting—Establish rapport
2. Ask, Analyze and Assess—Offer professional advice
3. Agreement—Clarify expectations

NAIL WRAP OVERLAY PREPARATION

After completing the consultation, it is advisable to ask the client to remove any jewelry from hands and wrists. **Require that hands be washed with liquid or foam soap**.

Products
- Liquid soap
- Antiseptic sanitizer
- Polish remover
- Cuticle remover
- Cuticle oil
- Nail adhesive
- Resin
- Accelerator
- Hand lotion or cream
- Nail preparation solution
- Polishes

Implements
- Nail brush
- Cuticle pusher
- Cuticle nippers
- Nail clippers
- Tip cutter
- Tweezers
- Small scissors
- Files
- Buffer

Supplies
- Cotton or lint-free wipes in a disinfected glass container
- Nail tips
- Towels
- Disposable towels
- Orangewood stick
- Fabric

Equipment
- Manicure table
- Table lamp
- Glass container
- Disinfection container filled with EPA-registered, broad spectrum (hospital-level) disinfectant
- Technician and client chairs

Basic Table Set-Up
- Clean and disinfect surface of table with an EPA-registered, broad spectrum (hospital-level) disinfectant.
- Place polishes on left side of table.
- Place all other products on right side of table in the order of use.
- Place disinfection container filled with an EPA-registered, broad spectrum (hospital-level) disinfectant on right side of table.
- Disinfect all implements properly before beginning.
- Place clean towel on table, making sure to cover client cushion, if there is one. Place all implements on towel.
- Place a covered trash can on the floor to right. If a trash can is not available, fasten a plastic bag to right side of table and discard the bag after every service.
- The drawer is used to store new materials in the original container or sealed bag. Never place used or unsanitized items in drawer. Store additional clean implements in a covered container in drawer.

NAIL WRAP OVERLAY PROCEDURE

With a nail wrap procedure, woven materials (fabrics or mesh) are applied to natural nails or nails with tips to add strength. Nail wraps are also good for quick nail repairs. Fiberglass, silk, linen and nylon are some examples of fabrics used in nail wraps. Note that the procedure below corresponds with the step-by-step technical images that follow.

4. Delivery - Meet client's expectations

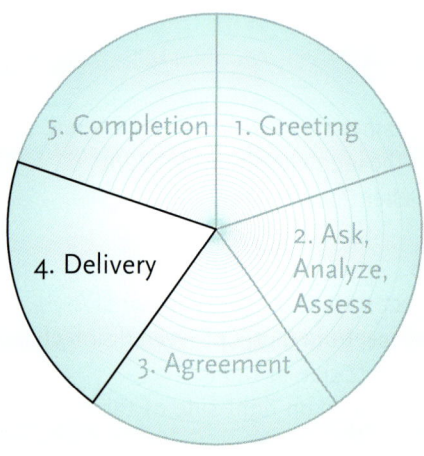

PREPARE NAILS

1. Prepare nails following **Basic Artificial Nail Preparation Procedure** on page 279
2. Apply tips, if desired, following **Nail Tip Application** on page 284

APPLY FABRIC

3. Size fabric and apply to nails
4. Trim fabric

APPLY RESIN

5. Apply resin to all nails on first hand
6. Apply accelerator to all nails on first hand

REPEAT APPLY RESIN (Steps 5-6), second hand

7. Apply resin to all nails on first hand
8. Apply accelerator to all nails on first hand

REPEAT APPLY RESIN (Steps 7-8), second hand

9. Apply resin to all nails on first hand
10. Apply accelerator to all nails on first hand

REPEAT APPLY RESIN (Steps 9-10), second hand

BALANCE

11. Balance nails following **Basic Artificial Nail Balancing Procedure** on page 288

FINISH

12. Finish nails following **Basic Artificial Nail Finishing Procedure** on page 290

NAIL WRAP OVERLAY

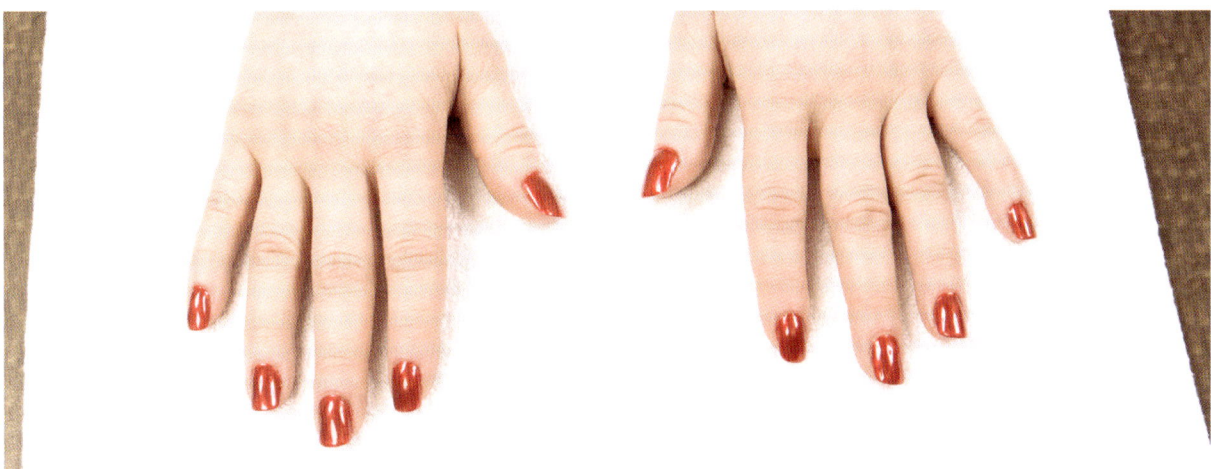

 A checkmark next to a step indicates an ideal time to check on your client's comfort, and to take extra safety precautions.

PREPARE NAILS

1. Prepare nails following Basic Artificial Nail Preparation Procedure on page 279.
   - ANALYZE
   - CUTICLE CARE
   - FILE

2. Apply tips, if desired, following Nail Tip Application on page 284.
   - PREPARE TIPS
   - APPLY TIPS
   - FILE TIPS

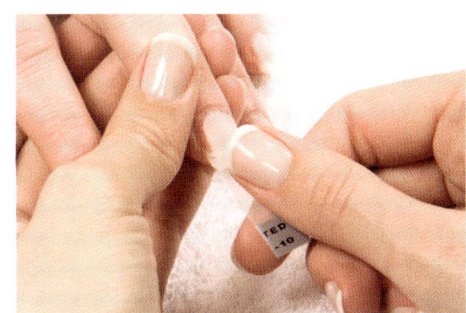

APPLY FABRIC

3. Size fabric and apply to nails.
   - Cut fabric to approximate width and length of nail.
   - Make sure fabric is slightly smaller (approximately 1/16" or 0.16 cm) than nail to help prevent lifting.
   - Apply coat of resin (adhesive) to nail.
   - Place fabric onto nail using your fingers or tweezers if necessary.
   - Use a small piece of plastic to smooth.
   - Repeat on all 10 nails.

NOTE: Although you can use your fingers to place the fabric onto the nail, avoid handling the fabric excessively to prevent contamination.

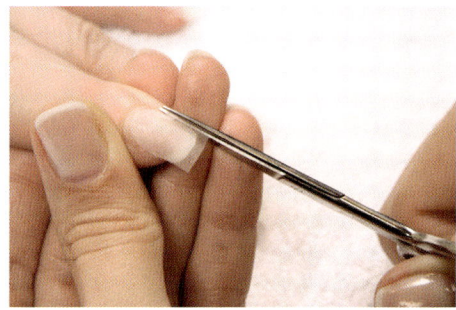

4. **Trim fabric with small scissors if necessary.**
   - Use caution not to cut skin while trimming with scissors.

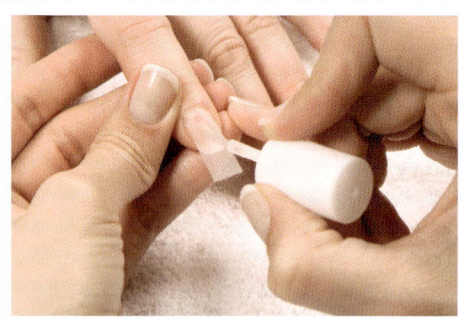

APPLY RESIN

5. **Apply resin to all nails on first hand.**
   - Cover entire nail plate with resin and seal free edge of nail.
   - Follow manufacturer's instructions on application procedure.

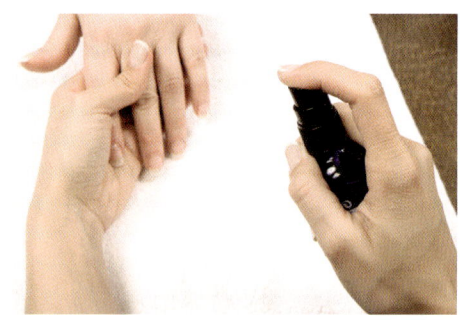

6. **Apply accelerator to all nails on first hand.**
   - Follow manufacturer's instructions for application.
   - File using downward stroke on free edge to remove any excess fabric if necessary.

REPEAT APPLY RESIN (Steps 5–6), second hand.

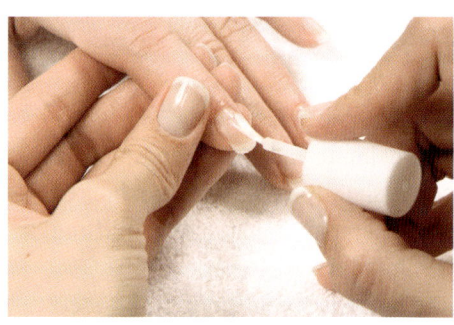

7. **Apply resin to all nails on first hand.**
   - Cover entire nail plate with resin and seal free edge of nail.
   - Follow manufacturer's instructions on application procedure.

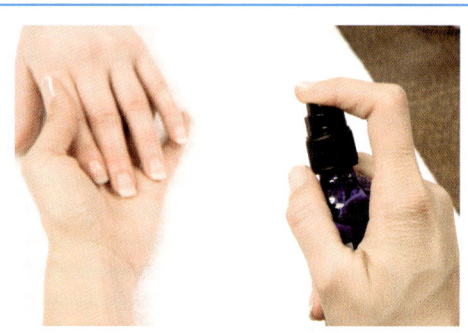

8. **Apply accelerator to all nails on first hand.**

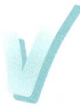

REPEAT APPLY RESIN (Steps 7–8), second hand.

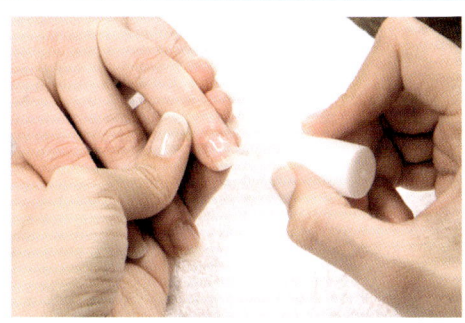

9. **Apply resin to all nails on first hand.**
   - Cover entire nail plate with resin and seal free edge of nail.
   - Follow manufacturer's instructions on application.

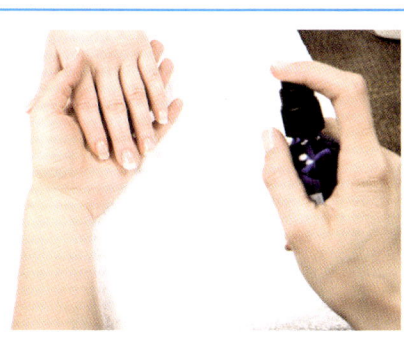

10. **Apply accelerator to all nails on first hand.**
    - Follow manufacturer's instructions for application.

REPEAT APPLY RESIN (Steps 9–10), second hand.

NOTE: Always follow manufacturer's instructions for application. While many manufacturers recommend three layers of resin, some may recommend fewer and some may recommend additional layers. Follow the same procedures to create each additional layer of resin.

BALANCE

11. Balance nails following Basic Artificial Nail Balancing Procedure on page 288.

FINISH

12. Finish nails following Basic Artificial Nail Finishing Procedure on page 290.

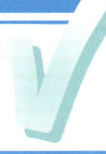

TWO-WEEK NAIL WRAP MAINTENANCE

A checkmark next to a step indicates an ideal time to check on your client's comfort, and to take extra safety precautions.

PREPARE NAILS

1. Prepare nails following Basic Artificial Nail Preparation Procedure on page 279.
   - ANALYZE
     - Check for cracks or any lifting or separation of product.
     - If cracks, lifting or separation are present, carefully file away product from area.
     - If necessary, completely remove product from nail following Nail Wrap Removal Procedure on page 307.

NOTE: Avoid removing lifted product with nippers or clippers. Doing so may damage the natural nail.

   - CUTICLE CARE

   - FILE
     - Blend "old product" with new growth using 180-grit file or higher to eliminate line of demarcation.
     - Thin entire nail; free edge and sidewalls should be thinnest.
     - Concentrate on product: Only remove shine on natural nail using 240-grit file.
     - Hold file flat against nail to prevent damaging natural nail.
     - Shape free edge and remove length. If natural nail is the same length as the enhancement, use 240-grit file or higher.

NOTE: Avoid trimming free edge with nail clippers. Doing so may create small cracks in the product and tip.

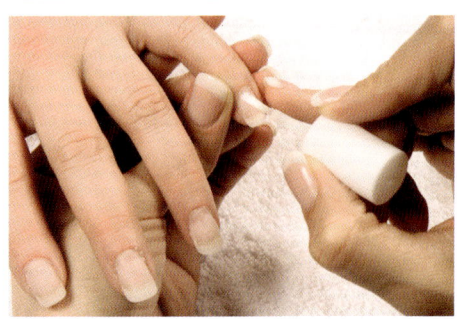

APPLY RESIN

2. Apply resin over the new growth area.
   - Apply to all nails on the first hand.
   - Follow manufacturer's instructions for application.

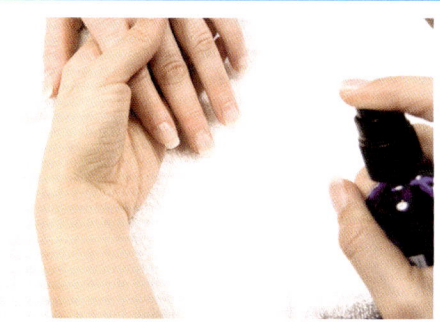

3. **Apply accelerator to all nails on first hand.**
   - Follow manufacturer's instructions for application.

REPEAT APPLY RESIN (Steps 2–3), second hand.

REPEAT APPLY RESIN (Steps 2–3), first hand.
- Apply resin to entire nail and seal free edge.

REPEAT APPLY RESIN (Steps 2–3), second hand.
- Follow manufacturer's instructions regarding the number of layers of resin and accelerator to be applied.

BALANCE

4. Balance nails following Basic Artificial Nail Balancing Procedure on page 288.

FINISH

5. Finish nails following Basic Artificial Nail Finishing Procedure on page 290.

9

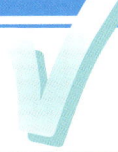

FOUR-WEEK NAIL WRAP MAINTENANCE

A checkmark next to a step indicates an ideal time to check on your client's comfort, and to take extra safety precautions.

PREPARE NAILS

1. Prepare nails following Basic Artificial Nail Preparation Procedure on page 279.
   - ANALYZE
     - Check for cracks or any lifting or separation of product.
     - If cracks, lifting or separation are present, carefully file away product from area.
     - If necessary, completely remove product from nail following Nail Wrap Removal Procedure on page 307.

NOTE: Avoid removing lifted product with nippers or clippers. Doing so may damage the natural nail.

   - CUTICLE CARE

   - FILE
     - Blend "old product" with new growth using 180-grit file or higher to eliminate line of demarcation.
     - Thin entire nail; free edge and sidewalls should be thinnest.
     - Concentrate on product: Only remove shine on natural nail using 240-grit file.
     - Hold file flat against nail to prevent damaging natural nail.
     - Shape free edge and remove length. If natural nail is the same length as the enhancement, use 240-grit file or higher.

NOTE: Avoid trimming free edge with nail clippers. Doing so may create small cracks in the product and tip.

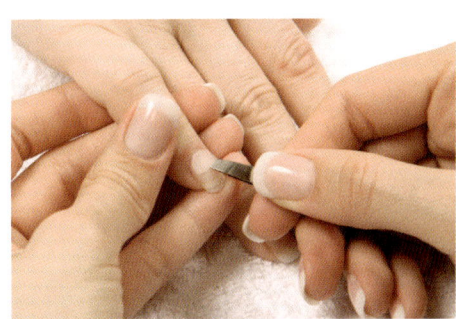

APPLY FABRIC

2. Size fabric and apply to nails.
   - Cut fabric to approximate width and length of new growth area of nail.
   - Make sure fabric is slightly smaller to help prevent lifting.
   - Apply coat of resin (adhesive) to nail.
   - Place fabric onto nail using tweezers if necessary.
   - Use a small piece of plastic to smooth.
   - Repeat on all 10 nails.

NOTE: Avoid touching fabric as much as possible to prevent contamination.

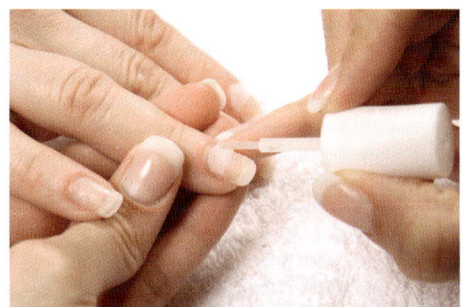

APPLY RESIN

3. **Apply resin over new growth area on first hand.**
   - Follow manufacturer's instructions for application.

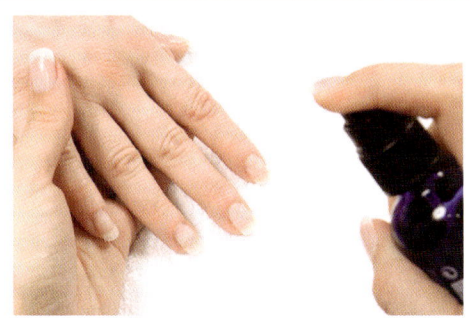

4. **Apply accelerator to all nails on first hand.**
   - Follow manufacturer's instructions for application.

REPEAT APPLY RESIN (Steps 3-4), second hand.

REPEAT APPLY RESIN (Steps 3-4), first hand.
- Apply resin to entire nail and seal free edge.

REPEAT APPLY RESIN (Steps 3-4), second hand.
- Follow manufacturer's instructions regarding the number of layers of resin and accelerator to be applied.

BALANCE

5. Balance nails following Basic Artificial Nail Balancing Procedure on page 288.

FINISH

6. Finish nails following Basic Artificial Nail Finishing Procedure on page 290.

NATURAL NAIL REPAIR WITH WRAP

A checkmark next to a step indicates an ideal time to check on your client's comfort, and to take extra safety precautions.

PREPARE NAIL

1. Prepare the nail following Basic Artificial Nail Preparation Procedure on page 279.
   - ANALYZE
   - CUTICLE CARE
   - FILE

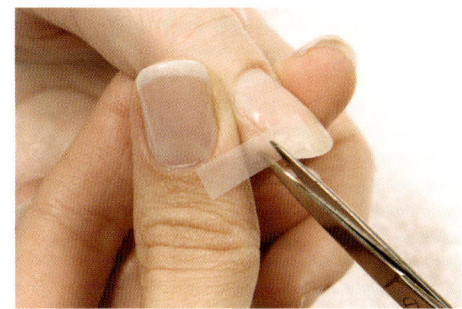

2. **Size fabric and apply to break.**
   - Cut fabric to the size and shape that will completely cover the broken area.
   - For a "stress strip," the fabric should be approximately 1/8" (0.32 cm) thick and the width of the nail to cover the weak area of the nail.
   - Apply coat of resin (adhesive) to nail.
   - Place fabric onto nail over the break using tweezers if necessary.
   - Use a small piece of plastic to smooth.

NOTE: Although you can use your fingers to place the fabric onto the nail, avoid handling fabric excessively to prevent contamination.

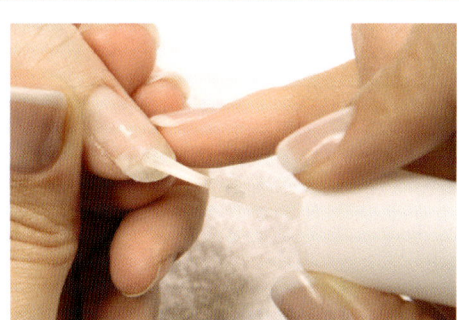

APPLY RESIN
3. **Apply resin to the nail.**
   - Cover the fabric completely.
   - Follow manufacturer's instructions for application.

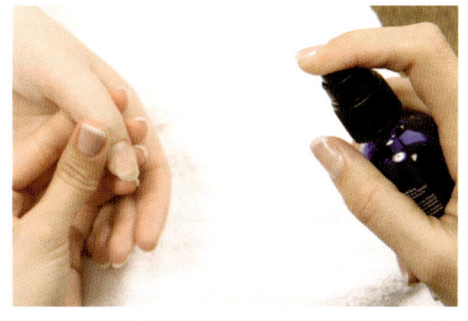

4. **Apply accelerator to the nail.**
   - Follow manufacturer's instructions for application.

REPEAT APPLY RESIN (Steps 3-4)

REPEAT APPLY RESIN (Steps 3-4)

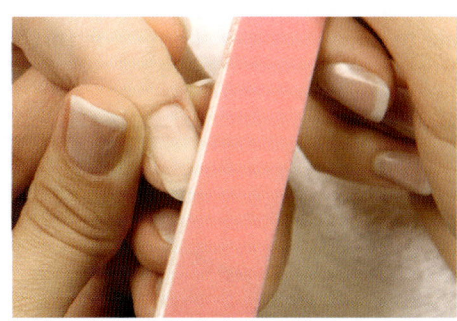

5. **Shape and refine.**
   - Use a buffer to refine the surface of the nail, blending the repair into the natural nail.

Proceed with desired service, such as a manicure or polish

NAIL WRAP REMOVAL

A checkmark next to a step indicates an ideal time to check on your client's comfort, and to take extra safety precautions.

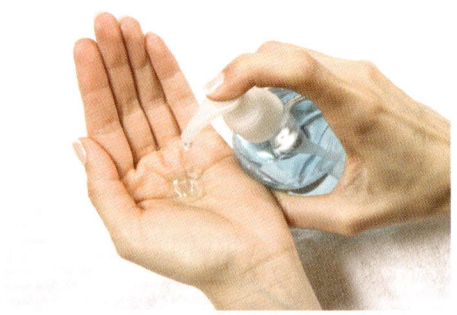

1. **Wash and sanitize your hands.**
   - Use liquid or foam soap.
   - Use waterless sanitizer or topical antiseptic if required by regulating agency.
   - Wear protective gloves if required by regulating agency.

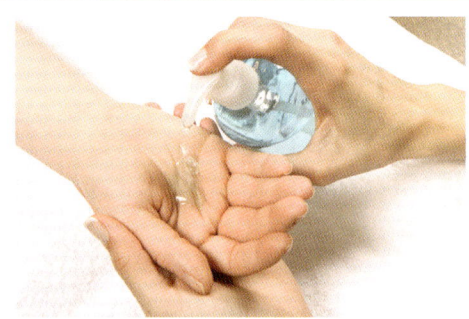

2. **Sanitize client's hands.**
   - Use waterless sanitizer or topical antiseptic if required by regulating agency.

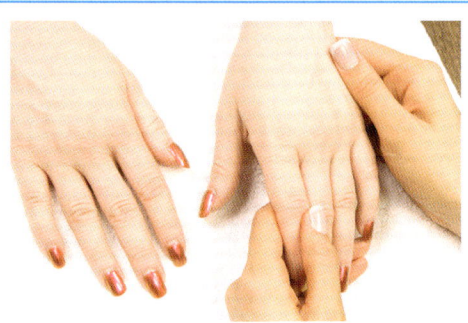

ANALYZE

3. **Perform visual analysis of hands.**
   - Continue with service if hands are free of any visible signs of diseases or disorders.

Skin: Signs to look for during analysis on hands include open skin, redness, swelling, discoloration or any other signs of an infection that would prevent the service from being performed.

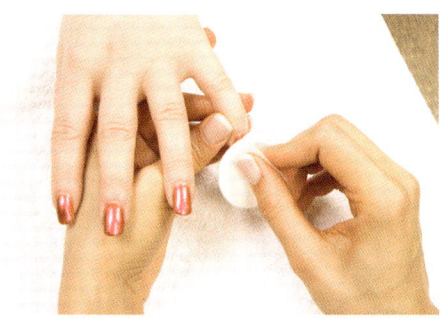

4. **Remove polish.**
   - Use a lint-free wipe or cotton saturated with polish remover on nail plate.
   - Let remover set for a few seconds.
   - Wipe toward free edge.
   - Remove all polish from each nail before moving to next nail.
   - Repeat on other hand.

9

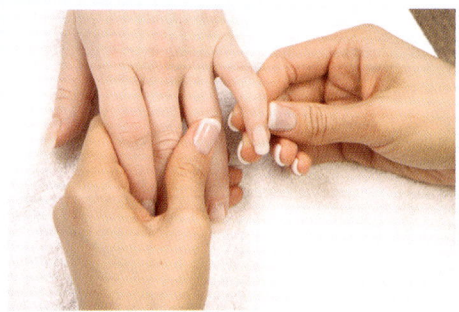

5. **Perform visual analysis of nails.**
   - Continue with service if nail plates are free of any visible signs of diseases or disorders.

Nails: Signs to look for during analysis on fingernails include discoloration, flaking, swelling, pain indicators, pus, detached nail plate, growth under the nail or any other signs of an infection that would prevent the service from being performed.

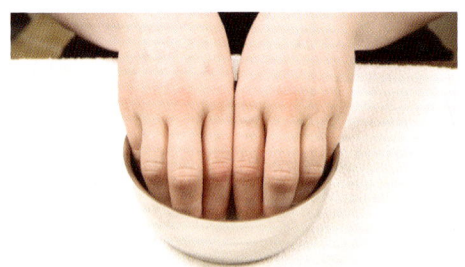

6. **Soak nails.**
   - Place all nails in a finger bowl (glass or metal) containing acetone or artificial nail product remover.
   - Completely submerge nails for approximately 10 minutes.

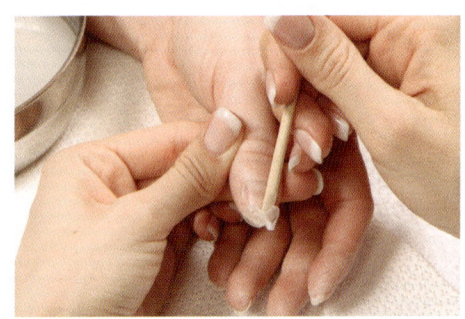

7. **Push product off.**
   - Remove first hand from bowl.
   - Use orangewood stick to push softened product toward free edge and off nail.
   - Replace nails in acetone if necessary.

NOTE: It may be necessary to soak nails for more than 10 minutes to completely remove product. Patience is sometimes required during this process.

NOTE: Avoid removing product with nippers or clippers. Doing so may damage the natural nail.

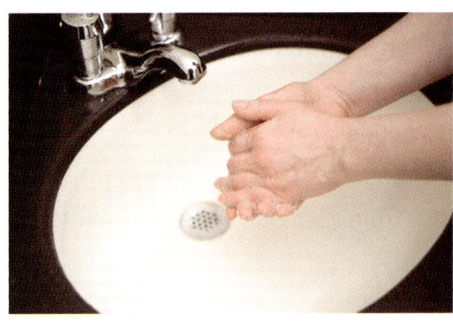

8. **Wash hands.**
   - Remove chemicals from the skin to prevent irritation.
   - Wash hands (yours and client's) with nail brush.

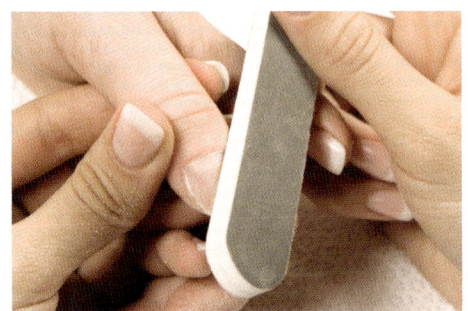

9. **Shape and buff nails.**
- Use file to shape free edge.
- Gently buff nails to remove any residue from softened product.

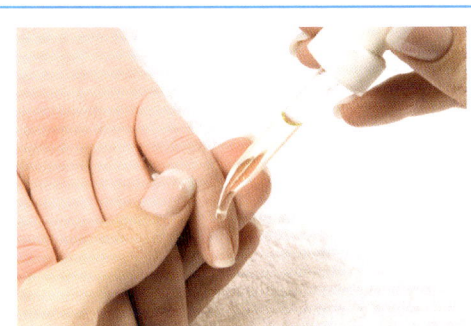

10. **Apply cuticle conditioner.**
- Use cotton-tipped orangewood stick, cotton swab or dropper.
- Apply to all 10 fingers.
- Gently massage conditioner into cuticle area.

9

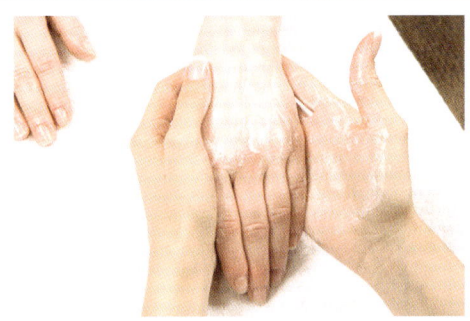

11. **Apply lotion or cream to client's hands.**
- Apply lotion to the hands using effleurage movements.

NOTE: You may recommend to your clients that they use a cuticle conditioner and lotion daily to prevent dryness from acetone.

Proceed with desired service.

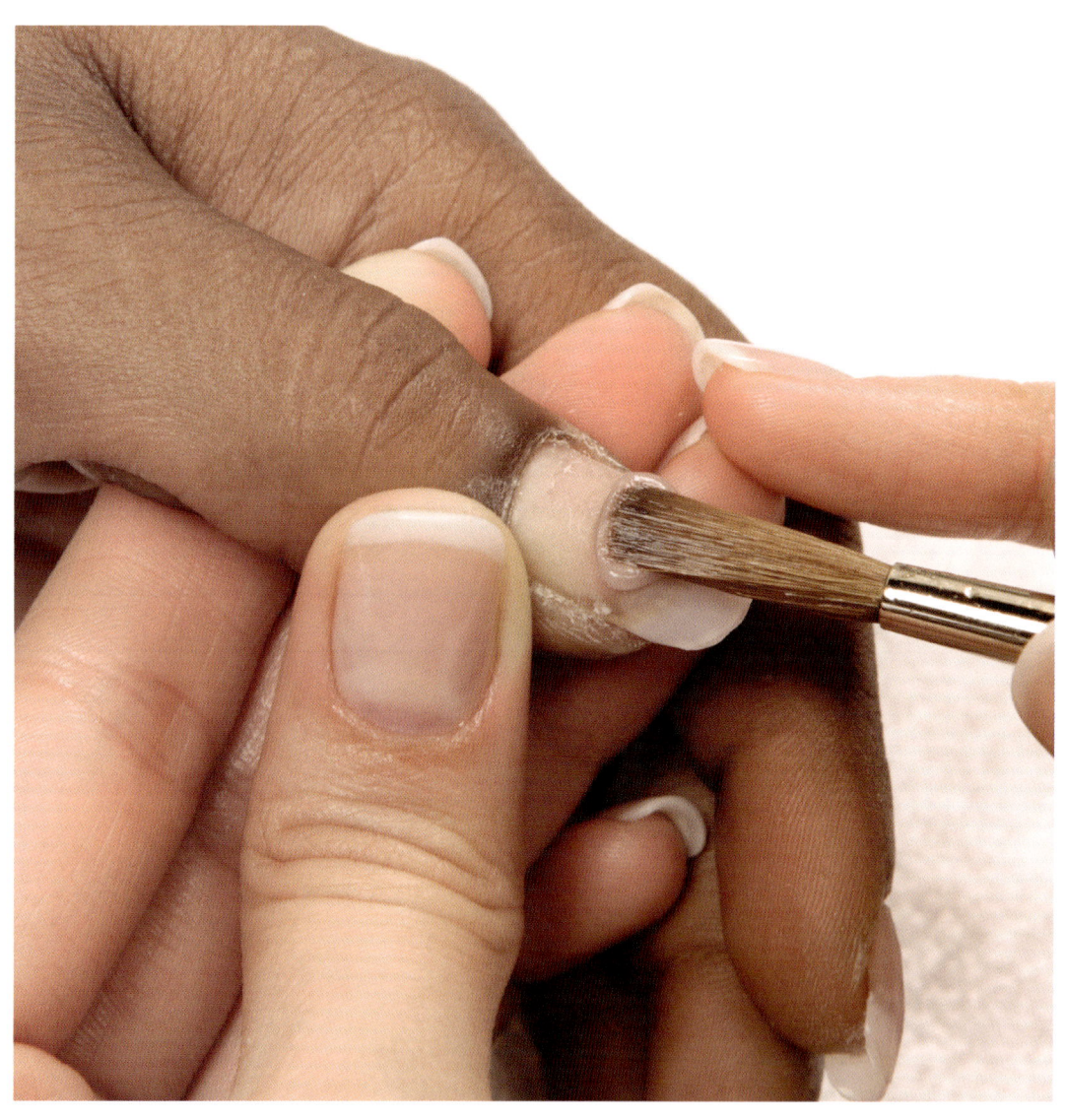

FIVE PHASES OF SERVICE

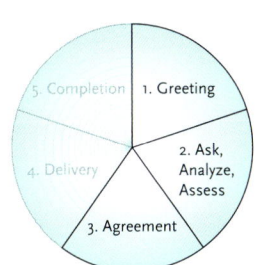

Preparing for a successful service involves the first Three Phases of Service:

1. Greeting—Establish rapport
2. Ask, Analyze and Assess—Offer professional advice
3. Agreement—Clarify expectations

ACRYLIC NAIL OVERLAY PREPARATION

After completing the consultation, it is advisable to ask the client to remove any jewelry from hands and wrists. **Require that hands be washed with liquid or foam soap**.

Products
- Liquid soap
- Antiseptic sanitizer
- Polish remover
- Cuticle remover
- Nail adhesive
- Nail preparation solution
- Cuticle oil
- Monomer
- Polymer
- Primer
- Dehydrator
- Polishes

Implements
- Nail brush
- Cuticle pusher
- Cuticle nippers
- Nail clippers
- Tip cutter
- Acrylic brush
- Files
- Buffer

Supplies
- Cotton or lint-free wipes in a disinfected glass container
- Nail tips
- Towels
- Disposable towels
- Orangewood stick

Equipment
- Manicure table
- Table lamp
- Glass container
- Disinfection container filled with EPA-registered, broad spectrum (hospital-level) disinfectant
- Technician and client chairs

Basic Table Set-Up
- Clean and disinfect surface of table with an EPA-registered, broad spectrum (hospital-level) disinfectant.
- Place polishes on left side of table.
- Place all other products on right side of table in order of use.
- Place disinfection container filled with an EPA-registered, broad spectrum (hospital-level) disinfectant on right side of table.
- Disinfect all implements properly before beginning.
- Place clean towel on table, making sure to cover client cushion, if there is one. Place all implements on towel.
- Place a covered trash can on floor to right. If a trash can is not available, fasten a plastic bag to right side of table and discard bag after every service.
- The drawer is used to store new materials in original container or sealed bag. Never place used or unsanitized items in drawer. Store additional clean implements in a covered container in drawer.

SINGLE-COLOR ACRYLIC NAIL OVERLAY PROCEDURE

Acrylic nails are applied using a mixture of monomer (acrylic liquid) and polymer (acrylic powder). Note that the procedure below corresponds with the step-by-step technical images that follow.

4. Delivery - Meet client's expectations

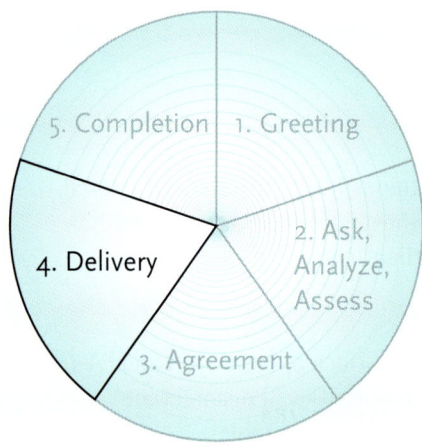

PREPARE NAILS

1. Prepare nails following **Basic Artificial Nail Preparation Procedure** on page 279

2. Apply nail tips, if desired, following **Nail Tip Application** on page 284

3. Apply primer

PREPARE PRODUCT

4. Prepare acrylic liquid and acrylic powder
5. Prepare brush

SCULPT ZONE 1

6. Pick up and apply first acrylic bead

SCULPT ZONE 2

7. Pick up and apply second acrylic bead

SCULPT ZONE 3

8. Pick up and apply third acrylic bead

REPEAT SCULPT ZONE 1, 2, AND 3 (Steps 6–8) on remaining nails

BALANCE

9. Balance nails following **Basic Artificial Nail Balancing Procedure** on page 288

FINISH

10. Finish nails following **Basic Artificial Nail Finishing Procedure** on page 290

SINGLE-COLOR ACRYLIC NAIL OVERLAY

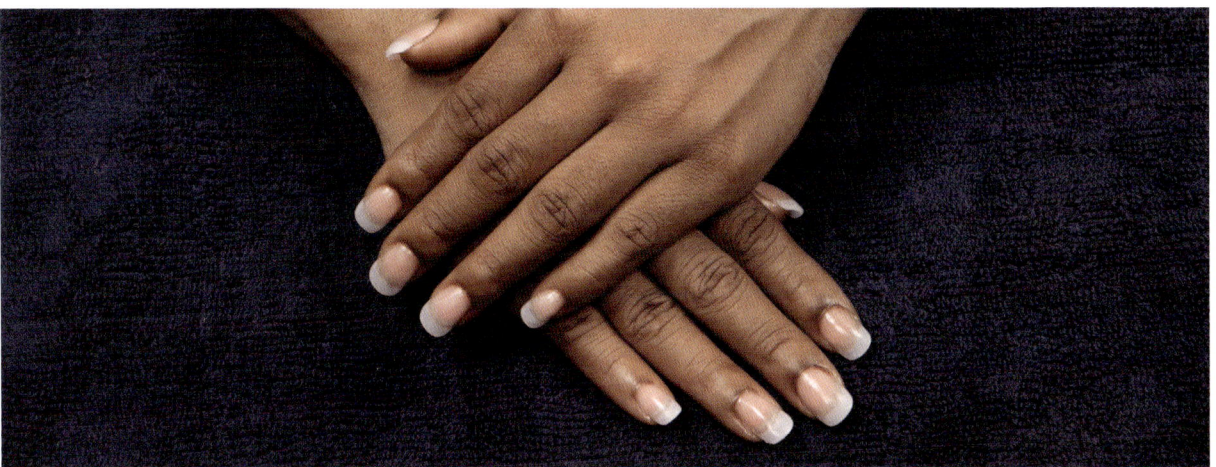

9

 A checkmark next to a step indicates an ideal time to check on your client's comfort, and to take extra safety precautions.

PREPARE NAILS

1. Prepare nails following Basic Artificial Nail Preparation Procedure on page 279.
   - ANALYZE
   - CUTICLE CARE
   - FILE

2. Apply nail tips, if desired, following Nail Tip Application on page 284.
   - PREPARE TIPS
   - APPLY TIPS
   - FILE TIPS

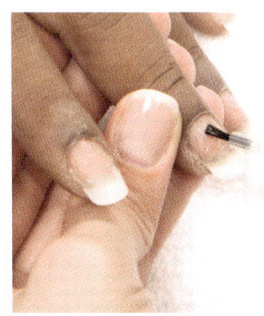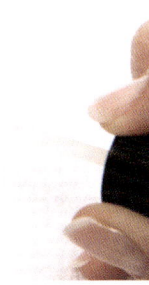

3. Apply primer if necessary according to manufacturer's instructions.
   - Apply primer only to natural nail.
   - Avoid allowing primer to touch skin.
   - Allow it to dry.

   NOTE: Some primers appear chalky white when dry.

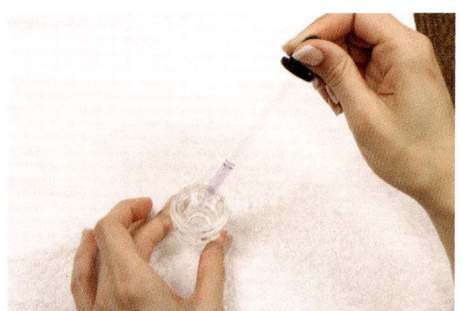

PREPARE PRODUCT

4. **Prepare acrylic liquid and acrylic powder.**
    *   Place small amount of acrylic liquid in dappen dish.
    *   Place small amount of acrylic powder in separate dappen dish.
    *   Refer to Forming an Acrylic Bead on page 269.

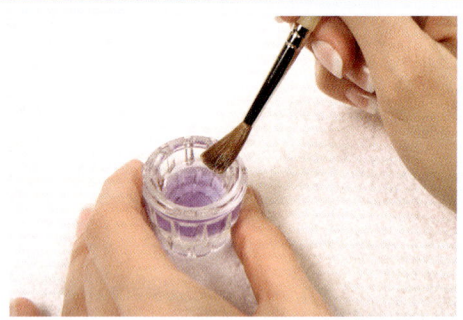

5. **Prepare brush.**
    *   Submerge brush completely into acrylic liquid pressing hairs flat against bottom. Move around to release air trapped in brush.
    *   When removing brush from dappen dish, wipe against sides to flatten brush on both sides.

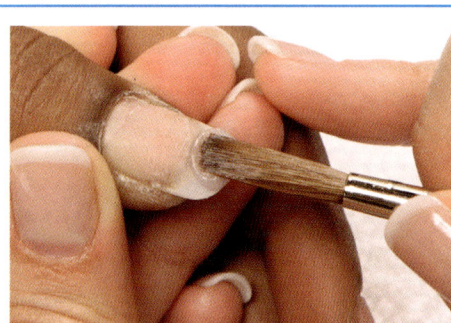

SCULPT ZONE 1

6. **Pick up and apply first acrylic bead.**
    *   Pick up a medium-sized bead of acrylic.
    *   Place bead on nail or tip to create Zone 1.
    *   Press middle of bead down holding brush parallel to nail.
    *   Press each side of bead down rotating angle of brush to follow the c-curve of nail.
    *   Continue working in this manner to distribute product in Zone 1.
    *   Distribute product so it is thinnest at free edge and thickest toward Zone 2.

NOTE: Avoid touching skin with brush or any product.

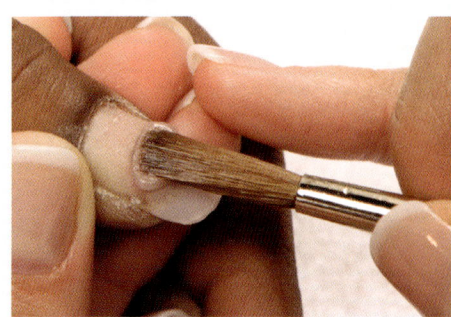

SCULPT ZONE 2

7. **Pick up and apply second acrylic bead.**
    *   Pick up a medium to large-sized bead of acrylic.
    *   Place it directly behind Zone 1.
    *   Hold brush at approximately 45° or slightly smaller angle.
    *   Press acrylic to distribute in same manner as in Step 6.
    *   Make sure product is thinnest at sidewalls.
    *   Blend remaining product into Zone 1.

NOTE: Avoid touching skin with brush or any product.

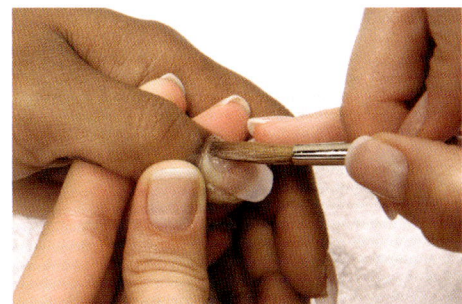

SCULPT ZONE 3

8. **Pick up and apply third acrylic bead.**
   - Pick up a small-sized bead of acrylic.
   - Place it directly behind Zone 2.
   - Hold the brush at a slightly higher angle than 45°.
   - Press acrylic to distribute it in the same manner as in Step 6.
   - Make sure product is thinnest at sidewalls and cuticle.
   - Blend remaining product into Zone 2.

NOTE: Avoid touching skin with brush or any product.

9

NOTE: When first beginning to work with acrylic it may be easier to use smaller beads. Always form Zone 1 first and work toward Zone 3. Distribute product in the same manner, pressing it from side to side. Place the next bead of acrylic directly behind the previous one and blend. Make sure to cover the entire nail without allowing the product to come into contact with the skin.

REPEAT SCULPT ZONE 1, 2, AND 3 (Steps 6–8) on remaining nails.
   - Work from little finger to thumb on each hand.

BALANCE

9. Balance nails following Basic Artificial Nail Balancing Procedure on page 288.

FINISH

10. Finish nails following Basic Artificial Nail Finishing Procedure on page 290.

PINK AND WHITE SCULPTURED ACRYLIC NAILS

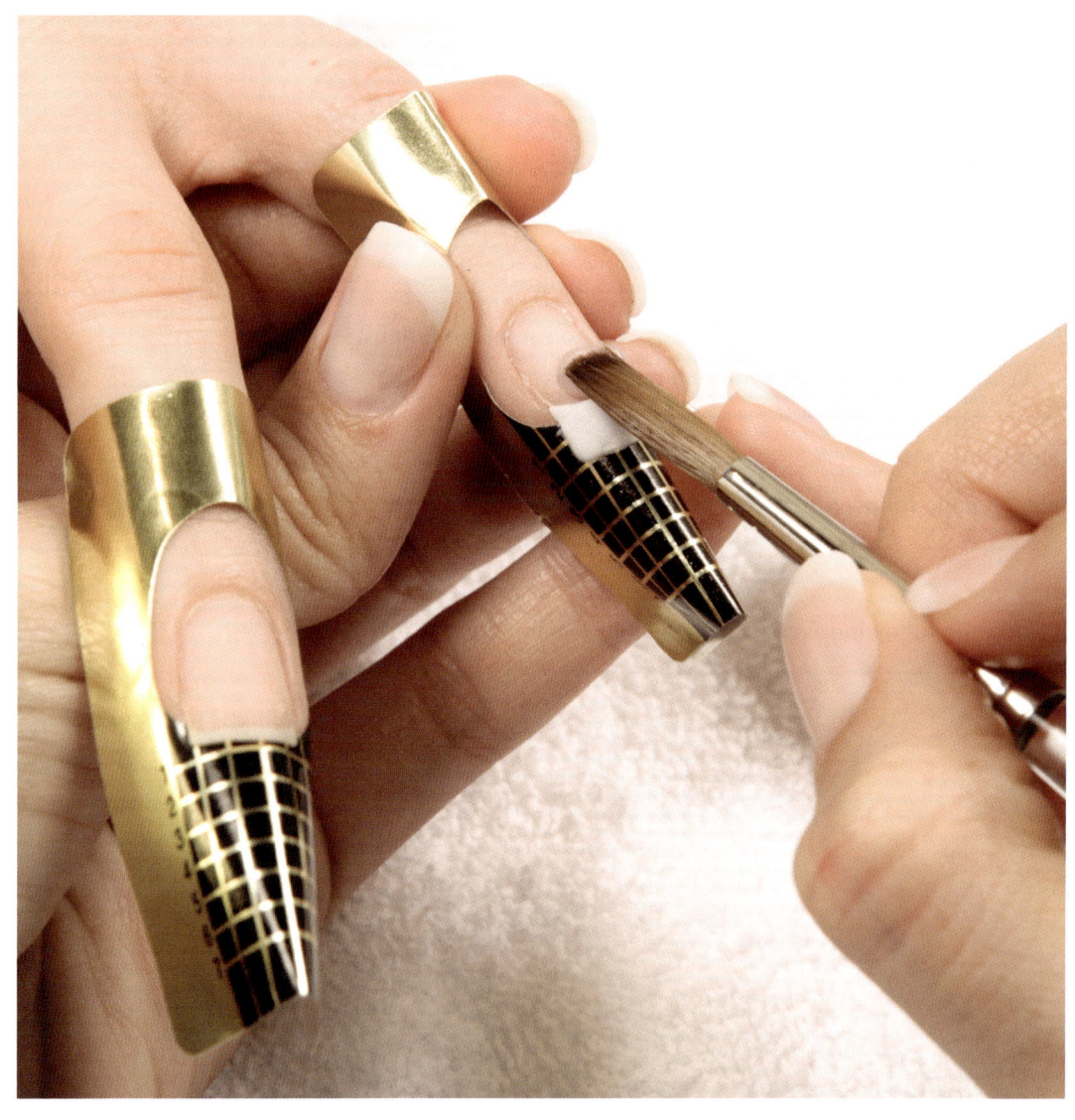

FIVE PHASES OF SERVICE

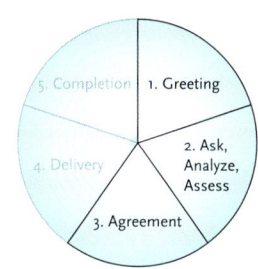

Preparing for a successful service involves the first Three Phases of Service:

1. Greeting—Establish rapport
2. Ask, Analyze and Assess—Offer professional advice
3. Agreement—Clarify expectations

SCULPTURED ACRYLIC NAIL PREPARATION

After completing the consultation, it is advisable to ask the client to remove any jewelry from hands and wrists. **Require that hands be washed with liquid or foam soap**.

Products
- Liquid soap
- Antiseptic sanitizer
- Polish remover
- Cuticle remover
- Nail adhesive
- Nail preparation solution
- Cuticle oil
- Monomer
- Polymer
- Primer
- Dehydrator
- Polishes

Implements
- Nail brush
- Cuticle pusher
- Cuticle nippers
- Nail clippers
- Tip cutter
- Acrylic brush
- Files
- Buffer

Supplies
- Cotton or lint-free wipes in a disinfected glass container
- Nail tips
- Towels
- Disposable towels
- Orangewood stick
- Nail forms

Equipment
- Manicure table
- Table lamp
- Glass container
- Disinfection container filled with EPA-registered, broad spectrum (hospital-level) disinfectant
- Technician and client chairs

Basic Table Set-Up
- Clean and disinfect surface of table with an EPA-registered, broad spectrum (hospital-level) disinfectant.
- Place polishes on left side of table.
- Place all other products on right side of table in order of use.
- Place disinfection container filled with an EPA-registered, broad spectrum (hospital-level) disinfectant on right side of table.
- Disinfect all implements properly before beginning.
- Place clean towel on table, making sure to cover client cushion, if there is one. Place all implements on towel.
- Place covered trash can on floor to right. If a trash can is not available, fasten a plastic bag to right side of table and discard bag after every service.
- The drawer is used to store new materials in original container or sealed bag. Never place used or unsanitized items in drawer. Store additional clean implements in a covered container in drawer.

PINK AND WHITE SCULPTURED ACRYLIC NAIL PROCEDURE

Pink and white sculptured nails are sometimes referred to as a "permanent French manicure." You can choose any color acrylic to apply over nail forms for sculptured nails. Note that the procedure below corresponds with the step-by-step technical images that follow.

4. Delivery - Meet client's expectations

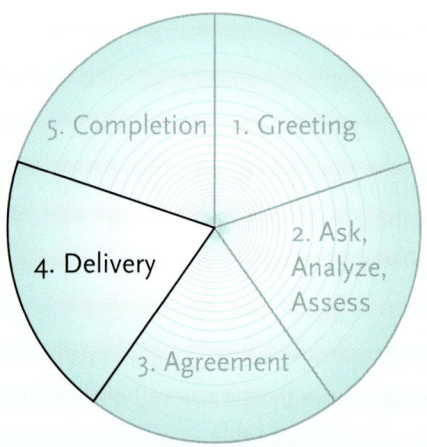

PREPARE NAILS

1. Prepare nails following **Basic Artificial Nail Preparation Procedure** on page 279

2. Apply forms

3. Apply primer

PREPARE PRODUCT

4. Prepare acrylic liquid and pink and white acrylic powder

5. Prepare brush

SCULPT ZONE 1

6. Pick up and apply white acrylic bead

SCULPT ZONE 2

7. Pick up and apply first pink acrylic bead

SCULPT ZONE 3

8. Pick up and apply second pink acrylic bead

REPEAT SCULPT ZONE 1, 2, AND 3 (Steps 6-8) on remaining nails

BALANCE

9. Balance nails following **Basic Artificial Nail Balancing Procedure** on page 288

FINISH

10. Finish nails following **Basic Artificial Nail Finishing Procedure** on page 290

PINK AND WHITE SCULPTURED ACRYLIC NAILS

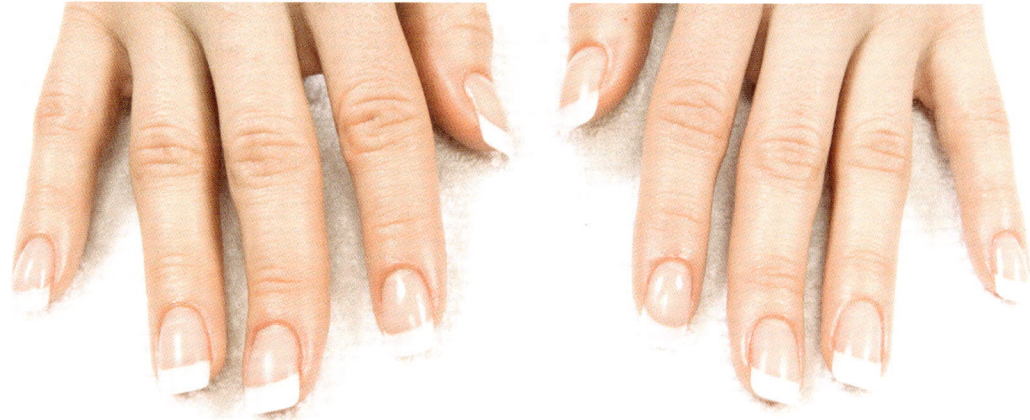

9

 A checkmark next to a step indicates an ideal time to check on your client's comfort, and to take extra safety precautions.

PREPARE NAILS

1. **Prepare nails following** Basic Artificial Nail Preparation Procedure **on page 279.**
   - ANALYZE
   - CUTICLE CARE
   - FILE

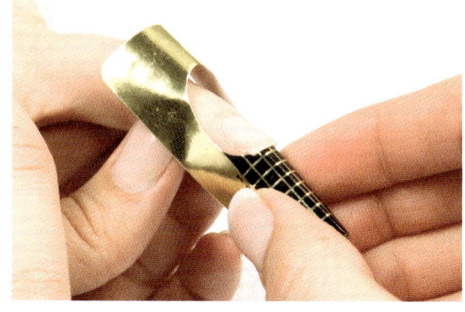

2. **Apply forms.**
   - Place form under free edge of each nail.
   - Pinch or roll form to match the natural c-curve.
   - Check to make sure each one fits snugly under free edge with no gap and is under both corners of nail.

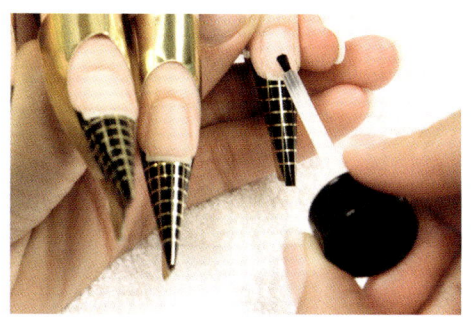

3. **Apply primer if necessary according to manufacturer's instructions.**
   - Apply primer only to natural nail.
   - Avoid allowing primer to touch skin.
   - Allow it to dry.

   NOTE: Some primers appear chalky white when dry.

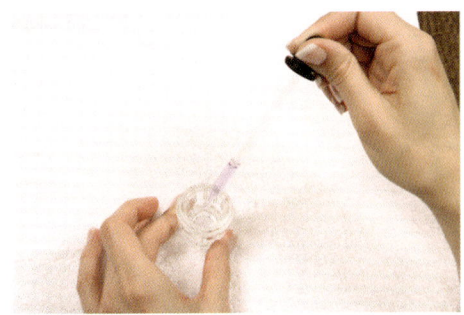

PREPARE PRODUCT

4. **Prepare acrylic liquid and pink and white acrylic powder.**
   - Place a small amount of acrylic liquid in a dappen dish.
   - Place a small amount of pink acrylic powder in a separate dappen dish.
   - Place a small amount of white acrylic powder in another dappen dish.
   - Refer to Forming an Acrylic Bead on page 269.

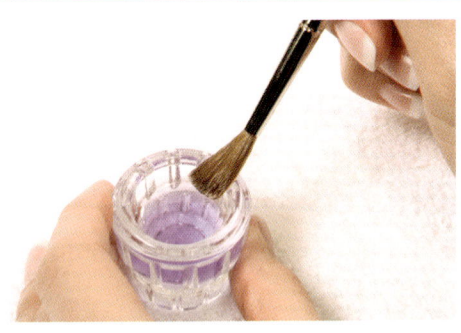

5. **Prepare brush.**
   - Submerge brush completely into acrylic liquid pressing hairs flat against bottom. Move around to release air trapped in brush.
   - When removing brush from dappen dish, wipe against sides to flatten brush on both sides.

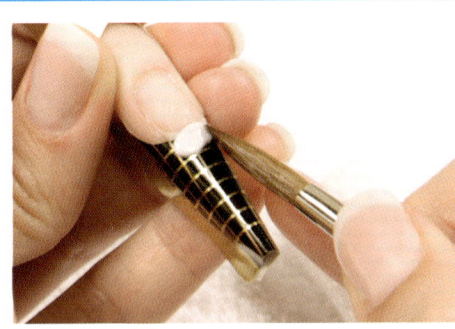

SCULPT ZONE 1

6. **Pick up and apply white acrylic bead.**
   - Pick up a medium-sized bead of white acrylic.
   - Place bead on form to create Zone 1.
   - Press middle of bead down holding brush parallel to nail.
   - Press each side of bead down rotating angle of brush to follow the c-curve of nail.
   - Continue working in this manner to distribute product in Zone 1.
   - Distribute product so it is thinnest at free edge and thickest toward Zone 2.
   - Create smile line by using small, light pressing motions.

NOTE: Avoid touching skin with brush or any product.

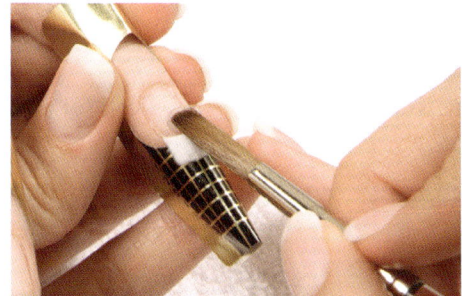

SCULPT ZONE 2

7. **Pick up and apply first pink acrylic bead.**

- Pick up a medium to large-sized bead of pink acrylic.
- Place it directly behind Zone 1.
- Hold brush at approximately 45°or slightly smaller angle.
- Press acrylic to distribute it in the same manner as in Step 6.
- Make sure product is thinnest at sidewalls.
- Blend remaining product into Zone 1.

NOTE: Avoid touching skin with brush or any product.

9

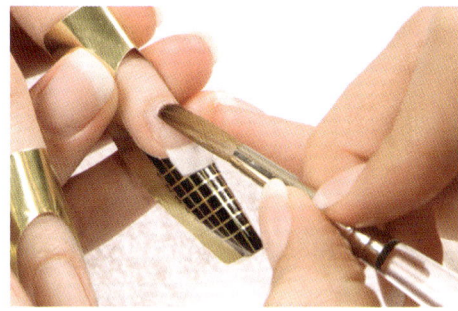

SCULPT ZONE 3

8. **Pick up and apply second pink acrylic bead.**

- Pick up a small-sized bead of pink acrylic.
- Place it directly behind Zone 2.
- Hold the brush at a slightly higher angle than 45°.
- Press acrylic to distribute it in the same manner as in Step 6.
- Make sure product is thinnest at sidewalls and cuticle.
- Blend remaining product into Zone 2.

NOTE: Avoid touching skin with brush or any product.

NOTE: When first beginning to work with acrylic, it may be easier to use smaller beads of acrylic. Always form Zone 1 first and work toward Zone 3. Distribute product in the same manner, pressing it from side to side. Place the next bead of acrylic directly behind the previous one and blend. Make sure to cover the entire nail.

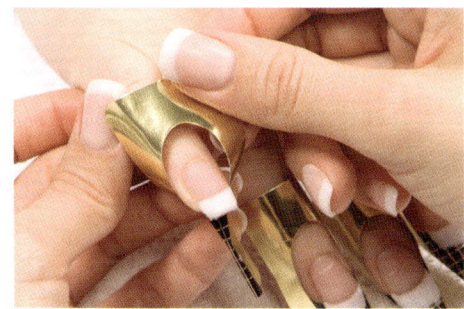

REPEAT SCULPT ZONE 1, 2 AND 3 (Steps 6–8) on remaining nails.

- Work from little finger to thumb on each hand.
- Remove forms when product is dry.

NOTE: To be sure that product is completely dry, use handle of brush to lightly tap surface of nail. If acrylic is dry it will make a clicking noise.

BALANCE

9. Balance nails following Basic Artificial Nail Balancing Procedure on page 288.

FINISH

10. Finish nails following Basic Artificial Nail Finishing Procedure on page 290.

TWO-WEEK ACRYLIC NAIL MAINTENANCE

A checkmark next to a step indicates an ideal time to check on your client's comfort, and to take extra safety precautions.

PREPARE NAILS

1. Prepare and balance nails following Basic Artificial Nail Preparation Procedure on page 279.

   • ANALYZE
      • Check for cracks or any lifting or separation of product.
      • If cracks, lifting or separation are present, carefully file away product from area.
      • If necessary, completely remove product from nail following Acrylic Nail Removal Procedure on page 327.

   NOTE: Avoid removing lifted product with nippers or clippers. Doing so may damage the natural nail.

   • CUTICLE CARE

   • FILE
      • Blend "old product" with new growth using a 180-grit file or higher to eliminate line of demarcation.
      • Thin the entire nail; free edge and sidewalls should be thinnest.
      • Concentrate on product: Only remove shine on natural nail using a 240-grit file.
      • Hold file flat against nail to prevent damaging natural nail.
      • Shape free edge and remove length. If natural nail is same length as the enhancement, use a 240-grit file or higher.
      • Remove oils and debris before proceeding.

   NOTE: Avoid trimming free edge with nail clippers. Doing so may create small cracks in the product.

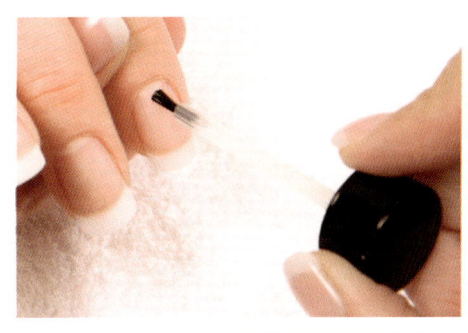

2. **Apply primer if necessary according to manufacturer's instructions.**
   • Apply primer only to natural nail.
   • Avoid allowing primer to touch skin.
   • Allow it to dry.

   NOTE: Some primers appear chalky white when dry.

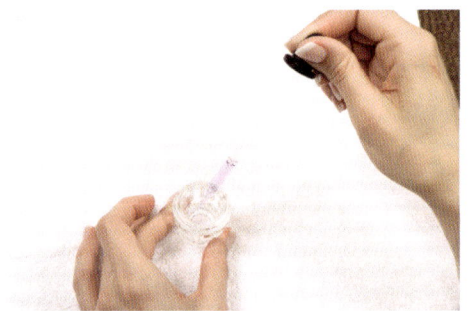

PREPARE PRODUCT

3. **Prepare acrylic liquid and acrylic powder.**
   - Place a small amount of acrylic liquid in a dappen dish.
   - Place a small amount of acrylic powder in another dappen dish.
   - Refer to Forming an Acrylic Bead on page **269**.

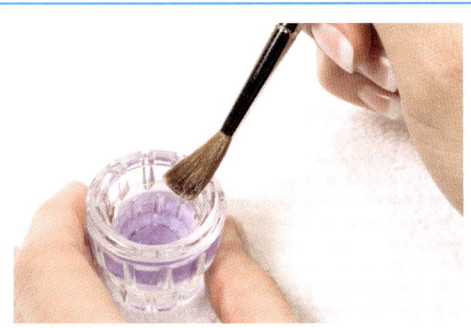

4. **Prepare brush.**
   - Submerge brush completely into acrylic liquid pressing hairs flat against bottom. Move around to release air trapped in brush.
   - When removing brush from dappen dish, wipe against sides to flatten brush on both sides.

9

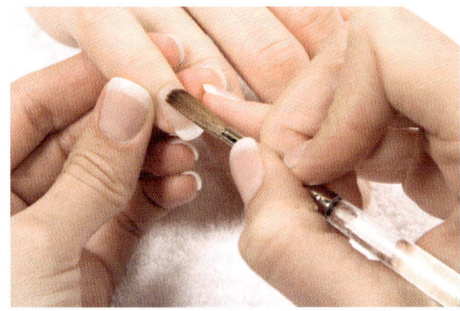

SCULPT ZONE 3

5. **Pick up and apply first acrylic bead.**
   - Pick up a small-sized bead of acrylic.
   - Place it directly behind Zone 2.
   - Hold the brush at a slightly higher angle than 45˚.
   - Press acrylic to distribute it.
   - Make sure product is thinnest at sidewalls and cuticle.
   - Blend remaining product into Zone 2.

NOTE: Repair any lifted or cracked areas of the nail at this time if necessary.

REPEAT SCULPT ZONE 3 (Step 5) on remaining nails.
- Work from little finger to thumb on each hand.

BALANCE
6. Balance nails following Basic Artificial Nail Balancing Procedure on page **288.**

FINISH
7. Finish nails following Basic Artificial Nail Finishing Procedure on page **290.**

FOUR–WEEK PINK AND WHITE ACRYLIC NAIL MAINTENANCE

A checkmark next to a step indicates an ideal time to check on your client's comfort, and to take extra safety precautions.

PREPARE NAILS

1. Prepare and balance nails following Basic Artificial Nail Preparation Procedure on page 279.

- **ANALYZE**
  - Check for cracks or any lifting or separation of product.
  - If cracks, lifting or separation are present, carefully file away product from area.
  - If necessary, completely remove product from nail following Acrylic Nail Removal Procedure on page 327.

NOTE: Avoid removing lifted product with nippers or clippers. Doing so may damage the natural nail.

- **CUTICLE CARE**

- **FILE**
  - Blend "old product" with new growth using a 180-grit file or higher to eliminate line of demarcation.
  - Thin the entire nail; free edge and sidewalls should be thinnest.
  - Concentrate on product: Only remove shine on natural nail using a 240-grit file.
  - Hold file flat against nail to prevent damaging natural nail.
  - Shape free edge and remove length. If natural nail is same length as the enhancement, use a 240-grit file or higher.
  - Remove oils and debris before proceeding.

NOTE: Avoid trimming free edge with nail clippers. Doing so may create small cracks in the product.

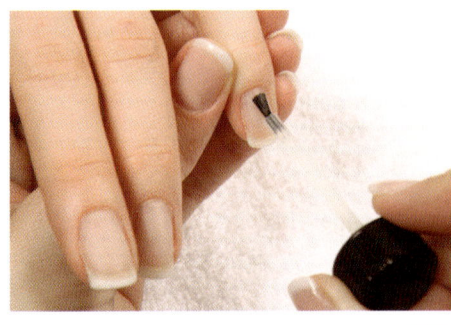

2. Apply primer if necessary according to manufacturer's instructions.
   - Apply primer only to natural nail.
   - Avoid allowing primer to touch skin.
   - Allow it to dry.

NOTE: Some primers appear chalky white when dry.

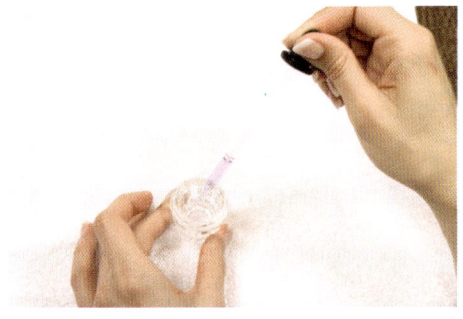

PREPARE PRODUCT

3. **Prepare acrylic liquid and pink and white acrylic powder.**
   - Place a small amount of acrylic liquid in a dappen dish.
   - Place a small amount of pink acrylic powder in a separate dappen dish.
   - Place a small amount of white acrylic powder in a separate dappen dish.
   - Refer to Forming an Acrylic Bead on page **269**.

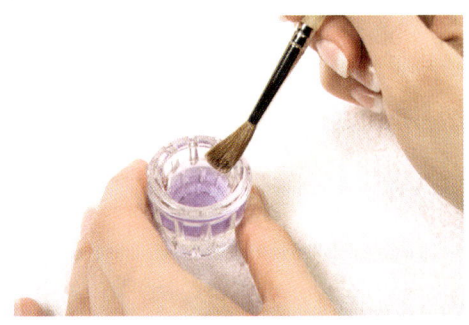

4. **Prepare brush.**
   - Submerge brush completely into acrylic liquid pressing hairs flat against bottom. Move around to release air trapped in brush.
   - When removing brush from dappen dish, wipe against sides to flatten brush on both sides.

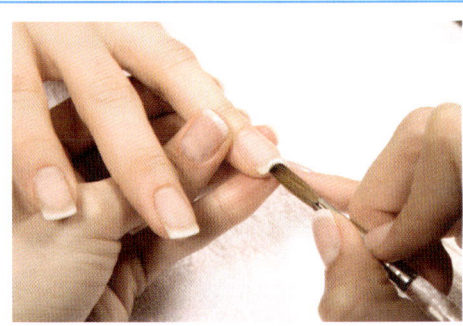

SCULPT ZONE 1

5. **Pick up and apply white acrylic bead.**
   - Pick up a medium-sized bead of white acrylic.
   - Place bead in Zone 1.
   - Press middle of bead down holding brush parallel to nail.
   - Press each side of bead down rotating angle of brush to follow the c-curve of nail.
   - Continue working in this manner to distribute product in Zone 1.
   - Distribute product so it is thinnest at free edge and thickest toward Zone 2.
   - Create smile line by using light and small pressing motions.

NOTE: Avoid touching skin with brush or any product.

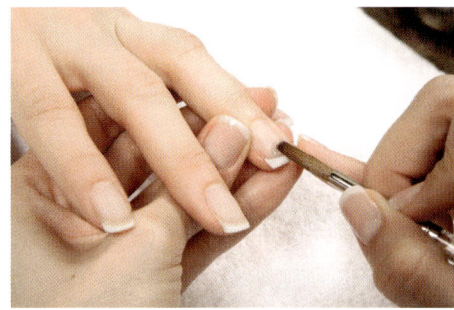

SCULPT ZONE 2

6. **Pick up and apply first pink acrylic bead.**
   - Pick up a medium to large-sized bead of pink acrylic.
   - Place it directly behind Zone 1.
   - Hold the brush at approximately 45° or slightly smaller angle.
   - Press acrylic to distribute it in the same manner as in Step 5.
   - Make sure product is thinnest at sidewalls.
   - Blend remaining product into Zone 1.

NOTE: Avoid touching skin with brush or any product.

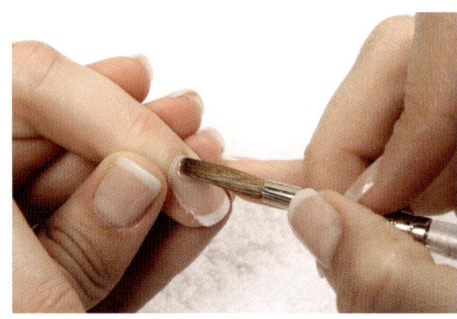

SCULPT ZONE 3

7. **Pick up and apply second pink acrylic bead.**
   - Pick up a small-sized bead of pink acrylic.
   - Place it directly behind Zone 2.
   - Hold the brush at a slightly higher angle than 45°.
   - Press acrylic to distribute it in the same manner as in Step 6.
   - Make sure product is thinnest at sidewalls and cuticle.
   - Blend remaining product into Zone 2.

NOTE: Avoid touching skin with brush or any product.

REPEAT SCULPT ZONE 1, 2 AND 3 (Steps 5–7) on remaining nails.
   - Work from little finger to thumb on each hand.

BALANCE

8. Balance nails following Basic Artificial Nail Balancing Procedure on page 288.

FINISH

9. Finish nails following Basic Artificial Nail Finishing Procedure on page 290.

ACRYLIC NAIL REMOVAL

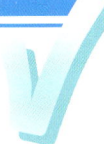

A checkmark next to a step indicates an ideal time to check on your client's comfort, and take extra safety precautions.

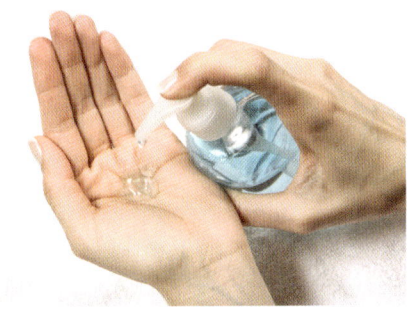

1. **Wash and sanitize your hands**
   - Use liquid or foam soap.
   - Use waterless sanitizer or topical antiseptic if required by regulating agency.
   - Wear protective gloves if required by regulating agency.

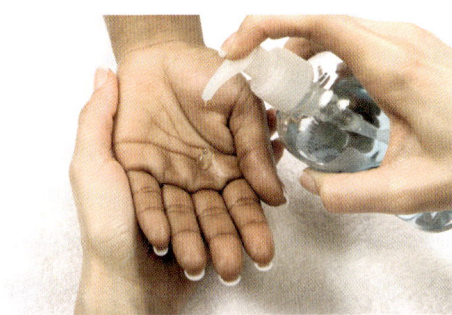

2. **Sanitize client's hands.**
   - Use waterless sanitizer or topical antiseptic if required by regulating agency.

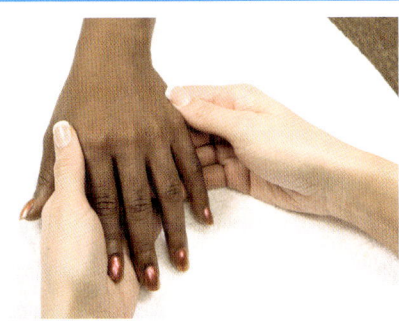

ANALYZE

3. **Perform visual analysis of hands.**
   - Continue with service if hands are free of any visible signs of diseases or disorders.

Skin: Signs to look for during analysis on hands include open skin, redness, swelling, discoloration or any other signs of an infection that would prevent the service from being performed.

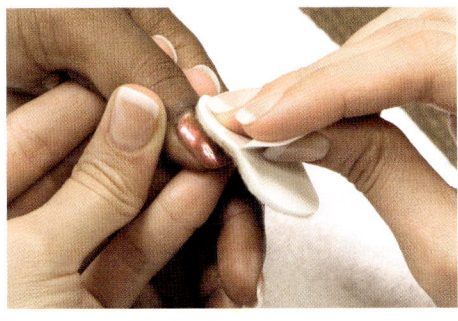

4. **Remove polish if necessary.**
   - Use a lint-free wipe or cotton saturated with polish remover on nail plate.
   - Let remover set for a few seconds.
   - Wipe toward free edge.
   - Remove all polish from each nail before moving to next nail.
   - Repeat on other hand.

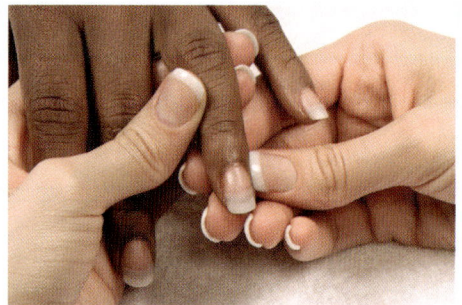

5. **Perform visual analysis of nails.**
   - Continue with service if nail plates are free of any visible signs of diseases or disorders.

Nails: Signs to look for during analysis on fingernails include discoloration, flaking, swelling, pain indicators, pus, detached nail plate, growth under the nail or any other signs of an infection that would prevent the service from being completed.

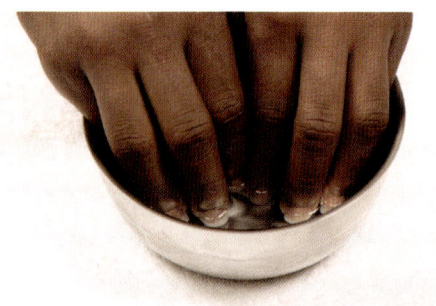

6. **Soak nails.**
   - Place all nails in a finger bowl (glass or metal) containing acetone or artificial product remover.
   - Completely submerge nails for approximately 20 minutes.

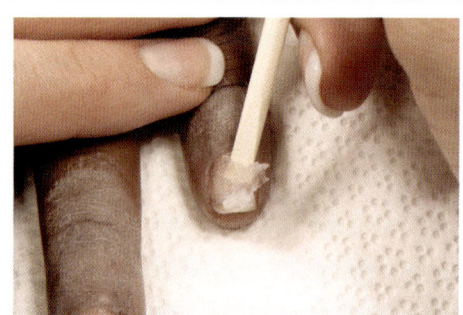

7. **Push product off.**
   - Remove first hand from finger bowl.
   - Use orangewood stick to push softened product toward free edge and off nail.
   - Replace nails in acetone if necessary.

NOTE: It may be necessary to soak nails for more than 20 minutes to completely remove product. Patience is sometimes required during this process.

NOTE: Avoid removing product with nippers or clippers. Doing so may damage the natural nail.

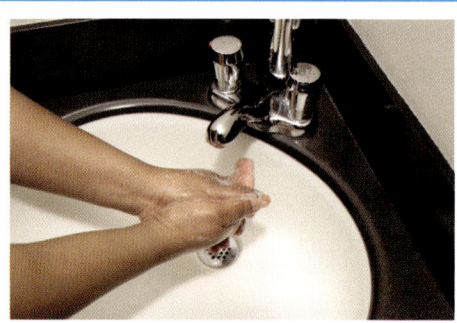

8. **Wash hands.**
   - Remove chemicals from skin to prevent irritation.
   - Wash hands (yours and client's) with nail brush.

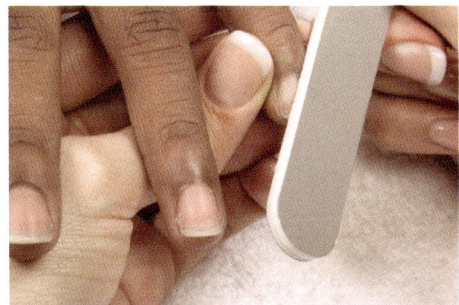

9. **Shape and buff nails.**

- Use file to shape free edge.
- Gently buff nails to remove any residue from softened product.

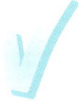

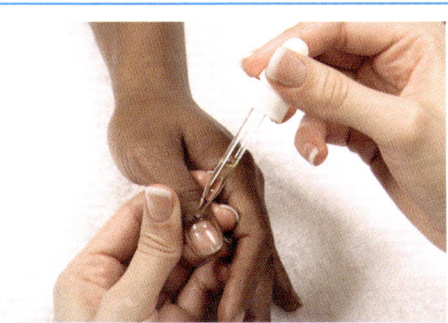

10. **Apply cuticle conditioner.**

- Use cotton-tipped orangewood stick, cotton swab or dropper.
- Apply to all 10 fingers.
- Gently massage conditioner into the cuticle area.

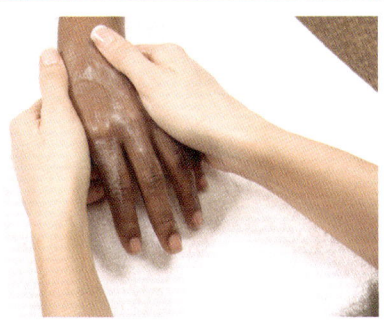

11. **Apply lotion or cream to client's hands.**

- Apply lotion to hands using effleurage movements.

NOTE: You may recommend to your clients that they use a cuticle conditioner and lotion daily to prevent dryness from acetone.

Proceed with desired service.

9

SINGLE–COLOR GEL OVERLAY

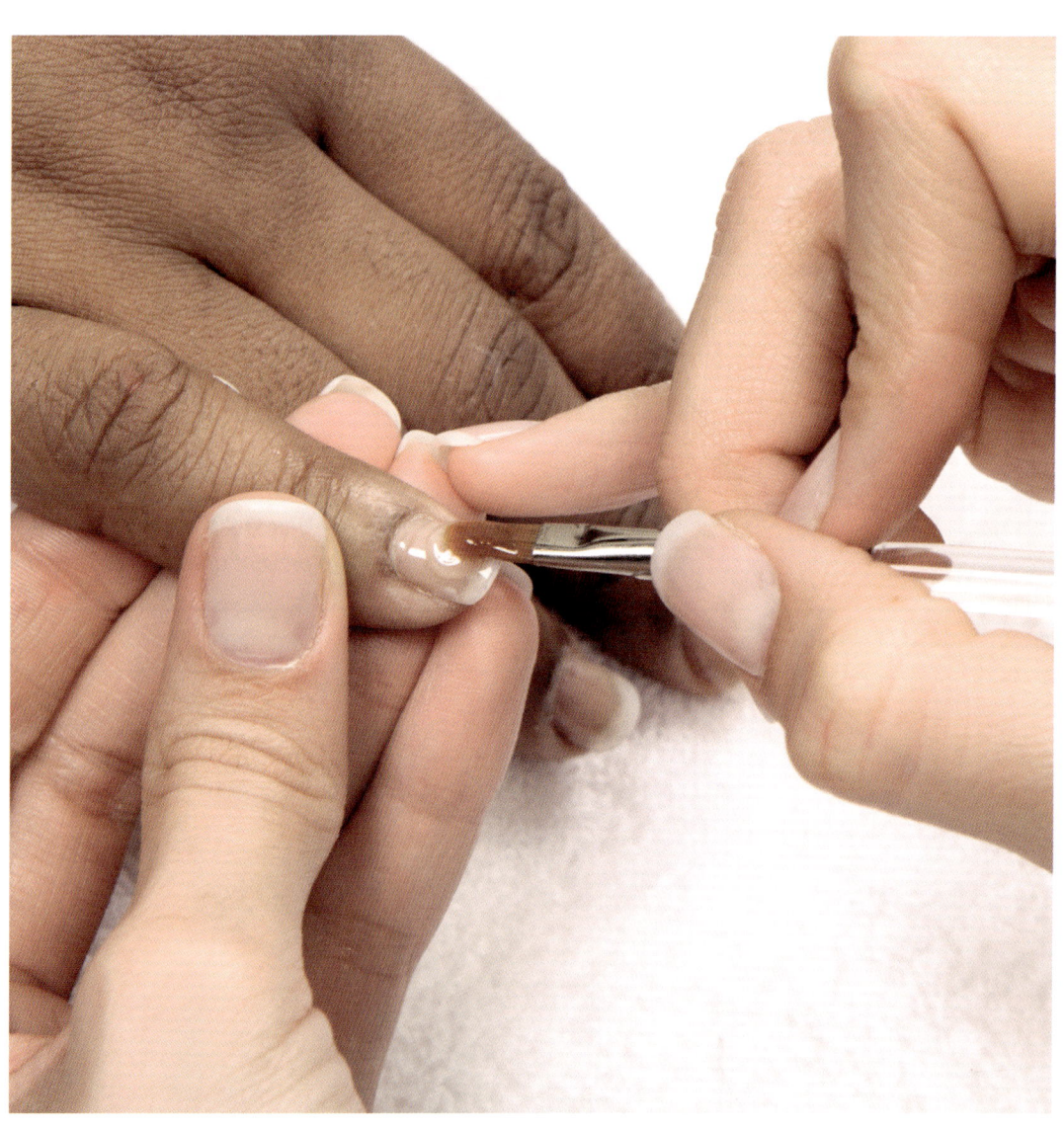

FIVE PHASES OF SERVICE

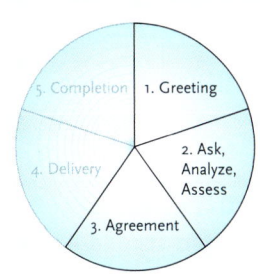

Preparing for a successful service involves the first Three Phases of Service:

1. Greeting—Establish rapport
2. Ask, Analyze and Assess—Offer professional advice
3. Agreement—Clarify expectations

GEL NAIL OVERLAY PREPARATION

9

After completing the consultation, it is advisable to ask the client to remove any jewelry from hands and wrists. **Require that hands be washed with liquid or foam soap.**

Products
- Liquid soap
- Antiseptic sanitizer
- Polish remover
- Cuticle remover
- Cuticle oil
- Nail adhesive
- Nail preparation solution
- Cuticle oil
- Gel
- Bonder or primer
- Sealer
- Dehydrator
- Polishes

Implements
- Nail brush
- Cuticle pusher
- Cuticle nippers
- Nail clippers
- Tip cutter
- Gel brush
- Files
- Buffer

Supplies
- Cotton or lint-free wipes in a disinfected glass container
- Nail tips
- Towels
- Disposable towels
- Orangewood stick

Equipment
- Manicure table
- Table lamp
- Glass container
- Disinfection container filled with EPA-registered, broad spectrum (hospital-level) disinfectant
- Technician and client chairs
- Curing light

Basic Table Set-Up
- Clean and disinfect surface of table with an EPA-registered, broad spectrum (hospital-level) disinfectant.
- Place polishes on left side of table.
- Place all other products on right side of table in order of use.
- Place disinfection container filled with an EPA-registered, broad spectrum (hospital-level) disinfectant on right side of table.
- Disinfect all implements properly before beginning.
- Place clean towel on table, making sure to cover client cushion, if there is one. Place all implements on towel.
- Place a covered trash can on floor to right. If a trash can is not available, fasten a plastic bag to right side of table and discard bag after every service.
- The drawer is used to store new materials in original container or sealed bag. Never place used or unsanitized items in drawer. Store additional clean implements in a covered container in drawer.

SINGLE-COLOR GEL NAIL OVERLAY PROCEDURE

The main difference between gel nails and acrylic nails is that gel nails don't harden or cure until they are exposed to an ultraviolet or halogen light. Note that the procedure below corresponds with the step-by-step technical images that follow.

4. Delivery - Meet client's expectations

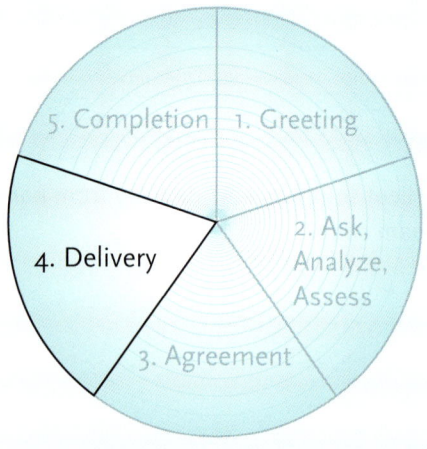

PREPARE NAILS
1. Prepare the nails following **Basic Artificial Nail Preparation Procedure** on page 279
2. Apply nail tips, if desired, following **Nail Tip Application** on page 284
3. Apply gel primer

SCULPT BASE LAYER
4. Apply first layer of gel on little finger through index finger of first hand
5. Cure nails

REPEAT SCULPT BASE LAYER (Steps 4–5) on little finger through index finger, second hand

REPEAT SCULPT BASE LAYER (Steps 4–5) on thumbs of both hands

SCULPT ZONE 1 AND 2
6. Apply second layer of gel on little finger through index finger of first hand
7. Cure nails

REPEAT SCULPT ZONE 1 AND 2 (Steps 6–7) on little finger through index finger, second hand

REPEAT SCULPT ZONE 1 AND 2 (Steps 6–7) on thumbs of both hands

BLEND
8. Apply third layer of gel on little finger through index finger, first hand
9. Cure nails

REPEAT BLEND (Steps 8–9) on little finger through index finger, second hand

REPEAT BLEND (Steps 8–9) on thumbs of both hands

10. Remove sticky residue

BALANCE
11. Balance nails following **Basic Artificial Nail Balancing Procedure** on page 288

SEAL GEL
12. Apply a finishing gel or sealer gel on little finger through index finger, first hand

REPEAT SEAL GEL (Step 12) on little finger through index finger, second hand

REPEAT SEAL GEL (Step 12) on thumbs of both hands

13. Remove sticky residue also known as the tacky layer

FINISH
14. Finish nails following **Basic Artificial Nail Finishing Procedure** on page 290

SINGLE-COLOR GEL NAIL OVERLAY

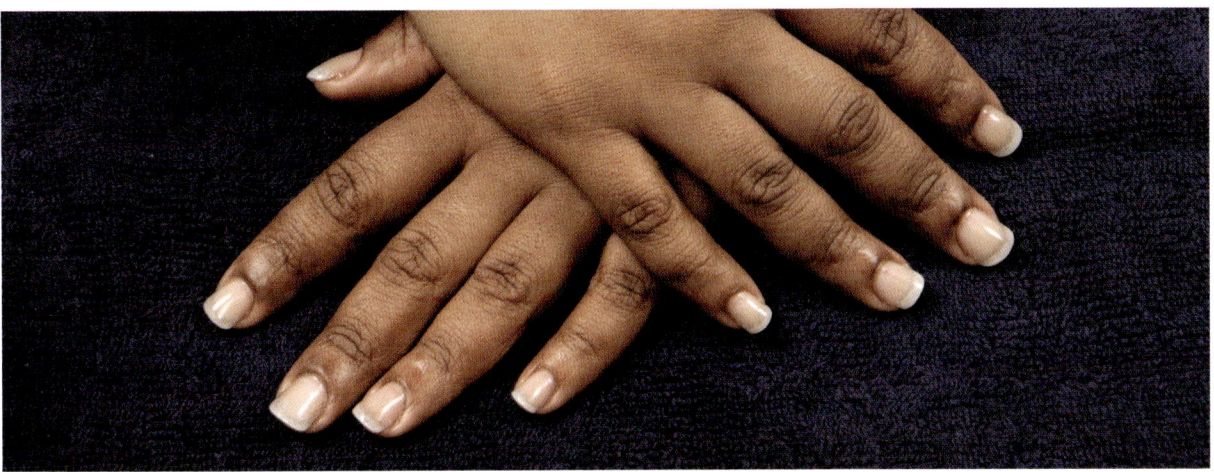

 A checkmark next to a step indicates an ideal time to check on your client's comfort, and to take extra safety precautions.

PREPARE NAILS

1. Prepare nails following Basic Artificial Nail Preparation Procedure on page 279.
   - ANALYZE
   - CUTICLE CARE
   - FILE

2. Apply nail tips, if desired, following Nail Tip Application on page 284.
   - PREPARE TIPS
   - APPLY TIPS
   - FILE TIPS

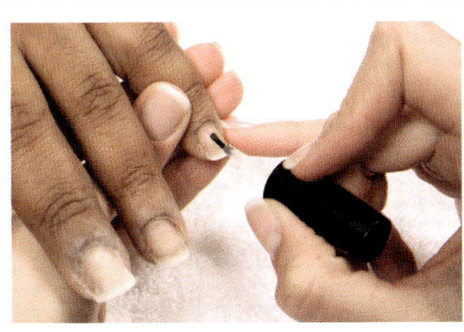

3. Apply gel primer if necessary according to manufacturer's instructions.
   - Apply gel primer only to natural nail.
   - Avoid allowing gel primer to touch skin.
   - Cure primer if necessary according to manufacturer's instructions.

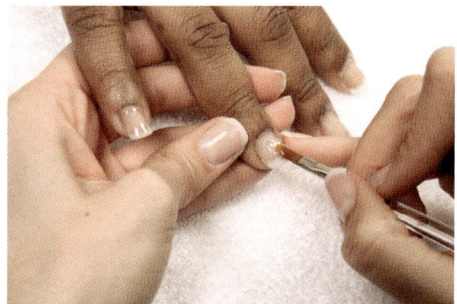

SCULPT BASE LAYER

4. **Apply first layer of gel on little finger through index finger of first hand.**
   - Obtain a small amount of gel using brush.
   - Place gel on nail.
   - Lightly brush into place.
   - Apply coat of gel to entire nail.

NOTE: Avoid touching skin with brush or any product.

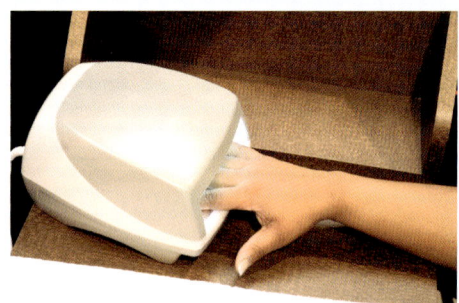

5. **Cure nails.**
   - Place fingers carefully under light.
   - Cure for manufacturer's recommended time.
   - Avoid tilting fingers; keep them as level as possible until gel is cured.
   - During curing time, move on to next step.

REPEAT SCULPT BASE LAYER (Steps 4–5) on little finger through index finger, second hand.
- Cure nails for recommended time.
- During curing time, move on to next step.

REPEAT SCULPT BASE LAYER (Steps 4–5) on thumbs of both hands.
- Cure thumbs of both hands.

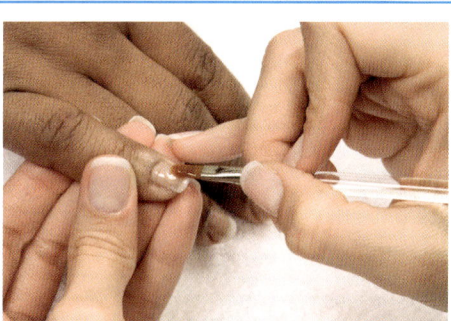

SCULPT ZONE 1 AND 2

6. **Apply second layer of gel on little finger through index finger, first hand.**
   - Obtain a small amount of gel using brush.
   - Place gel in Zone 2.
   - Lightly brush gel blending into Zone 1.
   - Make sure product is thinnest at sidewalls.

NOTE: Avoid touching skin with brush or any product.

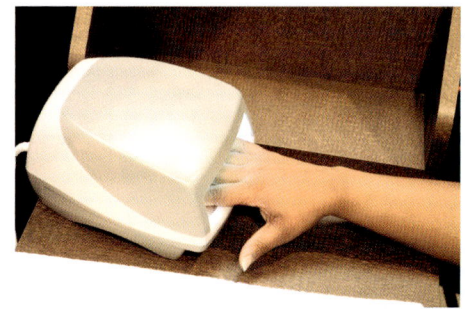

7. **Cure nails.**
   - Place fingers carefully under light.
   - Cure for manufacturer's recommended time.
   - Avoid tilting fingers; keep them as level as possible until gel is cured.
   - During curing time, move on to next step.

REPEAT SCULPT ZONE 1 AND 2 (Steps 6–7) on little finger through index finger, second hand.

- Cure nails for recommended time.
- During curing time, move on to next step.

REPEAT SCULPT ZONE 1 AND 2 (Steps 6–7) on thumbs of both hands.

- Cure thumbs on both hands.

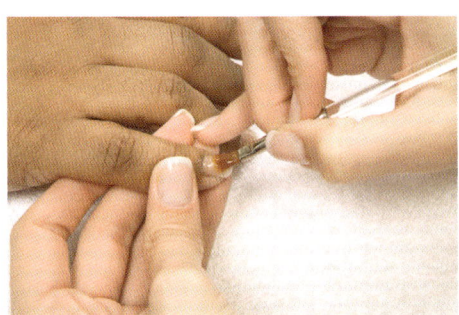

BLEND

8. **Apply third layer of gel on little finger through index finger, first hand.**

   - Obtain a small amount of gel using brush.
   - Place gel on nail.
   - Lightly brush into place.
   - Apply coat of gel to entire nail.
   - Fill in any uneven areas if necessary.

   NOTE: Avoid touching skin with brush or any product.

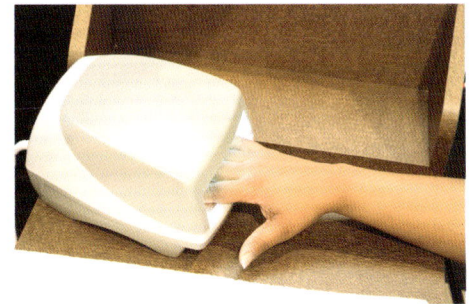

9. **Cure nails.**

   - Place fingers carefully under light.
   - Cure according to manufacturer's instructions.
   - Avoid tilting fingers; keep them as level as possible until gel is cured.
   - During curing time, move on to next step.

REPEAT BLEND (Steps 8–9) on little finger through index finger, second hand.

- Cure nails for recommended time.
- During curing time, move on to next step.

REPEAT BLEND (Steps 8–9) on thumbs of both hands.

- Cure thumbs of both hands.

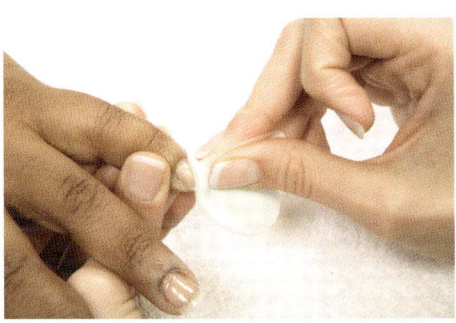

10. **Remove sticky residue.**

    - Using manufacturer's recommended product, remove sticky residue from all nails with a lint-free nail wipe.

BALANCE

11. Balance nails following Basic Artificial Nail Balancing Procedure on page 288.

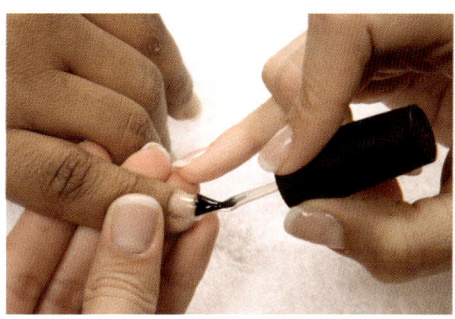

SEAL GEL

12. Apply a finishing gel or sealer gel little finger through index finger, first hand.
- Apply product to free edge to seal.
- Cure for recommended time.
- During curing time, move on to next step.

REPEAT SEAL GEL (Step 12) on little finger through index finger, second hand.
- Cure nails for recommended time.
- During curing time, move on to next step.

REPEAT SEAL GEL (Step 12) on thumbs of both hands.
- Cure thumbs of both hands.

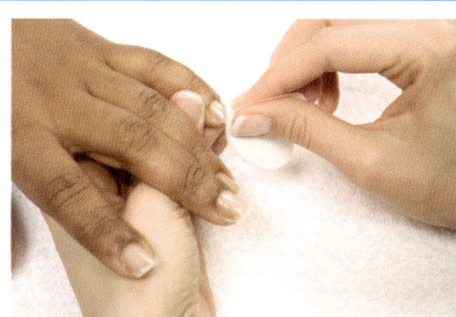

13. Remove sticky residue.
- Using the manufacturer's recommended product, remove sticky residue from all nails with a lint-free nail wipe.

FINISH

14. Finish nails following Basic Artificial Nail Finishing Procedure on page 290.

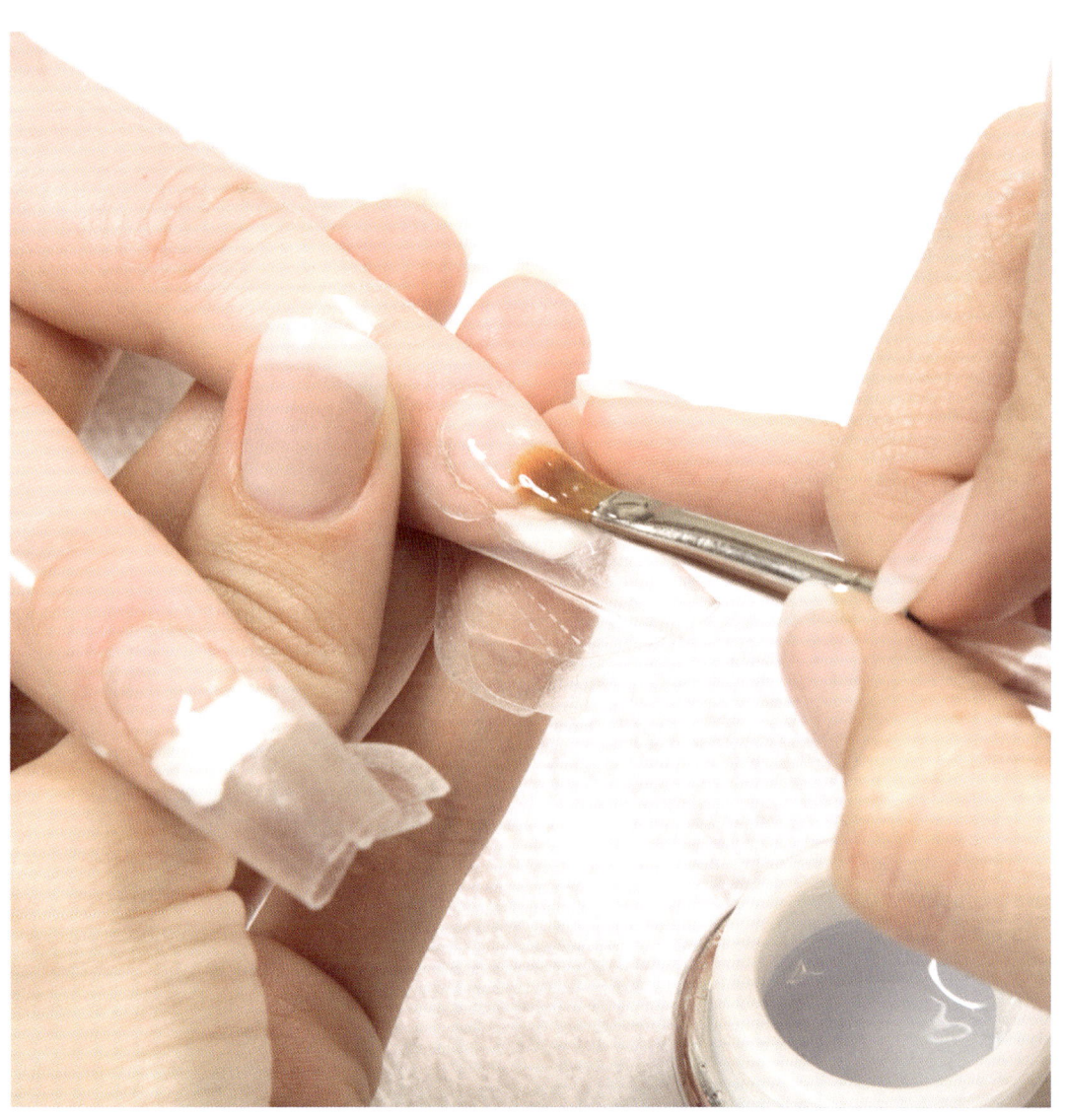

FIVE PHASES OF SERVICE

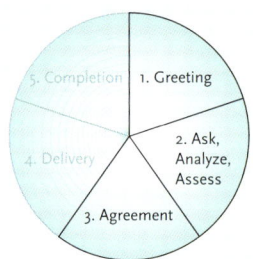

Preparing for a successful service involves the first Three Phases of Service:

1. Greeting—Establish rapport
2. Ask, Analyze and Assess—Offer professional advice
3. Agreement—Clarify expectations

SCULPTURED GEL NAIL PREPARATION

After completing the consultation, it is advisable to ask the client to remove any jewelry from hands and wrists. **Require that hands be washed with liquid or foam soap.**

Products
- Liquid soap
- Antiseptic sanitizer
- Polish remover
- Cuticle remover
- Cuticle oil
- Nail adhesive
- Nail preparation solution
- Cuticle oil
- Gel
- Bonder or primer
- Sealer
- Dehydrator
- Polishes

Implements
- Nail brush
- Cuticle pusher
- Cuticle nippers
- Nail clippers
- Tip cutter
- Gel brush
- Files
- Buffer

Supplies
- Cotton or lint-free wipes in a disinfected glass container
- Nail tips
- Towels
- Disposable towels
- Orangewood stick
- Nail forms

Equipment
- Manicure table
- Table lamp
- Glass container
- Disinfection container filled with EPA-registered, broad spectrum (hospital-level) disinfectant
- Technician and client chairs
- Curing light

Basic Table Set-Up
- Clean and disinfect surface of table with an EPA-registered, broad spectrum (hospital-level) disinfectant.
- Place polishes on left side of table.
- Place all other products on right side of table in order of use.
- Place disinfection container filled with an EPA-registered, broad spectrum (hospital-level) disinfectant on right side of table.
- Disinfect all implements properly before beginning.
- Place clean towel on table, making sure to cover client cushion, if there is one. Place all implements on towel.
- Place a covered trash can on floor to right. If a trash can is not available, fasten a plastic bag to right side of table and discard bag after every service.
- The drawer is used to store new materials in original container or sealed bag. Never place used or unsanitized items in drawer. Store additional clean implements in a covered container in drawer.

Since gel doesn't cure until it is exposed to light, it is important to keep the nails level in order to prevent the product from moving. Note that the procedure below corresponds with the step-by-step technical images that follow.

4. Delivery - Meet client's expectations

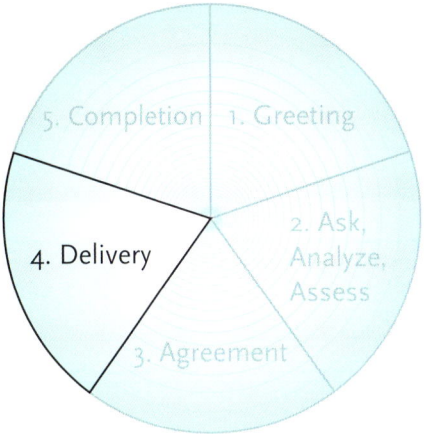

PREPARE NAILS
1. Prepare nails following the **Basic Artificial Nail Preparation Procedure** on page 279
2. Apply forms
3. Apply gel primer

SCULPT BASE LAYER
4. Apply first layer of pink gel on little finger through index finger of first hand
5. Cure nails

REPEAT SCULPT BASE LAYER (Steps 4–5) on little finger through index finger, second hand

REPEAT SCULPT BASE LAYER (Steps 4–5) on thumbs of both hands

SCULPT ZONE 2
6. Apply second layer of pink gel on little finger through index finger, first hand
7. Cure nails

REPEAT SCULPT ZONE 2 (Steps 6–7) on little finger through index finger, second hand

REPEAT SCULPT ZONE 2 (Steps 6–7) on thumbs of both hands

SCULPT ZONE 1
8. Apply white gel to Zone 1 on little finger through index finger, first hand
9. Cure nails

REPEAT SCULPT ZONE 1 (Steps 8–9) on little finger through index finger, second hand

REPEAT SCULPT ZONE 1 (Steps 8–9) on thumbs of both hands

BLEND
10. Apply clear layer of gel on little finger through index finger, first hand
11. Cure nails

REPEAT BLEND (Steps 10–11) on little finger through index finger, second hand

REPEAT BLEND (Steps 10–11) on thumbs of both hands

12. Remove nail forms
13. Remove sticky residue

BALANCE
14. Balance nails following **Basic Artificial Nail Balancing Procedure** on page 288

SEAL GEL
15. Apply a finishing gel or sealer gel on little finger through index finger, first hand

REPEAT SEAL GEL (Step 15) on little finger through index finger, second hand

REPEAT SEAL GEL (Step 15) on thumbs of both hands

16. Remove sticky residue

FINISH
17. Finish nails following **Basic Artificial Nail Finishing Procedure** on page 290

9

PINK AND WHITE SCULPTURED GEL NAILS

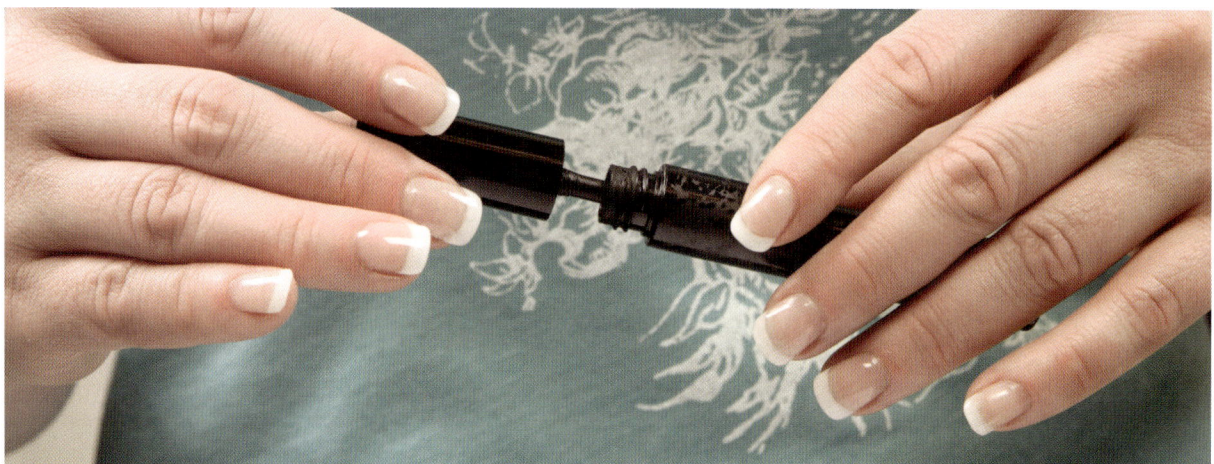

A checkmark next to a step indicates an ideal time to check on your client's comfort, and to take extra safety precautions.

PREPARE NAILS

1. Prepare nails following Basic Artificial Nail Preparation Procedure on page 279.
   - ANALYZE
   - CUTICLE CARE
   - FILE

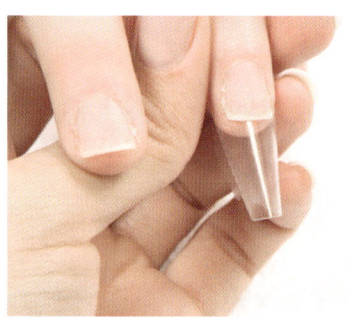

2. Apply forms.
   - Place form under free edge of each nail.
   - Pinch or roll form to match the natural c-curve.
   - Check to make sure it fits snugly under free edge with no gap and is under both corners of nail.

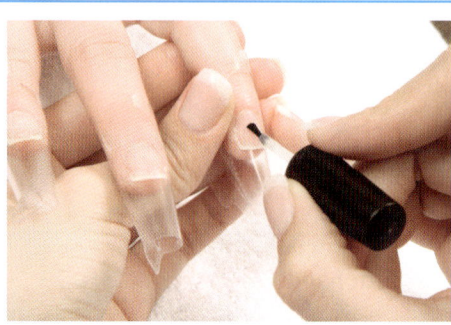

3. Apply gel primer if necessary according to manufacturer's instructions.
   - Apply gel primer only to the natural nail.
   - Avoid allowing gel primer to touch skin.
   - Cure primer if necessary according to manufacturer's instructions.

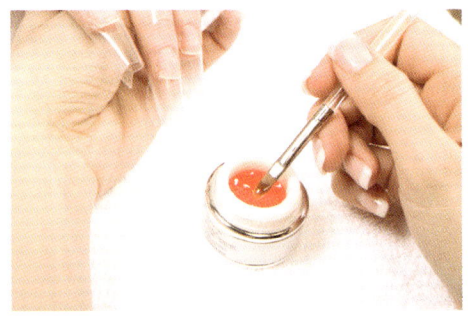

SCULPT BASE LAYER

4. **Apply first layer of pink gel on little finger through index finger, first hand.**
   - Obtain a small amount of gel using brush.
   - Place gel on nail.
   - Lightly brush into place.
   - Apply coat of gel to entire nail.

NOTE: Avoid touching skin with brush or any product.

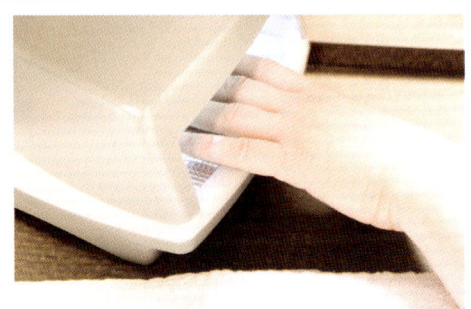

5. **Cure nails.**
   - Place fingers carefully under light.
   - Cure according to manufacturer's instructions.
   - Avoid tilting fingers; keep them as level as possible until gel is cured.
   - During curing time, move on to next step.

REPEAT SCULPT BASE LAYER (Steps 4–5) on little finger through index finger, second hand.
- Cure for recommended time.
- During curing time, move on to next step.

REPEAT SCULPT BASE LAYER (Steps 4–5) on thumbs of both hands.
- Cure thumbs of both hands.

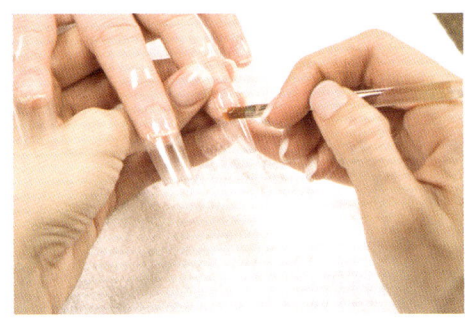

SCULPT ZONE 2

6. **Apply second layer of pink gel on little finger through index finger, first hand.**
   - Obtain a small amount of pink gel using brush.
   - Place gel in Zone 2.
   - Lightly brush gel, blending into Zone 1 and Zone 3.
   - Remove excess product from Zone 1 with brush to make a guide for smile line.
   - Make sure product is thinnest at sidewalls.

NOTE: Avoid touching skin with brush or any product.

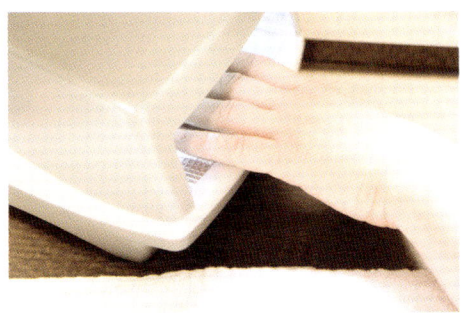

7. **Cure nails.**
   - Place fingers carefully under light.
   - Cure according to manufacturer's instructions.
   - Avoid tilting fingers; keep them as level as possible until gel is cured.
   - During curing time, move on to next step.

9

REPEAT SCULPT ZONE 2 (Steps 6–7) on little finger through index finger, second hand.

- Cure nails for recommended time.
- During curing time, move on to next step.

REPEAT SCULPT ZONE 2 (Steps 6–7) on thumbs of both hands.

- Cure thumbs of both hands.

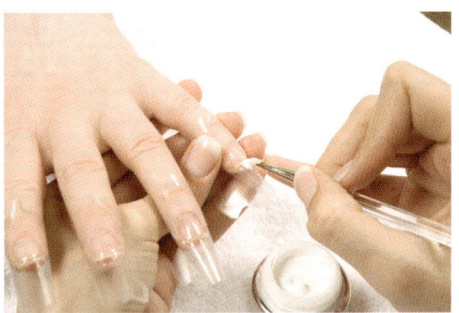

SCULPT ZONE 1

8. **Apply white gel to Zone 1 on little finger through index finger, first hand.**
   - Obtain a small amount of white gel using brush.
   - Place gel in Zone 1.
   - Lightly brush gel to create smile line.

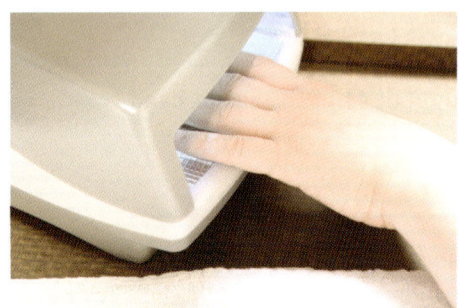

9. **Cure nails.**
   - Place fingers carefully under light.
   - Cure according to manufacturer's instructions.
   - Avoid tilting fingers; keep them as level as possible until gel is cured.

REPEAT SCULPT ZONE 1 (Steps 8–9) on little finger through index finger, second hand.

- Cure for recommended time.
- During the curing time, move on to next step.

REPEAT SCULPT ZONE 1 (Steps 8–9) on thumbs of both hands.

- Cure thumbs of both hands.

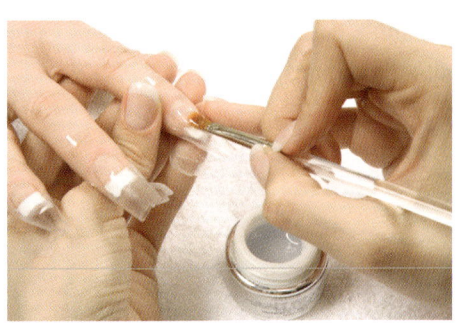

BLEND

10. **Apply clear layer of gel on little finger through index finger of first hand.**
    - Obtain a small amount of clear gel using brush.
    - Place gel on nail.
    - Lightly brush into place.
    - Apply coat of gel to entire nail.
    - Fill in any uneven areas if necessary.

NOTE: Avoid touching skin with brush or any product.

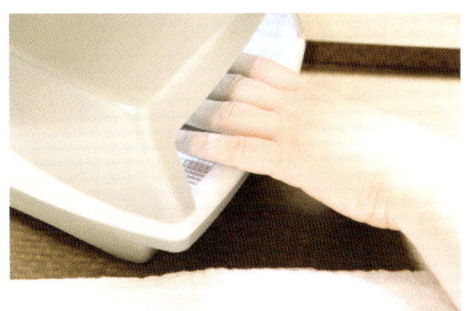

11. Cure nails.

- Place fingers carefully under light.
- Cure according to manufacturer's instructions.
- Avoid tilting fingers; keep them as level as possible until gel is cured.
- During curing time, move on to next step.

REPEAT BLEND (Steps 10–11) on little finger through index finger, second hand.

- Cure nails for recommended time.
- During curing time, move on to next step.

REPEAT BLEND (Steps 10–11) on thumbs of both hands.

- Cure thumbs of both hands.

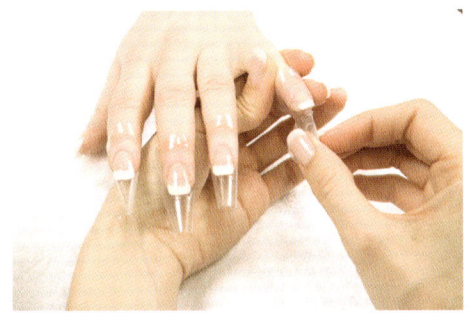

12. Remove nail forms.

- Remove forms after final layer of gel has been cured.

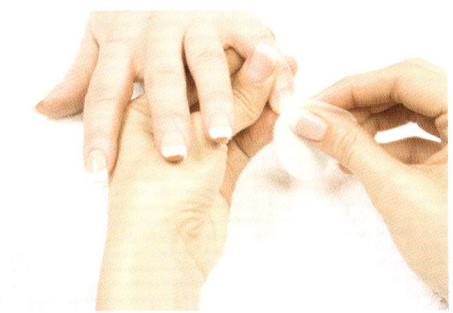

13. Remove sticky residue.

- Using the manufacturer's recommended product, remove sticky residue with a lint-free nail wipe.

BALANCE

14. Balance nails following Basic Artificial Nail Balancing Procedure on page 288.

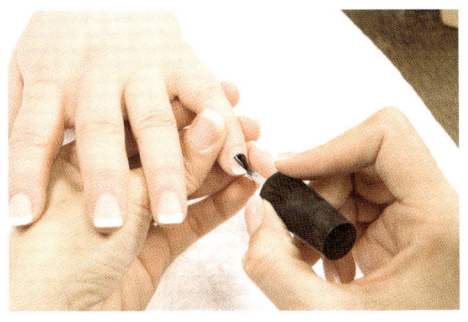

SEAL GEL

15. Apply a finishing gel or sealer gel on little finger through index finger, first hand.

- Apply product to free edge to seal.
- Cure for recommended time.
- During curing time, move on to next step.

REPEAT SEAL GEL (Step 15) on little finger through index finger, second hand.

- Cure for recommended time.
- During curing time, move on to next step.

REPEAT SEAL GEL (Step 15) on thumbs of both hands.

- Cure thumbs on both hands.

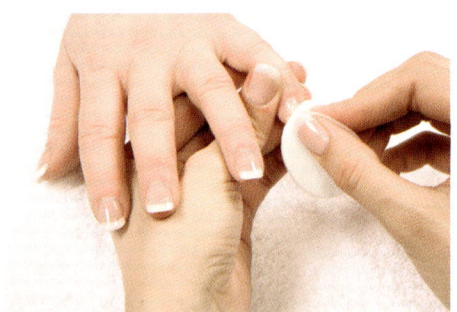

16. **Remove sticky residue.**
    - Using manufacturer's recommended product, remove sticky residue with a lint-free nail wipe.

FINISH

17. Finish nails following Basic Artificial Nail Finishing Procedure on page 290.

TWO-WEEK GEL NAIL MAINTENANCE

A checkmark next to a step indicates an ideal time to check on your client's comfort, and to take extra safety precautions.

PREPARE NAILS

1. Prepare and balance nails following Basic Artificial Nail Preparation Procedure on page 279.
   - ANALYZE
     - Check for cracks or any lifting or separation of product.
     - If cracks, lifting or separation are present, carefully file away product from area.
     - If necessary, completely remove product from nail following Gel Nail Removal Procedure on page 352.

NOTE: Avoid removing lifted product with nippers or clippers. Doing so may damage the natural nail.

   - CUTICLE CARE

   - FILE
     - Blend "old product" with new growth using a 180-grit file or higher to eliminate line of demarcation.
     - Thin the entire nail; free edge and sidewalls should be thinnest.
     - Concentrate on product: Only remove shine on natural nail using a 240-grit file.
     - Hold file flat against nail to prevent damaging natural nail.
     - Shape free edge and remove length. If natural nail is same length as the enhancement, use a 240-grit file or higher.
     - Remove oils and debris before proceeding.

NOTE: Avoid trimming free edge with nail clippers. Doing so may create small cracks in the product or tip.

NOTE: The last step before applying primer is always to use the manufacturer's recommended nail preparation solution.

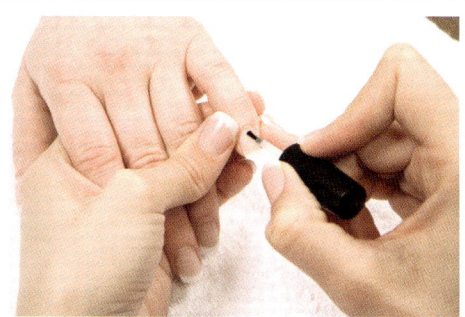

2. **Apply gel primer if necessary according to manufacturer's instructions.**
   - Apply gel primer only to natural nail.
   - Avoid allowing gel primer to touch skin.
   - Cure primer if necessary according to manufacturer's instructions.

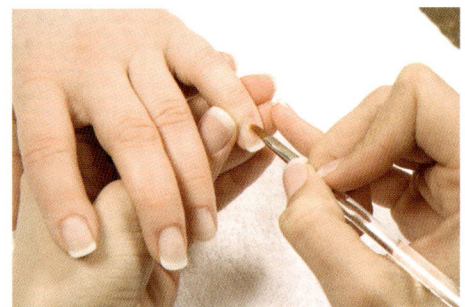

SCULPT ZONE 3

3. **Apply first layer of gel to new growth area on little finger through index finger of first hand.**
   - Obtain a small amount of gel using brush.
   - Place gel on nail.
   - Lightly brush into place.
   - Apply coat of gel to entire nail.

NOTE: Avoid touching skin with brush or any product.

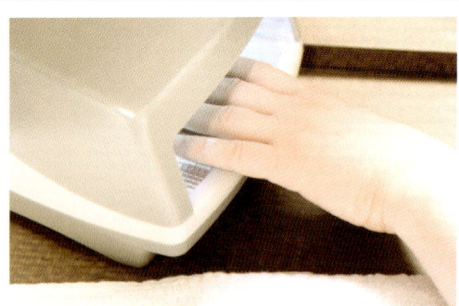

4. **Cure nails.**
   - Place fingers carefully under light.
   - Cure according to manufacturer's instructions.
   - Avoid tilting fingers; keep them as level as possible until gel is cured.
   - During curing time, move on to next step.

REPEAT SCULPT ZONE 3 (Steps 3–4) on little finger through index finger, second hand.
   - Cure nails for recommended time.
   - During curing time, move on to next step.

REPEAT SCULPT ZONE 3 (Steps 3–4) on thumbs of both hands.
   - Cure thumbs on both hands.

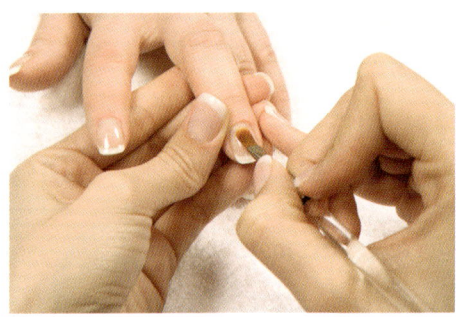

BLEND

5. **Apply second layer of gel on little finger through index finger, first hand.**
   - Obtain a small amount of gel using brush.
   - Place gel on nail.
   - Lightly brush into place.
   - Apply coat of gel to entire nail.
   - Fill in any uneven areas if necessary.

NOTE: Avoid touching skin with brush or any product.

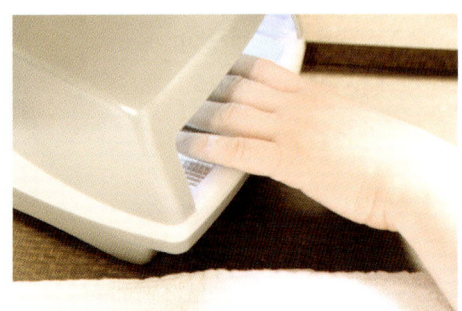

6. **Cure nails.**
   - Place fingers carefully under light.
   - Cure according to manufacturer's instructions.
   - Avoid tilting fingers; keep them as level as possible until gel is cured.
   - During curing time, move on to next step.

REPEAT BLEND (Steps 5–6) on little finger through index finger, second hand.

- Cure nails for recommended time.
- During curing time, move on to next step.

REPEAT BLEND (Steps 5–6) on thumbs of both hands.

- Cure thumbs on both hands.

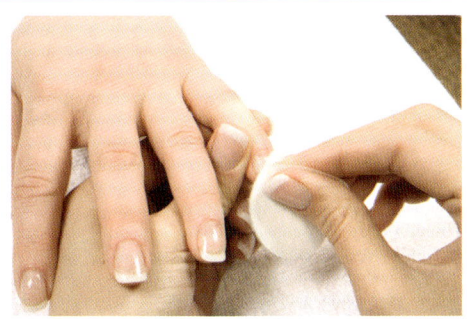

7. **Remove sticky residue.**
   - Using manufacturer's recommended product, remove the sticky residue from all nails with a lint-free nail wipe.

BALANCE

8. Balance nails following Basic Artificial Nail Balancing Procedure on page 288.

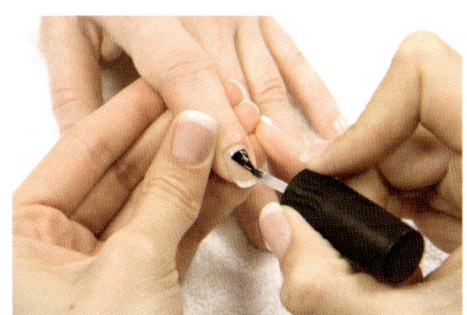

SEAL GEL

9. Apply a finishing gel or sealer gel on little finger through index finger of first hand.
   - Apply product to free edge to seal.
   - Cure for recommended time.
   - During the curing time, move on to next step.

REPEAT SEAL GEL (Step 9) on little finger through index finger, second hand.

- Cure nails for recommended time.
- During curing time, move on to next step.

REPEAT SEAL GEL (Step 9) on thumbs of both hands.

- Cure thumbs on both hands.

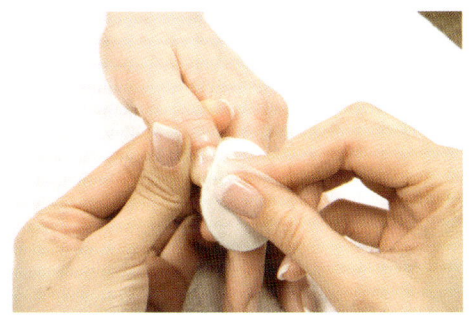

10. **Remove sticky residue.**
    - Using manufacturer's recommended product, remove sticky residue with a lint-free nail wipe.

FINISH

11. Finish nails following Basic Artificial Nail Finishing Procedure on page 290.

FOUR-WEEK PINK AND WHITE GEL NAIL MAINTENANCE

A checkmark next to a step indicates an ideal time to check on your client's comfort, and to take extra safety precautions.

PREPARE NAILS

1. Prepare and balance nails following Basic Artificial Nail Preparation Procedure on page 279.

- ANALYZE
  - Check for cracks or any lifting or separation of product.
  - If cracks, lifting or separation are present, carefully file away product from area.
  - If necessary, completely remove product from nail following Gel Nail Removal Procedure on page 352.

NOTE: Avoid removing lifted product with nippers or clippers. Doing so may damage the natural nail.

- CUTICLE CARE

- FILE
  - Blend "old product" with new growth using a 180-grit file or higher to eliminate line of demarcation.
  - Thin the entire nail; free edge and sidewalls should be thinnest.
  - Concentrate on product: Only remove shine on natural nail using a 240-grit file.
  - Hold file flat against nail to prevent damaging natural nail.
  - Shape free edge and remove length. If natural nail is same length as the enhancement, use a 240-grit file or higher.
  - Remove oils and debris before proceeding.

NOTE: Avoid trimming free edge with nail clippers. Doing so may create small cracks in the product.

NOTE: The last step before applying primer is always to use the manufacturer's recommended nail preparation solution.

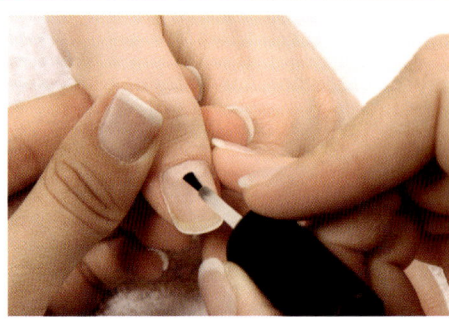

2. **Apply gel primer if necessary according to manufacturer's instructions.**
   - Apply gel primer only to natural nail.
   - Avoid allowing gel primer to touch skin.
   - Cure primer if necessary according to manufacturer's instructions.

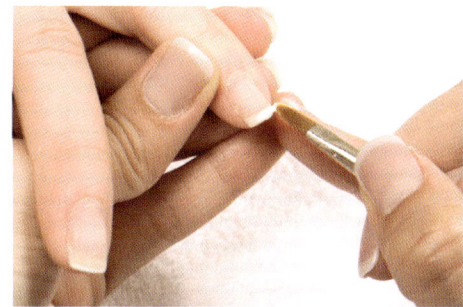

SCULPT ZONE 1

3. **Apply white gel to Zone 1 on little finger through index finger of first hand.**
   - Obtain a small amount of white gel using brush.
   - Place gel in Zone 1.
   - Lightly brush gel to create smile line.

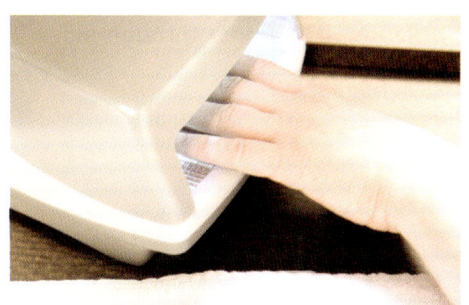

4. **Cure nails.**
   - Place fingers carefully under light.
   - Cure according to manufacturer's instructions.
   - Avoid tilting fingers; keep them as level as possible until gel is cured.

REPEAT SCULPT ZONE 1 (Steps 3–4) on little finger through index finger, second hand.
   - Cure nails for recommended time.
   - During curing time, move on to next step.

REPEAT SCULPT ZONE 1 (Steps 3–4) on thumbs of both hands.
   - Cure thumbs on both hands.

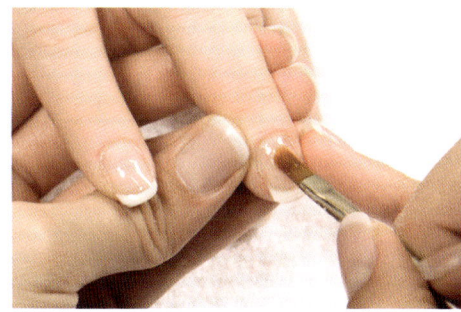

SCULPT ZONE 2

5. **Apply second layer of gel on little finger through index finger, first hand.**
   - Obtain a small amount of pink gel using brush.
   - Place gel in Zone 2.
   - Lightly brush gel blending into Zone 1 and Zone 3.
   - Remove excess product from Zone 1 with brush to make a guide for smile line.
   - Make sure product is thinnest at sidewalls.

NOTE: Avoid touching skin with brush or any product.

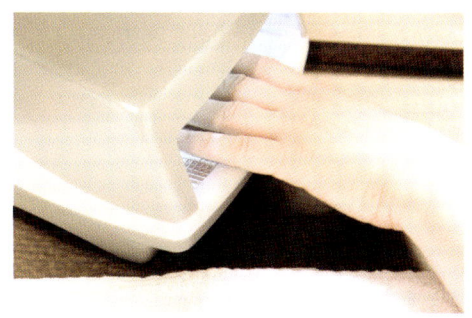

6. **Cure nails.**
   - Place fingers carefully under light.
   - Cure according to manufacturer's instructions.
   - Avoid tilting fingers; keep them as level as possible until gel is cured.
   - During curing time, move on to next step.

9

REPEAT SCULPT ZONE 2 (Steps 5–6) on little finger through index finger, second hand.
- Cure nails for recommended time.
- During curing time, move on to next step.

REPEAT SCULPT ZONE 2 (Steps 5–6) on thumbs of both hands.
- Cure thumbs on both hands.

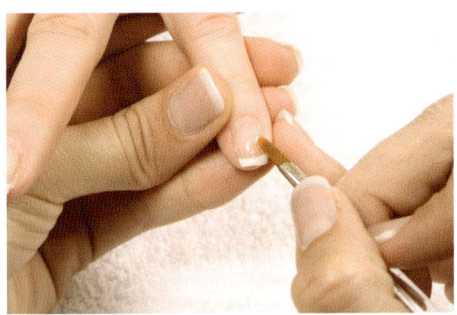

BLEND
7. **Apply third layer of gel on little finger through index finger of first hand.**
   - Obtain a small amount of gel using brush.
   - Place gel on nail.
   - Lightly brush into place.
   - Apply coat of gel to entire nail.
   - Fill in any uneven areas if necessary.

NOTE: Avoid touching the skin with brush or any product.

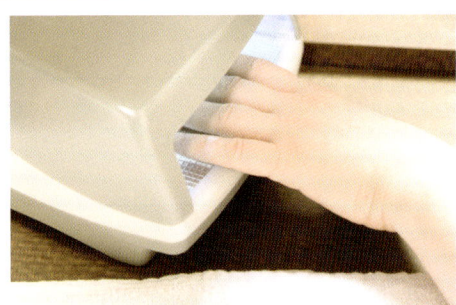

8. **Cure nails.**
   - Place fingers carefully under light.
   - Cure according to manufacturer's instructions.
   - Avoid tilting fingers; keep them as level as possible until gel is cured.
   - During curing time, move on to next step.

REPEAT BLEND (Steps 7–8) on little finger through index finger, second hand.
- Cure nails for recommended time.
- During curing time, move on to next step.

REPEAT BLEND (Steps 7–8) on thumbs of both hands.
- Cure thumbs on both hands.

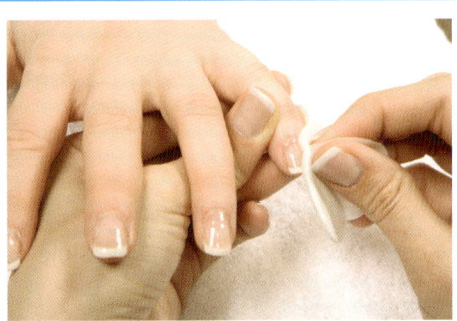

9. **Remove sticky residue.**
   - Using the manufacturer's recommended product remove the sticky residue from all nails with a lint-free nail wipe.

BALANCE
10. Balance nails following Basic Artificial Nail Balancing Procedure on page 288.

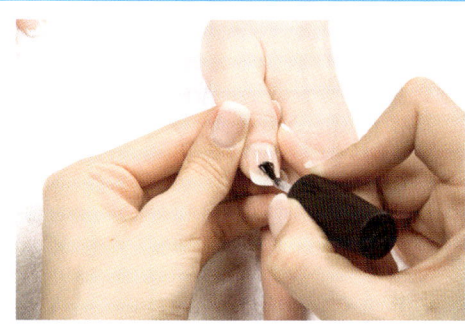

SEAL GEL
11. Apply a finishing gel or sealer gel on little finger through index finger, first hand.
- Apply product to free edge to seal.
- Cure for recommended time.
- During curing time, move on to next step.

REPEAT SEAL GEL (Step 11) on little finger through index finger, second hand.
- Cure nails for recommended time.
- During curing time, move on to next step.

REPEAT SEAL GEL (Step 11) on thumbs of both hands.
- Cure thumbs on both hands.

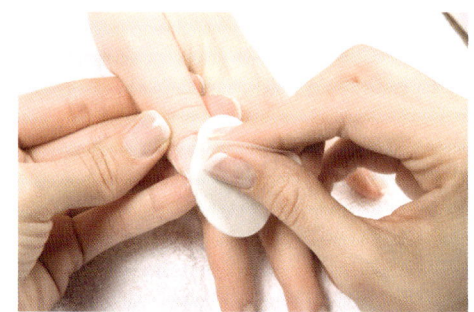

12. Remove sticky residue.
- Using manufacturer's recommended product remove residue from all nails with a lint-free nail wipe.

FINISH
13. Finish nails following Basic Artificial Nail Finishing Procedure on page 290.

9

GEL NAIL REMOVAL

A checkmark next to a step indicates an ideal time to check on your client's comfort, and take extra safety precautions.

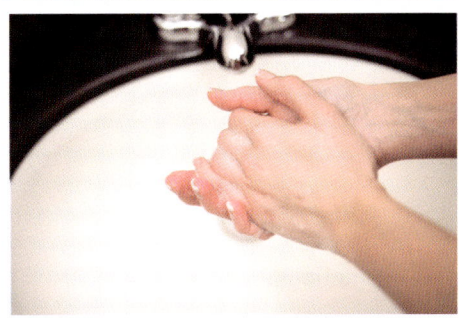

1. **Wash and sanitize your hands**
   - Use liquid or foam soap.
   - Wear protective gloves if required by regulating agency.
   - Use waterless sanitizer or topical antiseptic if required by regulating agency.

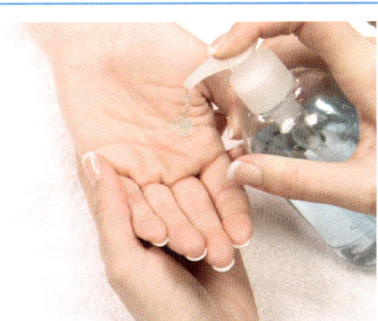

2. **Sanitize client's hands.**
   - Use waterless sanitizer or topical antiseptic if required by regulating agency.

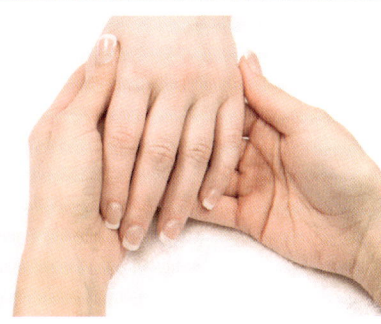

ANALYZE

3. **Perform visual analysis of hands.**
   - Continue with service if hands are free of any visible signs of diseases or disorders.

Skin: Signs to look for during analysis on hands include open skin, redness, swelling, discoloration or any other signs of an infection that would prevent the service from being performed.

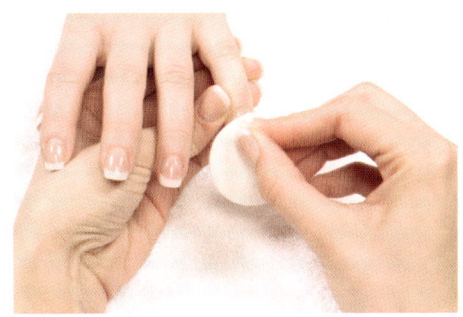

4. **Remove polish if necessary.**
   - Use a lint-free wipe or cotton saturated with polish remover on nail plate.
   - Let remover set for a few seconds.
   - Wipe toward free edge.
   - Remove all polish from each nail before moving to next nail.
   - Repeat on other hand.

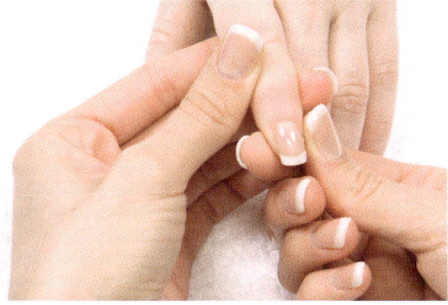

5. Perform visual analysis of nails.

- Continue with service if nail plates are free of any visible signs of diseases or disorders.

Nails: Signs to look for during analysis on fingernails include discoloration, flaking, swelling, pain indicators, pus, detached nail plate, growth under the nail or any other signs of an infection that would prevent the service from being performed.

9

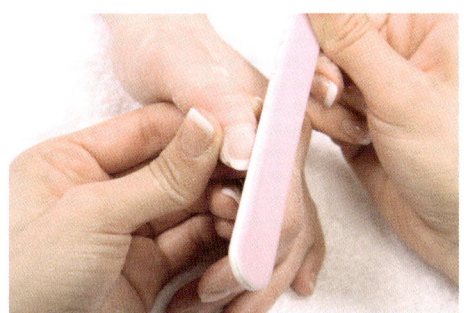

6. File product off carefully.

- Start with a lower grit file and work toward a higher grit file.
- Use caution not to file on natural nail.

NOTE: Avoid removing product with nippers or clippers. Doing so may damage the natural nail.

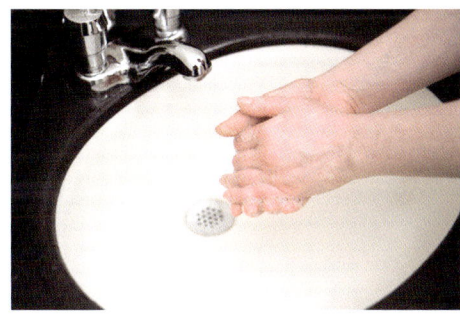

7. Wash hands.

- Wash hands (yours and client's) with nail brush.

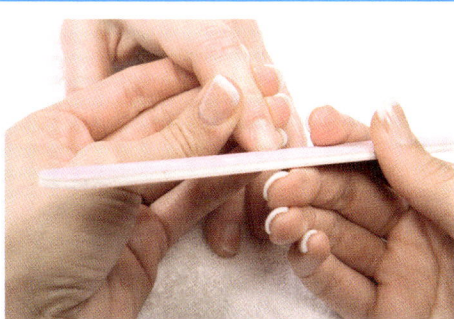

8. Shape and buff nails.

- Use file to shape free edge.
- Gently buff nails.

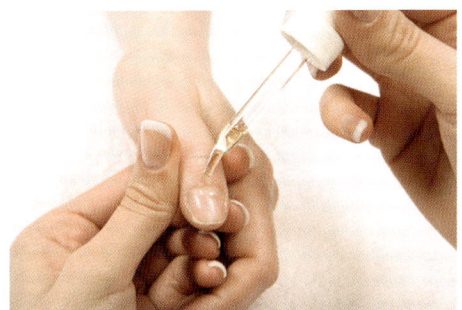

9. Apply a cuticle conditioner.
- Use cotton-tipped orangewood stick, cotton swab or dropper.
- Apply to all 10 fingers
- Gently massage conditioner into the cuticle area.

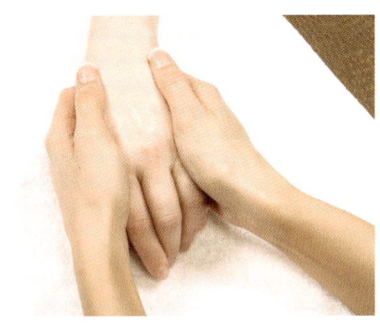

10. Apply lotion or cream to client's hands.
- Apply lotion to the hands using effleurage movements.

Proceed with desired service.

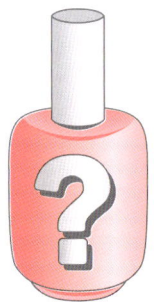

Which procedure do you see as the most challenging to perform as a nail technician and why?

NOTES

DECISION-MAKING SKILLS

Case Studies

The following situations are designed to help you build decision-making skills. Using your training to this point, review the following scenarios, then think through and describe how you would handle each challenge.

1. A client comes to you for an acrylic maintenance service after 3 1/2 weeks. Several of her nails are lifting and one is cracked. How would you proceed?

2. You are applying tips to your client's nails and are about to perform a nail wrap overlay service. She sees another client in the salon receiving an acrylic sculptured nail service. Your client asks why you aren't using "those things," referring to the nail forms. How would you explain the difference?

3. Your client has grown her nails to be all the same length but is afraid that they will break easily. What service would you recommend to strengthen and protect them?

Most clients come to you for the basic manicure and pedicure services you provide. Today, there is a wide range of specialty nail services—such as hot oil manicures, airbrushing and nail art—that are big business, and it's up to you to take advantage of it. Down the road, whether you are adding the final rhinestone to a nail design or using an electric file to balance an acrylic application, your advanced knowledge about specialty nail services will ultimately benefit your clients—and you.

VALUE

Although specialty nail services are in demand, not all nail technicians know how to provide them. The nail technician who goes above and beyond in learning about the intricacies of specialty nail services will have more to offer clients. This increases your value—and your income.

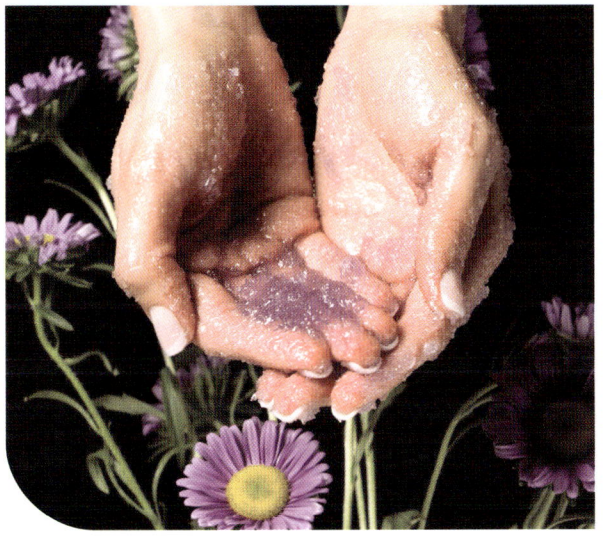

MAIN IDEA

While you build your clientele with manicure and pedicure services, you'll keep them coming back if you learn additional hand and foot services. As a professional nail technician, you can increase your knowledge—and your income—by learning how to perform paraffin wax services, design nail art or use advanced equipment such as an electric file or airbrush. Although these additional skills do require more training, learning about add-on services increases your value to your clients and shows you are a technician worth returning to. This chapter will introduce you to a variety of different services that you can learn more about when you enter the industry.

PLAN		OBJECTIVES
Add-On Services	• Exfoliation • Masks • Paraffin • Aromatherapy • Hot Oil Manicure • Reflexology	Describe the various hand and foot add-on services that can be offered to clients seeking nail services.
Nail Art	• Understanding Color • Freehand • Accents • Colored Acrylics and Gels	Explain the law of color and the relationship between the colors on the color wheel. Identify the different techniques for creating nail art.
Equipment	• Airbrush • Electric File • Nail Dryer	List and describe the types of electrical equipment that may be used in nail services.

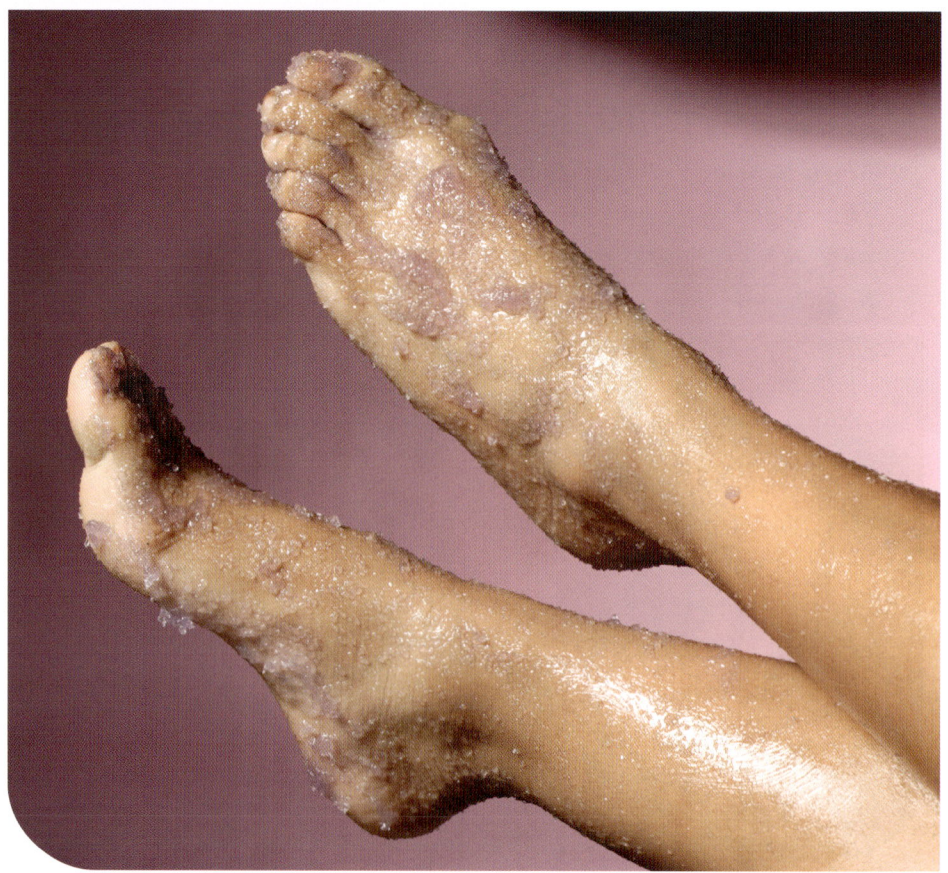

ADD-ON SERVICES

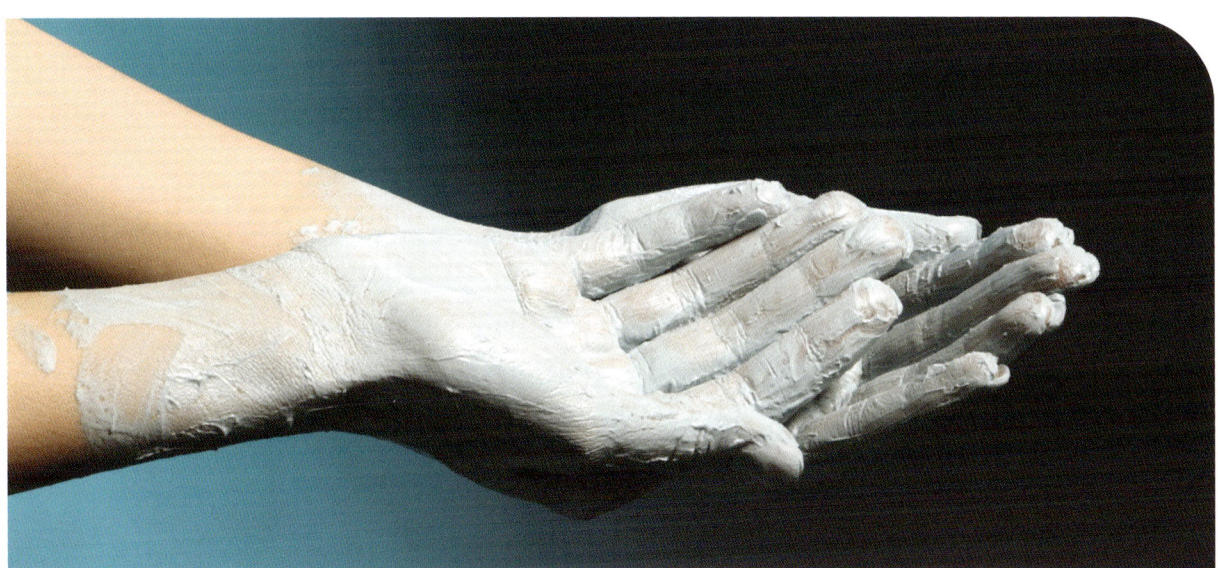

10

Have you ever heard of a spa manicure or pedicure? Do you know what makes them different from basic services? Generally, spa manicures and pedicures are ordinary manicures and pedicures with some extras, known as "add-on" services. Although add-on services can turn a basic service into a spa service, they are more involved and require more products and skills. While clients benefit when you can offer them additional ways to enhance the appearance and general health of their hands and feet, you also benefit by increasing the cost of the service, resulting in more money in your pocket!

Exfoliation

As mentioned in *Chapter 8, Natural Nail Services*, exfoliation is used to help remove dead skin cells from the surface of the skin. This helps keep the skin young and healthy looking. Using an exfoliant also increases circulation, improves the skin's ability to hold in moisture and smoothes the skin. **Mechanical** or **manual exfoliation** is the physical process of removing dead skin cells with a granular or abrasive product, such as a scrub.

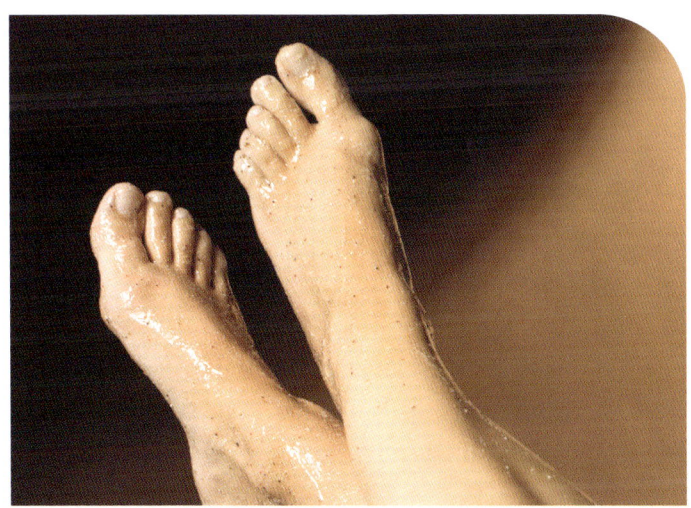

To specifically care for callused feet or rough areas of the hands, a chemical exfoliant can be used. **Chemical exfoliation** is the process of using natural substances, such as enzymes or alpha hydroxy acids, along with other ingredients to cause a chemical reaction to remove dead skin cells. These are used to soften the area and are usually followed by manual exfoliating with a foot file or paddle. Many manual exfoliators also contain a small amount of chemical exfoliant such as alpha hydroxy acids or sodium hydroxide.

Exfoliating scrubs have become one of the most popular hand and foot services available. They produce immediate results and are easy to add on to a regular manicure or pedicure service. **Scrubs** are exfoliants used to remove dead skin cells and produce soft, smooth, healthy skin. Another method of exfoliating is called **gomage**. In French, *gomage* means "to peel." This is an exfoliating method in which a layer of cream (gomage) is applied to the skin, allowed to dry, and is then rubbed away. This method causes friction that makes the cream bead up and fall away, taking dead surface skin cells with it. A product called sloughing lotion is used with the gomage technique and is commonly used for hand and foot services.

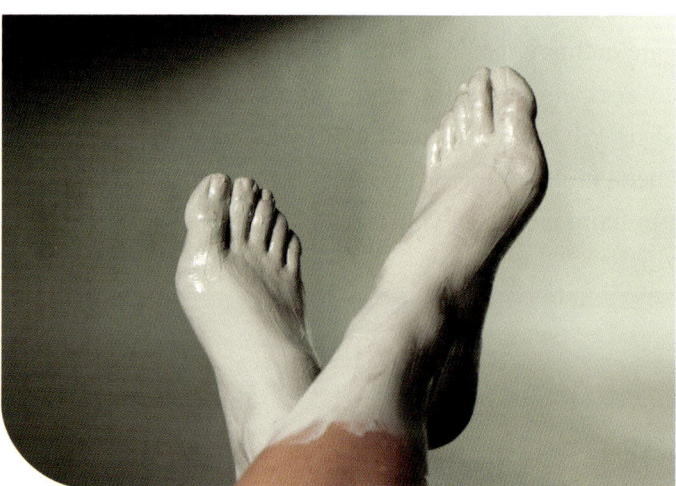

Masks

Masks for the hands and feet are typically cream, clay or gel products that are applied to the skin, allowed to dry for a period of time, and then removed. Different types of masks are used to provide the skin with a variety of necessary and desired benefits. Note that there are many mask options available to use during a hand or foot service. For instance, you may choose a hydrating mask to deeply condition the skin and help protect it from environmental stress; a cooling and rejuvenating mask that will help calm tired, sore muscles and keep the skin feeling refreshed; or a skin-softening mask that will target callused and extremely dry areas of the hands and feet. When it comes to choosing a mask, it is not just the type but the benefits it provides that will help you decide which is best for the skin.

Paraffin

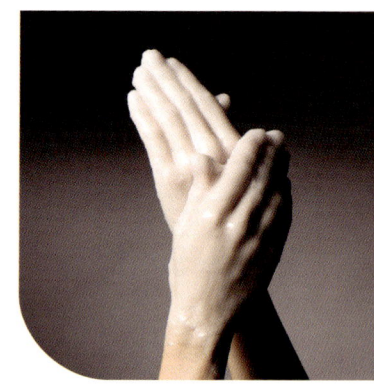

Paraffin is a type of wax that is frequently used for hand and foot services. It is warmed in an electric warmer and clients dip their hands and/or feet into the liquid. The heated wax is known to absorb and transfer heat to the area where it is applied. This helps soothe as well as moisturize the skin, leaving it soft and smooth. It also helps prepare the skin for other additional services such as masks and moisturizing creams or lotions. It is a simple, quick and inexpensive service to offer, and clients love it because they can see and feel the results right away.

Typically the client dips into the wax three to five times to build up a thick layer of the wax before allowing it to harden. As the wax hardens and cools, a plastic liner is applied to seal in the moisture, and a warming mitt or bootie goes over the liner to keep the wax warm longer to maximize the heat transfer aspect of the service.

To add a paraffin service to any natural or artificial nail service, the nail procedure is performed up until it's time to polish before having the client dip into the paraffin. Be sure to complete any repairs or re-balancing before the paraffin service.

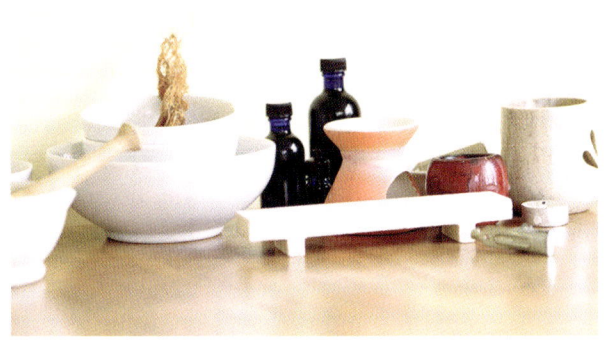

Aromatherapy

Aromatherapy is the controlled use of essential oils that are highly fragranced for specific outcomes. Derived solely from plant matter, they are also known as aromatherapy oils. The term aromatherapy comes from the two words: "aroma," meaning fragrance, and "therapy," meaning a healing treatment. Many salons and spas feature aromatherapy services and a large number of product lines carry aromatherapy items. While the general public focuses largely on the pleasing scent of an essential oil, in the salon or spa, fragrance is secondary. Oils can be stimulating, soothing, cleansing, calming, or antiseptic, to name a few!

As you continue to explore aromatherapy, you will encounter the phrase "carrier oil." A carrier oil is a neutral oil—most often grapeseed, almond, apricot kernel, jojoba or olive—used to dilute essential oils. To avoid severe irritation, all essential oils should be diluted before they are used on the skin. A carrier oil is the most common medium for dilution, but there are other options including lotions, creams, toners, cleansers, masks or even water if the essential oil is to be used in a bath, compress or oil diffuser.

Perhaps the easiest way to use fragrant essential oils is to add a calming or energizing oil to a room diffuser as part of the service. Specific essential oils or combinations of oils can be added to massage lotions and oils, masks, scrubs, paraffin or a hand or foot soak. However, when used in pure form, these oils can irritate the skin and cause adverse reactions, even when they are mixed with massage oil, a mask, paraffin or other preparation. Overexposure to certain oils by inhalation can produce a headache, nausea or fatigue. For this reason, it is imperative to study each oil's properties before use. It is also necessary to take each client's health history checking for allergies or previous reactions to aromatherapy oils.

It is recommended that you look up the effects of aromatherapy oils before using them on pregnant clients or clients with other health conditions.

ESSENTIAL OILS

Common essential oils used in hand and foot services include the following:

Oil	Effects
Bergamot	Soothing; antiseptic
Chamomile	Soothing; healing
Eucalyptus	Stimulating; antiseptic
Geranium	Stimulating; antiseptic
Lavender	Soothing; antiseptic
Peppermint	Stimulating; antiseptic
Rosemary	Stimulating; antiseptic
Tea Tree	Stimulating; antiseptic

An oil that is antiseptic helps prevent the growth of bacteria.

10

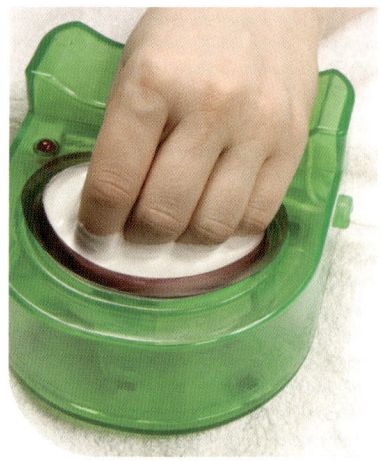

Hot Oil Manicure

A hot oil manicure is similar to a basic manicure. The main difference is that instead of soaking the hands and nails in water, cuticle oil is applied to the cuticle areas and then the fingers are placed in warm oil, lotion or cream that has been heated in an electric heating device. Unlike a basic manicure, when performing a hot oil manicure, the massage is performed once the warm oil, lotion or cream is applied. After the massage, the cuticles are cared for and the steps continue as in the Basic Manicure Procedure, *Chapter 8, Natural Nail Services*, page 205, skipping the massage steps since the massage is already done.

A hot oil manicure is highly moisturizing and replenishes dry skin and nails with much-needed moisture. This service is very beneficial for dry, aging or abused hands as well as dry or brittle nails. This service can be especially valuable to clients in the winter months when cold weather dehydrates the skin.

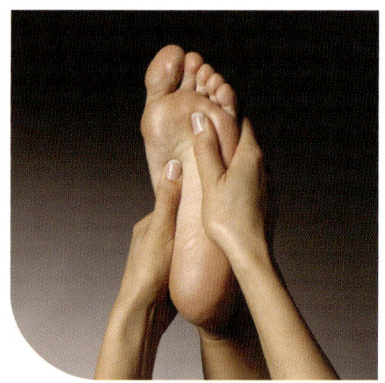

Reflexology

Spa services such as reflexology are highly popular with health-conscious clients. Though the origins of reflexology are attributed to the ancient Chinese, the early Egyptians and Indians also used forms of reflexology to soothe tired muscles and relieve pain. **Reflexology** is a massage method that uses pressure on specific points of the feet, hands and sometimes the ears to relieve tension and influence certain body conditions. According to professionals who practice reflexology, called **reflexologists**, distinct areas of the feet, hands and ears correspond with the body's internal organs. Reflexologists stimulate the appropriate area on the body to release body-bound energy blockages that cause stress, fatigue, irritability, pain and even disease. While reflexology can be performed by itself, it is frequently added to the massage element of manicures and pedicures.

Check with your state's regulating agency whether reflexology can be practiced in your state.

There are many ways to add-on to your basic manicure and pedicure services to turn them into much more. The more you "add-on" to your own education by learning about new ways to treat the hands and feet, the more your clients will return.

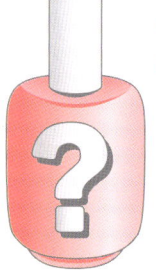

After learning about add-on services, which ones do you think you will enjoy the most and would be the most popular in the salon?

NAIL ART

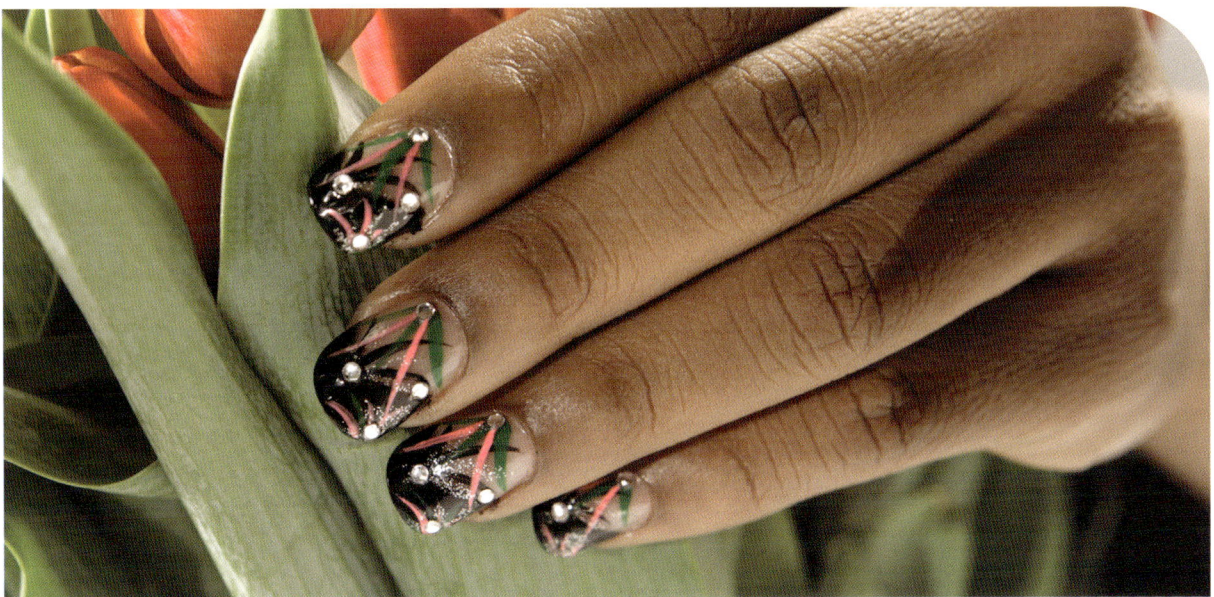

10

Nail art is a great way to add a special touch to any nail service. Adding designs or accents to freshly manicured nails offers your clients a unique way to express themselves. Depending on the desired effect, nail art can be as simple as adding a rhinestone to a freshly polished nail or as complex as a three-dimensional (3D) design sculpted with colored acrylic. Some clients may enjoy wearing nail art year round. For other clients, nail art may be a service they choose for holidays or special occasions. No matter what time of year or the occasion, nail art is a highly profitable and specialized service that you can use to attract new clients or introduce to existing clients.

Understanding Color

Understanding the relationships between colors will give you a good foundation for selecting the ones that complement and highlight your designs. As a nail artist, familiarity with the **law of color** is key to choosing colors for eye-pleasing nail designs. The law of color states that, out of all the colors of the universe, only three are pure. These three pure colors—red, yellow and blue—are referred to as **primary colors**. However, when they are mixed together in varying proportions, these primary colors create all other colors.

When primary colors are mixed together in equal proportions, they produce the three **secondary colors**: orange, green and violet. Orange contains equal amounts of red and yellow; green contains an equal mixture of blue and yellow; and violet contains equal proportions of red and blue.

Tertiary colors are the result of mixing primary colors with their neighboring secondary color in equal proportions. There are six tertiary colors: yellow-orange, yellow-green, blue-green, blue-violet, red-violet and red-orange. Mixing primary, secondary and tertiary colors in equal or unequal proportions makes colors such as brown and gray.

The Color Wheel

A color wheel is a tool in which the 12 colors (three primary, three secondary and six tertiary) are positioned in a circle. Their position on the wheel demonstrates the relationship of each color to the three primary colors of red, yellow and blue.

Color Vocabulary

- **Hue** is another term for color.
- **Tint** is a hue with white added.
- **Shade** is a hue with black added.
- **Value** is the lightness or darkness of a color.
- **Intensity** refers to the vibrancy of a color.
- **Tone** refers to the warmth or coolness of a color.

In order to achieve the greatest amount of contrast, complementary color schemes use colors that are opposite to each other on the color wheel.

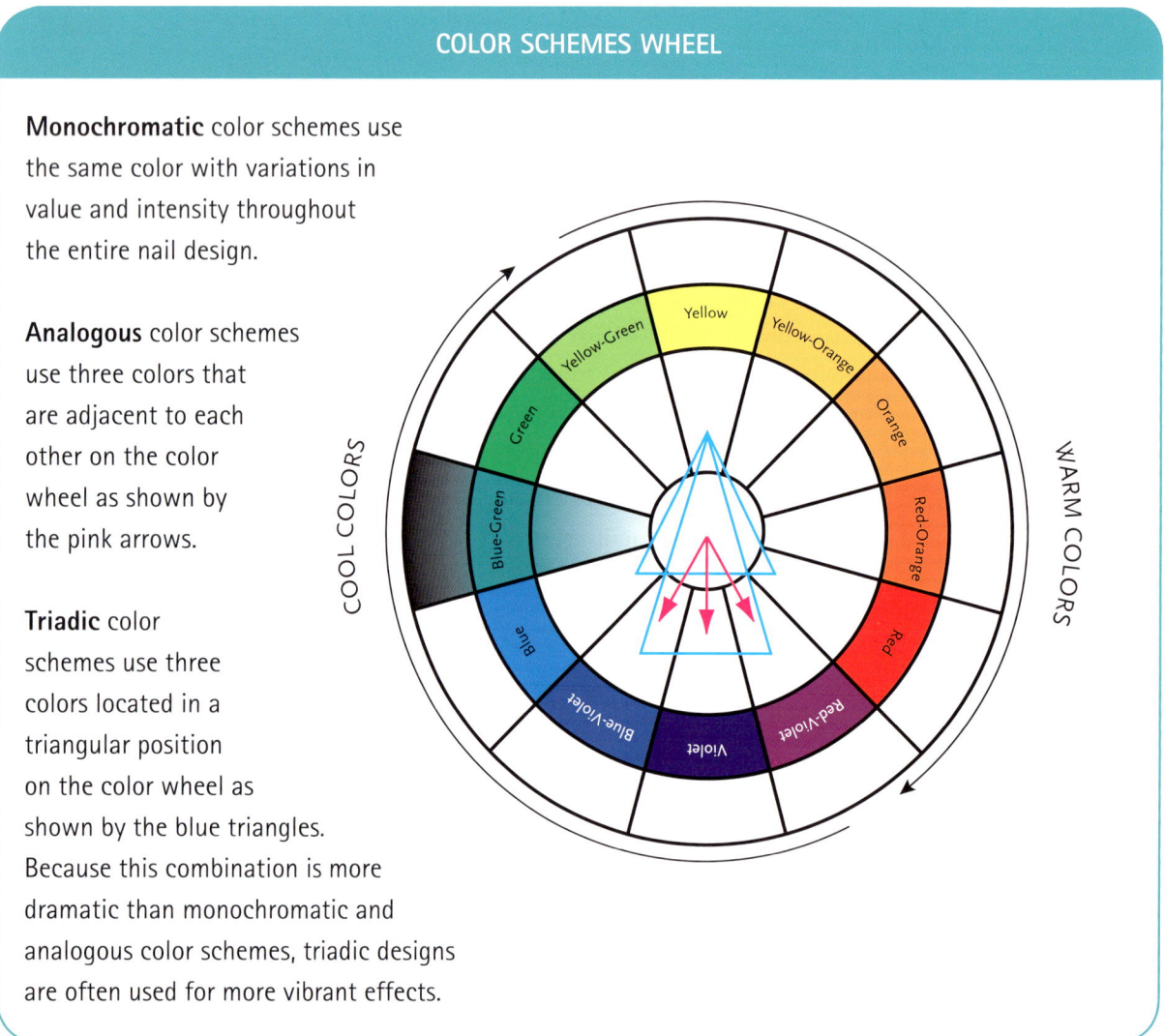

COLOR SCHEMES WHEEL

Monochromatic color schemes use the same color with variations in value and intensity throughout the entire nail design.

Analogous color schemes use three colors that are adjacent to each other on the color wheel as shown by the pink arrows.

Triadic color schemes use three colors located in a triangular position on the color wheel as shown by the blue triangles. Because this combination is more dramatic than monochromatic and analogous color schemes, triadic designs are often used for more vibrant effects.

Warm and cool are terms used to describe the tones of colors and the skin. Warm colors contain red or yellow tones within them and cool colors have more blue tones within them. Tones that are neither warm nor cool are considered neutral. Colors as well as skin tones are classified into the three color categories of warm, cool and neutral. In general, cool colors complement cooler skin tones, while warm colors complement warm skin tones.

Freehand

Freehand nail art, also called flat nail art, is the application of water-based paints or polish onto the surface of the nail using any variety of specialized brushes. With freehand nail art, the technician draws or paints designs onto the nails by hand without the use of stencils or any other guide.

Other than your own creativity, freehand nail art requires nothing more than polish or water-based paint and a brush. There are several types of brushes used to create freehand nail designs. By experimenting with a range of different brushes and a variety of techniques, such as the pressure applied and the position of the brush, you'll get a feel for what looks you can create using different freehand methods. The following is a list of brushes commonly used in freehand nail design and their recommended uses.

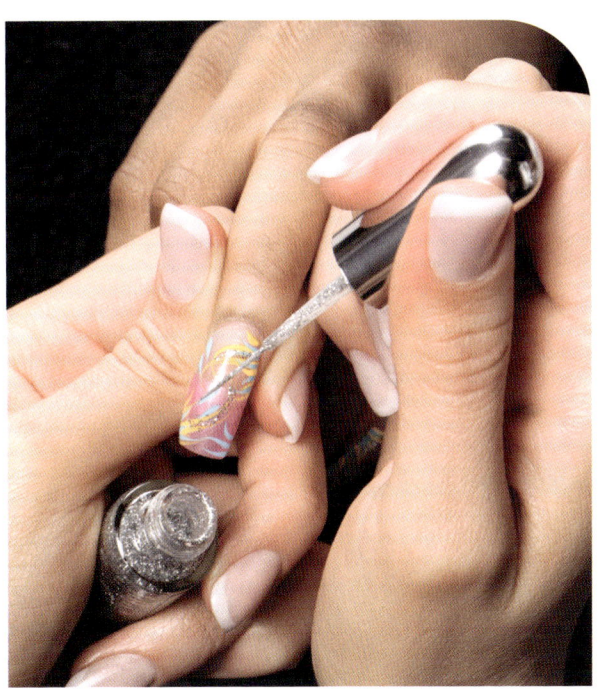

Some technicians refer to the combination of the pressure applied to the brush and the angle the brush is held as the "pull."

10

FREEHAND BRUSHES

The following brushes are commonly used in freehand nail art design.

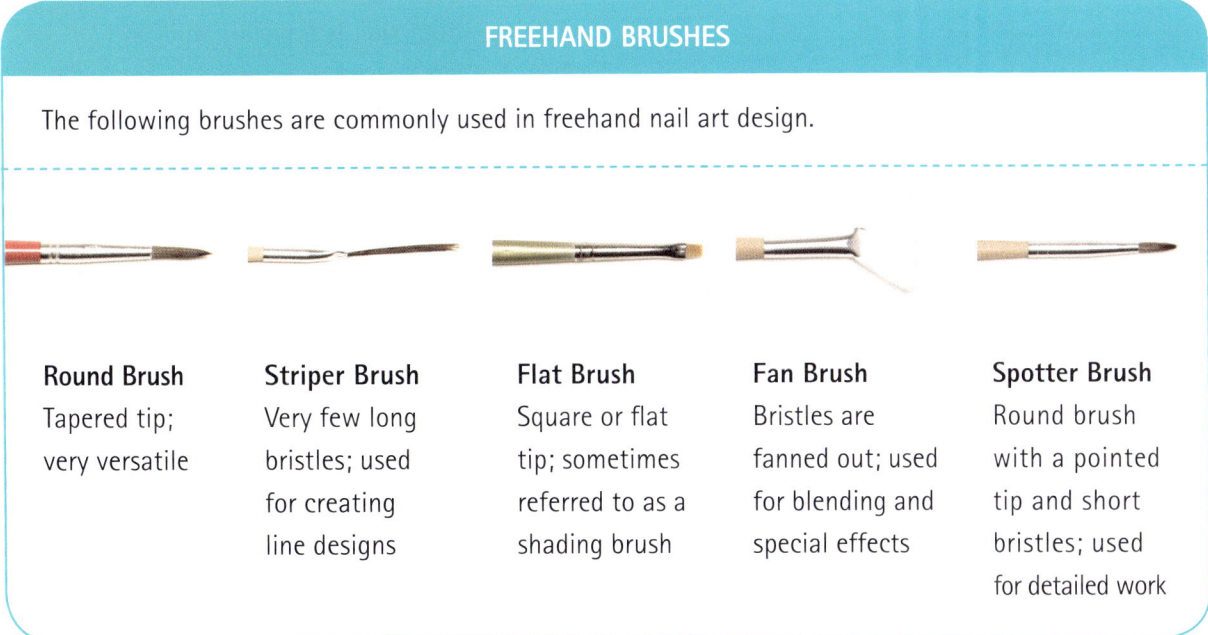

Round Brush	**Striper Brush**	**Flat Brush**	**Fan Brush**	**Spotter Brush**
Tapered tip; very versatile	Very few long bristles; used for creating line designs	Square or flat tip; sometimes referred to as a shading brush	Bristles are fanned out; used for blending and special effects	Round brush with a pointed tip and short bristles; used for detailed work

As you can see, there are several types of brushes designed specifically for creating nail art, but any synthetic fiber brush can be used.

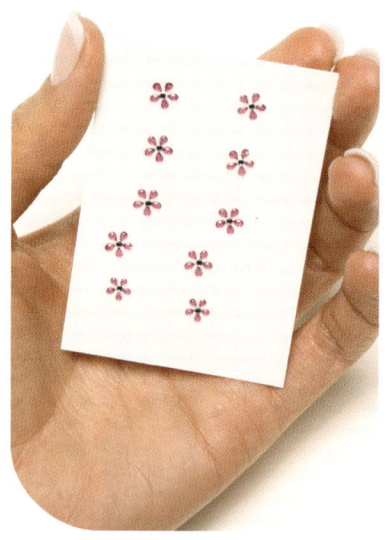

Accents

While freehand nail art requires just a brush, paint or polish, a steady hand and an imagination, other options for nail art include the addition of various accents. These additional design elements often give nail art a 3D effect and can be added to the surface of the nail, usually using an adhesive. There are several techniques for accentuating a freehand design or polish. Accents such as striping tape, nuggets, foil, appliqués and rhinestones are some examples that are often added to areas of the nail to create an even more dynamic nail design.

Striping Tape

Striping tape is a colored tape that comes on a roll or sheet that can be cut into various shapes, lengths or widths and added to any nail design. The tape has an adhesive backing that adheres to the nail until a clear polish, top coat or nail art sealer can be applied to seal the striping tape into the desired position.

The benefit of striping tape is that rather than trying to create perfectly straight lines freehand, it can be applied when the polish or nail design is completely dry. This creates a crisp, perfectly straight stripe on the nail. It is available in a wide variety of colors, including metallic silver and gold, which can appear much more vibrant than a thin line of metallic-colored polish applied freehand.

Nuggets

One way to add a textured effect to the surface of the nail is by applying nuggets, which are small pieces of foil applied to the nail with adhesive. Because it is a very thin, light-weight foil material, it must be handled with care. Nuggets come in a variety of colors, most commonly gold and silver, and can be added to the nail once the polish or design has dried completely. To place a nugget onto the nail, a nail adhesive is applied in the area where it is to be positioned. The adhesive must then be allowed to dry until it appears clear and feels tacky, meaning sticky. An orangewood stick or tweezers can be used to press the nugget into place. A clear polish or top coat is used to seal it.

Foiling

Foiling is another option for enhancing nails. Foil comes in rolls or pre-cut pieces in many different colors. One side of the foil is shiny while the other side is typically dull gray or silver. Foiling is used on completely dry nails. Again, a specially designed adhesive is applied to the nail. When it dries, it will turn clear, giving the nail a tacky feeling. The foil then is placed with the dull side against the nail and pressed into place using an orangewood stick or your finger. When the desired design is complete, it is sealed with a clear polish or top coat.

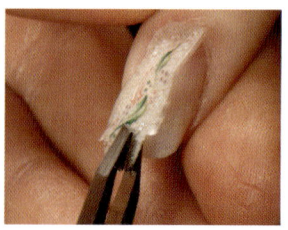

Appliqués

Appliqués are small, flat objects, such as stickers, that are applied to the nail. They are available in many different designs such as seasonal designs, characters and flowers. Typically, appliqués have an adhesive backing and they are placed on a dry nail and sealed with a clear top coat.

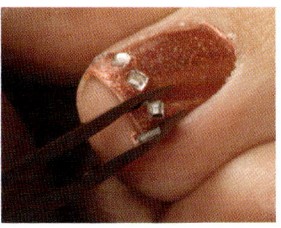

Rhinestones

Rhinestones are small pieces of plastic made to resemble gems that add a unique touch to any design or polished nail. They are available in many sizes, colors and shapes such as square, round, heart-shaped and even floral designs. A rhinestone has a flat back that is applied to the surface of the nail in the desired location with an adhesive and sealed with a clear top coat.

It takes practice and patience when first learning different designs. You can find many nail and beauty industry magazines that feature the latest in new, creative nail designs for inspiration.

Colored Acrylics and Gels

Colored acrylic and gel products are no different than ordinary acrylics and gels except that they

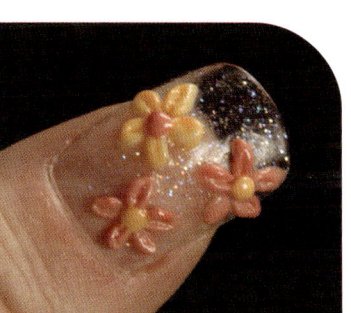

contain pigments that give them color. They can be used to create elaborate 3D designs or custom-blended to create color and used as an overlay or a "chip-proof polish."

These products are great for introducing nail art to your client. It can be as simple as adding sparkle to the pink or white of traditional acrylic or custom-blending a pink color to complement a skin tone. Color acrylics and gels can also be used to create nail art. The different colors can be used to sculpt a multi-colored nail design. You can sculpt a red tip, for example.

There are a few considerations to make when using colored acrylics or gels. For two-week and four-week maintenance or re-balancing, you'll want to remember the "recipe" or formula you originally mixed, so be sure to include that information on the client's record card. As mentioned previously, colored acrylics and gels can act as a chip-proof polish when applied in a thin layer over a thin clear acrylic or gel nail. This makes it easier to file off the top layer of product and still have the clear product underneath. This allows you to change the color without having to sculpt or build an entirely new nail.

Nail art takes beautiful nails one step further and lets you shine in the area of artistry. When you learn to understand the laws of color and combine your creativity with your manicure and pedicure skills, the results will thrill your clients. Nail art design definitely takes practice, but you will be rewarded by knowing you are a nail technician who goes above and beyond, and whose clients return to time and time again for this highly specialized service.

10

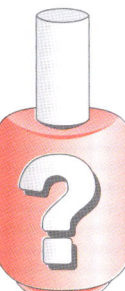

With the different options available for nail art designs, which do you think will be easiest to master? Which do you think will be most difficult?

EQUIPMENT

Equipment, as described in *Chapter 8, Natural Nail Services*, is considered to be permanent furniture or implements in the salon or spa. More advanced equipment is available other than the basic equipment necessary for nail services. Some of the options are an airbrush machine, an electric file and a drying station.

Purchasing additional equipment can be a very costly investment, so it is important to determine if the salon or spa will benefit from having it. Another thing to keep in mind is that using advanced equipment requires additional training in order to know how to use it properly. Not only does this ensure client safety and comfort, but it also educates the technicians on how to maintain the equipment and keep it in the best possible condition.

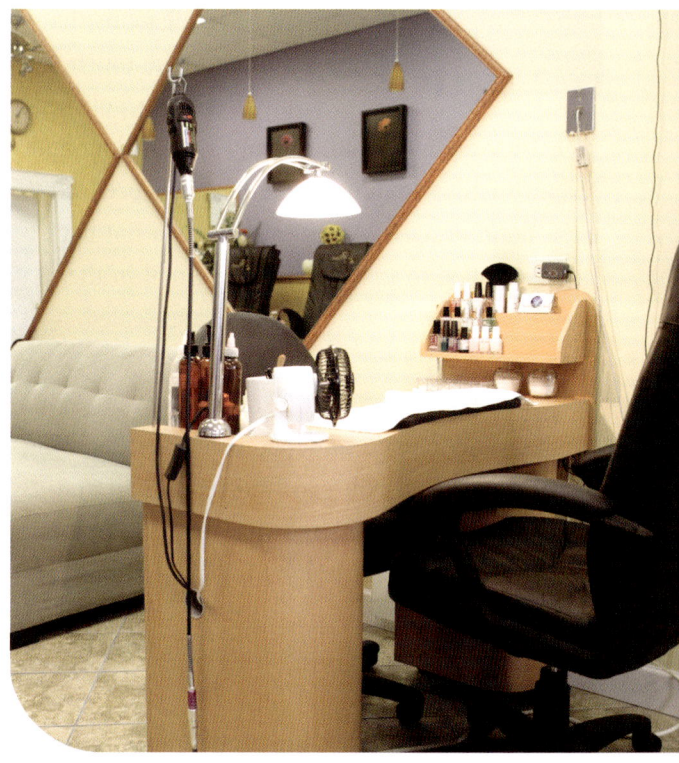

Airbrush

An **airbrush** is an electrically powered piece of equipment that is used to apply paint or polish to the nail without using a brush. It is a long, thin metal implement, sometimes referred to as a gun, that is held similar to the way you hold a pen. Paint is stored in the gun or attached to it. Air passes through it, forcing the paint out through the nozzle on the end of the gun and onto the nail in a fine, consistent mist.

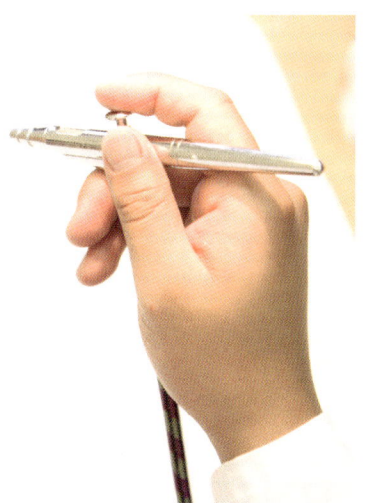

There are typically two types of airbrushes: a single action and a dual action.

- A single-action airbrush releases the air and paint at the same time. A valve controls the flow of the paint. To change the flow of the paint, the valve is adjusted by a knob usually located on the back of the handle.

- A dual-action airbrush allows the user to control the air and the paint separately. Air is released by pressing a lever down on the top of the airbrush. Pulling back on the lever releases the paint. Pulling the lever back farther releases more paint with the air. The dual action can be more difficult to learn but can allow the technician to apply the paint more quickly.

Although airbrushes are used to create many forms of art, it is especially important when creating nail art to use an airbrush specifically created for the nail industry. The equipment needed for airbrushing can be costly, but offering this service to clients can add to the final cost of the service. Before you know it, your investment in the equipment will have paid off. It is also wise to have a manufacturer's warranty to protect your investment.

Airbrushing Equipment

Using an airbrush requires more than just the airbrush implement itself. When purchasing airbrushing equipment, it is important that it comes with a compressor, moisture trap and hose.

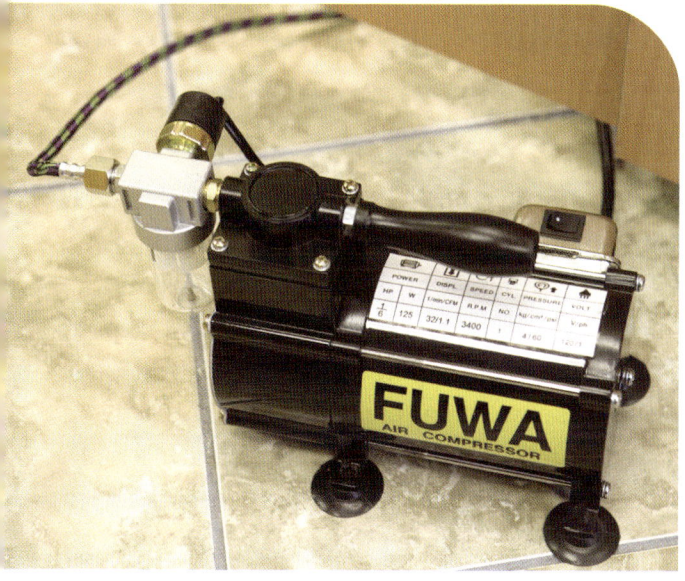

Compressor

A **compressor** is the source of the air pressure needed to push the paint out of the gun in a fine mist. Because there are several different options available, it's important to learn what will fit your needs and those of the salon or spa.

Although the least expensive way to provide airbrushing to your clients is by using canned compressed air, it is not as effective as using an air compressor. This is because there is a limited amount of air in each can and when the can is emptied, it has to be replaced with a new one.

This can be inconvenient, especially if it happens while you are in the middle of a service. It can also be more costly in the long run.

Another consideration to keep in mind when deciding to purchase an air compressor is the noise level. Some compressors are silent while others are about the same level as a hair dryer. The compressors most commonly used in the salon are generally those that are considered low-maintenance because they do not require oil to run. Silent compressors typically cost more, run on oil that needs to be changed regularly and require more maintenance.

Moisture Trap

A moisture trap is a reservoir that catches or collects moisture produced by the compressed air traveling through the gun. As the air comes out of the compressor it cools down, creating moisture. The humidity in the air also affects the amount of moisture produced. The moisture trap is necessary to prevent water from combining with the paint and air and ruining the nail design.

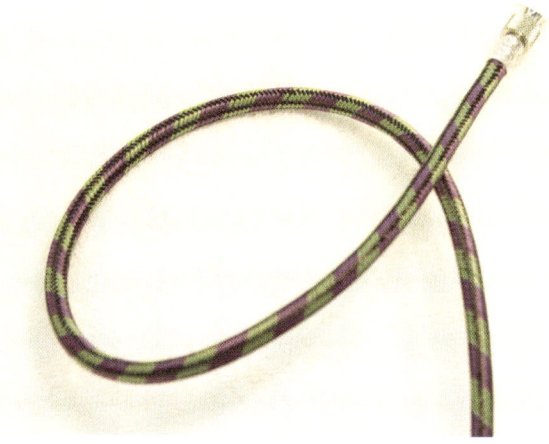

Hose

The airbrush is attached to the compressor with a hose. The hose is a flexible rubber or plastic tube through which the air travels from the compressor to the gun. The hose should be long enough for the technician to be able to work efficiently.

10

Airbrush Products and Supplies

Airbrush manufacturers require different products to use along with their equipment in order to provide the most effective and efficient service. As with any equipment, be sure to follow manufacturer's instructions on products used to remove the paint from the skin and to prep the nail.

There are several supplies available for you to use along with your airbrush that can enhance your service. Stencils are paper or plastic cut-outs that can be used with an airbrush to create more elaborate or detailed designs on the nail. Stencils are placed over the nail and the airbrush sprays over the entire surface of the nail. When the stencil is removed, only the design cut into the stencil appears on the nail. Stencils made of paper are not as long-lasting as plastic stencils, which can be cleaned and reused. Masking is another technique very similar to stenciling, used to isolate a specific area to be airbrushed.

You may use either water-based or acrylic-based nail paint with an airbrush. The paints are categorized as: translucent, opaque, metallic and opal. Translucent paints are the thinnest types of paint. Metallic and opal paints contain small flecks that can clog the airbrush more easily.

Airbrush Equipment Maintenance

To keep your airbrush in perfect working order, it is necessary to follow manufacturer's instructions on the maintenance and cleaning of the machine. The paint must be completely cleaned out before switching to another color of paint. To prevent paint from drying and clogging the airbrush, the entire hand piece should be completely cleaned at the end of every day.

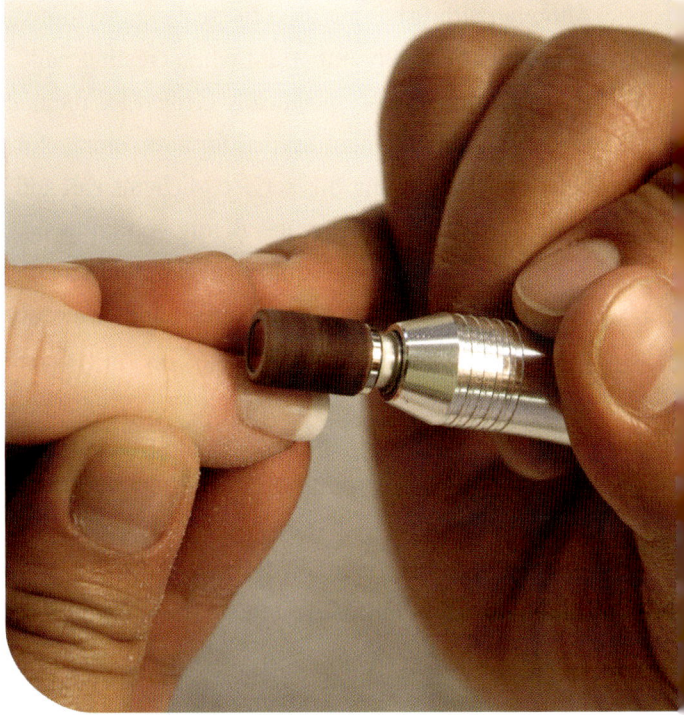

Electric File

As you already know, nail files are available with different levels of abrasives. You also know that different grit numbers or levels of abrasives are used to accomplish different steps in the filing and shaping process. What you may not know is that there are electric files available to make shaping and re-balancing quicker. Though it may shorten the overall filing time, it takes some time to master the technique.

An **electric file**, sometimes referred to as an e-file, is a machine with a motor and a hand piece that holds different abrasive pieces, called **bits**, that rotate to file the nail. It is important that only files created for this purpose are used on nails. There are two main types of electric files made specifically for use in the nail industry. The first is a **table file**, sometimes referred to as a **micro motor**. The second type is a **hand-held file**, also called a **hand-held micro motor**.

A table file has a small hand piece attached to a small box that contains the motor. Many table files come with an optional foot pedal to control the speed of the file. Even though this type of file is most commonly used, it tends to cost more than a hand-held file.

A hand-held file is a small hand piece that plugs directly into an electrical outlet. There is no separate box for the motor since the motor is within the hand piece. This can make it heavier to handle, but it is effective and less expensive.

Most electric files have a variety of operating features, such as a forward and reverse switch, a foot pedal speed control, small footprint (space taken by the file), digital display and light-weight hand pieces.

When looking for an electric file, it's important to consider the vibration level of the hand piece. High vibration can cause hand, wrist and arm problems.

Speed

The speed of an electric file refers to how fast the bit rotates. The speed is measured by **Revolutions Per Minute (RPM)**, which is the number of times the bit completes a rotation per minute. It is important to have a variable speed control in order to provide maximum control of the file. Most electric files range in speed from 1,000 RPM to 30,000 RPM. When working on natural nails, it is recommended to use a slower speed of approximately 4,000 RPM while a faster speed of around 12,000-15,000 RPM is recommended for artificial nails.

Torque

Torque is the amount of resistance in the file while the file bit is in motion. The torque is measured by pound per square inch. If there

is not enough torque, the file speed will vary when pressure is applied to the bit, which can cause the file to stall or stop. The file should work at a consistent speed and be able to file away acrylic, gels and wraps without slowing down or stalling.

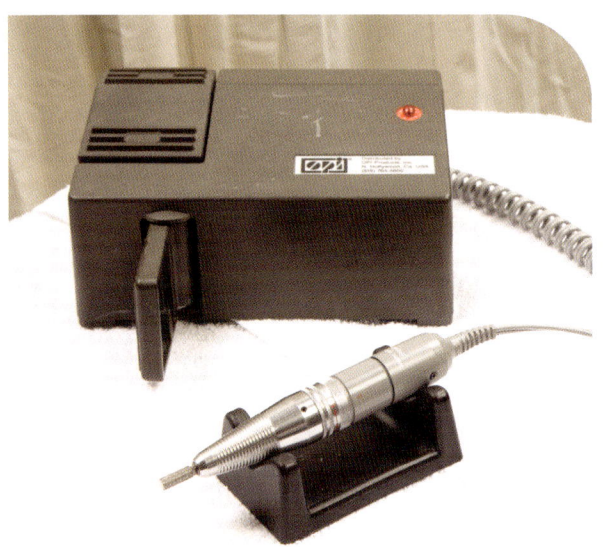

Electric File Bits

A **bit** is a removable abrasive tip that is part of every electric file. Each bit has a **shank**, or shaft, that is inserted into the end of the hand piece. The industry standard size for the shank of the bit is 3/32 of an inch. If the shank is a different size, it may be meant for a craft file or drill and should not be used. All bits should be concentric, or perfectly balanced. The bit will rotate on the nail unevenly with each rotation if it is unbalanced.

Rather than being distinguished by grit numbers like other files, electric file bits are available in extra-fine, fine, medium, coarse and extra-coarse. There are many different types of bits made of various materials.

10

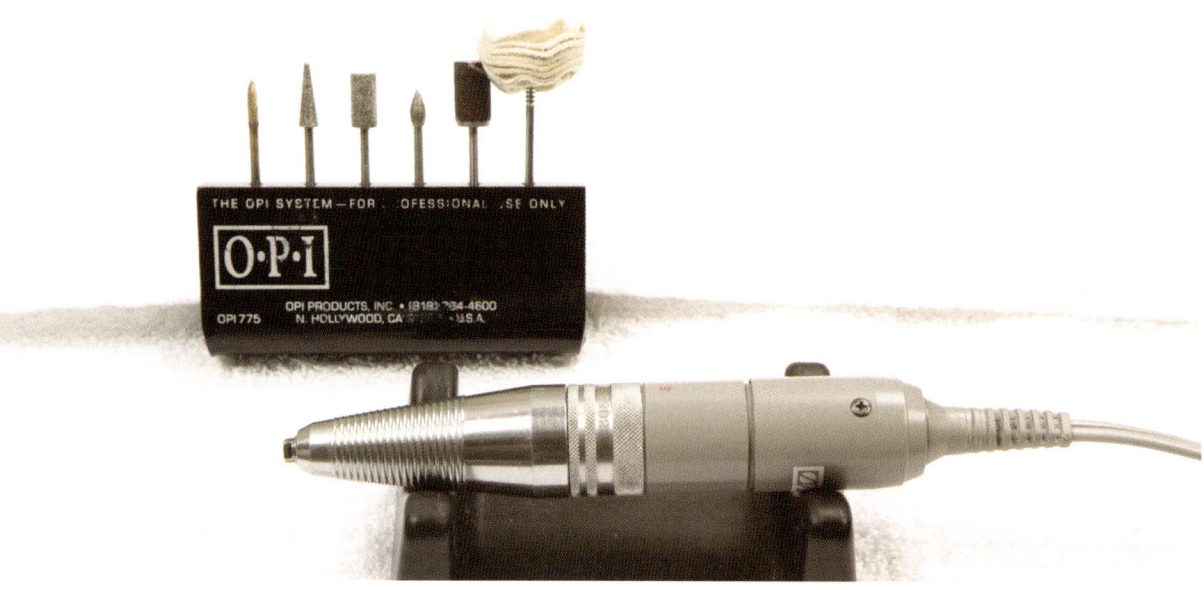

The following are some examples of the types of bits available:

1. **Carbide bits** are metal bits with small razor blade-type cuts known as flutes, which are designed to "shave" off the artificial product. They are cleaned with a scrub brush and disinfected after every client.
2. **Diamond bits** are metal bits with small diamond particles attached. They are cleaned with a scrub brush and disinfected after every client.
3. **Sanding bands** are paper files that are placed over a bit called a mandrel. Sanding bands are porous and cannot be properly disinfected. They must be discarded after each use.
4. **Buffing bits** are sometimes referred to as natural nail bits and are made from a synthetic rubberized material or from natural materials such as chamois. Because these bits are porous and cannot be properly disinfected, they must be discarded after each use. These are the only bits recommended for use on the natural nail.

The diamond and carbide bits also come in a variety of shapes designed to help the technician perform specific services. Some of the shapes available are cone, barrel, football and a specific backfill bit. Typically cone- and football-shaped bits are used for filing around the cuticle area, filing away cracks in the product, and cleaning underneath the nail. Barrel bits are commonly used for removing product that has lifted; they are used to shape the nail, shorten the nail, and also for backfills.

Basic Techniques for Electric Filing

It's important to seek hands-on education for an electric file. Make sure you are comfortable using the file before using it on a client. It is not advisable to use an electric file on a client before practicing on your own nails or with a friend.

Angle

The most important aspect of electric filing is making sure that the bit is only used flat against the nail and parallel to the nail when working on the top. Nail technicians should never hold the bit at an angle to the nail, since just as with a hand file, it may cause friction burns or "rings of fire." This occurs when the natural nail is over-filed, and a visible redness appears and the client may feel heat on the nail. When working on the free edge, the file should be held perpendicular (at a 90° angle) to the edge.

Pressure

The technician shouldn't have to apply pressure while using an electric file. If pressure is applied, this will cause more friction and create heat. Be sure to be in constant communication with your client to make sure that he or she alerts you to any heat or discomfort that may occur.

Movement

It is important to always keep the file moving around the surface of the nail and not stay in one area of the nail. The file should be lifted from the nail every few seconds to allow the nail to cool. One technique is to work from one side of the nail to the opposite and then lift the file and move back to the other side.

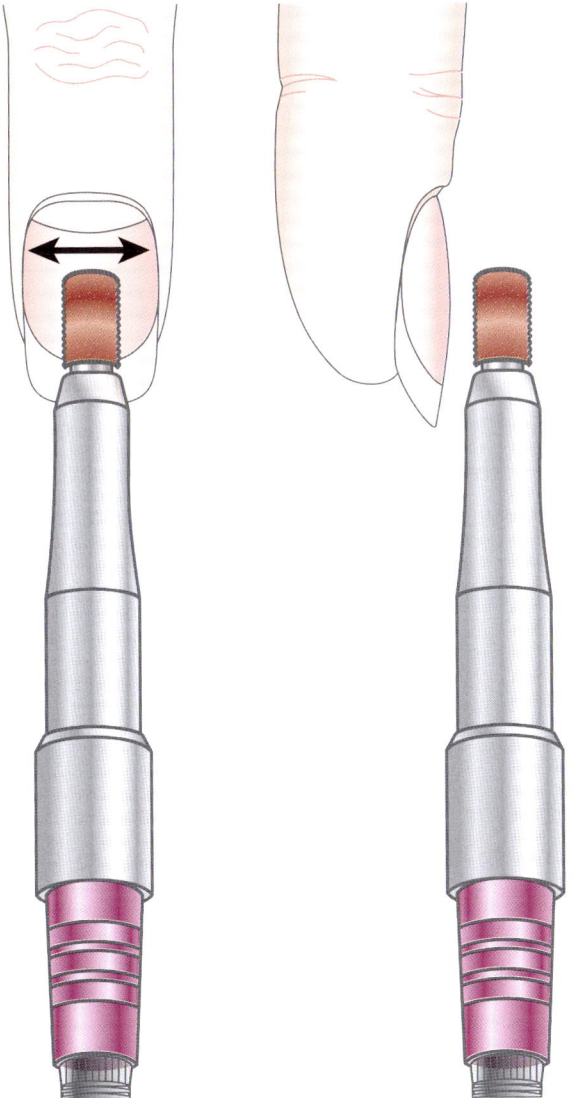

Using an electric file produces a larger amount of dust than hand filing, so wearing a dust mask and goggles to prevent dust from entering your body is for your protection.

Speed

The speed used with an electric file varies with each user. If the speed is just right, it will be easy to control and will move across the nail smoothly and evenly. If the speed is too fast, the bit may feel like it is skipping around, or getting caught in certain areas of the nail. The technician can tell the speed is too slow if the file is "bogging down" or stalling. Practice using different speeds to find what is comfortable for you. Remember though, it is not recommended to go above 4,000 RPM for natural nails or 15,000 RPM for artificial nails.

Sanitation and Disinfection of Electric Files

Electric files require the same sanitation and disinfection as all other equipment and implements. Sanitize or clean the bits with soap and water using a scrub brush to make sure all debris is removed after every client. Soak the bits in an EPA-registered broad spectrum (hospital-level) disinfectant for the recommended time. It is also important to clean the hand piece and machine by wiping it with a soft cloth and brush to remove any filings. Properly caring for your equipment will keep it in good working order.

Some regulating agencies require certification in order to use an electric file. Always follow your regulating agency guidelines on the use of advanced equipment such as this.

10

ELECTRIC FILING GUIDELINES

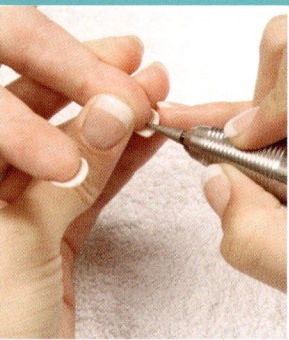

It is important that you receive the proper training in handling an electric file to protect you and your client.

To clean under the nail or to help define the c-curve of an enhancement, use a cone- or football-shaped bit:

- Turn the client's palm up or look down the front of the nail.
- Hold the bit parallel to the area being filed and move the file from one side to the other. Lift the file from the nail and begin again on the opposite side.
- Continue moving the file in this manner until the filing and shaping are complete.

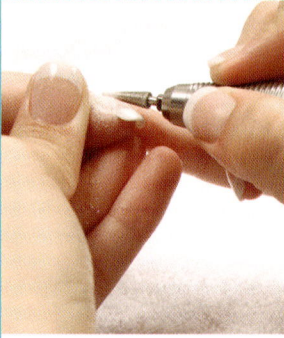

To prepare the enhancements for a fill, use a cone- or football-shaped bit:

- Hold the bit parallel to the area being filed.
- Work from one side of the nail to the other. Lift the file from the nail and begin again on the original side.
- Use caution: Do not allow the file bit to come into contact with the natural nail or skin.
- If cracks are present, use a small barrel bit and create a "groove" to expose the crack in order to replace the product.
- File the enhancement until the old product blends evenly with the natural nail.

If any lifting is present it may be necessary to use a barrel bit focusing on removing that area of the enhancement product. Avoid nipping or pulling the lifted product off the natural nail.

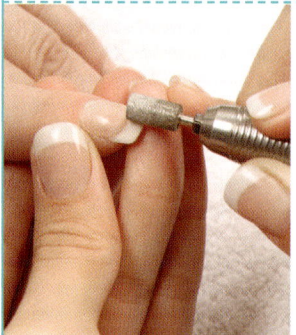

To prepare pink and white gel nails or acrylic nails for a four-week fill or backfill, use a barrel-shaped bit. Some manufacturers make a specific backfill bit that can also be used:

- Remove approximately 75% of the product from Zone 1.
- Work from one side of the nail to the other. Lift the file from the nail and begin again on the original side.

Be sure to remove enough product so that when the new smile line is created, the old product does not show through after filing and shaping.

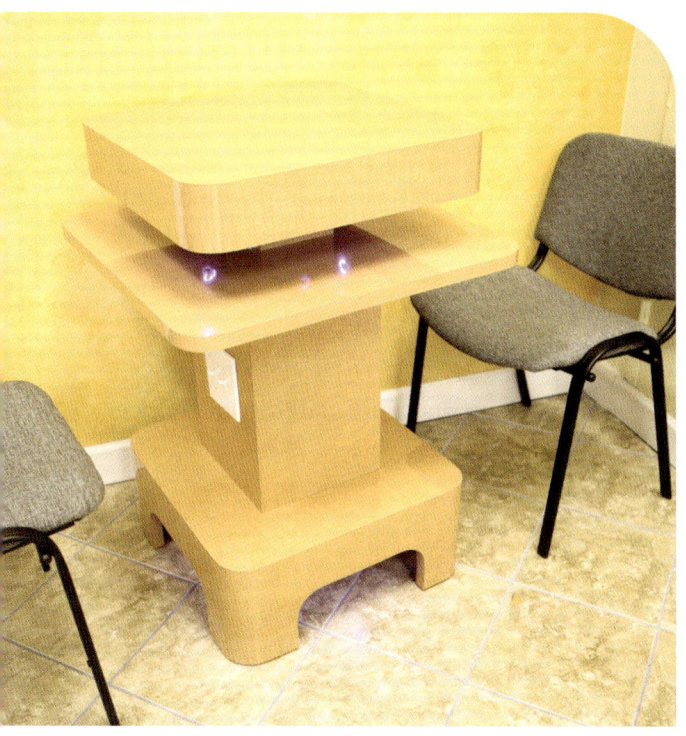

Nail Dryer

Nail dryers are commonly found in nail salons and spas. They are electrically powered devices that use air or light to dry the nails. Often salons and spas have an area designated as a drying station where clients sit after their service and place their hands and feet under the dryers. This ensures that clients leave with dry nails while allowing the nail technician to move on to the next client.

While some dryers use air to dry the nails, others have UV (ultraviolet) bulbs that dry or cure a UV-drying top coat. UV top coats act in the same way that UV gels do. They contain an activator that causes them to cure, or harden, under the appropriate light. When using a UV-drying top coat, it is important to use the manufacturer's recommended dryer and the required wattage. As always, it is important to properly disinfect the nail dryer after every client by wiping it down with an EPA-registered, broad spectrum (hospital-level) disinfectant.

As your career progresses as a nail technician, you will continue to learn about new equipment that can be used to enhance your services. By becoming familiar with the latest equipment available and seeking additional training on how to properly use it, you will add to your skills which will make you well-rounded. By being known as a nail technician who can efficiently use new equipment safely, you open the door to many opportunities and increased clientele. Add-on services are not required, but the nail technician who pursues advanced education with every new possibility in the industry is guaranteed a successful career.

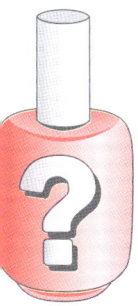

Which additional equipment do you think would be the most beneficial for the salon or spa that you plan to work in?

DECISION-MAKING SKILLS

Case Studies

The following situations are designed to help you build decision-making skills. Using your training to this point, review the following scenarios, then think through and describe how you would handle each challenge.

1. A new client comes in and mentions that her nails and cuticles are dry. What add-on service would you recommend for her? How would you explain the benefits of this additional service?

2. Most of your clients prefer to wear some sort of nail art. You are thinking about investing in an airbrush machine. What type of research would you do and why?

INDEX

Free edge, 132
Freehand brushes, 365
Freehand nail art, 365
French manicure, 217-218
French pedicure, 244
Friction, 186, 221
Fungal infections, 143
Furrows, 139, 142
Fuse, 79

G
Gases, 115
Gastrocnemius muscle, 97
Gel, 272-273
Gel brush, 272-273
Gel nail procedures
    four-week pink and white
        gel nail maintenance,
        348-351
    gel nail removal, 352-354
    pink and white sculptured
        gel nails, 337-344
    single-color gel nail overlay,
        330-336
    two-week gel nail
        maintenance, 345-347
Gel nails
    defined, 272
    essentials, 272-275
    light-cured, 176-177
    maintenance, 274-275
    removal, 275
General circulation, 100
General infection (systemic), 56
Glass container, 199, 201, 252
Glass file, 195, 197
Glutaraldehyde Based
    Formulations, 69
Gomage, 360
Grammar, 12
Granules, 146
Greeting Phase, 160, 173
Gross anatomy, 85

H
Habits, 17
Halitosis, 7
Hand and nail examination,
    136
Hand-held file, 370-371
Handwashing, 59
    procedure, 61
HBV (Hepatitis B Virus), 54
Health conditions, 166-167
Heart, 88, 95, 98
Heart attack, 99
Heat sterilization, 69
Heimlich Maneuver, 79
Hemoglobin, 99
Hepatitis B Virus (HBV), 54

Herpes Simplex, 151
Histology, 85
HIV (Human
    Immunodeficiency
    Virus), 54-55
Home care regimen, 176-177
Homeostasis, 103
Hormones, 110
Hose, 369
Hot oil manicure, 362
Human Immunodeficiency
    Virus (HIV), 54
Humerus bone, 93
Hydrochloric acid, 107
Hygiene
    personal, 7
    public, 7
Hyperkeratosis, 153
Hyponychium, 133

I
Image, 7
Immunity, 57
    natural, 57
    passive (acquired), 57
Income, 41
Infection
    general (systemic), 56
    local, 56
    pathogens, 55
    six signs of, 136
Infection control, 58-71
    procedures, 71
    vocabulary, 59
Inhalation, 75, 109
Inhibitors, 118
Initiator, 118
Insertion (muscle), 95
Insurance, 39
    malpractice, 39
    product liability, 39
    property or premise, 39
    worker's compensation, 39
Integumentary system, 89, 111
International Nail Technician's
    Association (INTA), 18
Interview, 26
Intestines, 88
Inventory, 44
Inventory control, 44
Involuntary muscle, 95
Iodophor Germicidal
    Solution, 69
Isopropyl alcohol, 69

J
Job
    benefits, 28
    cover letter, 26
    interview, 26-27

    resumé, 25
    work environment, 27

K
Keloids, 150
Keratin, 116, 134, 145
    hard, 145
    soft, 145
Keratinization, 146-147
Keratinize, 134
Kidneys, 88, 108
Koilonychia, 139, 142

L
Large intestine, 108
Larynx, 109
Law of color, 363
Lease, 38
Left atrium, 98
Left ventricle, 98
Lentigines,
    see also Macule, 149, 153
Lesions
    primary, 149-150
    secondary, 150
Leucocytes, 99
Leuconychia, 141-142
Leukoderma, 154
Lifelong learning
    comparison shopping, 31
    current periodicals, 31
    internet resources, 31
    seminars and classes, 30
    trade shows, 30
Ligaments, 95
Line of credit, 38
Lint-free nail wipes, 198
Liquids, 115
Liquid monomer, 125, 266-267
Liquid soap, 187
Liquid tissue, 88
Listening
    active, 15
    reflective, 15
Liver, 88, 108
Local infection, 56
Lunula, 132
Lungs, 88, 109
Lymph, 101
Lymph vascular system, 98, 101

M
Macule, 149, 153
Malpractice insurance, 39
Manicure
    children's, 220
    essentials, 187-201
    French, 217-218
    male, 219
    massage, 185-187

    procedure, 202-217
Manicure table, 199, 201
Mantle, 133
Marketing, 30
Masks, 360
Massage
    benefits of, 185-186
    contraindications, 187
    techniques, 186
Massage oil, 223-224
Material Safety Data Sheet
    (MSDS), 62-63
Matter, 115
Median nerve, 106
Medulla oblongata, 103
Melanin, 147-148, 153
Melanocytes, 147, 153
Melanoderma, 153
Melanoma, 154
Melanonychia, 141-142
Melanosomes, 147
Metabolism
    phases of, 87
Metabolic rate, 87
Metacarpals, 93
Metatarsal bones, 94
Metal file, 196-197
Methoxyethoxy Ethyl
    Methacrylate (MEM), 126
Methyl Methacrylate
    Monomer, 126
Microbiology, 51
Mitosis,
    of bacteria, 53
    of cells, 87, 147
Mixed nerves, 105
Moisture trap, 369
Moisturizing lotion, 190, 194,
    224
Mole, 154
Molecules, 117
Monomer, 118, 123
    see also Acrylic liquid,
        Liquid monomer
Motor nerves, 105
Movement, 373
Muscle
    foot, 97
    hand, 97
    lower leg, 97
    parts of, 95
    shoulder and arm, 96
    types of tissue, 95
Myology, 94

N
Naevus, 154
Nail
    composition of, 132-133
    growth of, 134

While this may be the end of this textbook, remember that it's not so much an ending as it is the beginning of your career in nail services. We encourage you to continue on a path of lifelong learning and to keep this book as a reference tool throughout your professional pursuits. BEST OF LUCK IN YOUR CAREER.

Sincerely,

The Staff of *Salon Fundamentals Nails*

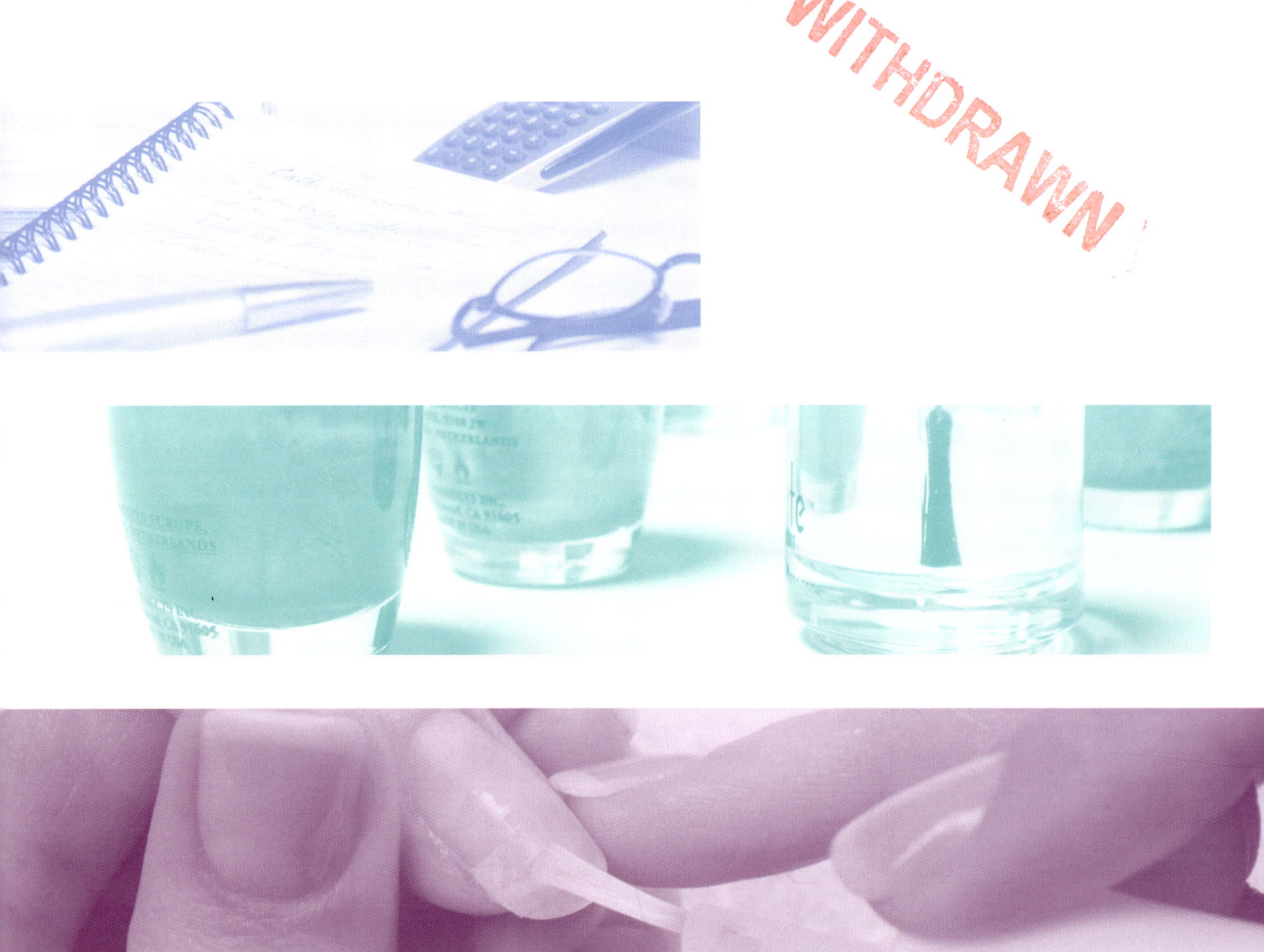